THE MEDICAL LETTER HANDBOOK OF ADVERSE DRUG INTERACTIONS

Edited by Richard B. Kim, M.D.
and Editors of The Medical Letter

PUBLISHED BY

The Medical Letter, Inc.
1000 Main Street
New Rochelle, New York 10801-7537

Copyright 2001
(ISBN 0-9660510-5-X)
(ISSN 0897-5418)

The Medical Letter, Inc.
1000 Main Street
New Rochelle, New York 10801-7537

800-211-2769

An adverse drug interaction program using the same database is also available from *The Medical Letter* for personal computers.

Visit our website at www.medletter.com

CONTENTS

Introduction 4
  Criteria for Listing Interactions 4
  Mechanisms of Interactions 5
  Recommendations 5

Adverse Interactions of Drugs 6

Foods Interacting With MAO Inhibitors 445

Index of Brand Names 447

THE MEDICAL LETTER HANDBOOK OF ADVERSE DRUG INTERACTIONS

This handbook offers a quick guide to possible adverse effects of drug interactions, with brief recommendations for precautionary measures. Pairs of interacting drugs are listed alphabetically, followed by the adverse interaction, its mechanism (in parentheses), references and recommendations for clinical management. These listings are usually based on clinical reports. Interactions listed for groups of drugs (such as "cephalosporins" or "antidepressants, tricyclic") may not have been reported for every drug in the group; known exceptions to the interaction are noted. The index on page 447 lists brand names with their generic equivalents, and indicates group headings for drugs not listed separately; brand names for combination products are generally not listed.

It is not possible to determine the frequency of most interactions. When an interaction is documented by one or two case reports rather than clinical studies or reports in many patients, the year of each report is given as some indication of frequency.

Reports of interactions between more than two drugs have begun to appear in the medical literature. Where these have been documented, they are noted in the comments under interacting pairs of drugs.

CRITERIA FOR LISTING INTERACTIONS — New adverse interactions are continually being reported; the absence of a listing in this table does not necessarily mean that drugs will not interact when given concurrently. Interactions extrapolated from animal studies or from interactions reported with related drugs, may not be included here. In the Index of Brand Names, drugs with no interactions listed are marked with a bullet (•).

Interactions between general anesthetics and drugs likely to be administered during surgery, such as autonomic drugs and local anesthetics, are not included. Interactions useful in therapy, such as the increased plasma concentration of penicillin with concurrent use of probenecid, are also not listed. Drug combinations should be looked up under their components.

Common additive effects, such as occur with use of two antihypertensive agents or two central-nervous-system depressants or two drugs that affect blood clotting, are generally not listed. Effects expected from the mechanism of a drug's action, such as that of potassium on digitalis glycosides or calcium on calcium-entry blockers, and useful antagonist effects, such as that between a poison and an antidote, are also not included. Most interactions of drugs with foods, beverages or other nutrients are not listed, but foods interacting with monoamine oxidase inhibitors are listed in a separate table on page 445.

MECHANISMS OF INTERACTIONS — Genetic differences can affect drug metabolism and interactions. Some drugs can interact by changing the metabolism of other drugs, either through inhibition or induction of any of several hepatic enzyme activities or through alterations in hepatic blood flow. Many drugs are metabolized by cytochrome P450 isozymes. A reference table of drugs and their CYP450 isoforms is available on the internet at www.drug-interactions.com. These isozymes are named according to a standard system, e.g. CYP3A4 or P4503A4. Drugs that are substrates or inhibitors for the same isozyme *in vitro* are likely to interact, but no interaction may be detectable, or it may not be clinically significant. Other drugs alter the binding of another drug to plasma proteins or tissue receptors, alter the distribution of drugs to active receptor sites, delay or enhance excretion, or cause additive or synergistic effects.

Elimination of a drug can also be affected by the P-glycoprotein membrane-bound transport system. Digoxin, for example, moves across cell membranes by a P-glycoprotein controlled process. Drugs such as quinidine that inhibit P-glycoprotein activity, can increase the serum concentration and toxicity of digoxin.

RECOMMENDATIONS — Monitoring is most important when one of the interacting drugs is stopped or started. Some experienced clinicians may prefer to monitor the patient's clinical status rather than follow serum concentrations of drugs. Concurrent use of drugs from the same group, e.g. aspirin and other NSAIDs, should be avoided.

(Updated through December 2000)

ADVERSE INTERACTIONS OF DRUGS

ABACAVIR, with:
  Alcohol
   Possible abacavir toxicity (probably decreased metabolism)
   > Manufacturer's package insert (abacavir); JA McDowell et al, Pharmacokinetic interaction of abacavir (1592U89) and ethanol in human immunodeficiency virus-infected adults. Antimicrob Agents Chemother, 44:1686, 2000

   Based on a study in patients; magnitude of effect may not be sufficient to produce toxicity in most patients

  Amprenavir
   Possible increased amprenavir effect (decreased metabolism; CYP3A4)
   > Manufacturer's package insert (amprenavir)

   One study in 4 subjects; monitor clinical status

Abciximab, no documented interactions, see page 4, Criteria for Listing Interactions

ACARBOSE, with:
  Anticoagulants, Oral
   Possible increased warfarin effect (mechanism not established)
   > AP Morreale and K Janetzky, Probable interaction of warfarin and acarbose. Am J Health Syst Pharm, 54:1551, 1997

   Single case report (1997)

  Digoxin
   Possible decreased digoxin effect (decreased absorption)
   > T Miura et al, Impairment of absorption of digoxin by acarbose. J Clin Pharmacol, 38:654, 1998; M Kusumoto et al, Lack of kinetic interaction between digoxin and voglibose. Eur J Clin Pharmacol, 55:79, 1999; H Ben-Ami et al, An interaction between digoxin and acarbose. Diabetes Care, 22:860, 1999

   Based on study in healthy subjects and two case reports (1999); monitor digoxin concentration and clinical status; voglibose may not interact

  Metformin
   Possible decreased metformin effect (decreased absorption)
   > SJ Scheen et al, Reduction of metformin acute bioavailability by the alpha-glucosidase inhibitor acarbose in normal man. Eur J Clin Invest, 23 suppl 1:A43, 1993

   Monitor blood glucose; based on study in healthy subjects

  Valproate
   Possible decreased effect of valproic acid (possibly decreased absorption)
   > JS Serrano et al, May acarbose impair valproate bioavailability? Methods Find Exper Clin Pharmacol, 18 suppl C:98, 1996

   Single case report (1996); monitor valproic acid concentration and clinical status

ACE inhibitors, see Angiotensin-converting enzyme (ACE) inhibitors

Acebutolol, see Beta-adrenergic blockers
Acenocoumarol, see Anticoagulants, oral
ACETAMINOPHEN, with:
Alcohol
Severe hepatotoxicity with therapeutic doses of acetaminophen in chronic alcoholics (probably increased formation of hepatotoxic acetaminophen metabolites [CYP2E1] and gluthathione depletion)

LB Seeff et al, Acetaminophen hepatotoxicity in alcoholics. Ann Intern Med, 104:399, 1986; HJ Zimmerman and WC Maddrey, Acetaminophen (paracetamol) hepatotoxicity with regular intake of alcohol: analysis of instances of therapeutic misadventure. Hepatology, 22:767, 1995; JT Slattery et al, The complex interaction between ethanol and acetaminophen. Clin Pharmacol Ther, 60:241, 1996; P Draganov et al, Alcohol-acetaminophen syndrome. Postgrad Med, 107:189, 2000; LF Prescott, Paracetamol, alcohol and the liver. Br J Clin Pharmacol, 49:291, 2000; KE Thummel et al, Ethanol and production of the hepatotoxic metabolite of acetaminophen in healthy adults. Clin Pharmacol Ther, 67:591, 2000; A Makin and R Williams, Paracetamol hepatotoxicity and alcohol consumption in deliberate and accidental overdose. QJM, 93:341, 2000

Incidence unknown; some have questioned validity of this interaction; until controversies are resolved, warn patients who abuse alcohol to limit acetaminophen use

Anticoagulants, oral
Increased anticoagulant effect of warfarin and possibly acenocoumarol or other oral anticoagulants (mechanism not established)

JJ Boeijinga et al, Interaction between paracetamol and coumarin anticoagulants. Lancet, 1:506, 1982; WR Bartle and JA Blakely, Potentiation of warfarin anticoagulation by acetaminophen. JAMA, 265:1260, 1991; RT Weibert, Warfarin-acetaminophen interaction. Int Pharmaceutical Abst, 31:2268, 1994; D Kwan et al, The effects of acute and chronic acetaminophen dosing on the pharmacodynamics and pharmacokinetics of (R)- and (S) warfarin. Clin Pharmacol Ther, 57:212, 1995; WR Bell, Acetaminophen and warfarin: undesirable synergy. JAMA, 279:702, 1998; D Kwan et al, The effects of acetaminophen on pharmacokinetics and pharmacodynamics of warfarin. J Clin Pharmacol, 39:68, 1999; H Bagheri et al, Potentiation of the acenocoumarol anticoagulant effect by acetaminophen. Ann Pharmacother, 33:506, 1999; KLA Shek et al, Warfarin-acetaminophen drug interaction revisited. Pharmacotherapy, 19:1153, 1999; MC Goldman et al, Warfarin-acetaminophen drug interaction: case report. ASHP Midyear Clinical Meeting, 34:P-432D, 1999; A Lo et al, New information on the acetaminophen — warfarin interaction. Can Pharm J, 132:35, 1999

Monitor INR or prothrombin time; patient susceptibility varies; acetaminophen effect dose-dependent; study in healthy subjects found no effect on warfarin with acetaminophen 4 g/day for 2 weeks (1999)

Antihistamines, H$_1$-blockers: astemizole, terfenadine
Torsades de pointes with terfenadine (mechanism not established)

PP Matsis and RN Easthope, Torsades de pointes ventricular tachycardia

(continued)

ACETAMINOPHEN, with: *(continued)*
    associated with terfenadine and paracetamol self medication. NZ Med J, 107:402, 1994

Single case report (1994); terfenadine is no longer available

Antihistamines, H$_1$-blockers: diphenhydramine
    Delayed absorption of acetaminophen (delayed gastric emptying)
        WO Tsang and AM Nadroo, An unusual case of acetaminophen overdose. Pediatr Emerg Care, 15:344, 1999

Peak acetaminophen serum concentrations may be later than expected in patients taking an overdose of acetaminophen/diphenhydramine (e.g., Tylenol PM)

Barbiturates
    Acetaminophen hepatic toxicity (mechanism not established)
        JH Pirotte, Apparent potentiation by phenobarbital of hepatotoxicity from small doses of acetaminophen. Ann Intern Med, 101:403, 1984

Case report in one epileptic maintained on barbiturates after taking acetaminophen for 6 months

Benzodiazepines
    Possible diazepam toxicity (mechanism not established)
        BA Mulley et al, Interactions between diazepam and paracetamol. J Clin Pharmacol, 3:25, 1978

Monitor clinical status

Beta-adrenergic blockers
    Decreased acetaminophen clearance with propranolol (decreased metabolism)
        OZ Baraka et al, The effect of propranolol on paracetamol metabolism in man. Br J Clin Pharmacol, 29:261, 1990

Clinical significance not established

Chloroquine
    Possible chloroquine toxicity (mechanism not established)
        RK Raina et al, The effect of aspirin, paracetamol and analgin on pharmacokinetics of chloroquine. Indian J Physiol Pharmacol, 37:229, 1993

Based on a study of 8 male subjects; monitor clinical status

Cholestyramine
    Decreased acetaminophen effect (decreased absorption)
        B Dordoni et al, Reduction of absorption of paracetamol by activated charcoal and cholestyramine: a possible therapeutic measure. Br Med J, 3:86, 1973

Take acetaminophen at least one hour before cholestyramine

Contraceptives, oral
    Possible decreased analgesic effect (increased metabolism)
        MC Mitchell et al, Effects of oral contraceptive steroids on acetaminophen metabolism and elimination. Clin Pharmacol Ther, 34:48, 1983

Monitor analgesia

    Possible ethinyl estradiol toxicity (decreased metabolism)
        SM Rogers et al, Paracetamol interaction with oral contraceptive steroids: increased plasma concentrations of ethinyloestradiol. Br J Clin Pharmacol,

ACETAMINOPHEN, with: *(continued)*
> 23:721, 1987

Clinical significance not established

Isoniazid

Acetaminophen toxicity (increase in toxic metabolites)
> R Murphy et al, Severe acetaminophen toxicity in a patient receiving isoniazid. Ann Intern Med, 113:799, 1990; JS Crippin, Acetaminophen Hepatotoxicity: potentiation by isoniazid. Am J Gastroenterol, 88:590, 1993;JY Chien et al, Influence of polymorphic N-acetyltransferase phenotype on the inhibition and induction of acetaminophen bioactivation with long-term isoniazid. Clin Pharmacol Ther, 61:24, 1997

Several case reports (1990—1993); interaction can be greater when acetaminophen is given 12 hours after isoniazid than if they are given simultaneously; avoid concurrent use

Mifepristone

Increased pain (mechanism not established)
> B Weber and J-E Fontan, Acetaminophen as a pain enhancer during voluntary interruption of pregnancy with mifepristone and sulprostone. Eur J Clin Pharmacol, 39:609, 1990

Avoid concurrent use; patients received mifepristone and sulprostone concurrently

Phenytoin

Possible increase in acetaminophen toxicity (probably enzyme induction)
> C Brackett and JD Bloch, Phenytoin as a possible cause of acetaminophen hepatotoxicity: case report and review of the literature. Pharmacotherapy, 20:229, 2000

Concomittant use of antiepileptics such as phenytoin with acetaminophen, may increase the risk of hepatic injury during prolonged or high dose acetaminophen therapy; avoid high doses of acetaminophen if possible; monitor liver function and clinical status, if continued acetaminophen therapy is required; in cases where acetaminophen poisoning is suspected, consider administering N-acetylcysteine even if plasma acetaminophen levels are below threshold values.

Probenecid

Possible acetaminophen toxicity (decreased metabolism and renal excretion)
> DR Abernethy et al, Probenecid impairment of acetaminophen and lorazepam clearance: direct inhibition of ether glucuronide formation. J Pharmacol Exp Ther, 234:345, 1985; F Kamali, The effect of probenecid on paracetamol metabolism and pharmacokinetics. Eur J Clin Pharmacol, 45:551, 1993

Avoid concurrent use

Sulfinpyrazone

Possible decreased acetaminophen effect (increased metabolism)
> JO Miners et al, Determinants of acetaminophen metabolism: effect of inducers and inhibitors of drug metabolism on acetaminophen's metabolic pathways. Clin Pharmacol Ther, 35:480, 1984

(continued)

ACETAMINOPHEN, with: *(continued)*
  Monitor clinical status
  Sulprostone
    Increased pain (mechanism not established)
      B Weber and J-E Fontan, Acetaminophen as a pain enhancer during voluntary interruption of pregnancy with mifepristone and sulprostone. Eur J Clin Pharmacol, 39:609, 1990
    Avoid concurrent use; patients received mifepristone and sulprostone concurrently
  Tobacco, smoking
    Decreased acetaminophen effect (increased metabolism)
      JC Mucklow et al, Environmental factors affecting paracetamol metabolism in London factory and office workers. Br J Clin Pharmacol, 10:67, 1980
    Monitor efficacy
  Zidovudine
    Granulocytopenia (mechanism not established)
      EM Steffe et al, The effect of acetaminophen on zidovudine metabolism in HIV-infected patients. J Acquir Immune Defic Syndr, 3:691, 1990
    Monitor white blood count; may be rare

    Hepatotoxicity (mechanism not established)
      K Shriner and MB Goetz, Severe hepatotoxicity in a patient receiving both acetaminophen and zidovudine. Am J Med, 93:94, 1992
    Single case report in cachectic AIDS patient (1992)

    Possible zidovudine toxicity (increased absorption)
      DM Burger et al, Short-term, combined use of paracetamol and zidovudine does not alter the pharmacokinetics of either drug. Ned J Med, 44:161, 1994; DM Burger et al, Pharmacokinetics of zidovudine and acetaminophen in a patient on chronic acetaminophen therapy. Ann Pharmacother, 28:327, 1994
    Single case report (1994); only after long-term use; clinical significance not established; no pharmacokinetic interaction noted with short-term combined use
Acetazolamide, see Carbonic anhydrase inhibitors
Acetohexamide, see Hypoglycemics, sulfonylurea
Acetophenazine, see Phenothiazines
Acetylcysteine, no documented interactions, see page 4, Criteria for Listing Interactions
ACITRETIN, with:
  Alcohol
    Possible increased teratogenic effect (increase conversion of acitretin to longer acting etretinate)
      FG Larsen et al, Conversion of acitretin to etretinate in psoriatic patients is influenced by ethanol. J Invest Dermatol, 100:623, 1993
    Avoid concurrent use
  Methotrexate
    Possible increased hepatotoxicity (additive)
      Manufacturer's package insert

ACITRETIN, with: *(continued)*
   Avoid concurrent use
  Progestins
    Decreased contraceptive effect with mini dose progestin (mechanism not established)
        P Berbis et al, Acitretin (RO10-1670) and oral contraceptives: interaction study. Arch Dermatol Res, 280:388, 1988
    Effect on other oral contraceptives unknown; use barrier contraception
  Tetracyclines
    Possible increased risk of pseudotumor cerebri (mechanism not established)
        Manufacturer's package insert
    Avoid concurrent use

Acrivastine, no documented interactions, see page 4, Criteria for Listing Interactions

ACYCLOVIR, with:
  Narcotics: meperidine and congeners
    Possible meperidine toxicity (decreased renal excretion)
        R Johnson et al, Adverse effects with acyclovir and meperidine. Ann Intern Med, 103:962, 1985
    Might also occur with other narcotics
  Probenecid
    Possible acyclovir toxicity (decreased renal excretion)
        OL Laskin et al, Effects of probenecid on the pharmacokinetics and elimination of acyclovir in humans. Antimicrob Agents Chemother, 21:804, 1982
    Significance not established, but high concentration of acyclovir can cause renal damage
  Theophyllines
    Possible theophylline toxicity (Probably decreased metabolism)
        Y Maeda et al, Inhibition of theophylline metabolism by aciclovir. Biol Pharm Bull, 19:1591, 1996
    Based on study in healthy subjects and case report (1996); monitor theophylline concentrations
  Zidovudine
    Severe drowsiness and lethargy (mechanism not established)
        MC Bach, Possible drug interaction during therapy with azidothymidine and acyclovir for AIDS. N Engl J Med, 316:547, 1987
    Single well-documented case report of 2 episodes (1987)

Adapalene, no documented interactions, see page 4, Criteria for Listing Interactions
Adefovir, no documented interactions, see page 4, Criteria for Listing Interactions

ADENOSINE, with:
  Digoxin
    Ventricular fibrillation
        N Mulla and PP Karpawich, Ventricular fibrillation following adenosine therapy for supraventricular tachycardia in a neonate with concealed Wolff-Parkinson-White syndrome treated with digoxin. Pediatr Emerg Care, 11:238, 1995

(continued)

ADENOSINE, with: *(continued)*
> *Based on single case report in neonate with Wolff-Parkinson-White syndrome (1995)*

Dipyridamole
> Possible adenosine toxicity (decreased metabolism secondary to decreased uptake)
>> AH Watt et al, Intravenous adenosine in the treatment of supraventricular tachycardia: a dose-ranging study and interaction with dipyridamole. Br J Clin Pharmacol, 21:227, 1986
>
> *Limit initial dose of adenosine to 1 mg*

Nicotine gum
> Increased chest pain and A-V block (possibly additive)
>> C Sylvén et al, Nicotine enhances angina pectoris-like chest pain and atrioventricular blockade provoked by intravenous bolus of adenosine in healthy volunteers. J Cardiovasc Pharmacol, 16:962, 1990
>
> *Study in healthy nonsmokers; avoid concurrent use*

Theophyllines
> Decreased adenosine effect (receptor antagonism)
>> DL Maxwell et al, Contrasting effects of two xanthines, theophylline and enprofylline, on the cardio-respiratory stimulation of infused adenosine in man. Acta Physiol Scand, 131:459, 1987
>
> *Based on a study of normal males*

Verapamil
> Increased adenosine effect (probably additive)
>> W-T Lai et al, Effects of verapamil, propranolol, and procainamide on adenosine-induced negative dromotropism in human beings. Am Heart J, 132:768, 1996
>
> *Based on study in patients; verapamil reduced the dose of adenosine required to produce AV nodal block*

Albuterol, see Sympathomimetic bronchodilators

ALCOHOL, with:

Abacavir - See Abacavir with Alcohol, page 6

Acetaminophen - See Acetaminophen with Alcohol, page 7

Acitretin - See Acitretin with Alcohol, page 10

Anticoagulants, oral
> Decreased anticoagulant effect with chronic alcohol abuse (increased metabolism)
>> RMH Kater et al, Increased rate of clearance of drugs from the circulation of alcoholics. Am J Med Sci, 258:35, 1969;
>
> *Monitor prothrombin time in chronic alcoholics*
>
> Increased anticoagulant effect of both oral anticoagulants and heparin with acute intoxication (decreased metabolism)
>> P Sandor et al, Effect of short- and long-term alcohol use on phenytoin kinetics in chronic alcoholics. Clin Pharmacol Ther, 30:390, 1981; EA Curry and DD Dunlop, Ethanol induced warfarin toxicity. ASHP Midyear Clinical Meeting, 33:P-178D, 1998

ALCOHOL, with: *(continued)*
Warn patients and monitor prothrombin time
Antidepressants, tricyclic
Toxicity of both drugs with amitriptyline or trazodone (decreased metabolism)
> M Linnoila et al, Effects of amitriptyline, desipramine, and zimelidine, alone and in combination with ethanol, on information processing and memory in healthy volunteers. Acta Psychiatr Scand, 68 suppl 308:175, 1983; P Dorian et al, Amitriptyline and ethanol: pharmacokinetic and pharmacodynamic interaction. Eur J Clin Pharmacol, 25:325, 1983; S J Warrington et al, An evaluation of possible interactions between ethanol and trazodone or amitriptyline. Br J Clin Pharmacol, 18:549, 1984; MC Hyatt and MA Bird, Amitriptyline augments and prolongs ethanol-induced euphoria. J Clin Psychopharmacol, 7:277, 1987

Avoid concurrent use; to some extent, zimelidine may partly counteract deleterious effects of alcohol on cognitive functions; the combination with amitriptyline can cause additive euphoria, which has led to abuse

Decreased imipramine and desipramine effect in alcoholics (mechanism not established)
> DA Ciraulo et al, Clinical pharmacokinetics of imipramine and desipramine in alcoholics and normal volunteers. Clin Pharmacol Ther, 43:508, 1988

Monitor imipramine and desipramine concentrations

Decreased cognitive function (probably additive)
> T Seppala et al, Effects of zimelidine, mianserin and amitriptyline on psychomotor skills and their interaction with ethanol; a placebo controlled cross-over study. Eur J Clin Pharmacol, 27:181, 1984; E Tanaka and S Misawa, Pharmacokinetic interactions between acute alcohol ingestion and single doses of benzodiazepines, and tricyclic and tetracyclic antidepressants - an update. J Clin Pharm Ther, 23:331, 1998

Avoid concurrent use

Antifungals, Griseofulvin
Disulfiram-like effect with flushing, nausea, vomiting, diarrhea (mechanism not established)
> DL Fett and LF Vukov, An unusual case of severe griseofulvin-alcohol interaction. Ann Emerg Med, 24:1, 1994

Single case report (1994); warn patients of possibility

Antifungals, imidazoles and triazoles
Possible disulfiram-like reaction with ketoconazole (mechanism not established)
> AJ Magnasco and LD Magnasco, Interaction of ketoconazole and ethanol. Clin Pharm, 5:522, 1986; RHB Meyboom and BW Pater, Overgevoeligheid voor alcoholische dranken tijdens behandeling met ketoconazol. Ned Tijdschr Geneeskd, 133:1463, 1989; RA Fazio et al, Ketoconazole treatment of *Candida esophagitis* – a prospective study of 12 cases. Am J Gastroenterol, 78:261 1983

Several case reports

(continued)

ALCOHOL, with: *(continued)*
Antihistamines, H$_2$-blockers
Increased alcohol effect with cimetidine, nizatidine, and ranitidine (possible inhibition of acetaldehyde metabolism in ALDH-1 deficiency)

> AW Jones, Histamine-2—receptor antagonists and serum ethanol levels. Ann Intern Med, 119:952, 1993; MD Cook et al, Effect of cimetidine on the pharmacokinetics of alcohol in social and chronic drinkers. Drug Invest, 7:84, 1994; E Baraona et al, Blood alcohol levels after prolonged use of histamine-2—receptor antagonists. Ann Intern Med, 121:73, 1994; A Mallat et al, Inhibition of gastric alcohol dehydrogenase activity by histamine H$_2$-receptor antagonists has no influence on the pharmacokinetics of ethanol after a moderate dose. Br J Clin Pharmacol, 37:208, 1994; E Baraona et al, Bioavailability of alcohol: role of gastric metabolism and its interaction with other drugs. Dig Dis, 12:351, 1994; AG Fraser, Is there an interaction between H$_2$-antagonists and alcohol? Drug Metab Drug Interact, 14:123, 1998

Small effect; clinical significance not established; patients should be warned of the possibility; famotidine may not interact

Barbiturates
Decreased sedative effect with chronic alcohol abuse (increased barbiturate metabolism)

> PS Misra, Increase of ethanol, meprobamate and pentobarbital metabolism after chronic ethanol administration in man and in rats. Am J Med, 51:346, 1971

Avoid concurrent use if possible

Increased CNS depression with acute intoxication (additive; decreased barbiturate metabolism)

> E Rubin et al, Inhibition of drug metabolism by acute ethanol intoxication: a hepatic microsomal mechanism. Am J Med, 49:801, 1970

Avoid concurrent use if possible

Benzodiazepines
Increased CNS depression (additive effects, possibly decreased metabolism of benzodiazepines)

> PV Desmond et al, Short-term ethanol administration impairs the elimination of chlordiazepoxide *(Librium)* in man. Eur J Clin Pharmacol, 18:275, 1980; H-P Willumeit et al, Alcohol interaction of lormetazepam, mepindolol sulphate and diazepam measured by performance on the driving simulator. Pharmacopsychiatry, 17:36, 1984; P Dorian et al, Triazolam and ethanol interaction: Kinetic and dynamic consequences. Clin Pharmacol Ther, 37:558, 1985; K Aranko et al, Interaction of diazepam or lorazepam with alcohol. Eur J Clin Pharmacol, 28:559, 1985; M Divoll and DJ Greenblatt, Alcohol does not enhance diazepam absorption. Pharmacology, 22:263, 1981; ARW Forrest et al, Fatal temazepam overdoses. Lancet, 2:226, 1986; M Linnoila et al, Effects of single doses of alprazolam and diazepam, alone and in combination with ethanol, on psychomotor and cognitive performance and on autonomic nervous system reactivity in healthy volunteers.

ALCOHOL, with: *(continued)*
> Eur J Clin Pharmacol, 39:21, 1990; T Kuitunen et al, Actions and interactions of hypnotics on human performance: single doses of zopiclone, triazolam and alcohol. Int Clin Psychopharmacol, 5 suppl 2:115, 1990; K Uemura and S Komura, Death caused by triazolam and ethanol intoxication. Am J Forensic Med Pathol, 16:66, 1995; CR Rush and RR Griffiths, Acute participant-rated and behavioral effects of alprazolam and buspirone, alone and in combination with ethanol, in normal volunteers. Exp Clin Psychopharmacol, 5:28, 1997; E Tanaka and S Misawa, Pharmacokinetic interactions between acute alcohol ingestion and single doses of benzodiazepines, and tricyclic and tetracyclic antidepressants - an update. J Clin Pharm Ther, 23:331, 1998

Since even small amounts of alcohol may impair driving ability in patients taking benzodiazepines, concurrent use should be avoided; clinical significance of possible zopiclone interaction has not been established

Anterograde amnesia with triazolam and possibly other benzodiazepines (mechanism not established)
> HH Morris, III and ML Estes, Traveler's amnesia; transient global amnesia secondary to triazolam. JAMA, 258:945, 1987; JL Lichtor et al, Alcohol after midazolam sedation: does it really matter? Anesth Analg, 72:661, 1991

Avoid concurrent use; midazolam and possibly other short-acting benzodiazepines given IV may not interact after 4 hours

Beta-adrenergic blockers
May block signs of delirium tremens
> RJ Zechnich, Beta-blockers can obscure diagnosis of delirium tremens. Lancet, 1:1071, 1982

Avoid beta-blockers in alcoholics

Decreased beta-blockade with propranolol (increased metabolism)
> BS Grabowski et al, Effects of acute alcohol administration on propranolol absorption. Int J Clin Pharmacol Ther Toxicol, 18:317, 1980; R Zaman et al, The effect of food and alcohol on the pharmacokinetics of acebutolol and its metabolite, diacetolol. Biopharm Drug Dispos, 5:91, 1984; R Maheswaran et al, The interaction of alcohol and β-blockers in arterial hypertension. J Clin Pharm Ther, 15:405, 1990

Reported only with propranolol, but warn patients taking any beta-blocker; acebutolol, oxprenolol and metoprolol may not interact; dosage should not be changed after short-term increased use of alcohol

Increased beta-blockade with sotalol (decreased elimination)
> RJ Zechnich, Beta-blockers can obscure diagnosis of delirium tremens. Lancet, 1:1071, 1982

Monitor clinical status

Bromocriptine
Possible bromocriptine toxicity (mechanism not established)
> J Ayres and MN Maisey, Alcohol increases bromocriptine's side effects. N Engl J Med, 302:806, 1980

(continued)

ALCOHOL, with: *(continued)*
Clinical evidence limited; warn patients

Caffeine
Caffeine may not affect or further decrease reaction time (synergism or antagonism)
> DJ Osborne and Y Rogers, Interactions of alcohol and caffeine on human reaction time. Aviat Space Environ Med, 54:528, 1983; O Azcona et al, Evaluation of the central effects of alcohol and caffeine interaction. Br J Clin Pharmacol, 40:393, 1995

Variable response; caffeine cannot be relied upon to reverse effects of alcohol on psychomotor performance

Cephalosporins
Disulfiram-like effect with cefamandole, cefoperazone, cefotetan, or moxalactam (probably inhibition of intermediary metabolism of alcohol)
> MK Buening et al, Disulfiram-like reaction to beta-lactams. JAMA, 245:2027, 1981; RM Elenbaas et al, On the disulfiram-like activity of moxalactam. Clin Pharmacol Ther, 32:347, 1982; S Umeda and T Arai, Disulfiram-like reaction to moxalactam after celiac plexus alcohol block. Anesth Analg, 64:377, 1985; SS Kline et al, Cefotetan-induced disulfiram-type reactions and hypoprothrombinemia. Antimicrob Agents Chemother, 31:1328, 1987; FG McMahon et al, Absence of disulfiram-type reactions to single and multiple doses of cefonicid: a placebo-controlled study. J Antimicrob Chemother, 20:913, 1987

Avoid alcohol and alcohol-containing medications; single case report on 2 occasions with cefonicid (1990)

Chloral hydrate
Prolonged hypnotic effect (synergism); adverse cardiovascular effects (mechanism not established)
> EM Sellers et al, Interaction of chloral hydrate and ethanol in man. I. Metabolism. Clin Pharmacol Ther, 13:37, 1972

Avoid concurrent use

Chlormethiazole
Chlormethiazole toxicity (decreased metabolism)
> GT McInnes, Chlormethiazole and alcohol: a lethal cocktail. Br Med J, 294:592, 1987

Avoid concurrent use

Cisapride
Possible increased alcohol effect (increased absorption)
> R Roine et al, Cisapride enhances alcohol absorption and leads to high blood alcohol levels. Gastroenterology, 102:A507, 1992; S Kechagias et al, Impact of gastric emptying on the pharmacokinetics of ethanol as influenced by cisapride. Br J Clin Pharmacol, 48:728, 1999

Warn patients; effect probably small in most people; cisapride is no longer marketed in the USA

Contraceptives, oral
Possible alcohol effect (decreased metabolism)
> MK Jones and BM Jones, Ethanol metabolism in women taking oral

ALCOHOL, with: *(continued)*
    contraceptives. Alcoholism (NY), 8:24, 1984
Caution patients

Cyclobenzaprine
    Increased CNS depression (additive)
        CL Winek, Jr et al, Drowning due to cyclobenzaprine and ethanol. Forensic Sci Int, 100:105, 1999
    Single fatal case report in intoxicated patient (1999)

Cycloserine
    Increased alcohol effect or convulsions (mechanism not established)
        AC Cohen, Pyridoxine in the prevention and treatment of convulsions and neurotoxicity due to cycloserine. Ann NY Acad Sci, 166:346, 1969; F Glass et al, Beobachtungen und untersuchungen uber die gemeinsame wirkung von alkohol und D-cycloserin. Arzneimittelforschung, 15:684, 1965
    Avoid concurrent use; warn patients

Cyclosporine
    Possible cyclosporine toxicity (probably decreased metabolism)
        MD Paul et al, The effect of ethanol on serum cyclosporine A levels in renal transplant recipients. Am J Kidney Dis, 10:133, 1987
    After acute intoxication in a renal transplant recipient with a history of alcoholism (1987); serum concentrations of cyclosporine in nonalcoholic renal transplant patients were not affected by ingestion of 50 ml of alcohol

Cytarabine
    Aggravation of pain from acral erythema caused by cytarabine (mechanism not established)
        KK Kampmann et al, Acral erythema secondary to high-dose cytosine arabinoside with pain worsened by cyclosporine infusions. Cancer, 63:2482, 1989
    Three case reports in patients receiving IV cyclosporine in an alcohol base; pain was controlled by slowing the infusion rate and giving analgesics

Disulfiram
    Single report (1988) of dyspareunia and male discomfort, when woman taking disulfiram and man intoxicated
        JD Chick, Disulfiram reaction during sexual intercourse. Br J Psychiatry, 152:438, 1988
    Avoid alcohol and alcohol-containing medications;

Felodipine
    Orthostatic hypotension (possible increased felodipine absorption)
        DG Bailey et al, Ethanol enhances the hemodynamic effects of felodipine. Clin Invest Med, 12:357, 1989; PJ Pentikäinen et al, Acute alcohol intake increases the bioavailability of felodipine. Clin Pharmacol Ther, 55:148, 1994
    Avoid concurrent use; based on study in 10 men with borderline hypertension

Guanadrel
    Increased sedation and orthostatic hypotension (additive)
        Manufacturer's package insert

(continued)

ALCOHOL, with: *(continued)*
Avoid concurrent use

Hypoglycemics, sulfonylurea

Decreased hypoglycemic effect with chronic alcohol abuse (increased metabolism)

    RMH Kater et al, Increased rate of clearance of drugs from the circulation of alcoholics. Am J Med Sci, 258:35, 1969

Avoid large amounts of alcohol

Increased or prolonged hypoglycemic effect with acute ingestion of alcohol, especially in fasting patients (suppression of gluconeogenesis)

    N Carulli et al, Alcohol-drugs interaction in man: alcohol and tolbutamide. Eur J Clin Invest, 1:421, 1971; MR Burge et al, Low-dose ethanol predisposes elderly fasted patients with type 2 diabetes to sulfonylurea-induced low blood glucose. Diabetes Care, 22:2037, 1999

Based on study in elderly type 2 diabetics given modest doses of ethanol under fasting conditions

Minor disulfiram-like symptoms, particularly with chlorpropamide (inhibition of intermediary metabolism of alcohol)

    L Groop et al, Roles of chlorpropamide, alcohol and acetaldehyde in determining the chlorpropamide-alcohol flush. Diabetologia, 26:34, 1984; SG Hartling et al, Interaction of ethanol and glipizide in humans. Diabetes Care, 10:683, 1987

Inform patients; unlikely with small amounts of alcohol with meals

Isoniazid

Increased incidence of hepatitis (mechanism not established)

    DE Kopanoff et al, Isoniazid-related hepatitis. Am Rev Respir Dis, 117:991, 1978

Incidence of serious consequences unknown

Possible decreased isoniazid effect in some alcoholics (increased metabolism)

    D Lester, The acetylation of isoniazid in alcoholics. Q J Studies Alcohol, 25:541, 1984

Do not use isoniazid alone for tuberculosis treatment in alcoholics

Isotretinoin

Decreased isotretinoin effect (mechanism not established)

    C Soria et al, Decreased isotretinoin efficacy during acute alcohol intake. Dermatologica, 182:203, 1991

Single case report (1991)

Ivermectin

Possible ivermectin toxicity (mechanism not established)

    EN Shu et al, Do alcoholic beverages enhance availability of ivermectin? Eur J Clin Pharmacol, 56:437, 2000

Based on study in healthy subjects; clinical importance not established; monitor clinical status

Lithium

Possible lithium effect (mechanism not established)

    RF Anton et al, Effect of acute alcohol consumption on lithium kinetics. Clin Pharmacol Ther, 38:52, 1985

ALCOHOL, with: *(continued)*
    Clinical significance not established; monitor lithium concentration
  Macrolide antibiotics
    Possible decreased erythromycin effect (decreased absorption)
      MI Morasso et al, Influence of alcohol consumption on erythromycin ethylsuccinate kinetics. Int J Clin Pharmacol Ther Toxicol, 28:426, 1990
    Based on studies in healthy subjects; avoid concurrent use
  Maprotiline
    Seizures, possibly due to maprotiline toxicity (mechanism not established)
      SK Strawn et al, Alcohol precipitation of maprotiline-associated seizures. South Med J, 81:1205, 1988
    Single case report (1988)
  Meprobamate
    Decreased sedative effect with chronic alcohol abuse (increased metabolism)
      PS Misra, Increase of ethanol, meprobamate and pentobarbital metabolism after chronic ethanol administration in man and in rats. Am J Med, 51:346, 1971
    Avoid meprobamate in alcoholics

    Increased CNS depression with acute intoxication (additive and decreased metabolism)
      E Rubin et al, Inhibition of drug metabolism by acute ethanol intoxication: a hepatic microsomal mechanism. Am J Med, 49:801, 1970
    Warn patients
  Metformin
    Lactic acidosis (additive)
      Manufacturer's package insert
    Avoid concurrent use
  Methotrexate
    Increased hepatotoxicity in chronic alcoholics (mechanism not established)
      Manufacturer's package insert; J Almeyda et al, Methotrexate, psoriasis and the liver. Br J Dermatol, 85:302, 1971; SH Pai et al, Severe liver damage caused by treatment of psoriasis with methotrexate. NY State J Med, 73:2585, 1973; H Zachariae, Alcohol interactions with drugs and its effect on the treatment of skin diseases. Clin Dermatol, 17:443, 1999
    Minimize alcohol intake; monitor hepatic function
  Metronidazole
    Mild disulfiram-like symptoms (possibly inhibition of intermediary metabolism of alcohol)
      AJ Giannini and DT De France, Metronidazole and alcohol – potential for combinative abuse. J Toxicol Clin Toxicol, 20:509, 1983; I Alexander, 'Alcohol-Antabuse' syndrome in patients receiving metronidazole during gynaecological treatment. Br J Clin Pract, 39:292, 1985; GL Plosker, Possible interaction between ethanol and vaginally administered metronidazole. Clin Pharm, 6:189, 1987; DP Harries et al, Metronidazole and alcohol: potential problems. Scot Med J, 35:179, 1990; DL Edwards et al, Disulfiram-like reaction associated with intravenous trimethoprim-sulfamethoxazole and

(continued)

ALCOHOL, with: *(continued)*
> metronidazole. Clin Pharm, 5:999, 1986; SJ Cina et al, Sudden death due to metronidazole/ethanol interaction. Am J Forensic Med Path, 17:343, 1996; KW Garey and KA Rodvold, Disulfiram reactions and anti-infective agents. Infect Med, 16:741, 1999; CS Williams and KR Woodcock, Do ethanol and metronidazole interact to produce a disulfiram-like reaction? Ann Pharmacother, 34:255, 2000
>
> *Vomiting rare; nausea mild or absent; excitement, giddiness, and flush found pleasant by some, have led to abuse; may occur with IV drugs containing alcohol; single report with vaginal metronidazole (1987); single report of severe metabolic acidosis and cardiovascular instability in an intoxicated man treated with IV metronidazole (1990); single report of fatality (1996); many patients have received combination without evidence of a disulfiram reaction*

Mianserin
> Toxicity of both drugs (decreased metabolism)
> > C Strömberg and MJ Mattila, Acute comparison of clovoxamine and mianserin, alone and in combination with ethanol, on human psychomotor performance. Pharmacol Toxicol, 60:374, 1987
>
> *Avoid concurrent use*

Mirtazapine
> Impaired motor function and cognition, and sedation (additive)
> > Manufacturer's package insert
>
> *Avoid concurrent use*

Narcotics: morphine-like
> Increased heroin effect (decreased metabolism; additive)
> > A Polettini et al, The role of alcohol abuse in the etiology of heroin-related deaths. Evidence for pharmacokinetic interactions between heroin and alcohol. J Anal Toxicol, 23:570, 1999
>
> *Based on study of heroin-related deaths*

Nicotinic acid
> Lactic acidosis (mechanism not established)
> > RA Schwab and BH Bachhuber, Delirium and lactic acidosis caused by ethanol and niacin coingestion. Am J Emerg Med, 9:363, 1991
>
> *Single case report (1991)*

Nifedipine
> Possible nifedipine toxicity (probably decreased metabolism)
> > S Qureshi et al, Effect of an acute dose of alcohol on the pharmacokinetics of oral nifedipine in humans. Pharm Res, 9:683, 1992
>
> *Avoid concurrent use; based on studies in healthy men*

Nitrates
> Possible hypotension with nitroglycerin (additive)
> > M Kupari et al, Does alcohol intensify the hemodynamic effects of nitroglycerin? Clin Cardiol, 7:382, 1984
>
> *Reported only when nitroglycerin was taken an hour or more after alcohol; warn patients*

ALCOHOL, with: *(continued)*
  Nonsteroidal anti-inflammatory drugs
    Bleeding with aspirin (additive)
      D Deykin et al, Ethanol potentiation of aspirin-induced prolongation of the bleeding time. N Engl J Med, 306:852, 1982; PR Pfau and GR Lichtenstein, NSAIDs and alcohol: Never the twain shall mix? Am J Gastroenterol, 94:3098, 1999
    Avoid large amounts of alcohol

    Acute renal failure with ibuprofen (mechanism not established)
      GN Elsasser et al, Reversible acute renal failure associated with ibuprofen ingestion and binge drinking. J Fam Pract, 27:221, 1988
    Single case report (1988)

    Increased bioavailability of alcohol after aspirin (decreased gastric oxidation)
      R Roine et al, Aspirin increases blood alcohol concentrations in humans after ingestion of ethanol. JAMA, 264:2406, 1990; O Melander et al, Pharmacokinetic interactions of alcohol and acetylsalicylic acid. Eur J Clin Pharmacol, 48:151, 1995; S Kechagias, Low-dose aspirin decreases blood alcohol concentrations by delaying gastric emptying. Eur J Clin Pharmacol, 53:241, 1997
    Normal men received 1 gm of aspirin with breakfast one hr before taking alcohol; not confirmed in subsequent report (1995); low-dose aspirin (75 mg) decreased blood alcohol in healthy subjects (1997)
  Olanzapine
    Increased orthostatic hypotensive effect of olanzapine (mechanism not established)
      Manufacturer's package insert (olanzapine)
    Avoid concurrent use
  Phenformin
    Lactic acidosis (synergism)
      HK Johnson and C Waterhouse, Relationship of alcohol and hyperlactatemia in diabetic subjects treated with phenformin. Am J Med, 45:98, 1968
    Avoid phenformin in alcoholics
  Phenothiazines
    Impaired motor coordination with chlorpromazine (probably additive); may occur with all phenothiazines
      GA Zirkle et al, Effects of chlorpromazine and alcohol on coordination and judgment. JAMA, 171:1496, 1959; VC Sutherland et al, Cerebral metabolism in problem drinkers under the influence of alcohol and chlorpromazine hydrochloride. J Appl Physiol, 15:189, 1960
    Warn patients, especially drivers
  Phenylbutazone
    Impaired motor coordination (probably additive)
      M Linnoila et al, Acute effect of antipyretic analgesics, alone or in combination with alcohol, on human psychomotor skills related to driving. Br J Clin Pharmacol, 1:477, 1974

(continued)

ALCOHOL, with: *(continued)*
> *Warn patients, especially drivers*

Phenytoin
> Decreased anticonvulsant effect with chronic alcohol abuse (increased metabolism); increased phenytoin toxicity with acute intoxication (decreased metabolism)
>> RMH Kater et al, Increased rate of clearance of drugs from the circulation of alcoholics. Am J Med Sci, 258:35, 1969; P Sandor et al, Effect of short- and long-term alcohol use on phenytoin kinetics in chronic alcoholics. Clin Pharmacol Ther, 30:390, 1981
>
> *Monitor phenytoin concentration in alcoholics; warn patients*

Prazosin
> Possible hypotension (additive)
>> Y Kawano et al, Interaction of alcohol and an α_1-blocker on ambulatory blood pressure in patients with essential hypertension. Am J Hypertens, 13:307, 2000
>
> *Based on a controlled study of hypertensive Japanese men; monitor blood pressure; avoid or limit alcohol intake*

Quetiapine
> Possibly increased cognitive and motor impairment (additive)
>> Manufacturer's package insert
>
> *Avoid concurrent use*

Tetracyclines
> Altered doxycycline effect (mechanism not established)
>> PJ Neuvonen et al, Effect of long-term alcohol consumption on the half-life of tetracycline and doxycycline in man. Int J Clin Pharmacol, 14:303, 1976; C Seitz et al, Influence of ethanol ingestion on tetracycline kinetics. Int J Clin Pharmacol Ther, 33:462, 1995
>
> *Increased metabolism with decreased effect reported in chronic alcoholics; increased absorption and increased serum concentration reported in normal subjects with acute ingestion*

Tizanidine
> CNS depression (additive)
>> Manufacturer's package insert
>
> *Warn patients of possible adverse effects*

Trimethoprim-sulfamethoxazole
> Possible disulfiram-like reaction (mechanism not established)
>> MW Heelon and M White, Disulfiram-cotrimoxazole reaction. Pharmacotherapy, 18:869, 1998
>
> *Two case reports (1998)*

Verapamil
> Prolonged intoxication (probably decreased metabolism)
>> LA Bauer et al, Verapamil inhibits ethanol elimination and prolongs the perception of intoxication. Clin Pharmacol Ther, 52:6, 1992
>
> *Based on study in young healthy men; avoid concurrent use*

Alendronate, no documented interactions, see page 4, Criteria for Listing Interactions

Alfentanil, see Narcotics: meperidine and congeners
Alglucerase, no documented interactions, see page 4, Criteria for Listing Interactions

ALKYLATING AGENTS, with:

Allopurinol
Possible toxicity of cyclophosphamide and possibly of other alkylating agents (mechanism not established)

    Boston Collaborative Drug Surveillance Program, Allopurinol and cytotoxic drugs. JAMA, 227:1036, 1974

Monitor for bone marrow depression

Azathioprine
Liver necrosis with azathioprine and cyclophosphamide given consecutively (mechanism not established)

    S Shaunak et al, Cyclophosphamide-induced liver necrosis: a possible interaction with azathioprine. Q J Med, 67:309, 1988

Avoid consecutive or concurrent use

Corticosteroids
Decreased dexamethasone effect with cylophosphamide (increased metabolism); cyclophosphamide toxicity (increased formation of major toxic metabolite phosphoramine mustard)

    MJ Moore et al, Rapid development of enhanced clearance after high-dose cyclophosphamide. Clin Pharmacol Ther, 44:622, 1988

Monitor clinical status; cyclophosphamide toxicity occurs within 24 hours after starting high-dose cyclophosphamide

Cyclosporine
Nephrotoxicity with melphalan (mechanism not established); seizures with combined busulfan and cyclophosphamide (mechanism not established)

    GR Morgenstern et al, Cyclosporin interaction with ketoconazole and melphalan. Lancet, 2:1342, 1982; AM Ghany et al, Cyclosporine-associated seizures in bone marrow transplant recipients given busulfan and cyclophosphamide preparative therapy. Transplantation, 52:310, 1991; DA Tweddle et al, Cyclosporin neurotoxicity after chemotherapy. BMJ, 318:1113, 1999

Monitor neurological and renal status

Digoxin
Decreased effect of digoxin tablets (decreased intestinal absorption)

    TD Bjornsson et al, Effects of high-dose cancer chemotherapy on the absorption of digoxin in two different formulations. Clin Pharmacol Ther, 39:25, 1986

Clinical significance not established; effect is negligible with digoxin capsules

Neuromuscular blocking agents
Prolonged neuromuscular blocking effect of succinylcholine with cyclophosphamide (inhibition of plasma cholinesterase); apnea with suxamethonium and cyclophosphamide (inhibition of plasma cholinesterase)

    EK Zsigmond and G Robins, The effect of a series of anti-cancer drugs on plasma cholinesterase activity. Can Anaesthesiol Soc J, 19:75, 1972; IR Walker et al, Cyclophosphamide, cholinesterase and anaesthesia. Aust N Z

(continued)

ALKYLATING AGENTS, with: *(continued)*
> J Med, 3:247, 1972

Measure plasma cholinesterase and decrease succinylcholine dosage accordingly; transfusion restores cholinesterase activity

Nonsteroidal anti-inflammatory drugs

Severe hyponatremia with low-dose IV cyclophosphamide and indomethacin (possibly synergism)
> MJ Webberley and JA Murray, Life-threatening acute hyponatraemia induced by low dose cyclophosphamide and indomethacin. Postgrad Med J, 65:950, 1989

Single case report (1989)

Ondansetron

Possible small alteration in cyclophosphamide effect (mechanism not established)
> PJ Cagnoni et al, Modification of the pharmacokinetics of high-dose cyclophosphamide and cisplatin by antiemetics. Bone Marrow Transplant, 24:1, 1999

Based on study in patients undergoing bone marrow transplant; clinical importance not established

Phenytoin

Possible decreased busulphan effect (increased metabolism)
> M Hassan et al, Influence of prophylactic anticonvulsant therapy on high-dose busulphan kinetics. Cancer Chemother Pharmacol, 33:181, 1993

Avoid concurrent use if possible

Thioguanine

Nodular regenerative hepatic hyperplasia with varices with busulfan (mechanism not established)
> Manufacturer's package insert; NS Key et al, Oesophageal varices associated with busulphan-thioguanine combination therapy for chronic myeloid leukaemia. Lancet, 2:1050, 1987

Requires confirmation

ALLOPURINOL, with:

Alkylating agents - See Alkylating agents with Allopurinol, page 23

Angiotensin-converting enzyme (ACE) inhibitors

Possible susceptibility to Stevens-Johnson syndrome and hypersensitivity reactions with captopril or enalapril (mechanism not established)
> DJ Pennell et al, Fatal Stevens-Johnson syndrome in a patient on captopril and allopurinol. Lancet, 1:463, 1984; A Samanta and AC Burden, Fever, myalgia, and arthralgia in a patient on captopril and allopurinol. Lancet, 1:679, 1984; S Ahmad, Allopurinol and enalapril, Chest, 108:586, 1995

Avoid concurrent use, if possible, especially in patients with renal failure

Antacids

Decreased allopurinol effect with aluminum hydroxide (decreased absorption)
> I Weissman and N Krivoy, Interaction of aluminum hydroxide and allopurinol in patients on chronic hemodialysis. Ann Intern Med, 107:787, 1987

Give aluminum hydroxide at least 3 hours before allopurinol

ALLOPURINOL, with: *(continued)*

Anticoagulants, oral

Increased anticoagulant effect (decreased metabolism)

> ES Vesell et al, Impairment of drug metabolism in man by allopurinol and nortriptyline. N Engl J Med, 283:1484, 1970; MD Rawlins and SE Smith, Influence of allopurinol on drug metabolism in man. Br J Pharmacol, 48:693, 1973

Monitor prothrombin time

Azathioprine

Azathioprine toxicity (decreased metabolism)

> IW Boyd, Allopurinol-azathioprine interaction. J Int Med, 229:386, 1991; DT Kennedy et al, Azathioprine and allopurinol: the price of an avoidable drug interaction. Ann Pharmacother, 30:951, 1996

Decrease azathioprine dosage and monitor clinical status

Cyclosporine

Cyclosporine toxicity (possibly decreased metabolism)

> SL Stevens and MH Goldman, Cyclosporine toxicity associated with allopurinol. South Med J, 85:1265, 1992

Single case report

Mercaptopurine

Mercaptopurine toxicity (decreased first-pass metabolism)

> GB Elion et al, Potentiation by inhibition of drug degradation: 6-substituted purines and xanthine oxidase. Biochem Pharmacol, 12:85, 1963; S Zimm et al, Inhibition of first-pass metabolism in cancer chemotherapy: interaction of 6-mercaptopurine and allopurinol. Clin Pharmacol Ther, 34:810, 1983

Decrease mercaptopurine dosage when given orally and monitor clinical status

Penicillins

Increased incidence of rash with ampicillin or penicillin (mechanism not established)

> H Jick and JB Porter, Potentiation of ampicillin skin reactions by allopurinol hyperuricemia. J Clin Pharmacol, 21:456, 1981; R Hoigne et al, Occurrence of exanthems in relation to aminopenicillin preparations and allopurinol. N Engl J Med, 316:1217, 1987

Monitor clinical status

Pyrazinamide

Failure of allopurinol to decrease hyperuricemia following pyrazinamide (accumulation of pyrazinoic acid, which inhibits urate excretion)

> C Lacroix et al, Interaction between allopurinol and pyrazinamide. Eur Respir J, 1:807, 1988

Avoid concurrent use

Theophyllines

Possible theophylline toxicity (decreased metabolism)

> RL Manfredi and ES Vesell, Inhibition of theophylline metabolism by long-term allopurinol administration. Clin Pharmacol Ther, 29:224, 1981

Monitor theophylline concentration

(continued)

ALLOPURINOL, with: *(continued)*
  Thiazide diuretics
    Allopurinol toxicity, rash (possibly decreased renal excretion in patients with impaired renal function)
      KR Hande, Evaluation of a thiazide – allopurinol drug interaction. Am J Med Sci, 292:213, 1986; W Löffler et al, Interaction of allopurinol and hydrochlorothiazide during prolonged oral administration of both drugs in normal subjects. Clin Investig, 72:1071, 1994; JX de Vries et al, Interaction of allopurinol and hydrochlorothiazide during prolonged oral administration of both drugs in normal subjects. Clin Investig, 72:1076, 1994
    Not reported with other diuretics; monitor renal and hepatic function; interaction minimal in normal subjects
  Vidarabine
    Vidarabine toxicity (decreased metabolism)
      HM Friedman and T Grasela, Adenine arabinoside and allopurinol – possible adverse drug interaction. N Engl J Med, 304:423, 1981
    Avoid concurrent use, if possible

ALPHA-ADRENERGIC BLOCKERS, with:
  Methyldopa
    Urinary incontinence with phenoxybenzamine (synergistic sympatholytic effects)
      PG Fernandez et al, Urinary incontinence due to interaction of phenoxybenzamine and p-methyldopa. Can Med Assoc J, 124:174, 1981
    Avoid concurrent use except to treat neurological bladder outlet obstruction

Alphacalcidol, see Vitamin D

Alpha-galactosidase, no documented interactions, see page 4, Criteria for Listing Interactions

Alprazolam, see Benzodiazepines

Alprostadil, no documented interactions, see page 4, Criteria for Listing Interactions

Alteplase, see Thrombolytics

ALTRETAMINE, with:
  Antidepressants, tricyclic
    Severe orthostatic hypotension with imipramine or amitriptyline (mechanism not established)
      HW Bruckner and SJ Schleifer, Orthostatic hypotension as a complication of hexamethylmelamine antidepressant interaction. Cancer Treat Rep, 67:516, 1983
    Case reports in older patients taking imipramine or amitriptyline; monitor blood pressure
  Monoamine oxidase inhibitors
    Severe orthostatic hypotension with phenelzine (mechanism not established)
      HW Bruckner and SJ Schleifer, Orthostatic hypotension as a complication of hexamethylmelamine antidepressant interaction. Cancer Treat Rep, 67:516, 1983
    One case report (1983) in older patient taking phenelzine; monitor blood pressure

Aluminum carbonate, see Antacids

Aluminum hydroxide, see Antacids
Aluminum phosphate, see Antacids
AMANTADINE, with:
Anticholinergics
Hallucinations, confusion, nightmares (mechanism not established)
> JU Postma and WV Tilburg, Visual hallucinations and delirium during treatment with amantadine (Symmetrel). J Am Geriatr Soc, 23:212, 1975

Decrease anticholinergic dosage before starting amantadine

Bupropion
Delirium and neurotoxicity (possibly synergism)
> I Liberzon et al, Bupropion and delirium. Am J Psychiatry, 147:1689, 1990; B Trappler and AM Miyashiro, Buproprion-amantadine-associated neurotoxicity. J Clin Psychiatry, 61:61, 2000

One case report of delirium (1990); 3 of 6 elderly patients given combination developed neurotoxicity such as agitation, tremors, confusion, ataxia, dizziness, vertigo (2000)

Monoamine oxidase inhibitors
Hypertension with phenelzine (mechanism not established)
> RA Jack and DG Daniel, Possible interaction between phenelzine and amantadine. Arch Gen Psychiatry, 41:726, 1984

Single case report (1984)

Thiazide diuretics
Amantadine toxicity with hydrochlorothiazide-triamterene combination (decreased renal excretion)
> TW Wilson and AH Rajput, Amantadine-Dyazide interaction. Can Med Assoc J, 129:974, 1983

Single case report (1983)

Triamterene
Amantadine toxicity with hydrochlorothiazide-triamterene combination (decreased renal excretion)
> TW Wilson and AH Rajput, Amantadine-Dyazide interaction. Can Med Assoc J, 129:974, 1983

Single case report (1983)

Trimethoprim-sulfamethoxazole
Amantadine toxicity (probably decreased renal excretion)
> KV Speeg et al, Case report: toxic delirium in a patient taking amantadine and trimethoprim-sulfamethoxazole. Am J Med Sci, 298:410, 1989

Single case report (1989); probably caused by trimethoprim

Amcinonide, no documented interactions, see page 4, Criteria for Listing Interactions

Amikacin, see Aminoglycoside antibiotics

AMILORIDE, with:
Angiotensin-converting enzyme (ACE) inhibitors
Hyperkalemia (additive)
> Manufacturer's package insert; TG Burnakis and HJ Mioduch, Combined therapy with captopril and potassium supplementation. Arch Intern Med, 144:2371, 1984; T-F Chiu et al, Rapid life-threatening hyperkalemia after

(continued)

AMILORIDE, with: *(continued)*
> addition of amiloride HCl/hydrochlorothiazide to angiotensin-converting enzyme inhibitor therapy. Ann Emerg Med, 30:612, 1997

May be more likely in patients with diabetes and/or renal impairment; monitor serum potassium; avoid concurrent use

Hypoglycemics, sulfonylurea
Hyponatremia with chlorpropamide and an amiloride-thiazide combination (additive)
> AM Zalin et al, Hyponatraemia during treatment with chlorpropamide and moduretic (amiloride plus hydrochlorothiazide). Br Med J, 289:659, 1984

Relative contribution of amiloride and thiazide to mild hyponatremia has not been evaluated

Magnesium sulfate
Hypermagnesemia (decreased renal excretion)
> DG Henderson, Amilorid og magnesium; alvorlig interaktion mellem amilorid og handkobsmedicin indeholdende magnesium. Ugeskr Laeger, 149:92, 1987

Avoid concurrent use

Penicillins
Modest reduction in amoxicillin bioavailability (possibly inhibition of the intestinal Na+-H+ exchange mechanism)
> J-F Westphal et al, Amoxicillin intestinal absorption reduction by amiloride: possible role of the Na+-H+ exchanger. Clin Pharmacol Ther, 57:257, 1995

Based on study in 8 healthy subjects; clinical significance not established.

Potassium
Hyperkalemia (additive)
> Manufacturer's package insert

Avoid potassium supplements

Quinidine
Proarrhythmic effects (mechanism not established)
> L Wang et al, Amiloride-quinidine interaction: adverse outcomes. Clin Pharmacol Ther, 56:659, 1994

Reported in all of 10 patients with inducible ventricular tachycardia on electrophysiologic study; avoid concurrent use

Thiazide diuretics
Hyponatremia (additive)
> PH Strykers et al, Hyponatremia induced by a combination of amiloride and hydrochlorothiazide. JAMA, 252:389, 1984; R Eastell and CJ Edmonds, Hyponatraemia associated with trimethoprim and a diuretic. Br Med J, 289:1658, 1984

Reported in elderly patients; monitor serum sodium; may be potentiated by trimethoprim

Trimethoprim
Trimethoprim may potentiate hyponatremia caused by concomitant use of amiloride with thiazide diuretics (additive)
> R Eastell and CJ Edmonds, Hyponatraemia associated with trimethoprim and a diuretic. Br Med J, 289:1658, 1984; TL Hart et al, Hyponatremia

AMILORIDE, with: *(continued)*
>> secondary to thiazide – trimethoprim interaction. Can J Hosp Pharm, 42:243, 1989
> *Monitor serum sodium*

Aminocaproic acid, no documented interactions, see page 4, Criteria for Listing Interactions

AMINOGLUTETHIMIDE, with:
> **Anabolic and androgenic steroids**
>> Decreased medroxyprogesterone effect (possibly increased metabolism)
>>> WA Van Deijk et al, Influence of aminoglutethimide on plasma levels of medroxyprogesterone acetate: its correlation with serum cortisol. Cancer Treat Rep, 69:85, 1985
>> *Monitor serum cortisol concentration as an index of adrenal suppression by medroxyprogesterone*
>
> **Anticoagulants, oral**
>> Decreased anticoagulant effect (increased metabolism)
>>> PF Bruning and JGM Bonfrer, Aminoglutethimide and oral anticoagulant therapy. Lancet, 2:582, 1983; E Lonning et al, Aminoglutethimide and warfarin. Cancer Chemother Pharmacol, 12:10, 1984
>> *Monitor prothrombin time*
>
> **Corticosteroids**
>> Decreased corticosteroid effect (increased metabolism)
>>> RJ Santen et al, Successful medical adrenalectomy with aminoglutethimide; role of altered drug metabolism. JAMA, 230:1661, 1974
>> *Large doses of dexamethasone (1.5 to 3 mg/day) may be required*
>
> **Digitoxin**
>> Possible decreased digitoxin effect (increased metabolism)
>>> E Lonning et al, Effect of aminoglutethimide on antipyrine, theophylline, and digitoxin disposition in breast cancer. Clin Pharmacol Ther, 36:796, 1984
>> *Monitor digitoxin concentration*
>
> **Tamoxifen**
>> Decreased tamoxifen effect (increased metabolism)
>>> EA Lien et al, Decreased serum concentrations of tamoxifen and its metabolites induced by aminoglutethimide. Cancer Res, 50:5851, 1990
>> *Avoid concurrent use*
>
> **Theophyllines**
>> Possible decreased theophylline effect (increased metabolism)
>>> E Lonning et al, Effect of aminoglutethimide on antipyrine, theophylline, and digitoxin disposition in breast cancer. Clin Pharmacol Ther, 36:796, 1984
>> *Avoid concurrent use*
>
> **Thiazide diuretics**
>> Hyponatremia (synergism)
>>> E Bork and M Hansen, Severe hyponatremia following simultaneous administration of aminoglutethimide and diuretics. Cancer Treat Rep, 70:689, 1986

(continued)

AMINOGLUTETHIMIDE, with: *(continued)*
Single case report (1986); monitor sodium concentration

AMINOGLYCOSIDE ANTIBIOTICS, with:

Antifungals, Amphotericin B

Nephrotoxicity (synergism)
> DN Churchill and J Seely, Nephrotoxicity associated with combined gentamicin-amphotericin B therapy. Nephron, 19:176, 1977

If concurrent use cannot be avoided, monitor renal function

Antifungals, imidazoles and triazoles

Possible decreased tobramycin effect with miconazole (mechanism not established)
> SM Hatfield et al, Miconazole-induced alteration in tobramycin pharmacokinetics. Clin Pharm, 5:415, 1986

Avoid concurrent use

Bumetanide

Ototoxicity (additive)
> Manufacturer's package insert

Avoid concurrent use, if possible

Cephalosporins

Nephrotoxicity (mechanism not established)
> JE Whiteley et al, A potential interaction between gentamicin and cephalexin. J Pharm Pharmacol, 30:201, 1978; JS Tobias et al, Severe renal dysfunction after tobramycin/cephalothin therapy. Lancet, 1:425, 1976; E Trvedegaard, Interaction between gentamicin and cephalothin as cause of acute renal failure. Lancet, 2:581, 1976

Avoid concurrent use in elderly patients or those with renal impairment

Cisplatin

Nephrotoxicity (mechanism not established)
> CF Stewart et al, The effect of cisplatin therapy on gentamicin pharmacokinetics. Drug Intell Clin Pharm, 18:512, 1984; ML Christensen et al, Evaluation of aminoglycoside disposition in patients previously treated with cisplatin. Ther Drug Monit, 11:631, 1989

Avoid concurrent use

Cyclosporine

Renal toxicity (possibly additive or synergism)
> JM Morales et al, Reversible acute renal toxicity by toxic sinergic effect between gentamicin and cyclosporine. Clin Nephrol, 29:272, 1988; PH Chandrasekar and SM Cronin, Nephrotoxicity in bone marrow transplant recipients receiving aminoglycoside plus cyclosporine or aminoglycoside alone. J Antimicrob Chemother, 27:845, 1991

Monitor serum concentration and/or renal status

Digoxin

Possible decreased digoxin effect with oral gentamicin or neomycin (decreased absorption)
> J Lindenbaum et al, Inhibition of digoxin absorption by neomycin. Gastroenterology, 71:399, 1976

AMINOGLYCOSIDE ANTIBIOTICS, with: *(continued)*
Monitor digoxin concentration; spacing doses will not avoid the interaction

Enflurane

Possible renal toxicity (mechanism not established)

> DJ Motuz et al, The increase in urinary alanine aminopeptidase excretion associated with enflurane anesthesia is increased further by aminoglycosides. Anesth Analg, 67:770, 1988

Avoid concurrent use, especially in patients with renal damage

Ethacrynic acid

Ototoxicity (additive)

> WD Meriwether et al, Deafness following standard intravenous dose of ethacrynic acid. JAMA, 216:795, 1971; RH Mathog and WJ Klein, Jr, Ototoxicity of ethacrynic acid and aminoglycoside antibiotics in uremia. N Engl J Med, 280:1223, 1969; J Prazma et al, Ethacrynic acid ototoxicity potentiation by kanamycin. Ann Otol Rhinol Laryngol, 83:111, 1974

Avoid concurrent use, if possible

Furosemide

Ototoxicity and nephrotoxicity (additive)

> DH Lawson et al, Effect of furosemide on the pharmacokinetics of gentamicin in patients. J Clin Pharmacol, 22:254, 1982; GH Schwartz et al, Ototoxicity induced by furosemide. N Engl J Med, 282:1413, 1970; JS Kaka et al, Tobramycin-furosemide interaction. Drug Intell Clin Pharm, 18:235, 1984

Avoid concurrent use, if possible

Gallium

Renal toxicity (additive)

> Manufacturer's package insert

Avoid concurrent use

Magnesium sulfate

Increased neuromuscular blockade (additive)

> CS L'Hommedieu et al, Potentiation of magnesium sulfate-induced neuromuscular weakness by gentamicin, tobramycin, and amikacin. J Pediatr, 102:629, 1983

Reported in one newborn treated with an aminoglycoside, whose mother took magnesium sulfate (1983)

Malathion

Possible respiratory depression (additive)

> United States Pharmacopeial Convention, *Drug Information for the Health Care Professional* (USP DI), Vol I, 18th ed., Rockville, MD: Authors, 1998, page 1914

Topical malathion not significantly absorbed unless skin damaged

Methotrexate

Decreased methotrexate effect with oral aminoglycosides (decreased absorption)

> MH Cohen et al, Effect of oral prophylactic broad spectrum nonabsorbable antibiotics on the gastrointestinal absorption of nutrients and methotrexate in small cell bronchogenic carcinoma patients. Cancer, 38:1556, 1976

(continued)

AMINOGLYCOSIDE ANTIBIOTICS, with: *(continued)*
> *Avoid concurrent use*

Neuromuscular blocking agents
> Increased neuromuscular blockade (additive)
>> AG Regan and PPV Perumbetti, Pancuronium and gentamicin interaction in patients with renal failure. Anesth Analg, 59:393, 1980; M Giala et al, Possible interaction of pancuronium and tubocurarine with oral neomycin. Anaesthesia, 37:776, 1982; BF Vanacker and J Van de Walle, The neuromuscular blocking action of vecuronium in normal patients and in patients with no renal function and interaction vecuronium-tobramycin in renal transplant patients. Acta Anaesthesiol Belg, 37:95, 1986; R Jedeikin et al, Prolongation of neuromuscular blocking effect of vecuronium by antibiotics. Anaesthesia, 42:858, 1987; JY Dupuis et al, Atracurium and vecuronium interaction with gentamicin and tobramycin. Can J Anaesthesiol, 36:407, 1989
>
> *Monitor neuromuscular status; atracurium may not be affected*

Nonsteroidal anti-inflammatory drugs
> Possible aminoglycoside toxicity in preterm infants with indomethacin given for patent ductus closure (decreased renal clearance)
>> Y Zarfin et al, Possible indomethacin – aminoglycoside interaction in preterm infants. J Pediatr, 106:511, 1985; RP Dean et al, Prophylactic indomethacin alters gentamicin pharmacokinetics in preterm infants <1250 grams. Pediatric Research, 35 (4 part 2):83A, 1994
>
> *Decrease aminoglycoside dosage before giving indomethacin and monitor concentration*
>
> Acute renal failure with ibuprofen and IV aminoglycosides (mechanism not established)
>> TA Kovesi et al, Transient renal failure due to simultaneous ibuprofen and aminoglycoside therapy in children with cystic fibrosis. N Engl J Med, 338:65, 1998
>
> *Four case reports in children with cystic fibrosis (1998)*

Penicillins
> Decreased aminoglycoside effect with high concentrations of carbenicillin, ticarcillin, or piperacillin (inactivation)
>> WA Kradjan and R Burger, *In vivo* inactivation of gentamicin by carbenicillin and ticarcillin. Arch Intern Med, 140:1668, 1980; CE Halstenson et al, Effect of concomitant administration of piperacillin on the dispositions of isepamicin and gentamicin in patients with end-stage renal disease. Antimicrob Agents Chemother, 36:1832, 1992; MSS Chow et al, *In vivo* inactivation of tobramycin by ticarcillin: a case report. JAMA, 247:658, 1982; GR Matzke et al, Effect of ticarcillin on gentamicin and tobramycin pharmacokinetics in a patient with end-stage renal disease. Pharmacotherapy, 4:158, 1984; CE Halstenson et al, Effect of concomitant administration of piperacillin on the dispositions of netilmicin and tobramycin in patients with end-stage renal disease. Antimicrob Agents Chemother, 34:128, 1990

AMINOGLYCOSIDE ANTIBIOTICS, with: *(continued)*
>> *Occurs in renal failure; monitor aminoglycoside concentration (freeze specimen to prevent in vitro inactivation); netilmicin may not interact*

> **Polymyxins**
>> Nephrotoxicity; increased neuromuscular blockade (additive)
>>> Manufacturer's package insert
>> *Avoid concurrent use*

> **Vancomycin**
>> Possible nephrotoxicity and ototoxicity (possibly additive)
>>> BF Farber end RC Moellering, Jr, Retrospective study of the toxicity of preparations of vancomycin from 1974 to 1981. Antimicrob Agents Chemother, 23:138, 1983; C Odio et al, Nephrotoxicity associated with vancomycin – aminoglycoside therapy in four children. J Pediatr, 105:491, 1984; MP Goren et al, Vancomycin does not enhance amikacin-induced tubular nephrotoxicity in children. Pediatr Infect Dis J, 8:278, 1989; DJ Pauly et al, Risk of nephrotoxicity with combination vancomycin-aminoglycoside antibiotic therapy. Pharmacotherapy, 10:378, 1990; MY Munar et al, The effect of tobramycin on the renal handling of vancomycin. J Clin Pharmacol, 31:618, 1991
>> *Avoid concurrent use; may be more likely in children; in one study in 14 children taking amikacin, vancomycin did not enhance nephrotoxicity*

Aminohippurate sodium, no documented interactions, see page 4, Criteria for Listing Interactions

Aminophylline, see Theophyllines

AMINOSALICYLIC ACID, with:
> **Probenecid**
>> Possible aminosalicylic acid toxicity (decreased renal excretion)
>>> WP Boger and FW Pitts, Influence of p-(Di-n-Propylsulfamyl)-benzoic acid, "Benemid," on para-aminosalicylic acid (PAS) plasma concentrations. Am Rev Tuberc, 61:862, 1950
>> *Avoid concurrent use*

> **Rifampin**
>> Decreased rifampin effect (decreased absorption)
>>> G Boman et al, Drug interaction: decreased serum concentrations of rifampicin when given with P.A.S. Lancet, 1:800, 1971
>> *Avoid concurrent use or give at least 8 hours apart*

AMIODARONE, with:
> **Amprenavir**
>> Possible serious or life-threatening toxicity with amiodarone (decreased metabolism; CYP3A4)
>>> Manufacturer's package insert (amprenavir)
>> *Monitor amiodarone concentration*

> **Anticoagulants, oral**
>> Increased anticoagulant effect (decreased metabolism)
>>> U Martinowitz et al, Interaction between warfarin sodium and amiodarone. N Engl J Med, 304:671, 1981; LD Heimark et al, The mechanism of the interaction between amiodarone and warfarin in humans. Clin Pharmacol

(continued)

AMIODARONE, with: *(continued)*
> Ther, 51:398, 1992; B Cheung et al, Insidiously evolving, occult drug interaction involving warfarin and amiodarone. BMJ, 312:107, 1996

Monitor prothrombin time; increases gradually and may persist for several months after stopping amiodarone

Benzodiazepines
Clonazepam toxicity (probable decreased metabolism)
> DM Witt et al, Amiodarone-clonazepam interaction. Ann Pharmacother, 27:1463, 1993

Single case report (1993)

Beta-adrenergic blockers
Bradycardia with atenolol; severe bradycardia and hypotension with metoprolol; cardiac arrest with propranolol (mechanism not established)
> J Leor et al, Amiodarone and beta-adrenergic blockers. Am Heart J, 116:206, 1988; JP Derrida et al, Amiodarone et propranolol: une association dangereuse? Nouvelle Pressé Méd, 8:1429, 1979; F Boutitie et al, Amiodarone interaction with β-blockers: analysis of the merged EMIAT (European Myocardial Infarct Amiodarone Trial) and CAMIAT (Canadian Amiodarone Myocardial Infarction Trial) databases. Circulation, 99:2268, 1999; H Krum et al, Efficacy and safety of carvedilol in patients with chronic heart failure receiving concomitant amiodarone therapy. J Card Fail, 4:281, 1998; EJ Eichhorn and MH Hamdan, β-blockade and amiodarone therapy: twin brothers from different parents. J Card Fail, 4:289, 1998

Single reports (1979,1988); 2 reports of cardiac arrest; monitor cardiac status; nonetheless, analysis of two large trials suggests that the combination is beneficial

Cholestyramine
Decreased amiodarone effect (decreased absorption)
> J Nitsch and B Luderitz, Beschleunigte elimination von amiodaron durch colestyramin. Deutsch Med Wochenschr, 111:1241, 1986

Avoid concurrent use

Contrast media
Fatal pulmonary failure; possible additive
> E Malden et al, Acute fatality following pulmonary angiography in a patient on an amiodarone regimen—a case report. Angiology, 44:152, 1993

Three fatal cases (1985, 1993)

Cyclosporine
Possible cyclosporine toxicity (decreased metabolism)
> DP Nicolau et al, Amiodarone-cyclosporine interaction in a heart transplant patient. J Heart Lung Transplant, 11:564, 1992; JG Preuner et al, Development of severe adverse effects after discontinuing amiodarone therapy in human heart transplant recipients. Transplant Proc, 30:3943, 1998

Monitor renal status and drug concentrations

Digoxin
Possible digoxin toxicity (mechanism not established)
> G Koren et al, Digoxin toxicity associated with amiodarone therapy in children. J Pediatr, 104:467, 1984; K Nademanee et al, Amiodarone-digoxin

AMIODARONE, with: *(continued)*
> interaction: clinical significance, time course of development, potential pharmacokinetic mechanisms and therapeutic implications. J Am Coll Cardiol, 4:111, 1984; HO Klein et al, Asystole produced by the combination of amiodarone and digoxin. Am Heart J, 113:399, 1987

Monitor digoxin concentration

Diltiazem
Sinus arrest and low cardiac output (additive effect on atrial node and myocardial contractility)
> TH Lee et al, Sinus arrest and hypotension with combined amiodarone – diltiazem therapy. Am Heart J, 109:163, 1985

Single case report (1985); monitor cardiac status

Dofetilide
Increased risk of arrhythmias (additive effect on QTc interval)
> Manufacturer's package insert (dofetilide)

Avoid concurrent use

Enflurane
Cardiovascular toxicity (mechanism not established)
> BA Liberman and SJ Teasdale, Anaesthesia and amiodarone. Can Anaesth Soc J, 32:629, 1985

Monitor cardiovascular status

Flecainide
Possible flecainide toxicity (probably decreased flecainide metabolism by CYP2D6)
> JF Leclercq et al, Flecainide acetate dose-concentration relationship in cardiac arrhythmias: influence of heart failure and amiodarone. Cardiovasc Drugs Ther, 4:1161, 1990; P Andrivet et al, Torsades de pointe with flecainide-amiodarone therapy. Intensive Care Med, 16:342, 1990; MJ Kantoch, Combination of amiodarone and flecainide. Am J Cardiol, 75:862, 1995

Monitor flecainide concentration; single case reports of torsades de pointes (1990) and QRS widening (1995)

Fluoroquinolones
Possible ventricular arrhythmia with grepafloxacin (possible additive effect on QTc interval; CYP3A4)
> Manufacturer's package insert

Theoretical; manufacturer recommends avoiding concurrent use

Grapefruit juice
Possible amiodarone toxicity (decreased metabolism; CYP3A4)
> CC Libersa et al, Dramatic inhibition of amiodarone metabolism induced by grapefruit juice. Br J Clin Pharmacol, 49:373, 2000

Based on study in healthy subjects with large amount of grapefruit juice; avoid concurrent use

Halothane
Cardiovascular toxicity (mechanism not established)
> BA Liberman and SJ Teasdale, Anaesthesia and amiodarone. Can Anaesth Soc J, 32:629, 1985

(continued)

AMIODARONE, with: *(continued)*
   Monitor cardiovascular status
  Indinavir
    Possible amiodarone toxicity (probably decreased metabolism)
      JJHM Lohman et al, Antiretroviral therapy increases serum concentrations of amiodarone. Ann Pharmacother, 33:645, 1999
    Singe case report (1999); monitor clinical status and amiodarone serum concentrations
  Isoflurane
    Cardiovascular toxicity (mechanism not established)
      BA Liberman and SJ Teasdale, Anaesthesia and amiodarone. Can Anaesth Soc J, 32:629, 1985
    Monitor cardiovascular status
  Lidocaine
    Seizures with IV lidocaine (probably decreased lidocaine metabolism)
      JB Siegmund et al, Amiodarone interaction with lidocaine. J Cardiovasc Pharmacol, 21:513, 1993; S Nattel et al, Absence of pharmacokinetic interaction between amiodarone and lidocaine. Am J Cardiol, 73:92, 1994
    Single case report (1993); no interaction was found when a single IV bolus dose of lidocaine was given to patients receiving amiodarone
  Lopinavir/Ritonavir
    Possible increased amiodarone toxicity (decreased metabolism)
      Manufacturer's package insert (*Kaletra*)
    Theoretical; avoid combination if possible; monitor amiodarone concentrations and clinical status
  Methotrexate
    Methotrexate toxicity (mechanism not established)
      NJ Reynolds et al, Methotrexate induced skin necrosis: a drug interaction with amiodarone? BMJ, 299:980, 1989
    Single case report (1989) in a patient with psoriasis
  Narcotics: dextromethorphan
    Possible dextromethorphan toxicity (decreased metabolism in extensive metabolizers)
      C Funck-Brentano et al, Influence of amiodarone on genetically determined drug metabolism in humans. Clin Pharmacol Ther, 50:259, 1991
    Monitor clinical status
  Narcotics: meperidine and congeners
    Cardiovascular toxicity with fentanyl (mechanism not established)
      BA Liberman and SJ Teasdale, Anaesthesia and amiodarone. Can Anaesth Soc J, 32:629, 1985
    Monitor cardiovascular status
  Phenytoin
    Phenytoin toxicity (decreased phenytoin metabolism)
      JM Gore et al, Interaction of amiodarone and diphenylhydantoin. Am J Cardiol, 54:1145, 1984; PE Nolan, Jr et al, Pharmacokinetic interaction between intravenous phenytoin and amiodarone in healthy volunteers. Clin Pharmacol Ther, 46:43, 1989; S Ahmad, Amiodarone and phenytoin: interaction.

AMIODARONE, with: *(continued)*
> J Am Geriatr Soc, 43:1449, 1995

Monitor phenytoin concentration and clinical status

Procainamide

Procainamide toxicity (mechanism not established)
> J Windle et al, Pharmacokinetic and electrophysiologic interactions of amiodarone and procainamide. Clin Pharmacol Ther, 41:603, 1987

Monitor procainamide concentration

Quinidine

Quinidine toxicity (mechanism not established)
> J Windle et al, Pharmacokinetic and electrophysiologic interactions of amiodarone and procainamide. Clin Pharmacol Ther, 41:603, 1987

Monitor quinidine concentration

Rifampin

Possible decreased amiodarone effect (probably increased metabolism)
> DG Zarembski et al, Impact of rifampin on serum amiodarone concentrations in a patient with congenital heart disease. Pharmacotherapy, 19:249, 1999

Single case report (1999)

Ritonavir

Possible amiodarone toxicity (decreased metabolism)
> Manufacturer's package insert (ritonavir)

Theoretical; listed as contraindicated in product information

Theophyllines

Possible theophylline toxicity (mechanism not established)
> J Soto et al, Possible theophylline-amiodarone interaction. DICP, 24:1115, 1990; A Hirsch et al, Interaction between theophylline (Theo) and amiodarone (Amio). Ann Allergy, 70:68, Jan 1993

Two case reports (1990, 1993)

Thyroid hormones

Decreased thyroxine (T_4) effect (decreased metabolism to T_3)
> JM Hershman et al, Thyroxine and triiodothyronine kinetics in cardiac patients taking amiodarone. Acta Endocrinol, 111:193, 1986

Switch to triiodothyronine (T_3)

Amitriptyline, see Antidepressants, tricyclic

AMLODIPINE, with:

Cyclosporine

Possible cyclosporine toxicity (probably decreased metabolism)
> TE Pesavento et al, Amlodipine increases cyclosporine levels in hypertensive renal transplant patients: results of a prospective study. J Am Soc Nephrol, 7:831, 1996; YC Schrama and HA Koomans, Interactions of cyclosporin A and amlodipine: blood cyclosporin A levels, hypertension and kidney function. J Hypertens, 16, suppl 4:S33, 1998

Single case report (1996) and study of 11 renal transplant patients; effect smaller than with verapamil or diltiazem

Amobarbital, see Barbiturates

AMODIAQUINE, with:
: **Phenothiazines**
    Possible chlorpromazine toxicity (decreased metabolism)
    : ROA Makanjuola et al, Effects of antimalarial agents on plasma levels of chlorpromazine and its metabolites in schizophrenic patients. Trop Geographic Med, 40:31, 1988
    Monitor chlorpromazine concentration

Amoxapine, see Antidepressants, tricyclic
Amoxicillin, see Penicillins
Amphetamine, see Sympathomimetic amines
Amphotericin B, see Antifungals, Amphotericin B
Ampicillin, see Penicillins

AMPRENAVIR, with:
: **Abacavir** - See Abacavir with Amprenavir, page 6
: **Amiodarone** - See Amiodarone with Amprenavir, page 33
: **Antacids**
    Possible decreased amprenavir effect (decreased absorption)
    : Manufacturer's package insert (amprenavir)
    Manufacturer recommends not taking amprenavir within one hour of antacid
: **Anticoagulants, oral**
    Possible increased anticoagulant effect
    : Manufacturer's package insert (amprenavir)
    Monitor INR
: **Antidepressants, tricyclic**
    Possible serious or life-threatening toxicity with tricyclic antidepressants (decreased metabolism; CYP3A4)
    : Manufacturer's package insert (amprenavir)
    Monitor antidepressant concentration
: **Antifungals, imidazoles and triazoles**
    Possible toxicity of antifungal and amprenavir (decreased metabolism; CYP3A4)
    : RE Polk et al, Pharmacokinetic interaction between ketoconazole and amprenavir after single doses in healthy men. Pharmacotherapy, 19:1378, 1999
    Single dose study in 12 healthy subjects; monitor clinical status
: **Antihistamines, H$_1$-blockers: astemizole, terfenadine**
    Possible serious or life-threatening toxicity with astemizole (decreased metabolism; CYP3A4)
    : Manufacturer's package insert (amprenavir)
    Avoid concurrent use; astemizole is no longer available
: **Benzodiazepines**
    Possible serious or life-threatening toxicity with midazolam or triazolam (decreased metabolism; CYP3A4)
    : Manufacturer's package insert (amprenavir)
    Avoid concurrent use

AMPRENAVIR, with: *(continued)*

Bepridil
Possible serious or life-threatening toxicity with bepridil (decreased metabolism; CYP3A4)
> Manufacturer's package insert (amprenavir)

Avoid concurrent use

Cisapride
Possible serious or life-threatening toxicity with cisapride (decreased metabolism; CYP3A4)
> Manufacturer's package insert (amprenavir)

Avoid concurrent use; cisapride is no longer marketed in the USA

Didanosine
Decreased amprenavir effect (decreased absorption)
> Manufacturer's package insert (amprenavir)

Manufacturer recommends not taking amprenavir within one hour of didanosine due to antacid content

Efavirenz
Possible decreased amprenavir effect (increased metabolism)
> BM Sadler et al, Pharmacokinetic drug interactions with amprenavir, 12th World AIDS Conference, Geneva Switzerland, 1998, Poster 12389; J Falloon et al, Combination therapy with amprenavir, abacavir, and efavirenz in human immunodeficiency virus (HIV)-infected patients failing a protease-inhibitor regimen: pharmacokinetic drug interactions and antiviral activity. Clin Infect Dis, 30:313, 2000

Monitor clinical status, amprenavir dose may need to be increased

Ergot alkaloids
Possible serious or life-threatening toxicity with ergotamine or dihydroergotamine (decreased metabolism; CYP3A4)
> Manufacturer's package insert (amprenavir)

Avoid concurrent use

Indinavir
Possible decreased indinavir effect (increased metabolism; CYP3A4) and increased amprenavir toxicity (decreased metabolism; CYP3A4)
> Manufacturer's package insert (amprenavir)

One study in 9 subjects; monitor clinical status

Lidocaine
Possible serious or life-threatening toxicity with lidocaine (decreased metabolism; CYP3A4)
> Manufacturer's package insert (amprenavir)

Monitor lidocaine concentration

Lopinavir/Ritonavir
Increased amprenavir toxicity (decreased metabolism)
> Manufacturer's package insert (*Kaletra*)

Doses of the combination may need to be adjusted

(continued)

AMPRENAVIR, with: *(continued)*

Quinidine
Possible serious or life-threatening toxicity with quinidine (decreased metabolism; CYP3A4)
> Manufacturer's package insert (amprenavir)

Monitor quinidine concentration

Rifabutin
Possible increased rifabutin toxicity (decreased metabolism)
> BM Sadler et al, Pharmacokinetic drug interactions with amprenavir, 12th World AIDS Conference, Geneva Switzerland, 1998, Poster 12389

Rifabutin dosage should be decreased

Rifampin
Decreased amprenavir effect (increased metabolism; CYP3A4)
> Manufacturer's package insert (amprenavir)

In one study in 11 subjects amprenavir concentration decreased by 90%; avoid concurrent use

Ritonavir
Possible amprenavir toxicity (probably decreased metabolism)
> BM Sadler et al, Pharmacokinetic (PK) drug-interaction between amprenavir (APV) and ritonavir (RTV) in HIV-seronegative subjects after multiple, oral dosing. 7th Conf Retrovir Opportun Infect, 2000, abstract 77

Based on study in healthy subjects; substantial increase in amprenavir plasma concentrations; monitor clinical status

Saquinavir
Possible decreased amprenavir effect (increased metabolism; CYP3A4)
> Manufacturer's package insert (amprenavir)

One study in 7 subjects; monitor clinical status

Sildenafil
Possible toxicity with sildenafil (decreased metabolism; CYP3A4)
> Manufacturer's package insert (amprenavir)

Reduce sildenafil dosage

Zidovudine
Possible increased zidovudine toxicity (decreased metabolism; CYP3A4)
> Manufacturer's package insert (amprenavir)

Single dose study in 12 subjects; monitor clinical status

AMRINONE, with:

Disopyramide
Severe hypotension (mechanism not established)
> Manufacturer's package insert

Single case report (1984)

ANABOLIC AND ANDROGENIC STEROIDS, with:

Aminoglutethimide - See Aminoglutethimide with Anabolic and androgenic steroids, page 29

Anticoagulants, oral
Bleeding with danazol (decreased hepatic synthesis of vitamin K-dependent clotting factors)
> IA Goulbourne and DAD Macleod, An interaction between danazol and

ANABOLIC AND ANDROGENIC STEROIDS, with: *(continued)*
>warfarin. Br J Obstet Gynaecol, 88:950, 1981; ML Meeks et al, Danazol increases the anticoagulant effect of warfarin. Ann Pharmacother, 26:641, 1992

Monitor prothrombin time

Increased anticoagulant effect (decreased metabolism)
>S Husted et al, Increased sensitivity to phenprocoumon during methyltestosterone therapy. Eur J Clin Pharmacol, 10:209, 1976; MS Edwards and JR Curtis, Decreased anticoagulant tolerance with oxymetholone. Lancet, 2:221, 1971; SM Lorentz and RT Weibert, Potentiation of warfarin anticoagulation by topical testosterone ointment. Clin Pharm, 4:332, 1985; JJ Schrogie and HM Solomon, The anticoagulant response to bishydroxycoumarin II. The effect of D-thyroxine, clofibrate, and norethandrolone. Clin Pharmacol Ther, 8:70, 1967; JC de Oya et al, Decreased anticoagulant tolerance with oxymetholone in paroxysmal nocturnal haemoglobinuria. Lancet, 2:259, 1971; PW Shaw and AM Smith, Possible interaction of warfarin and stanozolol. Clin Pharm, 6:500, 1987

Reported in many patients with oxymetholone, several patients with stanozolol, one patient with methyltestosterone, and one patient using testosterone vaginal ointment; monitor prothrombin time

Beta-adrenergic blockers
Possible decreased propranolol effect (increased metabolism)
>T Walle et al, Propranolol metabolism in normal subjects: association with sex steroid hormones. Clin Pharmacol Ther, 56:127, 1994

In one pharmacokinetic study, testosterone cypionate increased clearance of propranolol in 9 of 11 healthy men

Carbamazepine
Carbamazepine toxicity with danazol (decreased metabolism)
>JJ Zielinski et al, Clinically significant danazol – carbamazepine interaction. Ther Drug Monit, 9:24, 1987

Avoid concurrent use

Cyclosporine
Cyclosporine toxicity (decreased metabolism; CYP3A4)
>BB Moller and B Ekelund, Toxicity of cyclosporine during treatment with androgens. N Engl J Med, 313:1416, 1985; WB Ross et al, Cyclosporin interaction with danazol and norethisterone. Lancet, 1:330, 1986; E Goffin et al, Cyclosporine-methyltestosterone interaction. Nephron, 59:174, 1991; J Passfall et al, Pharmacokinetics of cyclosporin during administration of danazol. Nephrol Dial Transplant, 9:1807, 1994; J Borrás-Blasco et al, Possible cyclosporin-danazol interaction in a patient with aplastic anaemia. Am J Hematol, 62:63, 1999

Concurrent use is best avoided; if combination is used monitor cyclosporine serum concentrations and clinical status

Epoetin
Priapism (mechanism not established)
>K Sombolos et al, To the Editor. Am J Kidney Dis, 19:94, 1992

(continued)

ANABOLIC AND ANDROGENIC STEROIDS, with: *(continued)*
Single case report (1992)

HMG-CoA reductase inhibitors
Myopathy and rhabdomyolysis following danazol and lovastatin (probably decreased lovastatin metabolism by CYP3A4)
> M Dallaire and M Chamberland, Rhabdomyolyse sévère chez un patient recevant lovastatine, danazol et doxycycline. Can Med Assoc J, 150:1991, 1994

Single case report (1994)

Hypoglycemics, sulfonylurea
Increased hypoglycemic effect (mechanism not established)
> J Landon et al, The effect of anabolic steroids on blood sugar and plasma insulin levels in man. Metabolism, 12:924, 1963

Monitor blood glucose

Neuromuscular blocking agents
Resistance to neuromuscular blockade (mechanism not established)
> P Reddy et al, Resistance to muscle relaxants in a patient receiving prolonged testosterone therapy. Anesthesiology, 70:871, 1989

Single report (1989) in woman receiving prolonged testosterone therapy prior to total abdominal hysterectomy

Tacrolimus
Tacrolimus toxicity with danazol (probable decreased metabolism)
> R Shapiro et al, FK 506 interaction with danazol. Lancet, 341:1344, 1993

Single case report (1993); monitor tacrolimus concentration

Vitamin D
Hypercalcemia with alphacalcidol and danazol (mechanism not established)
> NC Hepburn et al, Danazol-induced hypercalcaemia in alphacalcidol-treated hypoparathyroidism. Postgrad Med J, 65:849, 1989

Single report (1989) of patient with hypothyroidism; monitor calcium concentration

ANAGRELIDE, with:

Sucralfate
Possible decreased anagrelide effect (decreased absorption)
> Manufacturer's package insert

Single case report (1997); the absorption of most drugs is not affected when given 2 hours before or 6 hours after sucralfate

Anastrozole, no documented interactions, see page 4, Criteria for Listing Interactions

ANGIOTENSIN-CONVERTING ENZYME (ACE) INHIBITORS, with:

Allopurinol
- See Allopurinol with Angiotensin-converting enzyme (ACE) inhibitors, page 24

Amiloride
- See Amiloride with Angiotensin-converting enzyme (ACE) inhibitors, page 27

Antacids
Possible decreased antihypertensive effect with captopril or fosinopril (decreased absorption)
> R Mantyla et al, Impairment of captopril bioavailability by concomitant

ANGIOTENSIN-CONVERTING ENZYME (ACE) INHIBITORS, with: *(continued)*
food and antacid intake. Int J Clin Pharmacol Ther Toxicol, 22:626, 1984
Clinical significance not established

Antidepressants, tricyclic
Clomipramine toxicity with enalapril (mechanism not established)
M Toutoungi, Potential effect of enalapril on clomipramine metabolism. Hum Psychopharmacol, 7:347, 1992
Several case reports; monitor clomipramine concentration

Antihistamines, H$_2$-blockers
Severe neuropathies with captopril and cimetidine (possibly additive)
AB Atkinson et al, Neurological dysfunction in two patients receiving captopril and cimetidine. Lancet, 2:36, 1980; C Richer et al, Cimetidine does not alter free unchanged captopril pharmacokinetics and biological effects in healthy volunteer. J Pharmacol, 17:338, 1986
Occurs in patients with renal impairment; monitor neurological function

Azathioprine
Anemia (mechanism not established)
J Gossmann et al, Anemia in renal transplant recipients caused by concomitant therapy with azathioprine and angiotensin-converting enzyme inhibitors. Transplantation, 56:585, 1993
Avoid concurrent use; observed in renal transplant patients

Blood transfusion
Possible increased risk of hypotensive transfusion reactions (mechanism not established)
K Quillen, Hypotensive transfusion reactions in patients taking angiotensin-converting-enzyme inhibitors. N Engl J Med, 343:1422, 2000
Based on series of 8 patients taking ACE inhibitors who received red cells or platelets

Bupivacaine
Possible increased risk of hypotension and bradycardia with captopril (mechanism not established)
NE Williams, Profound bradycardia and hypotension following spinal anaesthesia in a patient receiving an ACE inhibitor: an important
Single case report of patient receiving spinal anesthesia with bupivacaine; monitor clinical status

Capsaicin
Increased cough (mechanism not established)
JF Hakas, Jr, MT O'Hollaren and GA Porter, Topical capsaicin induces cough in patient receiving ACE inhibitor. Ann Allergy, 65:322, 1990
Single patient on ACE inhibitor developed cough only after starting topical capsaicin (1990)

COX-2 inhibitors
Decreased hypotensive effect (possibly decreased prostaglandin synthesis)
Manufacturer's package insert
In one study in hypertensive patients, rofecoxib given with benazeril increased blood pressure; monitor blood pressure

(continued)

ANGIOTENSIN-CONVERTING ENZYME (ACE) INHIBITORS, with: *(continued)*

Cyclopropane

Hypotension with captopril (additive)

Manufacturer's package insert

Monitor blood pressure

Cyclosporine

Renal failure in kidney transplant recipient with enalapril (mechanism not established)

BM Murray et al, Enalapril-associated acute renal failure in renal transplants: possible role of cyclosporine. Am J Kidney Dis, 16:66, 1990

Reported in 2 patients with normal renal arteries, but possible vasoconstriction by cyclosporine (1990)

Dextran sulfate

Hypotension, bradycardia, dyspnea, and flushing during apheresis with dextran sulfate columns (possible decreased metabolism of bradykinin generated through dextran sulfate release)

CJ Olbricht et al, Anaphylactoid reactions, LDL apheresis with dextran sulphate, and ACE inhibitors. Lancet, 340:908, 1992

Reported in two patients (1992); avoid concurrent use

Diltiazem

False positive captopril renography tests (probably additive, postglomerular vasodilation)

R Claveau-Tremblay et al, False-positive captopril renography in patients taking calcium antagonists. J Nucl Med, 39:1621, 1998

Stop diltiazem and other calcium-channel blockers before performing captopril-stimulated renography

Enflurane

Hypotension with captopril (additive)

Manufacturer's package insert

Monitor blood pressure

Epoetin

Possible reduction in erythropoietin effect (mechanism not established)

J Walter, Does captopril decrease the effect of human recombinant erythropoietin in haemodialysis patients? Nephrol Dial Transplant, 8:1428, 1993; MH Schwenk et al, Potential angiotensin-converting enzyme inhibitor—epoetin alfa interaction in patients receiving chronic hemodialysis. Pharmacotherapy, 18:627, 1998; IC Macdougall, The role of ACE inhibitors and angiotensin II receptor blockers in the response to epoetin. Nephrol Dial Transplant, 14:1836, 1999

Monitor hematogical parameters; conflicting reports; appears to be most likely when ACE inhibitor dose is high and epoetin dose is low

Ether

Hypotension with captopril (additive)

Manufacturer's package insert

Monitor blood pressure

ANGIOTENSIN-CONVERTING ENZYME (ACE) INHIBITORS, with: *(continued)*
Furosemide
Increased risk of renal failure, especially in patients with bilateral renal artery stenosis (mechanism not established)

> P Scanu et al, Reversible acute renal insufficiency with combination of enalapril and diuretics in a patient with a single renal-artery stenosis. Nephron, 45:321, 1987; M Packer et al, Functional renal insufficiency during long-term therapy with captopril and enalapril in severe chronic heart failure. Ann Intern Med, 106:346, 1987; AK Mandal et al, Diuretics potentiate angiotensin converting enzyme inhibitor-induced acute renal failure. Clin Nephrol, 42:170, 1994

Monitor blood pressure and renal function

Hypotension with enalaprilat; possible hypotension with enalapril (mechanism not established)

> Manufacturer's package insert

Monitor blood pressure and renal function

Decreased diuretic effect of furosemide with captopril (decreased proximal tubular secretion of furosemide)

> JS McLay et al, Acute effects of captopril on the renal actions of furosemide in patients with chronic heart failure. Am Heart J, 126:879, 1993

Monitor blood pressure and renal function; based on studies in healthy volunteers treated with high doses and patients with heart failure treated with conventional doses

Gold sodium thiomalate
Nitritoid reaction – flushing, fainting, nausea, and dizziness – with captopril, enalapril, or lisinopril (mechanism not established)

> LA Healey and MB Backes, Nitritoid reactions and angiotensin-converting-enzyme inhibitors. N Engl J Med, 321:763, 1989

Single case reports with captopril and lisinopril (1989); in 2 patients with enalapril (1989)

Halothane
Hypotension with captopril (additive)

> Manufacturer's package insert

Monitor blood pressure

Hypoglycemics, sulfonylurea
Increased hypoglycemic effect with captopril and enalapril (increased insulin effect)

> C Arauz-Pacheco et al, Hypoglycemia induced by angiotensin-converting enzyme inhibitors in patients with non-insulin-dependent diabetes receiving sulfonylurea therapy. Am J Med, 89:811, 1990; RMC Herings et al, Hypoglycaemia associated with use of inhibitors of angiotensin converting enzyme. Lancet, 345:1195, 1995; S Ahmad, Drug interaction induces hypoglycemia. J Fam Pract, 40:541, 1995; E Girardin and D Raccah, Interaction entre inhibiteurs de l'enzyme de conversion et sulfamides hypoglycémiants ou insuline. Presse Med, 27:1914, 1998; M Thamer et al, Association between antihypertensive drug use and hypoglycemia: a case-control

(continued)

ANGIOTENSIN-CONVERTING ENZYME (ACE) INHIBITORS, with: *(continued)*
> study of diabetic users of insulin or sulfonylureas. Clin Ther, 21:1387, 1999

May also occur with other ACE inhibitors; monitor blood glucose; one epidemiologic study found only enalapril to increase the risk of hypoglycemia

Insect venom extracts
> Anaphylactoid reaction during desensitization to insect venom (mechanism not established)
>> JM Tunon-de-Lara et al, ACE inhibitors and anaphylactoid reactions during venom immunotherapy. Lancet, 340:908, 1992
>
> *Reported in two patients on enalapril; no reaction when enalapril stopped 24 hours before desensitization (1992)*

Insulin
> Increased hypoglycemic effect with captopril and enalapril (probable increased insulin effect)
>> J McMurray and DM Fraser, Captopril, enalapril, and blood glucose. Lancet, 1:1035, 1986; RMC Herings et al, Hypoglycaemia associated with use of inhibitors of angiotensin converting enzyme. Lancet, 345:1195, 1995; E Girardin and D Raccah, Interaction entre inhibiteurs de l'enzyme de conversion et sulfamides hypoglycémiants ou insuline. Presse Med, 27:1914, 1998
>
> *May occur with other ACE inhibitors; monitor blood glucose*

Interferon
> Possible risk of severe granulocytopenia (mechanism not established)
>> M Casato et al, Granulocytopenia after combined therapy with interferon and angiotensin-converting enzyme inhibitors: evidence for a synergistic hematologic toxicity. Am J Med, 99:386, 1995
>
> *Three case reports, one with positive dechallenge and rechallenge (1995); avoid concurrent use*

Iron
> Possible toxicity with IV iron (mechanism not established)
>> G Rolla et al, Systemic reactions to intravenous iron therapy in patients receiving angiotensin converting enzyme inhibitor. J Allergy Clin Immunol, 93:1074, 1994
>
> *Reported in three patients receiving ferrigluconate (1994); monitor clinical status and discontinue iron infusion if reaction occurs*
>
> Decreased captopril effect (decreased absorption)
>> JP Schaefer et al, Ferrous sulphate interacts with captopril. Br J Clin Pharmacol, 46:377, 1998
>
> *Based on study in healthy subjects*

Isoflurane
> Hypotension with captopril (additive)
>> Manufacturer's package insert
>
> *Monitor blood pressure*

Lithium
> Lithium toxicity (possibly decreased renal excretion)
>> M Pulik and H Lida, Interaction lithium-inhibiteurs de l'enzyme de

ANGIOTENSIN-CONVERTING ENZYME (ACE) INHIBITORS, with: *(continued)*
conversion. Pressé Méd, 17:755, 1988; FJ Correa and AR Eiser, Angiotensin-converting enzyme inhibitors and lithium toxicity. Am J Med, 93:108, 1992; SS Chandragiri et al, Lithium, ACE inhibitors, NSAIDs, and verapamil: a possible fatal combination. Psychosomatic, 39:281, 1998

May occur with any ACE inhibitor; monitor lithium concentration

Nifedipine

False positive captopril renography tests (probably additive, postglomerular vasodilation)

R Claveau-Tremblay et al, False-positive captopril renography in patients taking calcium antagonists. J Nucl Med, 39:1621, 1998

Stop nifedipine and other calcium-channel blockers before performing captopril-stimulated renography

Nitrous oxide

Hypotension with captopril (additive)

Manufacturer's package insert

Monitor blood pressure

Nonsteroidal anti-inflammatory drugs

Decreased hypotensive effect (possibly decreased prostaglandin synthesis)

D Hall et al, Counteraction of the vasodilator effects of enalapril by aspirin in severe heart failure. J Am Coll Cardiol, 20:1549, 1992; SR Smith et al, Effect of low-dose aspirin on thromboxane production and the antihypertensive effect of captopril. J Am Soc Nephrol, 4:1133, 1993; MD Guazzi et al, Antihypertensive efficacy of angiotensin converting enzyme inhibition and aspirin counteraction. Clin Pharmacol Ther, 63:79, 1998; JJ Nawarskas et al, Effect of aspirin on blood pressure in hypertensive patients taking enalapril or losartan. Am J Hypertens, 12:784, 1999; JJ Nawarskas and SA Spinler, Update on the interaction between aspirin and angiotensin-converting enzyme inhibitors. Pharmacotherapy, 20:698, 2000; PR Conlin et al, Effect of indomethacin on blood pressure lowering by captopril and losartan in hypertensive patients. Hypertension, 36:461, 2000

Avoid concurrent use if possible; if combination used monitor blood pressure; low-dose aspirin (325 mg/d or less) may not interact

Aggravation of impaired renal function and induction of renal failure (probably additive)

MM Hawkins and CB Seelig, A case of acute renal failure induced by the co-administration of NSAIDs and captopril. NCMJ, 51:291, 1990; CB Seelig et al, Nephrotoxicity associated with concomitant ACE inhibitor and NSAID therapy. South Med J, 83:1144, 1990; C Badid et al, Anti-inflammatoire non stéroïdien et inhibiteur de l'enzyme de conversion: association dangereuse en période postopératoire. Ann Fr Anesth Reanim, 16:55, 1997; MC Thomas, Diuretics, ACE inhibitors and NSAIDs — the triple whammy. Med J Aust, 172:184, 2000

Avoid concurrent use

(continued)

ANGIOTENSIN-CONVERTING ENZYME (ACE) INHIBITORS, with: *(continued)*

Enalapril may antagonize favorable effect of aspirin on mortality after myocardial infarction (mechanism not established)

> KN Nguyen et al, Interaction between enalapril and aspirin on mortality after acute myocardial infarction: subgroup analysis of the cooperative new Scandinavian enalapril survival study II (Consensus II). Am J Cardiol, 79:115, 1997; J Leor et al, Aspirin and mortality in patients treated with angiotensin-converting enzyme inhibitors. J Am Coll Cardiol, 33:1920, 1999;

Based on retrospective study; another study found lower mortality with ACE inhibitors combined with low-dose aspirin than with ACE inhibitors without aspirin in patients with coronary artery disease

Possible worsening of congestive heart failure with aspirin (possibly decreased prostaglandin synthesis)

> JJ Nawarskas and SA Spinler, Does aspirin interfere with the therapeutic efficacy of angiotensin-converting enzyme inhibitors in hypertension or congestive heart failure? Pharmacotherapy, 18:1041, 1998; M Guazzi et al, Aspirin worsens exercise performance and pulmonary gas exchange in patients with heart failure who are taking angiotensin-converting enzyme inhibitors. Am Heart J, 138: 254, 1999; T Stys et al, Does aspirin attenuate the beneficial effects of angiotensin-converting enzyme inhibition in heart failure? Arch Intern Med, 160:1409, 2000; JJ Nawarskas and SA Spinler, Update on the interaction between aspirin and angiotensin-converting enzyme inhibitors. Pharmacotherapy, 20:698, 2000

Based on study of patients with CHF given aspirin 325 mg daily; more study needed to assess benefit-risk of aspirin-ACE inhibitor combinations in CHF; some have suggested use of clopidogrel in place of aspirin as an antiplatelet agent

Pergolide

Severe hypotension with lisinopril (mechanism not established)

> JC Kando et al, Pergolide-induced hypotension. DICP, 24:543, 1990

Single case report (1990)

Potassium

Hyperkalemia (additive)

> TG Burnakis and HJ Mioduch, Combined therapy with captopril and potassium supplementation. Arch Intern Med, 144:2371, 1984; KK Ray et al, Severe hyperkalaemia due to the concomitant use of salt substitutes and ACE inhibitors in hypertension: a potentially life threatening interaction. J Hum Hyperten, 13:717, 1999

Monitor serum potassium and clinical status

Probenecid

Possible enalapril or enalaprilat toxicity (decreased renal excretion of enalapril and its metabolite, enalaprilat)

> FH Noormohamed et al, Pharmacokinetic and pharmacodynamic actions of enalapril in humans: effect of probenecid pretreatment. J Pharmacol Exp Ther, 253:362, 1990

ANGIOTENSIN-CONVERTING ENZYME (ACE) INHIBITORS, with: *(continued)*
Monitor clinical status; based on studies in healthy men

Spironolactone
Hyperkalemia (additive)
> Manufacturer's package insert; TG Burnakis and HJ Mioduch, Combined therapy with captopril and potassium supplementation. Arch Intern Med, 144:2371, 1984

Avoid concurrent use; effect of spironolactone can persist for up to several months

Increased risk of renal failure with enalapril, especially in patients with unilateral or bilateral renal artery stenosis (mechanism not established)
> P Scanu et al, Reversible acute renal insufficiency with combination of enalapril and diuretics in a patient with a single renal-artery stenosis. Nephron, 45:321, 1987

Monitor renal function

Thiazide diuretics
Increased risk of renal failure with captopril or enalapril, especially in patients with bilateral renal artery stenosis (mechanism not established)
> ML Watson et al, Captopril/diuretic combinations in severe renovascular disease: a cautionary note. Lancet, 2:404, 1983; P Scanu et al, Reversible acute renal insufficiency with combination of enalapril and diuretics in a patient with a single renal-artery stenosis. Nephron, 45:321, 1987; AK Mandal et al, Diuretics potentiate angiotensin converting enzyme inhibitor-induced acute renal failure. Clin Nephrol, 42:170, 1994

Monitor blood pressure and renal function

Hypotension with captopril or enalaprilat, possible with enalapril, benazepril, fosinopril, or ramipril (mechanism not established)
> JS Budd and MAR Hoghton, Interaction of captopril and Dyazide causing hypotension and abdominal pain. Br Med J, 295:612, 1987

Monitor blood pressure; single case report with captopril (1987)

Aggravation of hyponatremia with bendroflumethiazide and enalapril (mechanism not established)
> JG Collier and DJ Webb, Severe thiazide-induced hyponatraemia during treatment with enalapril. Postgrad Med J, 63:1105, 1987

Single case report (1987)

Triamterene
Hyperkalemia (additive)
> Manufacturer's package insert; TG Burnakis and HJ Mioduch, Combined therapy with captopril and potassium supplementation. Arch Intern Med, 144:2371, 1984

Avoid concurrent use

Trimethoprim
Possible increased risk of hyperkalemia (additive)
> JF Bugge, Severe hyperkalaemia induced by trimethoprim in combination with an angiotensin-converting enzyme inhibitor in a patient with transplanted lungs. J Intern Med, 240:249, 1996

(continued)

ANGIOTENSIN-CONVERTING ENZYME (ACE) INHIBITORS, with: *(continued)*
Single case report (1996); monitor serum potassium
Verapamil
False positive captopril renography tests (probably additive, postglomerular vasodilation)
> R Claveau-Tremblay et al, False-positive captopril renography in patients taking calcium antagonists. J Nucl Med, 39:1621, 1998

Stop verapamil and other calcium-channel blockers before performing captopril-stimulated renography

Anisindione, see Anticoagulants, oral
Anistreplase, see Thrombolytics
ANTACIDS, with:
Allopurinol - See Allopurinol with Antacids, page 24
Amprenavir - See Amprenavir with Antacids, page 38
Angiotensin-converting enzyme (ACE) inhibitors - See Angiotensin-converting enzyme (ACE) inhibitors with Antacids, page 42
Antifungals, imidazoles and triazoles
Decreased ketoconazole and itraconazole effect (decreased absorption)
> RA Blum et al, Increased gastric pH and the bioavailability of fluconazole and ketoconazole. Ann Intern Med, 114:755, 1991; SG Lim et al, Short report: the absorption of fluconazole and itraconazole under conditions of low intragastric acidity. Aliment Pharmacol Ther, 7:317, 1993

Give 2 hours apart

Antihistamines, H$_2$-blockers
Decreased cimetidine, famotidine, nizatidine, and ranitidine effect (decreased absorption)
> WM Steinberg et al, Antacids inhibit absorption of cimetidine. N Engl J Med, 307:400, 1982; H Albin et al, Effect of aluminum phosphate on the bioavailability of cimetidine and prednisolone. Eur J Clin Pharmacol, 26:271, 1984; DW Shelly et al, Effect of concomitant antacid administration on plasma cimetidine concentrations during repetitive dosing. Drug Intell Clin Pharm, 20:792, 1986; GW Mihaly et al, High dose of antacid *(Mylanta II)* reduces bioavailability of ranitidine. Br Med J, 285:998, 1982; H Albin et al, Effect of aluminum phosphate on the bioavailability of ranitidine. Eur J Clin Pharmacol, 32:97, 1987; N Barzaghi et al, Impaired bioavailability of famotidine given concurrently with a potent antacid. J Clin Pharmacol, 29:670, 1989; MP Knadler et al, Absorption studies of the H$_2$-blocker nizatidine. Clin Pharmacol Ther, 42:514, 1987

Take at least one hour apart; absorption may return to normal with continued use; low dose of aluminum phosphate may not interfere; sorbitol and mannitol excipients may play a role

Antacid bezoar with large antacid doses and ranitidine (decreased gastric secretion)
> GL Burruss et al, Small bowel obstruction from an antacid bezoar: a ranitidine – antacid interaction? South Med J, 79:917, 1986

ANTACIDS, with: *(continued)*
Avoid excessive antacid intake

Benzodiazepines

Decreased oral clorazepate effect with single dose, but possibly not with chronic use (decreased absorption)

> RI Shader et al, Impaired absorption of desmethyldiazepam from clorazepate by magnesium aluminum hydroxide. Clin Pharmacol Ther, 24:308, 1978; RI Shader et al, Steady-state plasma desmethyldiazepam during long-term clorazepate use: effect of antacids. Clin Pharmacol Ther, 31:180, 1982; PD Kroboth et al, Effects of end stage renal disease and aluminum hydroxide on triazolam pharmacokinetics. Br J Clin Pharmacol, 19:839, 1985

Give as far apart as possible; could occur with other oral benzodiazepines; may not occur with triazolam

Beta-adrenergic blockers

Decreased oral atenolol, propranolol, or sotalol effect with calcium or aluminum antacid salts (decreased absorption)

> W Kirch et al, Interaction of atenolol with furosemide and calcium and aluminum salts. Clin Pharmacol Ther, 30:429, 1981; JH Dobbs et al, Effects of aluminum hydroxide on the absorption of propranolol. Curr Ther Res, 21:887, 1977; S Läer et al, Pharmacodynamically relevant interaction between D,L-sotalol and an antacid preparation (Maalox®). Circulation, 92, suppl I-194, 1995; S Läer et al, Interaction between sotalol and an antacid preparation. Br J Clin Pharmacol, 43:269, 1997

Give beta-blocker 2 hours before or 6 hours after antacid; monitor cardiovascular status

Cephalosporins

Possible decreased cefpodoxime or cefdinir effect with aluminum magnesium hydroxide (decreased absorption)

> GS Hughes et al, The effects of gastric pH and food on the pharmacokinetics of a new oral cephalosporin, cefpodoxime proxetil. Clin Pharmacol Ther, 46:674, 1989; manufacturer's package insert (cefdinir)

Give cefdinir or cefpodoxime 2 hours before or after antacids

Citrates

Aluminum toxicity in uremic patients with aluminum-containing antacids (increased absorption)

> JW Coburn et al, Calcium citrate markedly enhances aluminum absorption from aluminum hydroxide. Am J Kidney Dis, 17:708, 1991; J Main and MK Ward, Potentiation of aluminum absorption by effervescent analgesic tablets in a haemodialysis patient. BMJ, 304:1686, 1992

Avoid concurrent use in uremic patients

Corticosteroids

Decreased oral corticosteroid effect (decreased absorption)

> M Uribe et al, Decreased bioavailability of prednisone due to antacids in patients with chronic active liver disease and in healthy volunteers. Gastroenterology, 80:661, 1981

(continued)

ANTACIDS, with: *(continued)*
Give as far apart as possible; low dose of aluminum phosphate may not interfere

COX-2 inhibitors
Possible decreased rofecoxib effect (probably decreased absorption)
> Medical Letter, 41:59, 1999

Effect modest; give rofecoxib at least 2 hours before or 4 to 6 hours after antacids

Cyclosporine
Possible decreased cyclosporine effect (probably decreased absorption)
> M Ichisawa et al, The effect of dried aluminum hydroxide gel on the blood concentration of cyclosporine-A. Jpn J Hosp Pharm, 23:407, 1997

Based on study in pediatric patients; theoretically, interaction could be minimized by giving cyclosporine at least 2 hours before or 6 hours after aluminum-containing antacids

Delavirdine
Decreased delavirdine effect with aluminum-magnesium hydroxides (decreased absorption)
> Manufacturer's package insert

Give delavirdine 2 hours before or 4 to 6 hours after antacids

Digoxin
Decreased digoxin effect (decreased absorption)
> DD Brown and RP Juhl, Decreased bioavailability of digoxin due to antacids and kaolin-pectin. N Engl J Med, 295:1034, 1976; MD Allen et al, Effect of magnesium-aluminum hydroxide and kaolin-pectin on absorption of digoxin from tablets and capsules. J Clin Pharmacol, 21:26, 1981

Give as far apart as possible; use digoxin capsules rather than tablets and monitor digoxin concentration

Fluoride
Decreased fluoride effect with aluminum or calcium antacids (decreased absorption)
> H Spencer et al, Effect of aluminum hydroxide on fluoride metabolism. Clin Pharmacol Ther, 28:529, 1980; D Briançon et al, Comparative study of fluoride bioavailability following the administration of sodium fluoride alone and in combination with different calcium salts. J Bone Mineral Res, 5 suppl 1:S71, 1990; J-P Devogelaer et al, Bioavailability of enteric-coated sodium fluoride tablets as affected by the administration of calcium supplements at different time intervals. J Bone Mineral Res, 5 suppl 1:S75, 1990

Avoid concurrent use or give as far apart as possible; enteric-coated fluoride and calcium solutions may not interact; calcium antacids may not interact significantly

Fluoroquinolones
Decreased fluoroquinolone effect with aluminum, magnesium, or calcium antacids (decreased absorption)
> JJ Schentag et al, Time dependent interactions between antacids and quinolone antibiotics. Clin Pharmacol Ther, 43:135, 1988; S Flor et al, Effects of magnesium-aluminum hydroxide and calcium carbonate antacids

ANTACIDS, with: *(continued)*
> on bioavailability of ofloxacin. Antimicrob Agents Chemother, 34:2436, 1990; RW Frost et al, Effects of aluminum hydroxide and calcium carbonate antacids on the bioavailability of ciprofloxacin. Antimicrob Agents Chemother, 36:830, 1992; GR Granneman et al, Effect of antacid medication on the pharmacokinetics of temafloxacin. Clin Pharmacokinet, 22 suppl 1:83, 1992; J Shimada et al, Effect of antacid on absorption of the quinolone lomefloxacin. Antimicrob Agents Chemother, 36:1219, 1992; NRC Campbell et al, Norfloxacin interaction with antacids and minerals. Br J Clin Pharmacol, 33:115, 1992; P Lehto and KT Kivistö, Different effects of products containing metal ions on the absorption of lomefloxacin. Clin Pharmacol Ther, 56:477, 1994; manufacturer's package insert; T Motoya et al, Effects of milk and aluminium hydroxide on the absorption of norfloxacin, ciprofloxacin and tosufloxacin in healthy volunteers. J Appl Ther, 1:213, 1997; RD Johnson et al, Effect of Maalox on the oral absorption of sparfloxacin. Clin Ther, 20:1149, 1998

Avoid concurrent use, if possible; antacid given 2 to 4 hours after fluoroquinolone interacts less; fluoroquinolone was 70% bioavailable when given 4 hours after antacid; lomefloxacin and trovafloxacin minimally affected by calcium carbonate; tosufloxacin minimally affected by aluminum hydroxide; sparfloxacin may be somewhat less affected by antacids that other fluoroquinolones

Gabapentin
Possible decreased gabapentin effect (decreased absorption)
> JA Busch et al, Effect of *Maalox TC* on single-dose pharmacokinetics of gabapentin capsules in healthy subjects. Pharm Res, 9:S315, 1992

Clinical significance not established

Halofantrine
Possible decreased halofantrine effect with magnesium carbonate (decreased rate of absorption)
> SO Aideloje et al, Altered pharmacokinetics of halofantrine by an antacid, magnesium carbonate. Eur J Pharm Biopharm, 46:299, 1998

Based on study in healthy subjects which shows peak levels of halofantrine are lower with magnesium carbonate use. However, the AUCs were not significantly different. Separate dosing is advised.

Hypoglycemics, sulfonylurea
Possible hypoglycemia with glipizide, glibenclamide, or tolbutamide and magnesium antacids or sodium bicarbonate (increased absorption and accelerated insulin response)
> KT Kivistö and PJ Neuvonen, Enhancement of absorption and effect of glipizide by magnesium hydroxide. Clin Pharmacol Ther, 49:39, 1991; KT Kivistö and PJ Neuvonen, Differential effects of sodium bicarbonate and aluminum hydroxide on the absorption and activity of glipizide. Eur J Clin Pharmacol, 40:383, 1991; PJ Neuvonen and KT Kivistö, The effects of magnesium hydroxide on the absorption and efficacy of two glibenclamide preparations. Br J Clin Pharmacol, 32:215, 1991; KT Kivistö and PJ Neuvonen, Effect of magnesium hydroxide on the absorption and efficacy of tolbutamide and chlorpropamide. Eur J Clin Pharmacol, 42:675, 1992

(continued)

ANTACIDS, with: *(continued)*
Based on studies in healthy subjects; aluminum hydroxide may not interact; minimal effect when micronized glibenclamide was used

Iron

Decreased iron effect with carbonates (decreased absorption)
> MA O'Neil-Cutting and WH Crosby, The effect of antacids on the absorption of simultaneously ingested iron. JAMA, 255:1468, 1986; KL Wallace et al, Effect of magnesium hydroxide on iron absorption after ferrous sulfate. Ann Emerg Med, 34:685, 1999

Aluminum hydroxide and magnesium hydroxide do not interact; carbonates may not interact if ascorbic acid is present

Isoniazid

Decreased isoniazid effect with aluminum antacids (decreased absorption)
> A Hurwitz and DL Schlozman, Effects of antacids on gastrointestinal absorption of isoniazid in rat and man. Am Rev Respir Dis, 109:41, 1974; CA Peloquin et al, Pharmacokinetics of isoniazid under fasting conditions, with food, and with antacids. Int J Tuberc Lung Dis, 3:703, 1999

Conflicting reports; aluminum antacids may not interact with isoniazid when given without food

Metronidazole

Possible decreased metronidazole effect (decreased absorption)
> AM Molokhia and S Al-Rahman, Effect of concomitant oral administration of some adsorbing drugs on the bioavailability of metronidazole. Drug Devel Indust Pharm, 13:1229, 1987

Based on studies in 5 healthy volunteers; monitor metronidazole concentration or clinical status

Mycophenolate mofetil

Possible decreased mycophenolate effect (decreased absorption)
> Manufacturer's package insert

Monitor mycophenolate concentration

Nitrofurantoin

Possible decreased nitrofurantoin effect (decreased absorption)
> P Mannisto, The effect of crystal size, gastric content and emptying rate on the absorption of nitrofurantoin in healthy human volunteers. Int J Clin Pharmacol, 16:223, 1978

Give at least 6 hours apart

Nonsteroidal anti-inflammatory drugs

Decreased indomethacin effect (decreased absorption); but increased effect with sodium bicarbonate (increased absorption)
> JC Garnham et al, The different effects of sodium bicarbonate and aluminum hydroxide on the absorption of indomethacin in man. Postgrad Med J, 53:126, 1977

Clinical significance not established; small effects in healthy subjects

Mefenamic acid effect decreased with aluminum antacids (decreased absorption); but increased with magnesium antacids (increased absorption)
> PJ Neuvonen and KT Kivistö, Effect of magnesium hydroxide on the

ANTACIDS, with: *(continued)*
> absorption of tolfenamic and mefenamic acids. Eur J Clin Pharmacol, 35:495, 1988

Monitor clinical status

Decreased salicylate effect (increased renal excretion)
> G Levy et al, Decreased serum salicylate concentrations in children with rheumatic fever treated with antacid. N Engl J Med, 293:323, 1975; PD Hansten and WL Hayton, Effect of antacid and ascorbic acid on serum salicylate concentration. J Clin Pharmacol, 24:326, 1980

Monitor salicylate concentration

Nutrients, enteral preparations
Esophageal obstruction (precipitation of protein by aluminum)
> C Valli et al, Interaction of nutrients with antacids: a complication during enteral tube feeding. Lancet, 1:747, 1986

Avoid concurrent use if enteral preparations contain large percentage of high-molecular-weight peptides or proteins; low-molecular-weight peptides and amino acids do not precipitate

Penicillamine
Possible decreased penicillamine effect (decreased absorption)
> MA Osman et al, Reduction in oral penicillamine absorption by food, antacid, and ferrous sulfate. Clin Pharmacol Ther, 33:465, 1983

Clinical significance not established

Phenytoin
Decreased phenytoin effect with calcium-containing antacids (decreased absorption)
> VK Kulshrestha et al, Interaction between phenytoin and antacids. Br J Clin Pharmacol, 6:177, 1978; LS O'Brien et al, Failure of antacids to alter the pharmacokinetics of phenytoin. Br J Clin Pharmacol, 6:176, 1978

Give at least 2 hours apart; conflicting report

Pyrimethamine
Possible decreased pyrimethamine effect (decreased absorption)
> JC McElnay et al, In vitro experiments on chloroquine and pyrimethamine absorption in the presence of antacid constituents or kaolin. J Trop Med Hyg, 85:153, 1982

Give at least 4 hours apart

Quinidine
Possible quinidine toxicity (decreased renal excretion)
> RE Gerhardt et al, Quinidine excretion in aciduria and alkaluria. Ann Intern Med, 71:927, 1969; MB Zinn, Quinidine intoxication from alkali ingestion. Texas Med, 66:64, 1970

Monitor quinidine concentration

Quinine
Possible quinine toxicity (decreased renal excretion)
> HB Haag et al, The effect of urinary pH on the elimination of quinine in man. J Pharmacol Exp Ther, 79:136, 1943

(continued)

ANTACIDS, with: *(continued)*
Avoid concurrent use

Risedronate
Decreased risedronate effect (decreased absorption)
> Manufacturer's package insert (risedronate)

Antacids should be taken at a different time of the day

Sodium polystyrene sulfonate
Metabolic alkalosis (prevents neutralization of bicarbonate)
> PC Fernandez and PJ Kovnat, Metabolic acidosis reversed by the combination of magnesium hydroxide and a cation-exchange resin. N Engl J Med, 286:23, 1972; ET Schroeder, Alkalosis resulting from combined administration of a 'non-systemic' antacid and a cation-exchange resin. Gastroenterology, 56:868, 1969

Give sodium polystyrene sulfonate as an enema

Sympathomimetic amines
Pseudoephedrine toxicity (decreased renal excretion due to alkaline urine)
> RG Kuntzman et al, The influence of urinary pH on the plasma half-life of pseudoephedrine in man and dog and a sensitive assay for its determination in human plasma. Clin Pharmacol Ther, 12:62, 1971; DC Brater et al, Renal excretion of pseudoephedrine. Clin Pharmacol Ther, 28:690, 1980

Single report (1980)

Tetracyclines
Decreased oral tetracycline effect (decreased absorption)
> WH Barr et al, Decrease of tetracycline absorption in man by sodium bicarbonate. Clin Pharmacol Ther, 12:779, 1971; M Garty and A Hurwitz, Effect of cimetidine and antacids on gastrointestinal absorption of tetracycline. Clin Pharmacol Ther, 28:203, 1980

Avoid concurrent use or give at least 3 hours apart

Possible decreased IV doxycycline effect with oral aluminum hydroxide gel (mechanism not established)
> VX Nguyen et al, Effect of oral antacid administration on the pharmacokinetics of intravenous doxycycline. Antimicrob Agents Chemother, 33:434, 1989

Based on study in 6 healthy men; avoid concurrent use

Theophyllines
Possible theophylline toxicity with some long-acting preparations (increased absorption)
> KI Myhre and RA Walstad, The influence of antacid on the absorption of two different sustained-release formulations of theophylline. Br J Clin Pharmacol, 15:683, 1983

Monitor theophylline concentration; effect on Theo-Dur may not be clinically significant

Thiazide diuretics
Possible hypercalcemia with calcium antacids (decreased renal excretion)
> R Hakim et al, Severe hypercalcemia associated with hydrochlorothiazide and calcium carbonate therapy. Can Med Assoc J, 121:591, 1979; ML Gora

ANTACIDS, with: *(continued)*
> et al, Milk-alkali syndrome associated with use of chlorothiazide and calcium carbonate. Clin Pharm, 8:227, 1989

Two case reports (1979,1989); monitor serum calcium concentration

Thyroid hormones
Possible decreased levothyroxine effect with aluminum hydroxide, magnesium hydroxide, or calcium carbonate (decreased absorption)
> AD Sperber and Y Liel, Evidence for interference with the intestinal absorption of levothyroxine sodium by aluminum hydroxide. Arch Intern Med, 152:183, 1992; CR Schneyer, Calcium carbonate and reduction of levothyroxine efficacy. JAMA, 279:750, 1998; H Mersebach et al, Intestinal adsorption of levothyroxine by antacids and laxatives: case stories and *in vitro* experiments. Pharmacol Toxicol, 84:107, 1999; LE Butner et al, Calcium carbonate-induced hypothroidism. Ann Intern Med, 132:595, 2000; N Singh et al, Effect of calcium carbonate on the absorption of levothyroxine. JAMA, 283:2822, 2000; LE Butner et al, Calcium carbonate – induced hypothyroidism. Ann Intern Med, 132:595, 2000

Based on several case reports and study in 20 patients; monitor T4 or TSH concentration; give thyroxine 2 hours before or 4 to 6 hours after antacids

Ticlopidine
Possible decreased ticlopidine effect (decreased absorption)
> J Shah et al, Effect of food and antacid on absorption of orally administered ticlopidine hydrochloride. J Clin Pharmacol, 30:733, 1990

Monitor clinical effect or concentration of ticlopidine; based on study in 12 healthy men

Tiludronate
Decreased tiludronate effect with antacids containing calcium, aluminum or magnesium (decreased absorption)
> Manufacturer's package insert

The manufacturer recommends taking tiludronate 2 hours before or 2 hours after calcium-containing products, and 2 hours before aluminum- or magnesium-containing products

Ursodiol
Possible decreased ursodiol effect with aluminum antacids (decreased absorption)
> Manufacturer's package insert

Use alternative antacid

Valproate
Increased valproate concentration (increased absorption)
> CA May et al, Effects of three antacids on the bioavailability of valproic acid. Clin Pharm, 1:244, 1982

Clinical significance not established; give at least one hour apart

Vitamin C
Possible aluminum toxicity (possibly increased absorption)
> JL Domingo et al, Effect of ascorbic acid on gastrointestinal aluminum absorption. Lancet, 338:1467, 1991

(continued)

ANTACIDS, with: *(continued)*
> *Based on study in healthy volunteers*

Vitamin D
Possible bone toxicity with aluminum compounds (increased deposition of aluminum in bone, possibly due to increased absorption)
> G Colussi et al, Vitamin D treatment: a hidden risk factor for aluminum bone toxicity? Nephron, 47:78, 1987

Clinical significance not established

Anthralin, no documented interactions, see page 4, Criteria for Listing Interactions

ANTICHOLINERGICS, with:

Amantadine - See Amantadine with Anticholinergics, page 27

Antidepressants, tricyclic
Paralytic ileus and hyperthermia with benztropine (additive anticholinergic effects)
> Manufacturer's package insert

Monitor clinical status

Antihistamines, H_2-blockers
Decreased cimetidine effect with high doses of propantheline (decreased absorption)
> J Kanto et al, The effect of metoclopramide and propantheline on the gastrointestinal absorption of cimetidine. Br J Clin Pharmacol, 11:629, 1981

Avoid high doses of anticholinergics

Possible ranitidine toxicity with propantheline (increased absorption)
> KH Donn et al, The effects of antacid and propantheline on the absorption of oral ranitidine. Pharmacotherapy, 4:89, 1984

Clinical significance not established

Arbutamine
Possible interference with interpretation of arbutamine heart rate response with atropine (antagonism)
> Manufacturer's package insert

Avoid concurrent use of arbutamine with atropine or other anticholinergic drugs

Digoxin
Possible digoxin toxicity with propantheline (increased absorption)
> DD Brown et al, A steady-state evaluation of the effects of propantheline bromide and cholestyramine on the bioavailability of digoxin when administered as tablets or capsules. J Clin Pharmacol, 25:360, 1985

Monitor digoxin concentration; digoxin capsules affected less than tablets

Haloperidol
Decreased haloperidol effect with procyclidine (mechanism not established)
> JS Bamrah et al, Interactions between procyclidine and neuroleptic drugs; some pharmacological and clinical aspects. Br J Psychiatry, 149:726, 1986

Monitor haloperidol effect and, if necessary, concentration

Levodopa
Decreased levodopa effect (decreased absorption)
> M Contin et al, Combined levodopa-anticholinergic therapy in the

ANTICHOLINERGICS, with: *(continued)*
> treatment of Parkinson's disease; effect on levodopa bioavailability. Clin Neuropharmacol, 14:148, 1991

Monitor clinical status

Lithium

Nausea and vomiting with trihexyphenidyl (mechanism not established)
> CM Swartz and KJ Breen, Nausea from taking both lithium and trihexyphenidyl. Am J Psychiatry, 145:767, 1988

Avoid concurrent use; lithium citrate might be better tolerated if the effect is due to impaired emptying and prolonged mucosal contact with the drug

Phenothiazines

Paralytic ileus and hyperthermia with benztropine (additive anticholinergic effects)
> Manufacturer's package insert

Monitor clinical status

Decreased procyclidine effect (mechanism not established)
> JS Bamrah et al, Interactions between procyclidine and neuroleptic drugs; some pharmacological and clinical aspects. Br J Psychiatry, 149:726, 1986

Monitor phenothiazine effect and, if necessary, concentration

Selective serotonin reuptake inhibitors (SSRIs)

Delirium with benztropine and sertraline or paroxetine (mechanism not established)
> MJ Byerly et al, Delirium associated with a combination of sertraline, haloperidol, and benztropine. Am J Psychiatry, 153:965, 1996; SC Armstrong and SM Schweitzer, Delirium associated with paroxetine and benztropine combination. Am J Psychiatry, 154:581, 1997

Two case reports (1996 sertraline; 1997 paroxetine)

Sympathomimetic amines

Tachyarrhythmia with ritodrine and either atropine or glycopyrrolate (autonomic imbalance)
> JI Simpson and JP Giffin, A Glycopyrrolate-ritodrine drug-drug interaction. Can J Anaesth, 35:187, 1988; S Sheybany et al, Ritodrine in the management of fetal distress. Br J Obstet Gynaecol, 89:723, 1982

Avoid concurrent use

Trazodone

Urinary retention with isopropamide iodide (additive anticholinergic effects)
> CH Chan and RJ Ruskiewicz, Anticholinergic side effects of trazodone combined with another pharmacologic agent. Am J Psychiatry, 147:533, 1990

Single case report in a 69-year-old woman (1990)

ANTICHOLINESTERASES, with:

Beta-adrenergic blockers

Prolonged bradycardia and hypotension with atenolol or nadolol and neostigmine (sympathetic blockade); may also occur with physostigmine
> DC Seidl and DE Martin, Prolonged bradycardia after neostigmine administration in a patient taking nadolol. Anesth Analg, 63:365, 1984; DH Sprague, Severe bradycardia after neostigmine in a patient taking propranolol to

(continued)

ANTICHOLINESTERASES, with: *(continued)*
>control paroxysmal atrial tachycardia. Anesthesiology, 42:208, 1975; A Baraka and A Dajani, Severe bradycardia following physostigmine in the presence of beta-adrenergic blockade. Middle East J Anesthesiol, 7:291, 1984; J Eldor, Bradycardia after neostigmine in a patient receiving atenolol. Anaesthesia, 44:936, 1989

Multiple case reports; concurrent use should be avoided, if possible; shorter-acting beta-blockers such as propranolol and especially esmolol may cause a less severe reaction

Verapamil
Failure of neostigmine to reverse neuromuscular blockade (probably failure of acetylcholine secretion)
>JF van Poorten et al, Verapamil and reversal of vecuronium neuromuscular blockade. Anesth Analg, 63:155, 1984

Single case report (1984); decreased dosage of neuromuscular blocking agent may be indicated

ANTICOAGULANTS, ORAL, with:
Acarbose - See Acarbose with Anticoagulants, Oral, page 6
Acetaminophen - See Acetaminophen with Anticoagulants, oral, page 7
Alcohol - See Alcohol with Anticoagulants, oral, page 12
Allopurinol - See Allopurinol with Anticoagulants, oral, page 25
Aminoglutethimide - See Aminoglutethimide with Anticoagulants, oral, page 29
Amiodarone - See Amiodarone with Anticoagulants, oral, page 33
Amprenavir - See Amprenavir with Anticoagulants, oral, page 38
Anabolic and androgenic steroids - See Anabolic and androgenic steroids with Anticoagulants, oral, page 40

Antidepressants, tricyclic
Possible increased phenprocoumon effect with amitriptyline (mechanism not established)
>H Hampel et al, Modified anticoagulant potency of phenprocoumon during tricyclic antidepressant treatment: a potential drug-drug interaction. Pharmacopsychiatry, 28:183, 1995; H Hampel et al, Unstable anticoagulation in the course of amitriptyline treatment. Pharmacopsychiatry, 29:33, 1996

Based on observations in 4 patients, and a retrospective review of 7 patients; warfarin metabolized differently and may not interact

Antifungals, Griseofulvin
Decreased anticoagulant effect (mechanism not established)
>K Okino and RT Weibert, Warfarin-griseofulvin interaction. Drug Intell Clin Pharm, 20:291, 1986

Monitor prothrombin time

Antifungals, imidazoles and triazoles
Increased anticoagulant effect with fluconazole and ketoconazole (mechanism not established; probably decreased metabolism with fluconazole; CYP2C9)
>AG Smith, Potentiation of oral anticoagulants by ketoconazole. Br Med J, 288:188, 1984; LL Crussell-Porter et al, Low-dose fluconazole therapy potentiates the hypoprothrombinemic response of warfarin sodium. Arch Intern Med, 153:102, 1993; TL Seaton et al, Possible potentiation of warfarin by

ANTICOAGULANTS, ORAL, with: *(continued)*
>fluconazole. DICP, 24:1177, 1990; HD Kerr, Case report: Potentiation of warfarin by fluconazole. Am J Med Sci, 305:164, 1993; AM Baciewicz et al, Fluconazole-warfarin interaction. Ann Pharmacother, 28:1111, 1994; KW Ellis et al, Immediate potentiation of the hypoprothrombinemic response of warfarin by fluconazole. Infect Dis Clin Prac, 8:351, 1999

Effect more consistent with fluconazole than with ketoconazole or itraconazole; monitor INR/prothrombin time

Increased anticoagulant effect of warfarin or acenocoumarol with miconazole (decreased metabolism)
>RA O'Reilly et al, Mechanisms of the stereoselective interaction between miconazole and racemic warfarin in human subjects. Clin Pharmacol Ther, 51:656, 1992; P Pillans and DJ Woods, Interaction between miconazole oral gel and warfarin. NZ Med J, 109:346, 1996; S Ariyaratnam et al, Potentiation of warfarin anticoagulant activity by miconazole oral gel. BMJ, 314:349, 1997; M Ortín et al, Miconazole oral gel enhances acenocoumarol anticoagulant activity: a report of three cases. Ann Pharmacother, 33:175, 1999; M Marco and AJ Guy, Retroperitoneal haematoma and small bowel intramural haematoma caused by warfarin and miconazole interaction. Int J Oral Maxillofac Surg, 27:485, 1997; D Lansdorp et al, Potentiation of acenocoumarol during vaginal administration of miconazole. Br J Clin Pharmacol, 47:225, 1999; DJG Thirion and LAF Zanetti, Potentiation of warfarin's hypoprothrombinemic effect with miconazole vaginal suppositories. Pharmacotherapy, 20:98, 2000; M Silingardi et al, Miconazole oral gel potentiates warfarin anticoagulant activity. Thromb Haemost, 83:794, 2000

Monitor prothrombin time; numerous case reports with miconazole oral gel; three case reports with vaginal miconazole (1999, 2000)

Antifungals, terbinafine
Both warfarin toxicity (bleeding) and decreased warfarin effect reported with terbinafine (mechanism not established)
>JA Warwick and RJ Corrall, Serious interaction between warfarin and oral terbinafine. BMJ, 316:440, 1998; AK Gupta and CS Ross, Interaction between terbinafine and warfarin. Dermatology, 196:266, 1998; M Guerret et al, Evaluation of effects of terbinafine on single oral dose pharmacokinetics and anticoagulant actions of warfarin in healthy volunteers. Pharmacotherapy, 17:767, 1997; J Gantmacher et al and JA Warwick et al, Interaction between warfarin and oral terbinafine. BMJ, 317:205, 1998

Conflicting reports; monitor prothrombin time

Antihistamines, H$_2$-blockers
Increased anticoagulant effect (decreased metabolism)
>I Niopas et al, Further insight into the stereoselective interaction between warfarin and cimetidine in man. Br J Clin Pharmacol, 32:508, 1991; AM Baciewicz and PJ Morgan, Ranitidine-warfarin interaction. Ann Intern Med, 112:76, 1990; AF Shinn, Unrecognized drug interaction with famotidine and nizatidine. Arch Intern Med, 151:814, 1991; J Harenberg et al, Cimetidine

(continued)

ANTICOAGULANTS, ORAL, with: *(continued)*

does not increase the anticoagulant effect of phenprocoumon. Br J Clin Pharmacol, 14:292, 1982; I Niopas et al, The effect of cimetidine on the steady-state pharmacokinetics and pharmacodynamics of warfarin in humans. Eur J Clin Pharmacol, 55:399, 1999

Monitor prothrombin time; effect small in most patients; no interaction with phenprocoumon; more often with cimetidine; case reports with nizatidine and famotidine (1991) probably rare with ranitidine except at high dosage

Azathioprine

Possible decreased anticoagulant effect of warfarin (mechanism not established)

JD Singleton and L Conyers, Warfarin and azathioprine: an important drug interaction. Am J Med, 92:217, 1992

Single case report (1992); monitor prothrombin time

Barbiturates

Decreased anticoagulant effect (increased metabolism)

M Orme, Enantiomers of warfarin and phenobarbital. N Engl J Med, 295:1482, 1976; RA O'Reilly, Reply; MG MacDonald and DS Robinson, Clinical observations of possible barbiturate interference with anticoagulation. JAMA, 204:97, 1968

Avoid barbiturate hypnotics; stable anticoagulant dose can be established for epileptics on maintenance barbiturates

Beta-adrenergic blockers

Possible increased warfarin effect with propranolol; possible increased phenprocoumon effect with metoprolol (mechanism not established)

AK Scott et al, Interaction between warfarin and propranolol. Br J Clin Pharmacol, 17:559, 1984; H Spahn et al, Pharmacokinetic and pharmacodynamic interactions between phenprocoumon and atenolol or metoprolol. Br J Clin Pharmacol, 17:97S, 1984; SJ Warrington et al, Bisoprolol: studies of potential interactions with theophylline and warfarin in healthy volunteers. J Cardiovasc Pharmacol, 16 suppl 5:S164, 1990

Prothrombin time did not change; clinical significance not established; bisoprolol may not interact

Carbamazepine

Decreased anticoagulant effect (increased metabolism)

JM Hansen et al, Carbamazepine-induced acceleration of diphenylhydantoin and warfarin metabolism in man. Clin Pharmacol Ther, 12:539, 1971; EW Massey, Effect of carbamazepine on coumadin metabolism. Ann Neurol, 13:691, 1983; CE Denbow and HS Fraser, Clinically significant hemorrhage due to warfarin-carbamazepine interaction. South Med J, 83:981, 1990; T Böttcher et al, Carbamazepine-phenprocoumon interaction. Eur Neurol, 38:132, 1997; R Schlienger et al, Inhibition of phenprocoumon anticoagulation by carbamazepine. Eur Neuropsychopharmacol, 10:219, 2000

ANTICOAGULANTS, ORAL, with: *(continued)*
> Monitor prothrombin time; hemorrhage reported in one patient on warfarin after carbamazepine withdrawal (1990); two case reports of decreased phenprocoumon effect (1997; 2000)

Cephalosporins
> Possible anticoagulant effect with moxalactam, cefamandole, cefonicid, cefoperazone, cefotetan or cefmetazole (mechanism not established)
>> Anonymous, Moxalactam boxed warning about bleeding problems. FDA Drug Bull, 13:16, 1983; manufacturer's package insert; HR Freedy, Jr et al, Cefoperazone-induced coagulopathy. Drug Intell Clin Pharm, 20:281, 1986; W Rymer et al, Hypoprothrombinemia associated with cefamandole. Drug Intell Clin Pharm, 14:780, 1980; A Conjura et al, Cefotetan and hypoprothrombinemia. Ann Intern Med, 108:643, 1988; MP Garcia et al, Potenciación del efecto anticoagulante del acenocumarol por cefonicid. Revista Clinica Espanola, 199:620, 1999
>
> *Avoid concurrent use; also occurs with more than 20,000 U/day of heparin and moxalactam*

Chloral hydrate
> Increased anticoagulant effect (displacement from binding)
>> Boston Collaborative Drug Surveillance Program, Interaction between chloral hydrate and warfarin. N Engl J Med, 286:53, 1972; SA Cucinell et al, The effect of chloral hydrate on bishydroxycoumarin metabolism. JAMA, 197:366, 1966
>
> *Avoid concurrent use*

Chloramphenicol
> Increased dicumarol and probably warfarin effect (decreased metabolism; CYP2C9)
>> LK Christensen and L Skovsted, Inhibition of drug metabolism by chloramphenicol. Lancet, 2:1397, 1969; R Leone et al, Potential interaction between warfarin and ocular chloramphenicol. Ann Pharmacother, 33:114, 1999
>
> *Monitor prothrombin time if chloramphenicol must be used; single case report with ocular chloramphenicol and warfarin (1999)*

Cholestyramine
> Decreased anticoagulant effect (binding of drug in intestine)
>> E Jahnchen et al, Enhanced elimination of warfarin during treatment with cholestyramine. Br J Clin Pharmacol, 5:437, 1978
>
> *Avoid concurrent use, if possible, or give 6 hours apart and monitor prothrombin time*

Cisapride
> Increased anticoagulant effect (mechanism not established)
>> Manufacturer's package insert; MR Darlington, Hypoprothrombinemia induced by warfarin sodium and cisapride. Am J Health Syst Pharm, 54:320, 1997
>
> *Single case report (1997); monitor prothrombin time; cisapride is no longer marketed in the USA*

(continued)

ANTICOAGULANTS, ORAL, with: *(continued)*
  Clofibrate
    Increased anticoagulant effect (displacement from binding)
      RB Solomon and F Rosner, Massive hemorrhage and death during treatment with clofibrate and warfarin. NY State J Med, 73:2002, 1973; TD Bjornsson et al, Clofibrate displaces warfarin from plasma proteins in man: an example of a pure displacement interaction. J Pharmacol Exp Ther, 210:316, 1979
    Reduce anticoagulant dosage and monitor prothrombin time
  Clopidogrel
    Increased bleeding risk (additive)
      Manufacturer's package insert
    Theoretical; monitor clinical status and stool for occult blood
  Contraceptives, oral
    Decreased anticoagulant effect (increased factor VII and X; prothrombin may decrease, glucuronidation of phenprocoumon increases)
      E de Teresa et al, Interaction between anticoagulants and contraceptives: an unsuspected finding. Br Med J, 2:1260, 1979; H Mönig et al, Effect of oral contraceptive steroids on the pharmacokinetics of phenprocoumon. Br J Clin Pharmacol, 30:115, 1990
    Use alternative contraceptive
  Corticosteroids
    Possible increased bleeding risk with methylprednisolone and warfarin (mechanism not established)
      M Kaufman, Treatment of multiple sclerosis with high-dose corticosteroids may prolong the prothrombin time to dangerous levels in patients taking warfarin. Mult Scler, 3:248, 1997
    Two patients with multiple sclerosis taking high doses of methylprednisolone (1997); monitor prothrombin time
  COX-2 inhibitors
    Increased bleeding risk with warfarin (possibly decreased metabolism)
      Medical Letter, 41:59, 1999; TL Mersfelder and LR Stewart, Warfarin and celecoxib interaction. Ann Pharmacother, 34:325, 2000; A Karim et al, Celecoxib does not significantly alter the pharmacokinetics or hypoprothrombinemic effect of warfarin in healthy subjects. J Clin Pharmacol, 40:655, 2000
    Monitor prothrombin time; the effect appears to be small in most people; study in healthy sujects suggests that celecoxib does not affect the pharmacokinetics or hypoprothrombinemic response of warfarin
  Cyclosporine
    Decreased effects of both cyclosporine and warfarin (mechanism not established)
      DS Snyder, Interaction between cyclosporine and warfarin. Ann Intern Med, 108:311, 1988
    Single case report (1988)

ANTICOAGULANTS, ORAL, with: *(continued)*
    Increased acenocoumarol effect (mechanism not established)
        JM Campistol et al, Interaction between ciclosporin A and Sintrom. Nephron, 53:291, 1989
    Single case report (1989)

Dextrothyroxine
    Increased anticoagulant effect (mechanism not established)
        JJ Schrogie and HM Solomon, The anticoagulant response to bis-hydroxycoumarin. II The effect of D-thyroxine, clofibrate and norethandrolone. Clin Pharmacol Ther, 8:70, 1967; JC Owens et al, Effect of sodium dextrothyroxine in patients receiving anticoagulants. N Engl J Med, 266:76, 1962; HM Solomon and JJ Schrogie, Change in receptor site affinity: a proposed explanation for the potentiating effect of dextro-thyroxine on the anticoagulant response to warfarin. Clin Pharmacol Ther, 8:797, 1967
    Decrease anticoagulant dosage and monitor prothrombin time

Diazoxide
    Increased anticoagulant effect with IV diazoxide (possibly displacement from binding)
        EM Sellers and J Koch-Weser, Displacement of warfarin from human albumin by diazoxide and ethacrynic, mefenamic, and nalidixic acids. Clin Pharmacol Ther, 11:524, 1970
    Based on in vitro studies; monitor prothrombin time

Digoxin immune Fab
    Increased warfarin effect (mechanism not established)
        DB Hill, Drug interaction between digoxin immune Fab (Digibind) and warfarin. South Med J, 83:2S-31, 1990
    Single case report (1990)

Dipyridamole
    Possible bleeding (inhibition of platelet function)
        S Kalowski and P Kincaid-Smith, Interaction of dipyridamole with anticoagulants in the treatment of glomerulonephritis. Med J Aust, 2:164, 1973
    Avoid concurrent use, if possible

Disopyramide
    Increased anticoagulant effect (decreased metabolism)
        E Haworth and AK Burroughs, Disopyramide and warfarin interaction. Br Med J, 2:866, 1977
    Conflicting reports; avoid concurrent use, if possible

Disulfiram
    Increased anticoagulant effect (decreased metabolism)
        RA O'Reilly, Interaction of sodium warfarin and disulfiram (Antabuse) in man. Ann Intern Med, 78:73, 1973; E Rothstein, Warfarin effect enhanced by disulfiram (Antabuse). JAMA, 221:1052, 1972
    Avoid concurrent use, if possible

Dong Quai
    Possible increased bleeding risk (mechanism not established)
        RL Page II and JD Lawrence, Potentiation of warfarin by dong quai. Pharmacotherapy, 19:870, 1999; GR Ellis and MR Stephens, Chinese herbal

(continued)

ANTICOAGULANTS, ORAL, with: *(continued)*
remedy for menopausal symptoms. BMJ, 319:650, 1999
Two case reports of increased hypoprothrombinemic response to warfarin (1999); avoid concurrent use or monitor anticoagulation status carefully

Efavirenz
Possible decrease or increase in warfarin effect (enzyme induction or inhibition)
Manufacturer's package insert (efavirenz)
Monitor prothrombin time; theoretical

Ethacrynic acid
Increased anticoagulant effect (displacement from binding)
RJ Petrick et al, Interaction between warfarin and ethacrynic acid. JAMA, 231:843, 1975
Probably rare; monitor prothrombin time

Etoposide
Increased anticoagulant effect (possibly displacement from binding)
K Ward and JD Bitran, Warfarin, etoposide, and vindesine interactions. Cancer Treat Rep, 68:817, 1984
Monitor prothrombin time; case report in one patient also taking vindesine (1984)

Etretinate
Decreased anticoagulant effect of warfarin (mechanism not established)
LS Ostlere et al, Reduced therapeutic effect of warfarin caused by etretinate. Br J Dermatol, 124:505, 1991
Monitor prothrombin time; single case report (1991)

Felbamate
Increased anticoagulant effect with warfarin (decreased metabolism)
KA Tisdel et al, Warfarin-felbamate interaction: first report. Ann Pharmacother, 28:805, 1994
Single case report (1994); effect possibly due to withdrawal of phenobarbital and carbamazepine at the same time that felbamate was started

Fenofibrate
Increased anticoagulant effect with warfarin (mechanism not established)
KJ Ascah et al, Interaction between fenofibrate and warfarin. Ann Pharmacother, 32:765, 1998
Two well documented case reports (1998); monitor prothrombin time

Fluoroquinolones
Increased anticoagulant effect with ciprofloxacin, levofloxacin, norfloxacin, or ofloxacin; enoxacin, sparfloxacin, grepafloxacin, trovafloxacin and temafloxacin may not interact (mechanism not established)
AD McLeod and C Burgess, Drug interaction between warfarin and enoxacin. N Z Med J, 101:216, 1988; AK Kamada, Possible interaction between ciprofloxacin and warfarin. DICP, 24:27, 1990; ML Rocci, Jr et al, Norfloxacin does not alter warfarin's disposition or anticoagulant effect. J Clin Pharmacol, 30:728, 1990; JP Rindone et al, Hypoprothrombinemic effect of warfarin not influenced by ciprofloxacin. Clin Pharm, 10:136, 1991; E Millar et al, Temafloxacin does not potentiate the anticoagulant effect of warfarin in healthy subjects. Clin Pharmacokinet, 22 suppl 1:102, 1992; TM

ANTICOAGULANTS, ORAL, with: *(continued)*

Bianco et al, Potential warfarin-ciprofloxacin interaction in patients receiving long-term anticoagulation. Pharmacotherapy, 12:435, 1992; AM Baciewicz et al, Interaction of ofloxacin and warfarin. Ann Intern Med, 119:1223, 1993; RE Polk et al, Effect of ciprofloxacin on response to warfarin in anticoagulated adults. 34th Intersci Confer Antimicrob Agents Chemother, page 3, 1994; FE Mott et al, Ciprofloxacin and warfarin. Ann Intern Med, 111:542, 1989; S Liao et al, Absence of an effect of levofloxacin on warfarin pharmacokinetics and anticoagulation in male volunteers. J Clin Pharmacol, 36:1072, 1996; C Efthymiopoulos et al, Theophylline and warfarin interaction studies with grepafloxacin. Clin Pharmacokinet, 33:39, 1997; manufacturer's package insert; BK Brown, Warfarin and levofloxacin: report of a potential drug-drug interaction. ASHP Midyear Clinical Meeting, 34:P-431E, 1999; RJ Ellis et al, Ciprofloxacin-warfarin coagulopathy: a case series. Am J Hematol, 63:28, 2000

Monitor prothrombin time; 4 reports of hemorrhage (1989, 1991, 2000); appears to be large patient variability in the effect of norfloxacin and ciprofloxacin on anticoagulants; single case report with levofloxacin (1999); 66 cases reported to FDA (through 1997) but causal relationship difficult to evaluate in such cases

Fluorouracil

Increased anticoagulant effect with warfarin (mechanism not established)

RT Chlebowski et al, Clinical and pharmacokinetic effects of combined warfarin and 5-fluorouracil in advanced colon cancer. Cancer Res, 42:4827, 1982; T Wajima and P Mukhopadhyay, Possible interactions between warfarin and 5-fluorouracil. Am J Hematol, 40:238, 1992; MA Scarfe and MK Israel, Possible drug interaction between warfarin and combination of levamisole and fluorouracil. Ann Pharmacother, 28:464, 1994; MC Brown, Multisite mucous membrane bleeding due to a possible interaction between warfarin and 5-fluorouracil. Pharmacotherapy, 17:631, 1997; MC Brown, Interaction between warfarin and 5-fluorouracil, not between warfarin and levamisole. Clin Pharmacol Ther, 64:233, 1998; manufacturer's package insert (capecitabine); MC Brown, An adverse interaction between warfarin and 5-fluorouracil: a case report and review of the literature. Chemotherapy, 45:392, 1999; JM Kolesar et al, Warfarin–5-FU interaction—A consecutive case series. Pharmacotherapy, 19:1445, 1999; Z Aki et al, A patient with a prolonged prothrombin time due to an adverse interaction between 5-fluorouracil and warfarin. Am J Gastroenterol, 94:1093, 2000

Six case reports (1992, 1994, 1997, 1998, 1999 and 2000) in patients with colon, gastric, and lung cancer; five patients from a single institution developed increased INR (1999); previous study in 25 patients with colon cancer did not reveal interaction

Flutamide

Increased anticoagulant effect (mechanism not established)

Manufacturer's package insert

Monitor prothrombin time

(continued)

ANTICOAGULANTS, ORAL, with: *(continued)*
  Gemcitabine
    Possible increased warfarin effect (mechanism not established)
      SA Kinikar and JM Kolesar, Identification of a gemcitabine-warfarin interaction. Pharmacotherapy, 19:1331, 1999
    Single case report (1999); INR increase was modest; monitor anticoagulant response
  Gemfibrozil
    Increased warfarin effect (mechanism not established)
      S Ahmad, Gemfibrozil interaction with warfarin sodium (Coumadin). Chest, 98:1041, 1990; JP Rindone and H-C Keng, Gemfibrozil-warfarin drug interaction resulting in profound hypoprothrombinemia. Chest, 114:641, 1998
    Two case reports (1990, 1998)
  Ginkgo biloba
    Possible increased risk of hemorrhage (mechanism not established)
      M Rosenblatt and J Mindel, Spontaneous hyphema associated with ingestion of *Ginkgo biloba* extract. N Engl J Med, 336:1108, 1997; MK Matthews, Jr, Association of *Ginkgo biloba* with intracerebral hemorrhage. Neurology, 50:1933, 1998
    Case reports of ocular and cerebral hemorrhage; avoid concurrent use
  Ginseng
    Possible decreased warfarin effect (mechanism not established)
      K Janetzky and AP Morreale, Probable interaction between warfarin and ginseng. Am J Health Syst Pharm, 54:692, 1997
    Single case report (1997); causal relationship not established; monitor INR/prothrombin time and clinical status
  Glutethimide
    Decreased anticoagulant effect (increased metabolism)
      JA Udall, Clinical implications of warfarin interactions with five sedatives. Am J Cardiol, 35:67, 1975
    Use benzodiazepine hypnotic
  Grapefruit juice
    Possible increased anticoagulant effect with warfarin (mechanism not established)
      WR Bartle, Grapefruit juice might still be factor in warfarin response. Am J Health Syst Pharm, 56:676, 1999
    Single case report (1999); no effect seen in previous report of 10 patients on warfarin
  Green tea
    Possible decreased warfarin effect (antagonism)
      JR Taylor and VM Wilt, Probable antagonism of warfarin by green tea. Ann Pharmacother, 33:426, 1999
    Single case report (1999); green tea has a significant amount of vitamin K; limit green tea intake and monitor INR

ANTICOAGULANTS, ORAL, with: *(continued)*
HMG-CoA reductase inhibitors
Bleeding and increased hypoprothrombinemia with lovastatin and warfarin; possible increased anticoagulant effect with simvastatin or fluvastatin; atorvastatin and cerivastatin have minimal effect (decreased metabolism)

    S Ahmad, Lovastatin; warfarin interaction. Arch Intern Med, 150:2407, 1990; HS Hoffman, The interaction of lovastatin and warfarin. Conn Med, 56:107, 1992; E Grau et al, Simvastatin-oral anticoagulant interaction. Lancet, 347:405, 1996; A Keech et al, Three-year follow-up of the Oxford Cholesterol Study: assessment of the efficacy and safety of simvastatin in preparation for a large mortality study. Eur Heart J, 15:255, 1994; A Compton, Prolonged bleeding due to lovastatin-warfarin coadministration. J Pharm Prac, 8:5, 1995; LE Trilli et al, Potential interaction between warfarin and fluvastatin. Ann Pharmacother, 30:1399, 1996; R Stern et al, Atorvastatin does not alter the anticoagulant activity of warfarin. J Clin Pharmacol, 37:1062, 1997; manufacturer's package insert

Three case reports of bleeding (1990, 1995) and one case report of increased hypoprothrombinemia (1992) with lovastatin; three case reports with fluvastatin (1996); single case report and clinical study with simvastatin (1996); atorvastatin had minimal effects on warfarin in 12 patients; minimal effect with cerivastatin; monitor prothrombin time

Possible increased risk of rhabdomyolysis with simvastatin and warfarin (mechanism not established)

    A Mogyorósi et al, Rhabdomyolysis and acute renal failure due to combination therapy with simvastatin and warfarin. J Intern Med, 246:599, 1999

Single case report (1999); causal relationship not established; monitor clinical status

Hypoglycemics, sulfonylurea
Increased hypoglycemic effect with dicumarol (decreased metabolism)

    HM Solomon and JJ Schrogie, Effect of phenyramidol and bishydroxycoumarin on the metabolism of tolbutamide in human subjects. Metabolism, 16:1029, 1967; M Kristensen and JM Hansen, Accumulation of chlorpropamide caused by dicumarol. Acta Med Scand, 183:83, 1968; J Judis, Displacement of sulfonylureas from human serum proteins by coumarin derivatives and cortical steroids. J Pharm Sci, 62:232, 1973

Monitor blood glucose

Bruising and hematomas with warfarin (mechanism not established)

    SV Jassal, Letter, BMJ, 303:789, 1991

Monitor prothrombin time; single case report (1991)

Ifosfamide
Increased warfarin effect with ifosfamide and mesna (mechanism not established)

    G Hall et al, Intravenous infusions of ifosfamide/mesna and perturbation of warfarin anticoagulant control. Postgrad Med J, 66:860, 1990

Three case reports; patients received multiple drugs; monitor prothrombin time

(continued)

ANTICOAGULANTS, ORAL, with: *(continued)*

Indinavir
Possible decreased warfarin effect (possible increased metabolism)
> G Gatti et al, Influence of indinavir and ritonavir on warfarin anticoagulant activity. AIDS, 12:825, 1998

Single case report (1998); monitor prothrombin time

Influenza vaccine
Increased anticoagulant effect (possibly decreased metabolism)
> P Kramer et al, Effect of influenza vaccine on warfarin anticoagulation. Clin Pharmacol Ther, 35:416, 1984; JC Souto et al, Lack of effect of influenza vaccine on anticoagulation by acenocoumarol. Ann Pharmacother, 27:365, 1993

Conflicting reports; appears to be rare if it occurs at all

Interferon
Possible increased anticoagulant effect (probably decreased metabolism)
> Y Adachi et al, Potentiation of warfarin by interferon. BMJ, 311:292, 1995

Based on single case report (1995)

Isoniazid
Possible anticoagulant effect (decreased metabolism)
> AR Rosenthal et al, Interaction of isoniazid and warfarin. JAMA, 238:2177, 1977

Based on single case report (1977) and animal studies; monitor prothrombin time

Levocarnitine
Increased acenocoumarol effect (mechanism not established)
> E Martinez et al, Potentiation of acenocoumarol action by L-carnitine. J Intern Med, 23:94, 1993

Single case report (1993)

Lopinavir/Ritonavir
Possible increased or decreased warfarin effect (increased or decreased metabolism)
> Manufacturer's package insert (*Kaletra*)

Monitor prothrombin time

Macrolide antibiotics
Increased anticoagulant effect with erythromycin or clarithromycin and warfarin or acenocoumarol (possibly decreased metabolism); dirithromycin may not interact with warfarin
> K Bachmann et al, The effect of erythromycin on the disposition kinetics of warfarin. Pharmacology, 28:171, 1984; E Grau et al, Erythromycin – oral anticoagulants interaction. Arch Intern Med, 146:1639, 1986; G Lane, Increased hypoprothrombinemic effect of warfarin possibly induced by azithromycin. Ann Pharmacother, 30:884, 1996; E Grau et al, Interaction between clarithromycin and oral anticoagulants. Ann Pharmacotherapy, 30:1495, 1996; VS Watkins et al, Drug interactions of macrolides: emphasis on dirithromycin. Ann Pharmacother, 31:349, 1997; B Sanchez et al, Clarithromycin-oral anticoagulants interaction: report of five cases. Clin Drug Invest, 13:220, 1997; KC Oberg, Delayed elevation of international

ANTICOAGULANTS, ORAL, with: *(continued)*
>
> normalized ratio with concurrent clarithromycin and warfarin therapy. Pharmacotherapy, 81:386, 1998; DR Foster and NL Milan, Potential interaction between azithromycin and warfarin. Pharmacotherapy, 19:902, 1999; MJ Gooderham et al, Concomitant digoxin toxicity and warfarin interaction in a patient receiving clarithromycin. Ann Pharmacother, 33:796, 1999; E Grau et al, Macrolides and oral anticoagulants: a dangerous association. Acta Haematol, 102:113, 1999
>
> *Multiple cases with erythromycin and clarithromycin; two cases with azithromycin (1996, 1999) but a causal relationship was not established; monitor INR or prothrombin time*
>
> **Mercaptopurine**
>
> Possible decreased anticoagulant effect (mechanism not established)
>> MA Fernandez et al, Acenocoumarol and 6-mercaptopurine: an important drug interaction. Haematologica, 84:664, 1999
>
> *Single case report (1999); monitor INR or prothrombin time*
>
> **Mesalamine**
>
> Decreased warfarin effect (mechanism not established)
>> MA Marinella, Mesalamine and warfarin therapy resulting in decreased warfarin effect. Ann Pharmacother, 32:841, 1998
>
> *Single case report (1998); monitor prothrombin time*
>
> **Mesna**
>
> Increased warfarin effect with ifosfamide and mesna (mechanism not established)
>> G Hall et al, Intravenous infusions of ifosfamide/mesna and perturbation of warfarin anticoagulant control. Postgrad Med J, 66:860, 1990
>
> *Three case reports; patients received multiple drugs; monitor prothrombin time (1990)*
>
> **Metronidazole**
>
> Increased anticoagulant effect (decreased metabolism)
>> RA O'Reilly, The stereoselective interaction of warfarin and metronidazole in man. N Engl J Med, 295:354, 1976
>
> *Monitor prothrombin time*
>
> **Mianserin**
>
> Decreased anticoagulant effect with acenocoumarin (mechanism not established)
>> D Baettig et al, Interaction between mianserin and acenocoumarin. Int J Clin Pharmacol Ther, 32:165, 1994
>
> *Single case report (1994); patients was also receiving amiodarone*
>
> **Mitotane**
>
> Decreased anticoagulant effect (possibly increased metabolism)
>> PG Cuddy and LS Loftus, Influence of mitotane on the hypoprothrombinemic effect of warfarin. South Med J, 79:387, 1986
>
> *Single case report (1986); monitor prothrombin time*
>
> **Moricizine**
>
> Increased anticoagulant effect with warfarin (mechanism not established)
>> MD Serpa et al, Moricizine-warfarin: a possible drug interaction. Ann

ANTICOAGULANTS, ORAL, with: *(continued)*
Pharmacother, 26:127, 1992; IH Benedek et al, Effect of moricizine on the pharmacokinetics and pharmacodynamics of warfarin in healthy volunteers. J Clin Pharmacol, 32:558, 1992

Single case report, 3 others reported to the manufacturer (1991); single dose study in healthy men showed no clinically significant interaction

Nalidixic acid
Increased anticoagulant effect (displacement from binding)
J Leor et al, Interaction between nalidixic acid and warfarin. Ann Intern Med, 107:601, 1987

Monitor prothrombin time; possibly rare

Narcotics: methadone and congeners
Increased anticoagulant effect (possibly decreased metabolism)
JL Justice and SS Kline, Analgesics and warfarin; a case that brings up questions and cautions. Postgrad Med, 83:217, 1988

Several reports with an acetaminophen-propoxyphene combination; monitor prothrombin time

Narcotics: tramadol
Bleeding into skin with warfarin (mechanism not established)
ML Scher et al, Potential interaction between tramadol and warfarin. Ann Pharmacother, 31:646, 1997; JK Boeijinga et al, Is there interaction between tramadol and phenprocoumon? Lancet, 350:1552, 1997; JK Boeijinga et al, Lack of interaction between tramadol and coumarins. J Clin Pharmacol, 38:966, 1998; JR Sabbe et al, Tramadol-warfarin interaction. Pharmacotherapy, 18:871, 1998

Case reports of hemorrhagic blisters (1997) and ecchymoses (1998) with warfarin; controlled trial in 19 patients showed no interaction with phenprocoumon

Nonsteroidal anti-inflammatory drugs
Increased bleeding risk (inhibition of platelets, ulcerogenic effect; other mechanisms)
RA O'Reilly et al, Impact of aspirin and chlorthalidone on the pharmacodynamics of oral anticoagulant drugs in man. Ann NY Acad Sci, 179:173, 1971; F Littleton, Jr, Warfarin and topical salicylates, JAMA, 263:2888, 1990; JA Beirne et al, Gastrointestinal blood loss caused by tolmetin, aspirin, and indomethacin. Clin Pharmacol Ther, 16:821, 1974; RS Rhodes et al, A warfarin-piroxicam drug interaction. Drug Intell Clin Pharm, 19:556, 1985; JF Koren et al, AC Santopolo, Tolmetin – warfarin interaction. Am J Med, 82:1278, 1987; N Win et al, Azapropazone and warfarin. BMJ, 302:969, 1991; F Michot et al, A double-blind clinical trial to determine if an interaction exists between diclofenac sodium and the oral anticoagulant acenocoumarol (nicoumalone). J Int Med Res, 3:153, 1975; TYK Chan et al, Adverse interaction between warfarin and indomethacin. Drug Saf, 10:267, 1994; R Day and D Quinn, Adverse interaction between warfarin and indomethacin. Drug Saf, 11:21, 1994; JC Ermer et al, Concomitant etodolac affects neither the unbound clearance nor the pharmacologic effect of warfarin. Clin Pharmacol Ther, 55:305, 1994; JP Loftin and ES Vesell, Interaction between sulindac and warfarin: different results in

ANTICOAGULANTS, ORAL, with: *(continued)*
>normal subjects and in an unusual patient with a potassium-losing renal tubular defect. J Clin Pharmacol, 19:733, 1979; MJ Serlin et al, Interaction between diflunisal and warfarin. Clin Pharmacol Ther, 28:493, 1980; MF Flessner and H Knight, Prolongation of prothrombin time and severe gastrointestinal bleeding associated with combined use of warfarin and ketoprofen. JAMA, 259:353, 1988; C Mieszczak and K Winther, Lack of interaction of ketoprofen with warfarin. Eur J Clin Pharmacol, 44:205, 1993; SC Fagan et al, Safety of combination aspirin and anticoagulation in acute ischemic stroke. Ann Pharmacother, 28:441, 1994; TYK Chan, Ann Pharmacother, 29:1274, 1995; M Ramanathan, Warfarin – topical salicylate interactions: case reports. Med J Malaysia, 50:278, 1995; D Türck et al, Lack of interaction between meloxicam and warfarin in healthy volunteers. Eur J Clin Pharmacol, 51:421, 1997; T Chan, Prolongation of prothrombin time with the use of indomethacin and warfarin. Br J Clin Pract, 51:177, 1997; ME Ernst and LM Buys, Reevaluating the safety of concurrent warfarin and ibuprofen therapy: a case report. J Pharm Technol, 13:244, 1997; UP Masche et al, No clinically relevant effect of lornoxicam intake on acenocoumarol pharmacokinetics and pharmacodynamics. Eur J Clin Pharmacol, 54:865, 1999; UP Masche et al, Opposite effects of lornoxicam co-administration on phenprocoumon pharmacokinetics and pharmacodynamics. Eur J Clin Pharmacol, 54:857, 1999; A Pardo et al, A placebo-controlled study of interaction between nabumetone and acenocoumarol. Br J Clin Pharmacol, 47:441, 1999; AL Gulløv et al, Bleeding during warfarin and aspirin therapy in patients with atrial fibrillation. Arch Intern Med, 159:1322, 1999; VC Dennis et al, Potentiation of oral anticoagulation and hemarthrosis associated with nabumetone. Pharmacotherapy, 20:234, 2000; JD Joss and RF LeBlond, Potentiation of warfarin anticoagulation associated with topical methyl salicylate. Ann Pharmacother, 34:729, 2000

Monitor prothrombin time and for occult blood in stool and urine; the effect of aspirin is prolonged and concurrent use should be avoided unless additive effect is desired; diclofenac, meloxicam, and naproxen may not interact; ketoprofen (100 mg b.i.d.) and etodolac (200 mg b.i.d.) did not interact with warfarin in studies in healthy men; single case report of hemorrhage in 62-year-old man taking 25 mg of ketoprofen t.i.d. (1988); three case reports of bleeding with topical methylsalicylate (1995; 2000); single case report of GI bleeding with indomethacin (1997); single case report of prolonged prothrombin time and bleeding in an elderly patient taking ibuprofen (1998); lornoxicam may not affect pharmacokinetics of acenocoumarol, but may decrease anticoagulant effect of phenprocoumon; nabumetone may not affect pharmacokinetics of acenocoumarol

Nutrients, enteral preparations
Decreased anticoagulant effect (possibly increased vitamin K content or adsorption of anticoagulant)
>AJM Watson et al, Enteral feeds may antagonise warfarin. Br Med J, 288:557, 1984; R Michaelson et al, Inhibition of the hypoprothrombinemic effect of warfarin (Coumadin) by Ensure Plus, a dietary supplement. Clin

ANTICOAGULANTS, ORAL, with: *(continued)*

Bull, 10:171, 1980; AY Dubourg, Enteral feeds may antagonise warfarin. Br Med J, 289:630, 1984; DA Petretich, Reversal of Osmolite-warfarin interaction by changing warfarin administration time. Clin Pharm, 9:93, 1990

Use a preparation with low vitamin K content; in one patient there was no interaction when warfarin was given 3 hours before Osmolite was started

Omeprazole

Increased anticoagulant effect with warfarin (decreased metabolism of R-warfarin)

T Sutfin et al, Stereoselective interaction of omeprazole with warfarin in healthy men. Ther Drug Monit, 11:176, 1989; S Ahmad, Omeprazole-warfarin interaction. South Med J, 84:674, 1991; P Unge et al, A study of the interaction of omeprazole and warfarin in anticoagulated patients. Br J Clin Pharmacol, 34:509, 1992; EM Vreeburg et al, Lack of effect of omeprazole on oral acenocoumarol anticoagulant therapy. Scand J Gastroenterol, 32:991, 1997; JNJM de Hoon et al, No effect of short-term omeprazole intake on acenocoumarol pharmacokinetics and pharmacodynamics. Br J Clin Pharmacol, 44:399, 1997

Conflicting case reports; study in 35 patients found no significant clinical effect on warfarin; acenocoumarol does not appear to interact

Penicillins

Decreased anticoagulant effect with warfarin and nafcillin or dicloxacillin (increased metabolism)

GD Qureshi et al, Warfarin resistance with nafcillin therapy. Ann Intern Med, 100:527, 1984; RL Davis et al, Warfarin-nafcillin interaction. J Pediatr, 118:300, 1991; AT Mailloux et al, Potential interaction between warfarin and dicloxacillin. Ann Pharmacother, 30:1402, 1996; T Bandrowsky et al, Amoxicillin-related postextraction bleeding in an anticoagulated patient with tranexamic acid rinses. Oral Surg Oral Med Oral Pathol Oral Radio Endod, 82:610, 1996; AM Baciewicz et al, Probable nafcillin-warfarin interaction. J Pharm Technol, 15:5, 1999

Monitor prothrombin time; might occur with other penicillins

Increased anticoagulant effect with warfarin or acenocoumarol and amoxicillin (decreased metabolism)

J Soto et al, Probable acenocoumarol-amoxycillin interaction. Acta Haematol, 90:195, 1993

Single case report with acenocoumarol (1993) and warfarin (1996)

Pentosan

Increased bleeding risk with warfarin (additive)

Manufacturer's package insert

Other oral anticoagulants may be similarly affected; monitor prothrombin time

Phenformin

Increased bleeding risk (phenformin increases fibrinolytic activity)

TJ Hamblin, Interaction between warfarin and phenformin. Lancet, 2:1323, 1971

ANTICOAGULANTS, ORAL, with: *(continued)*
  Monitor for occult blood in stool and urine
 Phenylbutazone
  Increased anticoagulant effect (decreased metabolism and displacement from binding sites)
   RA O'Reilly and G Levy, Pharmacokinetic analysis of potentiating effect of phenylbutazone on anticoagulant action of warfarin in man. J Pharm Sci, 59:1258, 1970; C Banfield et al, Phenylbutazone-warfarin interaction in man. Br J Clin Pharmacol, 16:669, 1983
  Serious risk; avoid concurrent use
 Phenytoin
  Phenytoin toxicity (decreased metabolism)
   JW Taylor et al, Oral anticoagulant-phenytoin interactions. Drug Intell Clin Pharm, 14:669, 1980; PK Panegyres and RH Rischbieth, Fatal phenytoin warfarin interaction. Postgrad Med J, 67:98, 1991
  Monitor phenytoin concentration

  Both increased and decreased effects of anticoagulants have been reported (mechanism not established)
   JW Taylor et al, Oral anticoagulant-phenytoin interactions. Drug Intell Clin Pharm, 14:669, 1980; PK Panegyres and RH Rischbieth, Fatal phenytoin warfarin interaction. Postgrad Med J, 67:98, 1991
  Monitor prothrombin time; single report of fatal hemorrhage (1991)
 Proguanil
  Bleeding (mechanism not established)
   G Armstrong et al, Warfarin potentiated by proguanil. BMJ, 303:789, 1991
  Single case report (1991)
 Propafenone
  Increased warfarin effect (probably decreased metabolism)
   RE Kates et al, Interaction between warfarin and propafenone in healthy volunteer subjects. Clin Pharmacol Ther, 42:305, 1987
  Monitor prothrombin time; based on study in healthy men
 Propylthiouracil
  Increased anticoagulant effect (decreased catabolism of vitamin K dependant clotting factors)
   PD Hansten, Oral anticoagulants and drugs which alter thyroid function, Drug Intell Clin Pharm, 14:331, 1990
  Effect should last only until metabolic state stabilizes
 Quetiapine
  Possible increased anticoagulant effect (mechanism not established)
   T Rogers et al, Possible interaction between warfarin and quetiapine. J Clin Psychopharmacol, 19:382, 1999
  Single case report (1999); the patient was also taking phenytoin, its possible role in the interaction is unknown; monitor INR/prothrombin time
 Quinidine
  Increased anticoagulant effect (mechanism not established)
   J Koch-Weser, Quinidine-induced hypoprothrombinemic hemorrhage in

ANTICOAGULANTS, ORAL, with: *(continued)*
>patients on chronic warfarin therapy. Ann Intern Med, 68:511, 1968; IM Sopher and SC Ming, Fatal corpus luteum hemorrhage during anticoagulant therapy. Obstet Gynecol, 37:695, 1971

Probably rare; monitor prothrombin time

Quinine
Increased anticoagulant effect (mechanism not established)
>J Koch-Weser, Quinidine-induced hypoprothrombinemic hemorrhage in patients on chronic warfarin therapy. Ann Intern Med, 68:511, 1968

Occurs only occasionally; monitor prothrombin time

Raloxifene
Possible decreased warfarin effect (mechanism not established)
>Manufacturer's package insert

Monitor prothrombin time

Rifampin
Decreased anticoagulant effect (increased metabolism)
>LD Heimark et al, The mechanism of the warfarin-rifampin drug interaction in humans. Clin Pharmacol Ther, 42:388, 1987; PR Casner, Inability to attain oral anticoagulation: warfarin-rifampin interaction revisited. South Med J, 89:1200, 1996

Monitor prothrombin time

Ritonavir
Decreased or increased warfarin effect (possible alteration in metabolism)
>G Gatti et al, Influence of indinavir and ritonavir on warfarin anticoagulant activity. AIDS, 12:825, 1998; KR Knoell et al, Potential interaction involving warfarin and ritonavir. Ann Pharmacother, 32:1299, 1998; G Newshan and P Tsang, Ritonavir and warfarin interaction. AIDS, 13:1788, 1999

Two case reports of decreased warfarin effect (1998) and one case of increased warfarin effect (1999); monitor prothrombin time

Saint John's wort
Possible decreased effect of warfarin and phenprocoumon (probably enzyme induction)
>Q-Y Yue et al, Safety of St John's wort. Lancet, 355:576, 2000

Based on several case reports; monitor INR/prothrombin time

Saquinavir
Increased anticoagulant effect with warfarin (possibly decreased metabolism)
>MR Darlington, Hypoprothrombinemia during concomitant therapy with warfarin and saquinavir. Ann Pharmacother, 31:647, 1997

Single case report (1997)

Selective serotonin reuptake inhibitors (SSRIs)
Bleeding with warfarin and paroxetine (mechanism not established)
>SJ Bannister et al, Evaluation of the potential for interactions of paroxetine with diazepam, cimetidine, warfarin, and digoxin. Acta Psychiatr Scand, 80 suppl 350:102, 1989

Monitor clinical status; prothrombin time may not be elevated; based on study in healthy men

ANTICOAGULANTS, ORAL, with: *(continued)*
> Possible increased anticoagulant effect with fluoxetine (mechanism not established)
>> S Woolfrey et al, Fluoxetine-warfarin interaction. BMJ, 307:241, 1993; CP Alderman et al, Abnormal platelet aggregation associated with fluoxetine therapy. Ann Pharmacother, 26:1517, 1992; HC Hanger and F Thomas, Fluoxetine and warfarin interactions. NZ Med J, 108:157, 1995; LA Dent and MW Orrock, Warfarin-fluoxetine and diazepam-fluoxetine interaction. Pharmacotherapy, 17:170, 1997; MA Ford et al, Lack of effect of fluoxetine on the hypoprothrombinemic response of warfarin. J Clin Psychopharmacol, 17:110, 1997; manufacturer's package insert
>
> *Several case reports, especially in the elderly; monitor prothrombin time; prothrombin time was not affected in 6 anticoagulated patients given fluoxetine 20 mg once per day; citalopram also had no effect on warfarin pharmacokinetics*
>
> Possible increased anticoagulant effect with sertraline (mechanism not established)
>> G Apseloff et al, Effect of sertraline on protein binding of warfarin. Clin Pharmacokinet, 32 suppl 1:37, 1997
>
> *Monitor prothrombin time*
>
> Possible increased anticoagulant effect with fluvoxamine (possibly decreased metabolism; CYP2C9)
>> A Hemeryck et al, Inhibition of CYP2C9 by selective serotonin reuptake inhibitors: in vitro studies with tolbutamide and (s)-warfarin using human liver microsomes. Eur J Clin Pharmacol, 54:947, 1999; KB Yap and ST Low, Interaction of fluvoxamine with warfarin in an elderly woman. Singapore Med J, 40:480, 1999
>
> *Based on single case report (1999) and in vitro study*
>
> **Spironolactone**
>
> Decreased anticoagulant effect (hemoconcentration)
>> RA O'Reilly, Spironolactone and warfarin interaction. Clin Pharmacol Ther, 27:198, 1980
>
> *Monitor prothrombin time*
>
> **Sucralfate**
>
> Decreased anticoagulant effect (decreased absorption)
>> PJ Neuvonen et al, Clinically significant sucralfate-warfarin interaction is not likely. Br J Clin Pharmacol, 20:178, 1985; SE Braverman and MT Marino, Sucralfate – warfarin interaction. Drug Intell Clin Pharm, 22:913, 1988; RL Talbert et al, Effect of sucralfate on plasma warfarin concentration in patients requiring chronic warfarin therapy. Drug Intell Clin Pharm, 19:456, 1985; AM Rey and JG Gums, Altered absorption of digoxin, sustained-release quinidine, and warfarin with sucralfate administration. DICP Ann Pharmacother, 25:745, 1991

(continued)

ANTICOAGULANTS, ORAL, with: *(continued)*
Several case reports; sometimes observed at initiation of anticoagulation but not when added once anticoagulation has been established; may occur even when drugs taken 2 hours apart; negative studies have been reported in healthy subjects and patients

Sulfinpyrazone
Increased anticoagulant effect (decreased metabolism)
> S Toon et al, The warfarin-sulfinpyrazone interaction: stereochemical considerations. Clin Pharmacol Ther, 39:15, 1986; LD Heimark et al, The effect of sulfinpyrazone on the disposition of pseudoracemic phenprocoumon in humans. Clin Pharmacol Ther, 42:312, 1987; M He et al, Inhibition of (S)-warfarin metabolism by sulfinpyrazone and its metabolites. Drug Metab Dispos, 23:659, 1995

Monitor prothrombin time; phenprocoumon does not interact

Sulfonamides
Increased anticoagulant effect (decreased metabolism and displacement from binding sites)
> TH Self et al, Interaction of sulfisoxazole and warfarin. Circulation, 52:528, 1975; LJ Sioris et al, Potentiation of warfarin anticoagulation by sulfisoxazole. Arch Intern Med, 140:546, 1980

Monitor prothrombin time initially; highly variable patient response

Sympathomimetic amines
Increased anticoagulant effect with methylphenidate (decreased metabolism)
> Manufacturer's package insert *(Ritalin)*

Monitor prothrombin time

Tamoxifen
Increased anticoagulant effect (possibly decreased metabolism); possible decreased antineoplastic effect of tamoxifen (altered metabolism)
> P Tenni et al, Life threatening interaction between tamoxifen and warfarin. BMJ, 298:93, 1989; LD Ritchie and SMT Grant, Tamoxifen-warfarin interaction: the Aberdeen hospitals drug file. BMJ, 298:1253, 1989

Monitor prothrombin time; pending further investigation, heparin is preferred when neoplasms are treated with tamoxifen

Tetracyclines
Increased anticoagulant effect (mechanism not established)
> Y Caraco and A Rubinow, Enhanced anticoagulant effect of coumarin derivatives induced by doxycycline coadministration. Ann Pharmacother, 26:1084, 1992; EA Danos, Apparent potentiation of warfarin activity by tetracycline. Clin Pharm, 11:806, 1992

Monitor prothrombin time

Thiabendazole
Increased anticoagulant effect with acenocoumarol (mechanism not established)
> P Henri et al, Imputation d'une hypocoagulabilité à l'interaction tiabendazole-acénocoumarol. Therapie, 48:583, 1993

Single case report; monitor prothrombin time (1993)

ANTICOAGULANTS, ORAL, with: *(continued)*

Thyroid hormones
Increased anticoagulant effect (increased clotting factor catabolism)
>PD Hansten, Oral anticoagulants and drugs which alter thyroid function. Drug Intell Clin Pharm, 14:331, 1980

Monitor prothrombin time; anticoagulant effect should be constant when patients are euthyroid on stable thyroid replacement dosage

Ticlopidine
Increased plasma R-warfarin concentrations (decreased metabolism)
>BE Gidal et al, Evaluation of a potential enantioselective interaction between ticlopidine and warfarin in chronically anticoagulated patients. Ther Drug Monit, 17:33, 1995

Monitor prothrombin time

Tolterodine
Possible increased warfarin anticoagulant effect (mechanism not established)
>VJ Colucci and MP Rivey, Tolterodine-warfarin drug interaction. Ann Pharmacother, 33:1173, 1999

Two case reports (1999); monitor INR or prothrombin time and for evidence of bleeding

Toremifene
Possible increased anticoagulant effect (possibly decreased metabolism)
>Manufacturer's package insert

Theoretical; monitor prothrombin time

Trastuzumab
Possible increased bleeding risk (mechanism not established)
>MJ Nissenblatt and GI Karp, Bleeding risk with trastuzumab (Herceptin) treatment. JAMA, 282:2299, 1999

Causal relationship not established; monitor INR/prothrombin time and clinical status

Trazodone
Possible decreased warfarin effect (mechanism not established)
>NL Small and KA Giamonna, Interaction between warfarin and trazodone. Ann Pharmacother, 34:734, 2000

Three case reports (2000); monitor INR/prothrombin time and clinical status

Triclofos sodium
Increased anticoagulant effect (displacement from binding)
>EM Sellers et al, Enhancement of warfarin-induced hypoprothrombinaemia by triclofos. Clin Pharmacol Ther, 13:911, 1972

Avoid concurrent use

Trimethoprim-sulfamethoxazole
Increased anticoagulant effect (decreased metabolism)
>RA O'Reilly and CH Motley, Racemic warfarin and trimethoprim-sulfamethoxazole interaction in humans. Ann Intern Med, 91:34, 1979

Monitor prothrombin time; sulfonamides also interact

(continued)

ANTICOAGULANTS, ORAL, with: *(continued)*

Troglitazone

Possible increased anticoagulant effect with warfarin (mechanism not established)

BK Plowman and AP Morreale, Possible troglitazone-warfarin interaction. Am J Health Syst Pharm, 55:1071, 1998

Single case report (1998); troglitazone is no longer available

Valproate

Transient increase in anticoagulant effect (probably displacement from binding)

SK Guthrie et al, Hypothesized interaction between valproic acid and warfarin. J Clin Psychopharmacol, 15:138, 1995

Single case report (1995)

Vitamin A

Increased anticoagulant effect with large doses (mechanism not established)

JJ Schrogie, Coagulopathy and fat-soluble vitamins. JAMA, 232:19, 1975

Monitor prothrombin time

Vitamin C

Decreased anticoagulant effect (mechanism not established)

R Hume et al, Interaction of ascorbic acid and warfarin. JAMA, 219:1479, 1972; G Rosenthal, Interaction of ascorbic acid and warfarin. JAMA, 1671, 1971

Occurs only occasionally; monitor prothrombin time

Vitamin E

Increased anticoagulant effect (mechanism not established)

JJ Corrigan, Jr and FI Marcus, Coagulopathy associated with vitamin E ingestion. JAMA, 230:1300, 1974; JJ Corrigan, Jr, The effect of vitamin E on warfarin-induced vitamin K deficiency. Ann NY Acad Sci, 393:361, 1982; JM Kim and RH White, Effect of vitamin E on the anticoagulant response to warfarin. Am J Cardiol, 77:545, 1996

Variable; conflicting reports; monitor prothrombin time

Zafirlukast

Increased anticoagulant effect (decreased metabolism; CYP2C9)

Manufacturer's package insert; A Morkunas and K Graeme, Zafirlukast-warfarin drug interaction with gastrointestinal bleeding. J Toxicol Clin Toxicol, 35:501, 1997; DL Vargo et al, Effect of zafirlukast on prothrombin time and area under the curve of warfarin. J Clin Pharmacol, 37:858, 1997; A Van Hecken et al, Effect of montelukast on the pharmacokinetics and pharmacodynamics of warfarin in healthy volunteers. J Clin Pharmacol, 39:495, 1999

Monitor prothrombin time; single case of GI bleeding (1997); preliminary study in healthy subjects showed small increase in prothrombin time; study in healthy subjects found no effect of montelukast on warfarin response

Zileuton

Possible increased anticoagulant effect of warfarin (decreased metabolism)

WM Awni et al, Pharmacodynamic and stereoselective pharmacokinetic interactions between zileuton and warfarin in humans. Clin Pharmacokinet, 29 suppl 2:67, 1995

ANTICOAGULANTS, ORAL, with: *(continued)*
   Monitor prothrombin time

ANTIDEPRESSANTS, TRICYCLIC, with:
  Alcohol - See Alcohol with Antidepressants, tricyclic, page 13
  Altretamine - See Altretamine with Antidepressants, tricyclic, page 26
  Amprenavir - See Amprenavir with Antidepressants, tricyclic, page 38
  Angiotensin-converting enzyme (ACE) inhibitors - See Angiotensin-converting enzyme (ACE) inhibitors with Antidepressants, tricyclic, page 43
  Anticholinergics - See Anticholinergics with Antidepressants, tricyclic, page 58
  Anticoagulants, oral - See Anticoagulants, oral with Antidepressants, tricyclic, page 60
  Antifungals, imidazoles and triazoles
    Possible nortriptyline or amitriptyline toxicity with fluconazole (probably decreased metabolism)
      RH Gannon and ML Anderson, Fluconazole-nortriptyline drug interaction. Ann Pharmacother, 26:1456, 1992; RE Morrison et al, A fluconazole/amitriptyline drug interaction in three male adults. Clin Infect Dis, 24:270, 1997; E Spina et al, Effect of ketoconazole on the pharmacokinetics of imipramine and desipramine in healthy subjects. Br J Clin Pharmacol, 43:315, 1997; ST Dorsey and LA Bilbo, Prolonged QT interval and torsades de pointes caused by the combination of fluconazole and amitriptyline. Am J Emerg Med, 18:227, 2000
    Single case report with nortriptyline (1992); four cases with amitriptyline (1997; 2000); monitor clinical status and antidepressant concentration; the clinical significance of the effect with ketoconazole has not been established
  Antifungals, terbinafine
    Possible nortriptyline toxicity (possible decreased metabolism)
      P-HM van der Kuy and PM Hooymans, Nortriptyline intoxication induced by terbinafine. BMJ, 316:441, 1998
    Single case report (1998); positive rechallenge
  Antihistamines, H$_2$-blockers
    Possible antidepressant toxicity with cimetidine (decreased metabolism)
      PA Shapiro, Cimetidine-imipramine interaction: case report and comments. Am J Psychiatry, 141:152, 1984; SA Henauer and LE Hollister, Cimetidine interaction with imipramine and nortriptyline. Clin Pharmacol Ther, 35:183, 1984; SH Curry et al, Cimetidine interaction with amitriptyline. Eur J Clin Pharmacol, 29:429, 1985; ME Miller et al, Psychosis in association with combined cimetidine and imipramine treatment. Psychosomatics, 28:217, 1987; DL Sutherland et al, The influence of cimetidine versus ranitidine on doxepin pharmacokinetics. Eur J Clin Pharmacol, 32:159, 1987; E Steiner and E Spina, Differences in the inhibitory effect of cimetidine on desipramine metabolism between rapid and slow debrisoquin hydroxylators. Clin Pharmacol Ther, 42:278, 1987
    Monitor antidepressant concentration

(continued)

ANTIDEPRESSANTS, TRICYCLIC, with: *(continued)*
Arbutamine
Possible interference with interpretation of arbutamine heart rate response (antagonism)
> Manufacturer's package insert

Avoid concurrent use

Baclofen
Increased loss of muscle tone and inability to stand (mechanism not established)
> MJ Silverglat, Baclofen and tricyclic antidepressants: possible interaction. JAMA, 246:1659, 1981

Single report (1981); monitor muscle tone

Memory loss (mechanism not established)
> R Sandyk and MA Gillman, Baclofen-induced memory impairment. Clin Neuropharmacol, 8:294, 1985

Monitor mental status

Barbiturates
Decreased antidepressant effect (increased metabolism)
> B Alexanderson et al, Steady-state plasma levels of nortriptyline in twins: influence of genetic factors and drug therapy. Br Med J, 4:764, 1969; C von Bahr et al, Time course of enzyme induction in humans: effect of pentobarbital on nortriptyline metabolism. Clin Pharmacol Ther, 64:18, 1998

Avoid concurrent use unless barbiturate essential as anticonvulsant

Benzodiazepines
Possible decreased desipramine effect with clonazepam (mechanism not established)
> RF Deicken, Clonazepam-induced reduction in serum desipramine concentration. J Clin Psychopharmacol, 8:71, 1988; L Bertilsson et al, Alprazolam does not inhibit the metabolism of nortriptyline in depressed patients or inhibit the metabolism of desipramine in human liver microsomes. Ther Drug Monit, 10:231, 1988; DJ Buysse et al, Does lorazepam impair the antidepressant response to nortriptyline and psychotherapy? J Clin Psychiatry, 58:426, 1997

Single case report (1988); alprazolam and lorazepam (in the elderly) do not appear to interact with nortriptyline

Increased impairment of skills related to driving with amitriptyline and diazepam (additive)
> H Moskowitz and M Burns, The effects on performance of two antidepressants, alone and in combination with diazepam. Prog Neuropsychopharmacol Biol Psychiatry, 12:783, 1988; M Mattila et al, Actions and interactions of psychotropic drugs on human performance and mood: single doses of ORG 3770, amitriptyline, and diazepam. Pharmacol Toxicol, 65:81, 1989; EJ Antal et al, A multi-center study to evaluate the pharmacokinetic and clinical interactions between alprazolam and imipramine. J Pharmacokinet Biopharm, 19:93S, 1991

ANTIDEPRESSANTS, TRICYCLIC, with: *(continued)*
> *Warn patients taking either drug alone or in combination of the risk of driving; alprazolam and imipramine have been used in combination without adverse effects*

Possible serotonin syndrome with clomipramine plus alprazolam (mechanism not established)
> JL Cano-Muñoz et al, Possible serotonin syndrome following the combined administration of clomipramine and alprazolam. J Clin Psychiatry, 56:122, 1995

Single case report (1995)

Beta-adrenergic blockers
Possible imipramine toxicity (decreased metabolism)
> DJ Hermann et al, Comparison of verapamil, diltiazem, and labetalol on the bioavailability and metabolism of imipramine. J Clin Pharmacol, 32:176, 1992; DW Gillette and LP Tannery, Beta blocker inhibits tricyclic metabolism. J Am Acad Child Adolesc Psychiatry, 33:2, 1994

Monitor imipramine concentration; based on study in healthy men, also reported in a boy and girl aged 9 receiving propranolol

Bethanidine
Decreased antihypertensive effect (blockade of uptake at target site)
> JR Mitchell et al, Guanethidine and related agents II Antagonism by drugs which inhibit the norepinephrine pump in man. J Clin Invest, 49:1596, 1970

Use alternative antihypertensive

Brimonidine
Possible cardiovascular toxicity or decreased brimonidine effect (mechanism not established)
> Manufacturer's package insert

Monitor clinical status

Bupropion
Possible imipramine and desipramine toxicity (possibly decreased metabolism)
> MU Shad and SH Preskorn, A possible bupropion and imipramine interaction. J Clin Psychopharmacol, 17:118, 1997

Single case report (1997)

Increased seizure risk (additive)
> Manufacturer's package insert

Use only with caution; monitor clinical status

Carbamazepine
Possible toxicity of both drugs (possibly decreased metabolism and accumulation of cardiotoxic metabolites of tricyclics); possible decreased antidepressant effect (increased metabolism)
> I Lesser, Carbamazepine and desipramine: a toxic reaction. J Clin Psychiatry, 45:360, 1984; RJ Baldessarini et al, Anticonvulsant cotreatment may increase toxic metabolites of antidepressants and other psychotropic drugs. J Clin Psychopharmacol, 8:381, 1988; CS Brown et al, Possible influence of carbamazepine on plasma imipramine concentrations in children with attention deficit hyperactivity disorder. J Clin Psychopharmacol,

ANTIDEPRESSANTS, TRICYCLIC, with: *(continued)*
>
> 10:359, 1990; E Leinonen et al, Effects of carbamazepine on serum antidepressant concentrations in psychiatric patients. J Clin Psychopharmacol, 11:313, 1991; K Brøsen and P Kragh-Sørensen, Concomitant intake of nortriptyline and carbamazepine. Ther Drug Monit, 15:258, 1993; M Jerling et al, The use of therapeutic drug monitoring data to document kinetic drug interactions: an example with amitriptyline and nortriptyline. Ther Drug Monit, 16:1, 1994; Y Iwata et al, Carbamazepine augmentation of clomipramine in the treatment of refractory obsessive-compulsive disorder. J Clin Psychiatry, 61:528, 2000
>
> *Monitor serum concentration of both drugs; monitor cardiovascular status if concentrations of tricyclic metabolites cannot be obtained; combination of clomipramine and carbamazepine has been used to advantage in a patient with obsessive-compulsive disorder*

Cholestyramine

Decreased doxepin effect (decreased absorption)
> DS Geeze et al, Doxepin-cholestyramine interaction. Psychosomatics, 29:233, 1988
>
> *Single case report (1988); patient had hemigastrectomy*

Clonidine

Decreased antihypertensive effect (mechanism not established)
> RH Briant et al, Interaction between clonidine and desipramine in man. Br Med J, 1:522, 1973; L Lacomblez et al, Suppression de l'effet antihypertenseur de la clonidine par la clomipramine. Rev Med Interne, 9:291, 1988
>
> *Beta-blockers, diuretics or, in some patients, methyldopa can be used as alternatives*

Clozapine

Possible antidepressant toxicity with nortriptyline (possibly decreased metabolism)
> T Smith and J Riskin, Effect of clozapine on plasma nortriptyline concentration. Pharmacopsychiatry, 27:41, 1994
>
> *Single case report (1994); monitor clinical status and adjust antidepressant dosage if needed*

Contraceptives, oral

Possible antidepressant toxicity (decreased metabolism)
> DR Abernethy et al, Imipramine disposition in users of oral contraceptive steroids. Clin Pharmacol Ther, 35:792, 1984; KRR Krishnan et al, Tricyclic-induced akathisia in patients taking conjugated estrogens. Am J Psychiatry, 141:696, 1984
>
> *Demonstrated in women taking low-dose estrogen contraceptives or estrogen alone; monitor clinical status*

Cyproheptadine

Severe anticholinergic symptoms with cyproheptadine and desipramine (probably additive)
> EB Pontius, Case report of an anticholinergic crisis associated with cyproheptadine treatment of desipramine-induced inorgasmia. J Clin Psychopharmacol, 8:230, 1988

ANTIDEPRESSANTS, TRICYCLIC, with: *(continued)*
Single case report (1988)

Debrisoquine
Decreased antihypertensive effect (blockade of uptake at target site)
> JR Mitchell et al, Guanethidine and related agents II Antagonism by drugs which inhibit the norepinephrine pump in man. J Clin Invest, 49:1596, 1970

Use alternative antihypertensive

Diltiazem
Possible imipramine toxicity (decreased metabolism)
> DJ Hermann et al, Comparison of verapamil, diltiazem, and labetalol on the bioavailability and metabolism of imipramine. J Clin Pharmacol, 32:176, 1992

Monitor imipramine concentration; based on study in healthy men

Disulfiram
Organic brain syndrome (decreased metabolism)
> DA Ciraulo et al, Pharmacokinetic interaction of disulfiram and antidepressants. Am J Psychiatry, 142:1373, 1985

Monitor mental status

Dofetilide
Increased risk of arrhythmias (additive effect on QTc interval)
> Manufacturer's package insert (dofetilide)

Avoid concurrent use

Ergot alkaloids
Serotonin syndrome (additive)
> NT Mathew et al, Serotonin syndrome complicating migraine pharmacotherapy. Cephalalgia, 16:323, 1996

Single case report (1996)

Estrogens
Possible antidepressant toxicity with estrogens or oral contraceptives (mechanism not established)
> KRR Krishnan et al, Tricyclic-induced akathisia in patients taking conjugated estrogens. Am J Psychiatry, 141:696, 1984

Case reports suggest estrogen facilitation of akathisia; monitor clinical status

Fluoroquinolones
Possible ventricular arrhythmia with grepafloxacin (possible additive effect on QTc interval; CYP3A4)
> Manufacturer's package insert

Theoretical; manufacturer recommends avoiding concurrent use

Guanadrel
Decreased antihypertensive effect (blockade of guanadrel uptake at target site)
> Manufacturer's package insert

Use alternative antihypertensive

Guanethidine
Decreased antihypertensive effect (blockade of uptake at target site)
> JR Mitchell et al, Guanethidine and related agents II Antagonism by drugs which inhibit the norepinephrine pump in man. J Clin Invest, 49:1596, 1970; AWD Leishman et al, Antagonism of guanethidine by imipramine. Lancet,

ANTIDEPRESSANTS, TRICYCLIC, with: *(continued)*
1:112, 1963

Use alternative antihypertensive

Guanfacine

Decreased antihypertensive effect of guanfacine with amitriptyline or imipramine (mechanism not established)

> M Buckley and J Feely, Antagonism of antihypertensive effect of guanfacine by tricyclic antidepressants. Lancet, 337:1173, 1991

Avoid concurrent use

Haloperidol

Possible desipramine toxicity (decreased metabolism)

> GC Mahr et al, A grand mal seizure associated with desipramine and haloperidol. Can J Psychiatry, 32:463, 1987

Single case report of a seizure (1987)

Hypoglycemics, sulfonylurea

Hypoglycemia with doxepin and tolazamide or nortriptyline and chlorpropamide (mechanism not established)

> BL True et al, Profound hypoglycemia with the addition of a tricyclic antidepressant to maintenance sulfonylurea therapy. Am J Psychiatry, 144:1220, 1987

Two case reports (1987); monitor blood glucose

Levodopa

Decreased levodopa effect with imipramine (decreased absorption)

> JP Morgan et al, Imipramine-mediated interference with levodopa absorption from the gastrointestinal tract in man. Neurology, 25:1029, 1975

Monitor clinical status

Lithium

Increased incidence of tremor; bipolar patients may develop temporary refractory mania (mechanism not established)

> LH Price et al, Manic symptoms following addition of lithium to antidepressant treatment. J Clin Psychopharmacol, 4:361, 1984; LH Price, Lithium augmentation in tricyclic-resistant depression, in EL Extein, ed, *Treatment of Tricyclic-Resistant Depression*, Washington, DC: American Psychiatric Press, 1989, page 49; H Kojima et al, Serotonin syndrome during clomipramine and lithium treatment. Am J Psychiatry, 150:12, 1993

Combination generally well tolerated but, if not, adverse effects may require discontinuing tricyclic

Possible increase risk of cardiomyopathy with imipramine

> A Dietrich et al, Cardiac toxicity in an adolescent following chronic lithium and imipramine therapy. J Adolesc Health, 14:394, 1992

Single case report (1992)

Marijuana, smoking

Marked sinus tachycardia (additive)

> WVR Vieweg and JR Hillard, Adverse interactions of cannabis with psychotropic medicines. Psychiatr Med, 4:69, 1986

ANTIDEPRESSANTS, TRICYCLIC, with: *(continued)*
   Warn patients to avoid concurrent use
   Modafinil
      Clomipramine toxicity (decreased metabolism)
         Manufacturer's package insert (modafinil)
      Single case reported by manufacturer (1998)
   Monoamine oxidase inhibitors
      Serotonin syndrome - delirium, coma, hyperpyrexia, convulsions, mania (mechanism not established); single case report of disseminated intravascular coagulation (1987)
         K White and G Simpson, Combined MAOI-tricyclic antidepressant treatment: a reevaluation. J Clin Psychopharmacol, 1:264, 1981; RM Tackley and B Tregaskis, Fatal disseminated intravascular coagulation following a monoamine oxidase inhibitor/tricyclic interaction. Anaesthesia, 42:760, 1987; O Spigset et al, Serotonin syndrome caused by a moclobemide-clomipramine interaction. BMJ, 306:248, 1993; TA Stern et al, Catastrophic illness associated with the combination of clomipramine, phenelzine, and chlorpromazine. Ann Clin Psychiatry, 4:81, 1992; PK Gillman, Serotonin syndrome treated with chlorpromazine. J Clin Psychopharmacol, 17:128, 1997; BSH Chan et al, Serotonin syndrome resulting from drug interactions. MJA, 169:523, 1998
      Although the combination may be tolerated when both drugs are started together, a drug-free interval of at least one week is recommended when transferring from a tricyclic to an MAOI and a 2-week interval when transferring from an MAOI to a tricyclic; reported with both MAO A and MAO B inhibitors; serotonin syndrome from tranylcypromine plus clomipramine successfully treated in two patients with intramuscular chlorpromazine
   Narcotics: methadone and congeners
      Possible amitriptyline, doxepin and nortriptyline toxicity with propoxyphene (decreased metabolism)
         M Jerling et al, The use of therapeutic drug monitoring data to document kinetic drug interactions: an example with amitriptyline and nortriptyline. Ther Drug Monit, 16:1, 1994
      Avoid concurrent use of doxepin and proproxyphene when patient on methadone
      Possible desipramine toxicity with methadone (probably decreased metabolism)
         DR Abernethy et al, Impairment of hepatic drug oxidation by propoxyphene. Ann Intern Med, 97:223, 1982; TR Kosten et al, Desipramine and its 2-hydroxy metabolite in patients taking or not taking methadone. Am J Psychiatry, 147:1379, 1990; M Jerling et al, The use of therapeutic drug monitoring data to document kinetic drug interactions: an example with amitriptyline and nortriptyline. Ther Drug Monit, 16:1, 1994
      Monitor desipramine concentration

(continued)

ANTIDEPRESSANTS, TRICYCLIC, with: *(continued)*

Narcotics: pentazocine
Possible respiratory depression with amitriptyline and pentazocine (additive)
> U Saarialho-Kere et al, Parenteral pentazocine: effects on psychomotor skills and respiration, and interactions with amitriptyline. Eur J Clin Pharmacol, 35:483, 1988

Monitor respiratory status

Nifedipine
Failure to respond to nortriptyline (mechanism not established)
> FJ Hullett et al, Depression associated with nifedipine-induced calcium channel blockade. Am J Psychiatry, 145:1277, 1988

Single case report (1988)

Nitrates
Decreased nitrate effect (failure to dissolve)
> LJ Robbins, Dry mouth and delayed dissolution of sublingual nitroglycerin. N Engl J Med, 309:985, 1983

Antidepressant caused dry mouth

Nonsteroidal anti-inflammatory drugs
Possible desipramine toxicity with ibuprofen (mechanism not established)
> DW Gillette, Desipramine and ibuprofen. J Am Acad Child Adolesc Psychiatry, 37:1129, 1998

Single case report (1998)

Olanzapine
Possible increased risk of seizures (mechanism not established)
> D Deshauer et al, Seizures caused by possible interaction between olanzapine and clomipramine. J Clin Psychopharmacol, 20:283, 2000

Two case reports (2000); monitor clinical status

Oxybutynin
Possible decreased clomipramine effect (possibly increased metabolism)
> M Grözinger et al, Oxybutynin enhances the metabolism of clomipramine and dextrorphan possibly by induction of a cytochrome P450 isoenzyme. J Clin Psychopharmocol, 19:287, 1999

Single case report (1999); monitor clinical status

Phenothiazines
Antidepressant toxicity (decreased metabolism)
> M Linnoila et al, Interaction between antidepressants and perphenazine in psychiatric inpatients. Am J Psychiatry, 139:1329, 1982; J Hirschowitz et al, Thioridazine effect on desipramine plasma levels. J Clin Psychopharmacol, 3:376, 1983; PE Cook et al, Imipramine – flupenthixol decanoate interaction. Can J Psychiatry, 31:235, 1986; TE Wilens and TA Stern, Ventricular tachycardia associated with desipramine and thioridazine. Psychosomatics, 31:100, 1990; TE Wilens et al, Adverse cardiac effects of combined neuroleptic ingestion and tricyclic antidepressant overdose. J Clin Psychopharmacol, 10:51, 1990; TA Stern et al, Catastrophic illness associated with the combination of clomipramine, phenelzine, and chlorpromazine. Ann Clin Psychiatry, 4:81, 1992; K Linnet, Comparison of the kinetic interactions of the neuroleptics perphenazine and zuclopenthixol with tricyclic

ANTIDEPRESSANTS, TRICYCLIC, with: *(continued)*
> antidepressives. Ther Drug Monit, 17:308, 1995; BH Mulsant et al, The effects of perphenazine on the concentration of nortriptyline and its hydroxymetabolites in older patients. J Clin Psychopharmacol, 17:318, 1997

Monitor antidepressant concentration and clinical status

> False increase in imipramine and desipramine HPLC determinations with thioridazine (chemical interference); true increase in imipramine concentration (decreased metabolism)
>> GL Maynard and P Soni, Thioridazine interferences with imipramine metabolism and measurement. Ther Drug Monit, 18:729, 1996

Enzyme immunoassay or silica column HPLC may not be affected; monitor clinical status and imipramine concentration

Phenytoin

> Phenytoin toxicity with imipramine (mechanism not established)
>> E Perucca and A Richens, Interaction between phenytoin and imipramine. Br J Clin Pharmacol, 4:485, 1977

Monitor phenytoin concentration

> Decreased desipramine effect (possibly increased metabolism)
>> BS Fogel and S Haltzman, Desipramine and phenytoin: a potential drug interaction of therapeutic relevance. J Clin Psychiatry, 48:387, 1987

Two case reports (1987); monitor desipramine concentration

Potassium

> Jejunal ulceration with wax-matrix potassium chloride tablets (possibly decreased motility caused by amitriptyline)
>> DL Bronson and RL Gamelli, Jejunal ulceration and stricture due to wax-matrix potassium chloride tablets and amitriptyline. J Clin Pharmacol, 27:788, 1987

Single case report (1987); soluble or easily dispersed potassium supplements are preferred

Propafenone

> Possible desipramine toxicity (decreased metabolism)
>> MR Katz, Raised serum levels of desipramine with the antiarrhythmic propafenone. J Clin Psychiatry, 52:432, 1991

Single case report (1991); monitor desipramine concentration

Quinidine

> Possible desipramine, imipramine, or nortriptyline (in extensive metabolizers) toxicity (decreased metabolism)
>> K Brøsen and LF Gram, Quinidine inhibits the 2-hydroxylation of imipramine and desipramine but not the demethylation of imipramine. Eur J Clin Pharmacol, 37:155, 1989; B Pfandl et al, Stereoselective inhibition of nortriptyline hydroxylation in man by quinidine. Xenobiotica, 22:721, 1992; E Steiner et al, Inhibition of desipramine 2-hydroxylation by quinidine and quinine. Clin Pharmacol Ther, 43:577, 1988

Based on study in healthy volunteers; avoid concurrent use

(continued)

ANTIDEPRESSANTS, TRICYCLIC, with: *(continued)*
  Rifampin
   Decreased nortriptyline effect (probably increased metabolism)
    JM Bebchuk and DE Stewart, Drug interaction between rifampin and nortriptyline: a case report. Int J Psychiatry Med, 21:183, 1991; T Self et al, Case report: interaction of rifampin and nortriptyline. Am J Med Sci, 311:80, 1996
   Two case reports (1991, 1996); monitor nortriptyline concentration
  Ritonavir
   Possible desipramine toxicity (probably decreased metabolism)
    Manufacturer's package insert (ritonavir)
   Monitor clinical status; theoretical; listed as contraindicated in product information
  Selective serotonin reuptake inhibitors (SSRIs)
   Tricyclic toxicity with fluoxetine, fluvoxamine, paroxetine, sertraline or citalopram; tricyclic aggravation of depression with desipramine and fluoxetine (decreased metabolism; CYP 2D6)
    IR Bell and JO Cole, Fluoxetine induces elevation of desipramine level and exacerbation of geriatric nonpsychotic depression. J Clin Psychopharmacol, 8:447, 1988; SH Preskorn et al, Serious adverse effects of combining fluoxetine and tricyclic antidepressants. Am J Psychiatry, 147:532, 1990; J Westermeyer, Fluoxetine-induced tricyclic toxicity: extent and duration. J Clin Pharmacol, 31:388, 1991; K Brosen et al, Inhibition by paroxetine of desipramine metabolism in extensive but not in poor metabolizers of sparteine. Eur J Clin Pharmacol, 44:349, 1993; RB Lydiard et al, Interactions between sertraline and tricyclic antidepressants. Am J Psychiatry, 150:1125, 1993; E Spina et al, Effect of fluvoxamine on the pharmacokinetics of imipramine and desipramine in healthy subjects. Ther Drug Monit, 15:243, 1993; E Seifritz et al, Increased trimipramine plasma levels during fluvoxamine comedication. Eur Neuropsychopharmacol, 4:15, 1994; A El-Yazigi et al, Steady-state kinetics of fluoxetine and amitriptyline in patients treated with a combination of these drugs as compared with those treated with amitriptyline alone. J Clin Pharmacol, 35:17, 1995; AE Balant-Gorgia et al, Metabolic interaction between fluoxetine and clomipramine: a case report. Pharmacopsychiatry, 29:38, 1996; P Conus et al, Pharmacokinetic fluvoxamine-clomipramine interaction with favorable therapeutic consequences in therapy-resistant depressive patient. Pharmacopsychiatry, 29:108, 1996; LJ Albers et al, Paroxetine shifts imipramine metabolism. Psychiatry Res, 59:189, 1996; SH Preskorn and B Baker, Fatality associated with combined fluoxetine-amitriptyline therapy. JAMA, 277:1682, 1997; F Benazzi, Venlafaxine-fluoxetine-nortriptyline interaction. J Psychiatry Neurosci, 22:278, 1997; LK Solai et al, Effect of sertraline on plasma nortriptyline levels in depressed elderly. J Clin Psychiatry, 58:440, 1997; K-L Paul, Anticholinergic delirium possibly associated with protriptyline and fluoxetine. Ann Pharmacother, 31:1260, 1997; manufacturer's package insert; EF Skjelbo and K Brøsen, Interaktion imellem paroxetin og clomipramin som mulig årsag til indlæggelse på medicinsk afdeling. Ugeskr Laeger,

ANTIDEPRESSANTS, TRICYCLIC, with: *(continued)*

160:5665, 1998; LF Gram et al, Citalopram: interaction studies with levomepromazine, imipramine, and lithium. Ther Drug Monit, 15:18, 1993; Z-H Xu et al, Inhibition of imipramine N-demethylation by fluvoxamine in Chinese young men. Acta Pharmacologica Sinica, 17:399, 1996; AJ Levitt et al, Do depressed subjects who have failed both fluoxetine and a tricyclic antidepressant respond to the combination? J Clin Psychiatry, 60:613, 1999; E Haffen et al, Citalopram: an interaction study with clomipramine in a patient heterozygous for CYP2D6 genotype. Pharmacopsychiatry, 32:232, 1999; S Leucht et al, Effect of adjunctive paroxetine on serum levels and side-effects of tricyclic antidepressants in depressive inpatients. Psychopharmacology, 147:378, 2000; AK Ashton, Lack of desipramine toxicity with citalopram. J Clin Psychiatry, 61:144, 2000

Monitor clinical status and tricyclic antidepressant concentration, especially when combined with potent CYP2D6 inhibitors (fluoxetine, paroxetine); adverse effects can occur as long as 5 weeks after discontinuing fluoxetine; based on a study of 18 male subjects, there was no effect of sertraline on desipramine concentration after one week; fluvoxamine improved clomipramine response in one patient; fluoxetine has been used with desipramine or imipramine for resistant depression; fatality reported with fluoxetine and amitriptyline; citalopram did not affect imipramine concentration, but increased concentration of its metabolite desipramine

Serotonin syndrome with fluoxetine and clomipramine or sertraline and amitriptyline (probably additive)

CP Alderman and PC Lee, Comment: serotonin syndrome associated with combined sertraline-amitriptyline treatment. Ann Pharmacother, 30:1499, 1996; M Molaie, Serotonin syndrome presenting with migrainelike stroke. Headache, 37:519, 1997

Single case reports with fluoxetine and clomipramine (1997) and sertraline and amitriptyline (1996)

Sympathomimetic amines

Hypertension, hypertensive crisis with epinephrine, norepinephrine, or phenylephrine (inhibition of norepinephrine uptake by neurons)

AJ Boakes et al, Interactions between sympathomimetic amines and antidepressant agents in man. Br Med J, 1:311, 1973; D Kadar, Amitriptyline and isoproterenol: fatal drug combination. Can Med Assoc J, 112:556, 1975

Avoid concurrent use

Cognitive mood disturbances with methylphenidate and imipramine in children (mechanism not established)

CS Grob and JT Coyle, Suspected adverse methylphenidate – imipramine interactions in children. J Dev Behav Pediatr, 7:265, 1986

Avoid concurrent use

Possible increased imipramine effect (possible inhibition of imipramine metabolism)

DL Fogelson, Fenfluramine and the cytochrome P450 system. Am J Psychiatry, 154:436, 1997

(continued)

ANTIDEPRESSANTS, TRICYCLIC, with: *(continued)*
Single case report (1997)

Increased toxicity with desipramine and methylphenidate (possibly decreased desipramine metabolism)
> CS Pataki et al, Side effects of methylphenidate and desipramine alone and in combination in children. J Am Acad Child Adolesc Psychiatry, 32:1065, 1993

Monitor clinical status

Tamoxifen

Possible decrease in doxepin effect (mechanism not established)
> JW Jefferson, Tamoxifen-associated reduction in tricyclic antidepressant levels in blood. J Clin Psychopharmacol, 15:223, 1995

Single case report (1995)

Tetracyclines

Localized hemosiderosis with amitriptyline and minocycline (possibly synergism)
> RSW Basler and CS Goetz, Synergism of minocycline and amitriptyline in cutaneous hyperpigmentation. J Am Acad Dermatol, 12:577, 1985; RSW Basler and PW Kohnen, Localized hemosiderosis as a sequela of acne. Arch Dermatol, 114:1695, 1978

Avoid concurrent use

Tobacco, smoking

Decreased antidepressant effect (increased metabolism)
> JM Perel et al, Pharmacodynamics of imipramine in depressed patients. Psychopharmacol Bull, 11:16, 1975;

Monitor antidepressant concentration; reported with imipramine, but might occur with other tricyclics

Possible toxicity with nortriptyline (possibly displacement from binding)
> PJ Perry et al, Effects of smoking on nortriptyline plasma concentrations in depressed patients. Ther Drug Monit, 8:279, 1986

Monitor nortriptyline concentration and maintain at minimal effective dosage; total concentration may be in the therapeutic range, but free concentration elevated

Trimethoprim-sulfamethoxazole

Recurrence of depression (mechanism not established)
> S Brion et al, Interaction entre le cotrimoxazole et les antidépresseurs. L'Encéphale, 13:123, 1987

Monitor mental status

Troleandomycin

Possible imipramine toxicity (decreased metabolism)
> J-S Wang et al, Effect of troleandomycin on the pharmacokinetics of imipramine in Chinese: the role of CYP3A. Br J Clin Pharmacol, 44:195, 1997

Based on study in healthy subjects; monitor clinical status and adjust imipramine dose as needed

ANTIDEPRESSANTS, TRICYCLIC, with: *(continued)*
Valproate
Possible desipramine toxicity (mechanism not established)
> AB Joseph and BA Wroblewski, Potentially toxic serum concentrations of desipramine after discontinuation of valproic acid. Brain Injury, 7:463, 1993

Single case report (1993) of elevation of desipramine concentration on valproate withdrawal

Amitriptyline and nortriptyline toxicity (decreased metabolism)
> C Fu et al, Valproate/Nortriptyline interaction. J Clin Psychopharmacol, 14:205, 1994; SL Wong et al, Effects of divalproex sodium on amitriptyline and nortriptyline pharmacokinetics. Clin Pharmacol Ther, 60:48, 1996

Report of two cases (1994); confirmed by a study in normal men and women

Possible clomipramine toxicity (mechanism not established)
> C Fehr et al, Increase in serum clomipramine concentrations caused by valproate. J Clin Psychopharmacol, 20:493, 2000

Single case report (2000); monitor clomipramine concentrations and clinical status

Valpromide
Possible amitriptyline toxicity (decreased metabolism)
> G Bertschy et al, Interaction valpromide-amitriptyline: augmentation de la biodisponibilité de l'amitriptyline et de la nortriptyline par le valpromide. L'Encéphale, 16:43, 1990; S Vandel et al, Valpromide increases the plasma concentrations of amitriptyline and its metabolite nortriptyline in depressive patients. Ther Drug Monit, 10:386, 1988

Monitor clinical status and amitriptyline concentration

Venlafaxine
Possible increased risk of serotonin syndrome (additive)
> NK Perry, Venlafaxine-induced serotonin syndrome with relapse following amitriptyline. Postgrad Med J, 76:254, 2000

Single case report (2000); causal relationship not established; monitor clinical status

Verapamil
Possible imipramine toxicity (decreased metabolism)
> DJ Hermann et al, Comparison of verapamil, diltiazem, and labetalol on the bioavailability and metabolism of imipramine. J Clin Pharmacol, 32:176, 1992

Monitor imipramine concentration; based on study in healthy men

Zolpidem
Hallucinations with desipramine (additive)
> CJ Elko et al, Zolpidem-associated hallucinations and serotonin reuptake inhibition: a possible interaction. Clin Toxicol, 36:195, 1998

Single case report (1998)

ANTIFUNGALS, AMPHOTERICIN B, with:
Aminoglycoside antibiotics - See Aminoglycoside antibiotics with Antifungals, Amphotericin B, page 30

(continued)

ANTIFUNGALS, AMPHOTERICIN B, with: *(continued)*
Cyclosporine
Toxicity (mechanism not established)
> MS Kennedy et al, Acute renal toxicity with combined use of amphotericin B and cyclosporine after marrow transplantation. Transplantation, 35:211, 1983; ME Ellis et al, Is cyclosporin neurotoxicity enhanced in the presence of liposomal amphotericin B? J Infect, 29:106, 1994

Avoid concurrent use, if possible

Digitoxin
Possible digitoxin toxicity (hypokalemia)
> RP Miller and JH Bates, Amphotericin B toxicity. A follow-up report of 53 patients. Ann Intern Med, 71:1089, 1969; WG Cushard, Jr et al, Blastomycosis of bone. Treatment with intramedullary amphotericin B. J Bone Joint Surg, 51A:704, 1969

Monitor potassium concentration

Digoxin
Possible digoxin toxicity (hypokalemia)
> RP Miller and JH Bates, Amphotericin B toxicity. A follow-up report of 53 patients. Ann Intern Med, 71:1089, 1969; WG Cushard, Jr et al, Blastomycosis of bone. Treatment with intramedullary amphotericin B. J Bone Joint Surg, 51A:704, 1969

Monitor potassium concentration

Flucytosine
Granulocytopenia and thrombocytopenia (decreased renal clearance of flucytosine)
> K Shindo et al, Granulocytopenia and thrombocytopenia associated with combination therapy of amphotericin B and low-dose flucytosine in a patient with cryptococcal meningitis. DICP, 23:672, 1989; A Vermes et al, Flucytosine: a review of its pharmacology, clinical indications, pharmacokinetics, toxicity and drug interactions. J Antimicrob Chemother, 46:171, 2000

Single case report (1989); monitor clinical status

Gallium
Renal toxicity (additive)
> Manufacturer's package insert

Avoid concurrent use

Neuromuscular blocking agents
Increased neuromuscular blockade (hypokalemia)
> RP Miller and JH Bates, Amphotericin B toxicity. A follow-up report of 53 patients. Ann Intern Med, 71:1089, 1969; WG Cushard, Jr et al, Blastomycosis of bone. Treatment with intramedullary amphotericin B. J Bone Joint Surg, 51A:704, 1969

Monitor potassium concentration and neuromuscular status

ANTIFUNGALS, GRISEOFULVIN, with:
Alcohol - See Alcohol with Antifungals, Griseofulvin, page 13

ANTIFUNGALS, GRISEOFULVIN, with: *(continued)*

Anticoagulants, oral - See Anticoagulants, oral with Antifungals, Griseofulvin, page 60

Contraceptives, oral

Decreased contraceptive effect (increased metabolism)

> CPH vanDijke and JCP Weber, Interaction between oral contraceptives and griseofulvin. Br Med J, 288:1125, 1984

Use alternative contraceptive

Cyclosporine

Possible decreased cyclosporine effect (mechanism not established)

> SH Abu-Romeh and A Rashed, Ciclosporin A and griseofulvin: another drug interaction. Nephron, 58:237, 1991

Single case report (1991); patient also taking several other drugs

Nonsteroidal anti-inflammatory drugs

Decreased aspirin effect (mechanism not established)

> KR Phillips et al, Griseofulvin significantly decreases serum salicylate concentrations. Pediatr Infect Dis J, 12:350, 1993

Single case report (1993)

Theophyllines

Possible decreased theophylline effect (probably increased metabolism)

> BB Rasmussen et al, Griseofulvin and fluvoxamine interactions with the metabolism of theophylline. Ther Drug Monit, 19:56, 1997

Based on study in healthy subjects and case report (1997); monitor theophylline serum concentrations

ANTIFUNGALS, IMIDAZOLES AND TRIAZOLES, with:

Alcohol - See Alcohol with Antifungals, imidazoles and triazoles, page 13

Aminoglycoside antibiotics - See Aminoglycoside antibiotics with Antifungals, imidazoles and triazoles, page 30

Amprenavir - See Amprenavir with Antifungals, imidazoles and triazoles, page 38

Antacids - See Antacids with Antifungals, imidazoles and triazoles, page 50

Anticoagulants, oral - See Anticoagulants, oral with Antifungals, imidazoles and triazoles, page 60

Antidepressants, tricyclic - See Antidepressants, tricyclic with Antifungals, imidazoles and triazoles, page 81

Antihistamines, H_1-blockers: astemizole, terfenadine

Prolonged QT and torsades de pointes with ketoconazole, itraconazole, oxiconazole, or fluconazole and terfenadine or astemizole (decreased H_1 blocker metabolism)

> Manufacturer's package insert (astemizole); M Zimmerman et al, Torsades de pointes after treatment with terfenadine and ketoconazole. Eur Heart J, 13:1002, 1992; PK Honig et al, Terfenadine-ketoconazole interaction. JAMA, 269:1513, 1993; S Pohjola-Sintonen et al, Torsades de pointes after terfenadine-itraconazole interaction. BMJ, 306:186, 1993; JK Crane and H-T Shih, Syncope and cardiac arrhythmia due to an interaction between itraconazole and terfenadine. Am J Med, 95:445, 1993; LR Cantilena et al, Fluconazole alters terfenadine pharmacokinetics and electrocardiographic pharmacodynamics. Am Soc Clin Pharmacol Ther, 57:185, 1995; JS Griffith,

ANTIFUNGALS, IMIDAZOLES AND TRIAZOLES, with: *(continued)*
Interaction between terfenadine and topical antifungal agents. Am Fam Physician, 51:1396, 1995; RA Lefebvre et al, Influence of itraconazole on the pharmacokinetics and electrocardiographic effects of astemizole. Br J Clin Pharmacol, 43:319, 1997; W-C Tsai et al, Combined use of astemizole and ketoconazole resulting in torsade de pointes. J Formos Med Assoc, 96:144, 1997

Use antihistamine other than terfenadine or astemizole; single case with oxiconazole (1995); astemizole and terfenadine are no longer available

Antihistamines, H_1-blockers: Loratadine
Possible loratadine toxicity with ketoconazole (decreased metabolism)
A Van Peer et al, Ketoconazole inhibits loratadine metabolism in man. Allergy, 48 (suppl 16):34, 1993; MD Brannan et al, Effects of various cytochrome P450 inhibitors on the metabolism of loratadine. Clin Pharmacol Ther, 57,193, 1995

Clinical significance not established; loratadine does not appear to cause ventricular arrhythmias as has been reported with terfenadine and astemizole

Antihistamines, H_2-blockers
Decreased ketoconazole and itraconazole effect with cimetidine or ranitidine (decreased absorption)
RA Blum et al, Increased gastric pH and the bioavailability of fluconazole and ketoconazole. Ann Intern Med, 114:755, 1991; SC Piscitelli et al, Effects of ranitidine and sucralfate on ketoconazole bioavailability. Antimicrob Agents Chemother, 35:1765, 1991; D Lange et al, Effect of a cola beverage on the bioavailability of itraconazole in the presence of H_2 blockers. J Clin Pharmacol, 37:535, 1997; manufacturer's package insert

Avoid concurrent use; coadministration of itraconazole and an acidic solution, e.g. carbonated beverage, can prevent this interaction; theoretically, itraconazole oral solution would be less affected than capsules by H_2-receptor antagonists

Benzodiazepines
Possible chlordiazepoxide toxicity with ketoconazole (decreased metabolism)
MW Brown et al, Effect of ketoconazole on hepatic oxidative drug metabolism. Clin Pharmacol Ther, 37:290, 1985

Clinical significance not established, but concurrent use is best avoided

Midazolam toxicity with ketoconazole, itraconazole or fluconazole (decreased metabolism; CYP3A4)
KT Olkkola et al, Midazolam should be avoided in patients receiving the systemic antimycotics ketoconazole or itraconazole. Clin Pharmacol Ther, 55:481, 1994; JT Backman et al, The area under the plasma concentration-time curve for oral midazolam is 400-fold larger during treatment with itraconazole than with rifampicin. Eur J Clin Pharmacol, 54:53, 1998; YWF Lam et al, In vivo inhibition of midazolam disposition by ketoconazole and fluoxetine, and comparison to in vitro prediction. Clin Pharmacol Ther, 65:143, 1999; J Ahonen et al, Interaction between fluconazole and midazolam in intensive care patients. Acta Anaesthesiol Scand, 43:509, 1999; SM

ANTIFUNGALS, IMIDAZOLES AND TRIAZOLES, with: *(continued)*
>Tsunoda et al, Differentiation of intestinal and hepatic cytochrome P450 3A activity with use of midazolam as an in vivo probe: Effect of ketoconazole. Clin Pharmacol Ther, 66:461, 1999

Avoid concurrent use; based on studies in normal subjects and patients; effect greater with oral than parenteral midazolam

Triazolam toxicity with ketoconazole or itraconazole (decreased metabolism)
>A Varhe et al, Oral triazolam is potentially hazardous to patients receiving systemic antimycotics ketoconazole or itraconazole. Clin Pharmacol Ther, 56:601, 1994; DJ Greenblatt et al, Interaction of triazolam and ketoconazole. Lancet, 345:191, 1995; PJ Neuvonen et al, The effect of ingestion time interval on the interaction between itraconazole and triazolam. Clin Pharmacol Ther, 60:326, 1996; DJ Greenblatt et al, Ketoconazole inhibition of triazolam and alprazolam clearance: differential kinetic and dynamic consequences. Clin Pharmacol Ther, 64:237, 1998

Avoid concurrent use; based on studies in normal male and female subjects

Possible decrease in diazepam effect with itraconazole (probably decreased metabolism)
>J Ahonen et al, The effect of the antimycotic itraconazole on the pharmacokinetics and pharmacodynamics of diazepam. Fundam Clin Pharmacol, 10:314, 1996

Based on single dose diazepam study in healthy subjects; clinical significance not established

Possible alprazolam toxicity with ketoconazole or itraconazole (decreased metabolism; CYP3A4)
>DJ Greenblatt et al, Ketoconazole inhibition of triazolam and alprazolam clearance: differential kinetic and dynamic consequences. Clin Pharmacol Ther, 64:237, 1998; N Yasui et al, Effect of itraconazole on the single oral dose pharmacokinetics and pharmacodynamics of alprazolam. Psychopharmacology, 139:269, 1998

Based on studies in healthy subjects; monitor clinical status

Bupivacaine

Possible increased bupivacaine effect (probably decreased metabolism)
>VJ Palkama et al, Effect of itraconazole on the pharmacokinetics of bupivacaine enantiomers in healthy volunteers. Br J Anaesth, 83:659, 1999

Based on study in healthy subjects; clinical importance not established; effect modest (25% reduction in clearance); monitor clinical status

Buspirone

Possible buspirone toxicity with itraconazole (decreased metabolism; CYP3A4)
>KT Kivistö et al, Buspirone concentrations are greatly increased by erythromycin and itraconazole. Eur J Clin Pharmacol, 52:A134, 1997; KT Kivistö et al, Interactions of buspirone with itraconazole and rifampicin: effects on the pharmacokinetics of the active 1-(2-pyrimidinyl)-piperazine metabolite of buspirone. Pharmacol Toxicol, 84:94, 1999

(continued)

ANTIFUNGALS, IMIDAZOLES AND TRIAZOLES, with: *(continued)*
Avoid concurrent use; based on study in healthy subjects; ketoconazole likely to produce similar effect

Caffeine

Possible caffeine toxicity with fluconazole (decreased metabolism)
> DE Nix et al, The effect of fluconazole on the pharmacokinetics of caffeine in young and elderly subjects. Clin Pharmacol Ther, 51:183, 1992

Monitor cardiovascular status and possibly limit caffeine intake; based on study in both young and elderly healthy men

Carbamazepine

Decreased itraconazole effect (probably increased metabolism)
> RM Tucker et al, Interaction of azoles with rifampin, phenytoin, and carbamazepine: in vitro and clinical observations. Clin Infect Dis, 14:165, 1992

In patients receiving rifampin and/or carbamazepine and/or phenytoin

Possible carbamazepine toxicity with ketoconazole or fluconazole (decreased metabolism; CYP3A4)
> E Spina et al, Elevation of plasma carbamazepine concentrations by ketoconazole in patients with epilepsy. Ther Drug Monit, 19:535, 1997; DR Nair and HH Morris, Potential fluconazole-induced carbamazepine toxicity. Ann Pharmacother, 33:790, 1999

Monitor clinical status and serum carbamazepine concentration; itraconazole likely to interact as well

Cisapride

Possible ventricular arrhythmias with fluconazole, itraconazole, ketoconazole and miconazole; fatalities have occurred (decreased cisapride metabolism; CYP3A4)
> Manufacturer's package insert; EL Michalets and CR Williams, Drug interactions with cisapride. Clin Pharmacokinet, 39:49, 2000

Based on cases reported to the manufacturer and an in vitro study using human hepatic microsomes; avoid concurrent use; cisapride is no longer marketed in the USA

Contraceptives, oral

Decreased contraceptive effect with fluconazole, itraconazole, and ketoconazole (mechanism not established)
> PI Pillans and MJ Sparrow, Pregnancy associated with a combined oral contraceptive and itraconazole. NZ Med J, 106:436, 1993

Single case reports with itraconazole and ketoconazole; three reports with fluconazole (1993)

Menstrual disturbances with itraconazole and possible decreased contraceptive effect (possible decreased estrogen metabolism)
> RHB Meyboom et al, Disturbance of withdrawal bleeding during concomitant use of itraconazole and oral contraceptives. NZ Med J, 110:300, 1997; EP Van Puijenbroek et al, Verstoring van de pilcyclus tijdens het gelijktijdig gebruik van itraconazol en orale anticonceptiva. Ned Tijdschr Geneeskd, 142:146, 1998

ANTIFUNGALS, IMIDAZOLES AND TRIAZOLES, with: *(continued)*
  Avoid concurrent use
 Corticosteroids
  Possible toxicity of prednisone, methylprednisolone or budesonide with ketoconazole or itraconazole; might occur with other corticosteroids (decreased metabolism; CYP3A4, possibly decreased transport; p-glycoprotein)
   RJ Kandrotas et al, Ketoconazole effects on methylprednisolone disposition and their joint suppression of endogenous cortisol. Clin Pharmacol Ther, 42:465, 1987; RM Zürcher et al, Impact of ketoconazole on the metabolism of prednisolone. Clin Pharmacol Ther, 45:366, 1989; SK Yamashita et al, Lack of pharmacokinetic and pharmacodynamic interactions between ketoconazole and prednisolone. Clin Pharmacol Ther, 49:558, 1991; H Linthoudt et al, The association of itraconazole and methylprednisolone may give rise to important steroid-related side effects. J Heart Lung Transplant, 15:1165, 1996; T Varis et al, Plasma concentrations and effects of oral methylprednisolone are considerably increased by itraconazole. Clin Pharmacol Ther, 64:363, 1998; T Varis et al, Itraconazole decreases the clearance and enhances the effects of intravenously administered methylprednisolone in healthy volunteers. Pharmacol Toxicol, 85:29, 1999; T Varis et al, The effect of itraconazole on the pharmacokinetics and pharmacodynamics of oral prednisolone. Eur J Clin Pharmacol, 56:57, 2000; J Seidegård, Reduction of the inhibitory effect of ketoconazole on budesonide pharmacokinetics by separation of their time of administration. Clin Pharmacol Ther, 68:13, 2000
  Monitor corticosteroid effect; methylprednisolone and budesonide appear to be more affected than prednisone; effect on prednisolone appears to be small
 COX-2 inhibitors
  Possible celecoxib toxicity with fluconazole (decreased metabolism; CYP2C9)
   Manufacturer's package insert
  Manufacturer recommends beginning celecoxib at lowest recommended dosage in patients taking fluconazole
 Cyclosporine
  Renal toxicity with fluconazole, itraconazole, ketoconazole and miconazole (decreased presystemic cyclosporine metabolism)
   S Hariharan et al, The effect of diltiazem on cyclosporin A (CYA) bioavailability in patients treated with CYA and ketoconazole. J Am Soc Nephrol, 3:861, 1992 abs 106P; MR First et al, Cyclosporine-ketoconazole interaction. Transplantation, 55:1000, 1993; DM Canafax et al, Interaction between cyclosporine and fluconazole in renal allograft recipients. Transplantation, 51:1014, 1991; D Trenk et al, Time course of cyclosporin/itraconazole interaction. Lancet, 2:1335, 1987; MR Kramer et al, Cyclosporine and itraconazole interaction in heart and lung transplant recipients. Ann Intern Med, 113:327, 1990; RE Girardet et al, Concomitant administration of cyclosporine and ketoconazole for three and a half years in one heart transplant recipient. Transplantation, 48:887, 1989; DY Gomez et al, The effects of ketoconazole on the intestinal metabolism and bioavailability of cyclosporine. Clin Pharmacol Ther, 58:15, 1995; A Keogh et al, Ketoconazole to

(continued)

ANTIFUNGALS, IMIDAZOLES AND TRIAZOLES, with: *(continued)*
> reduce the need for cyclosporine after cardiac transplantation. N Engl J Med, 333:628, 1995; CL Osowski et al, Evaluation of the drug interaction between intravenous high-dose fluconazole and cyclosporine or tacrolimus in bone marrow transplant patients. Transplantation, 61:1268, 1996; P Jensen et al, Effect of oral terbinafine treatment on cyclosporin pharmacokinetics in organ transplant recipients with dermatophyte nail infection. Acta Derm Venereol, 76:280, 1996; AJ McLachlan and SE Tett, Effect of metabolic inhibitors on cyclosporine pharmacokinetics using a population approach. Ther Drug Monit, 20:390, 1998; A Foradori et al, Modification of the pharmacokinetics of cyclosporine A and metabolites by the concomitant use of Neoral and diltiazem or ketoconazol in stable adult kidney transplants. Transplant Proc, 30:1685, 1998; WK Sergent et al, Pharmacokinetics of the interaction between itraconazole oral solution and cyclosporine in stable post-liver transplant recipients. ASHP Midyear Clinical Meeting, 33:CR-19, 1998; K Sud et al, Unpredictable cyclosporin-fluconazole interaction in renal transplant recipients. Nephrol Dial Transplant, 14:1698, 1999; E Cohen et al, Cyclosporin drug-interaction-induced rhabdomyolysis. A report of two cases in lung transplant recipients. Transplantation, 70:119, 2000

Monitor cyclosporine concentrations and clinical status; renal toxicity may be prolonged after drugs are stopped; the combination has been used to reduce cyclosporine costs without toxicity with careful monitoring; postmortem studies in one patient revealed subclinical rejection; concomitant diltiazem may increase toxicity; terbinafine effect probably not clinically significant; microemulsionated formulation (Neoral) also interacts

Gingival hyperplasia (mechanism not established)
> S Veraldi and S Menni, Severe gingival hyperplasia following cyclosporin and ketoconazole therapy. Int J Dermatol, 27:730, 1988

Single case report (1988)

Delavirdine
Possible delavirdine toxicity with ketoconazole (probably decreased metabolism)
> Manufacturer's package insert

Based on population pharmacokinetic data from patients; monitor clinical status

Didanosine
Possible decreased didanosine effect with ketoconazole (decreased absorption)
> CA Knupp et al, A pharmacokinetic interaction study between didanosine (DDI) and ketoconazole (KET) in HIV patients. Clin Pharmacol Ther, 51:155, 1992 abs PII-37

No interaction if given 2 hours apart

Decreased itraconazole effect and probable decreased ketoconazole effect (decreased absorption – itraconazole requires low pH; didanosine buffered at pH 7-8)
> F Moreno et al, Itraconazole-didanosine excipient interaction. JAMA, 269:1508, 1993; DB May et al, Effect of simultaneous didanosine

ANTIFUNGALS, IMIDAZOLES AND TRIAZOLES, with: *(continued)*
>administration on itraconazole absorption in healthy volunteers. Pharmacotherapy, 14:509, 1994
>
>*Relapse of cryptococcal meningitis in HIV patients treated with itraconazole; do not give didanosine simultaneously with itraconazole or ketoconazole*

Digoxin
>Digoxin toxicity (visual and gastrointestinal) with itraconazole (decreased clearance; inhibition of transport, P-glycoprotein)
>>J Rex, Itraconazole-digoxin interaction. Ann Intern Med, 116:525, 1992; KL McClean and GJ Sheehan, Interaction between itraconazole and digoxin. Clin Infect Dis, 18:259, 1994; LA Cone et al, Itraconazole-related amaurosis and vomiting due to digoxin toxicity. West J Med, 165:322, 1996; CP Alderman and PD Allcroft, Digoxin-itraconazole interaction: possible mechanisms. Ann Pharmacother, 31:438, 1997; M Mochizuki et al, Serum itraconazole and hydroxyitraconazole concentrations and interaction with digoxin in a case of chronic hypertrophic pachymenigitis caused by *Aspergillus flavus*. Jpn J Med Mycol, 41:33, 2000
>
>*Monitor digoxin concentration and clinical status; interaction did not occur in one patient on low doses of both drugs (2000)*

Dofetilide
>Increased risk of arrhythmias with ketoconazole (decreased renal excretion of dofetilide)
>>Manufacturer's package insert (dofetilide)
>
>*Avoid concurrent use*

Donepezil
>Possible donepezil toxicity (mechanism not established)
>>PJ Tiseo et al, Concurrent administration of donepezil HCl and ketoconazole: assessment of pharmacokinetic changes following single and multiple doses. Br J Clin Pharmacol, 46 (suppl 1):30, 1998
>
>*Based on a study in healthy subjects; clinical significance not established*

Felodipine
>Possible felodipine toxicity with itraconazole (decreased metabolism; CYP3A4)
>>PJ Neuvonen and R Suhonen, Itraconazole interacts with felodipine. J Am Acad Dermatol, 33:134, 1995; K-M Jalava et al, Itraconazole greatly increases plasma concentrations and effects of felodipine. Clin Pharmacol Ther, 61:410, 1997
>
>*Based on two well-documented cases (1995) and study in healthy subjects*

Grapefruit juice
>Possible decreased itraconazole effect (probably decreased absorption)
>>SR Penzak et al, Grapefruit juice decreases the systemic availability of itraconazole capsules in healthy volunteers. Ther Drug Monit, 21:304, 1999
>
>*Based on study in healthy subjects; avoid concurrent use*

Haloperidol
>Possible haloperidol toxicity with itraconazole (probably decreased metabolism)
>>N Yasui et al, Effects of itraconazole on the steady-state plasma concentrations of haloperidol and its reduced metabolite in schizophrenic patients:

(continued)

ANTIFUNGALS, IMIDAZOLES AND TRIAZOLES, with: *(continued)*
   In vivo evidence of the involvement of CYP3A4 for haloperidol metabolism.
   J Clin Psychopharmacol, 19:149, 1999
   Based on study of schizophrenic patients; monitor clinical status

HMG-CoA reductase inhibitors

Rhabdomyolysis with lovastatin or simvastatin, and itraconazole, ketoconazole and probably fluconazole (decreased lovastatin and simvastatin metabolism; CYP3A4)

   RS Lees and AM Lees, Rhabdomyolysis from the coadministration of lovastatin and the antifungal agent itraconazole. N Engl J Med, 333:664, 1995; PJ Neuvonen and K-M Jalava, Itraconazole drastically increases plasma concentrations of lovastatin and lovastatin acid. Clin Pharmacol Ther, 60:54, 1996; M Horn, Coadministration of itraconazole with hypolipidemic agents may induce rhabdomyolysis in healthy individuals. Arch Dermatol, 132:1254, 1996; MF Segaert et al, Drug-interaction-induced rhabdomyolysis. Nephrol Dial Transplant, 11:1846, 1996; PJ Neuvonen et al, Simvastatin but not pravastatin is very susceptible to interaction with the CYP3A4 inhibitor itraconazole. Clin Pharmacol Ther, 63:332, 1998; KT Kivistö et al, Different effects of itraconazole on the pharmacokinetics of fluvastatin and lovastatin. Br J Clin Pharmacol, 46:49, 1998; T Kantola et al, Differential effects of itraconazole on fluvastatin and lovastatin pharmacokinetics. Eur J Clin Pharmacol, 52:A134, 1997; MB Bottorf, Distinct drug-interaction profiles for statins. Am J Health Syst Pharm, 56:1019, 1999; V Fischer et al, The 3-hydroxy-3-methylglutaryl coenzyme a reductase inhibitor fluvastatin: effect on human cytochrome P-450 and implications for metabolic drug interactions. Drug Metab Dispos, 27:410, 1999; W Jacobsen et al, Comparison of cytochrome P-450-dependent metabolism and drug interactions of the 3-hydroxy-3-methylglutaryl-CoA reductase inhibitors lovastatin and pravastatin in the liver. Drug Metab Dispos, 27:173, 1999; R Gilad and Y Lampl, Rhabdomyolysis induced by simvastatin and ketoconazole treatment. Clin Neuropharmacol, 22:295, 1999
   Avoid concurrent use; fluvastatin and pravastatin unlikely to interact

Possible atorvastatin or cerivastatin toxicity with itraconazole (decreased metabolism; CYP3A4)

   T Kantola et al, Effect of itraconazole on the pharmacokinetics of atorvastatin. Clin Pharmacol Ther, 64:58, 1998; T Kantola et al, Effect of itraconazole on cerivastatin pharmacokinetics. Eur J Clin Pharmacol, 54:851, 1999
   Clinical significance not established; ketoconazole and fluconazole may also interact; fluvastatin and pravastatin unlikely to interact

Hypoglycemics, sulfonylurea

Hypoglycemic coma with fluconazole and glipizide (possible decreased metabolism)

   JP Fournier et al, Coma hypoglycémique chez une patiente traitée par glipizide et fluconazole: une possible interaction? Therapie, 47:433, 1992
   Single case report (1992)

ANTIFUNGALS, IMIDAZOLES AND TRIAZOLES, with: *(continued)*

Hypoglycemia with tolbutamide and ketoconazole (decreased metabolism)
> YSR Krishnaiah et al, Interaction between tolbutamide and ketoconazole in healthy subjects. Br J Clin Pharmacol, 37:205, 1994

Based on a study of seven normal subjects

Severe hypoglycemia with miconazole and glibenclamide (mechanism not established)
> E Loupi et al, Interactions medicamenteuses et miconazole. Therapie, 37:437, 1982

Avoid concurrent use

Indinavir

Possible indinavir, and ketoconazole or itraconazole toxicity (probable decreased metabolism; CYP3A)
> Manufacturer's package insert; S DeWit et al, Effect of fluconazole on indinavir pharmacokinetics in human immunodeficiency virus-infected patients. Antimicrob Agents Chemother, 42:223, 1998; AR MacKenzie-Wood et al, Med J Aust, 170:46, 1999; SE Bellibas, Indinavir-fluconazole interaction. Antimicrob Agents Chemother, 43:432, 1999

Conflicting reports as to clinical significance; monitor concentration of both drugs when possible; fluconazole is a weaker inhibitor of CYP3A than ketoconazole or itraconazole

Irbesartan

Possible irbesartan toxicity (decreased metabolism; CYP2C9)
> SJ Kovacs et al, Steady state (SS) pharmacokinetics (PK) of irbesartan alone and in combination with fluconazole (F). Clin Pharmacol Ther, 65:132, 1999

Based on study in healthy subjects; monitor clinical status

Isoniazid

Decreased ketoconazole effect (decreased blood concentration)
> D Engelhard et al, Interaction of ketoconazole with rifampin and isoniazid. N Engl J Med, 311:1681, 1984

Avoid concurrent use, if possible; if not, monitor ketoconazole concentration

Lidocaine

Possible oral lidocaine toxicity with itraconazole (probably decreased first-pass metabolism; CYP3A4)
> MH Isohanni et al, Effect of erythromycin and itraconazole on the pharmacokinetics of oral lignocaine. Pharmacol Toxicol, 84:143, 1999

Based on study in healthy subjects; monitor clinical status; theoretically ketoconazole and, to a lesser extent, fluconazole would interact similarly

Lopinavir/Ritonavir

Possible ketoconazole or itraconazole toxicity (decreased metabolism)
> Manufacturer's package insert (*Kaletra*)

Avoid high dose (>200 mg/day) ketoconazole and itraconazole

Losartan

Possible losartan toxicity with fluconazole (decreased metabolism; CYP2C9)
> DJ Kazierad et al, Effect of fluconazole on the pharmacokinetics of

(continued)

ANTIFUNGALS, IMIDAZOLES AND TRIAZOLES, with: *(continued)*
>
> eprosartan and losartan in healthy male volunteers. Clin Pharmacol Ther, 62:417, 1997; K-M Kaukonen et al, Fluconazole but not itraconazole decreases the metabolism of losartan to E-3174. Eur J Clin Pharmacol, 53:445, 1998
>
> *Based on study in healthy subjects; monitor clinical status; itraconazole may not interact*

Macrolide antibiotics
>
> Possible enhanced clarithromycin effect with itraconazole (decreased metabolism)
>
>> B Auclair et al, Potential interaction between itraconazole and clarithromycin. Pharmacotherapy, 19:1439, 1999
>>
>> *Based on study in 3 patients treated for Mycobacterium avium complex (MAC) infection; clinical importance not established*

Narcotics: meperidine and congeners
>
> Alfentanil toxicity with fluconazole (decreased metabolism; CYP3A4)
>
>> VJ Palkama et al, The effect of intravenous and oral fluconazole on the pharmacokinetics and pharmacodynamics of intravenous alfentanil. Anesth Analg, 87:190, 1998; VJ Palkama et al, The CYP3A4 inhibitor itraconazole has no effect on the pharmacokinetics of i.v. fentanyl. Br J Anaesth, 81:598, 1998
>>
>> *Based on study in healthy subjects; both oral and IV fluconazole had a similar effect; monitor clinical status; itraconazole had no effect on IV fentanyl in 10 healthy subjects*

Narcotics: methadone and congeners
>
> Possible methadone toxicity with fluconazole (probably decreased metabolism)
>
>> MN Cobb et al, The effect of fluconazole on the clinical pharmacokinetics of methadone. Clin Pharmacol Ther, 63:655, 1998
>>
>> *Based on study of subjects on methadone maintenance; clinical significance not established*

Nifedipine
>
> Possible nifedipine toxicity (probably decreased metabolism due to CYP3A inhibition)
>
>> B Kremens et al, Loss of blood pressure control on withdrawal of fluconazole during nifedipine therapy. Br J Clin Pharmacol, 47:707, 1999
>>
>> *Single case report of loss of blood pressure control with discontinuation of fluconazole therapy (1999)*

Nisoldipine
>
> Possible increased nisoldipine toxicity (decreased metabolism; CYP3A4)
>
>> R Heinig et al, The effect of ketoconazole on the pharmacokinetics, pharmacodynamics and safety of nisoldipine. Eur J Clin Pharmacol, 55:57, 1999
>>
>> *Based on study in healthy subjects; marked increase in nisoldipine concentrations; monitor clinical status; avoid concommitant use of CYP3A inhibitors*

Omeprazole
>
> Decreased ketoconazole and itraconazole effect (decreased pH dependency absorption)
>
>> TWF Chin et al, Effects of an acidic beverage (coca-cola) on absorption of

ANTIFUNGALS, IMIDAZOLES AND TRIAZOLES, with: *(continued)*
> ketoconazole. Antimicrob Agents Chemother, 39:1671, 1995; S Jarura-
> tanasirikul and S Sriwiriyajan, Effect of omeprazole on the pharmacokine-
> tics of itraconazole. Eur J Clin Pharmacol, 54:159, 1998
>
> *Based on studies in healthy subjects; concurrent cola beverage improved absorption; effect likely with all proton-pump inhibitors*
>
> Possible omeprazole toxicity with ketoconazole (decreased metabolism)
> > Y Böttiger et al, Inhibition of the sulfoxidation of omeprazole by ketocona-
> > zole in poor and extensive metabolizers of S-mephenytoin. Clin Pharmacol
> > Ther, 62:384, 1997
> >
> > *Based on study in normal subjects; effect greater in patients deficient in CYP2C19*

Paclitaxel
> Possible paclitaxel toxicity (probably decreased metabolism; CYP3A4)
> > JD Schwartz et al, Potential interaction of antiretroviral therapy with pacli-
> > taxel in patients with AIDS-related Kaposi's sarcoma. AIDS, 13:283, 1999
> >
> > *Single case report (1999); patient also received two other CYP3A4 inhibitors (delavirdine, saquinavir); theoretically, itraconazole and ketoconazole would also interact*

Phenytoin
> Phenytoin toxicity with fluconazole or miconazole (decreased metabolism)
> > RA Blum et al, Effect of fluconazole on the disposition of phenytoin. Clin
> > Pharmacol Ther, 49:420, 1991; PE Rolan et al, Phenytoin intoxication during
> > treatment with parenteral miconazole. Br Med J, 287:1760, 1983
> >
> > *Monitor phenytoin concentration*
>
> Decreased itraconazole effect (possibly increased metabolism)
> > RM Tucker et al, Interaction of azoles with rifampin, phenytoin, and carba-
> > mazepine: in vitro and clinical observations. Clin Infect Dis, 14:165, 1992
> >
> > *In patients receiving rifampin and/or carbamazepine and/or phenytoin*
>
> Altered effects of ketoconazole and/or phenytoin (possible metabolic effects)
> > Manufacturer's package insert (ketoconazole)
> >
> > *Monitor serum concentrations*

Pimozide
> Increased pimozide toxiciity with itraconazole (decreased metabolism)
> > Manufacturer's package insert (itraconazole)
> >
> > *Avoid concurrent use of itraconazole and pimozide*

Quinidine
> Possible quinidine toxicity (decreased metabolism; CYP3A4 and decreased bili-
> ary and renal excretion; P-glycoprotein)
> > RM McNulty et al, Transient increase in plasma quinidine concentrations
> > during ketoconazole-quinidine therapy. Clin Pharm, 8:222, 1989; K-M Kau-
> > konen et al, Itraconazole increases plasma concentrations of quinidine. Clin
> > Pharmacol Ther, 62:510, 1997; P Damkier et al, Effect of diclofenac,
> > disulfiram, itraconazole, grapefruit juice and erythromycin on the pharma-
> > cokinetics of quinidine. Br J Clin Pharmacol, 48:829, 1999; manufacturer's
> > package insert (itraconazole)

(continued)

ANTIFUNGALS, IMIDAZOLES AND TRIAZOLES, with: *(continued)*
Single case report with ketoconazole (1989); two studies in healthy subjects with itraconazole; monitor quinidine concentration; avoid concurrent use of itraconazole and quinidine

Rabeprazole
Possible decreased ketoconazole effect (decreased absorption)
> Manufacturer's package insert (rabeprazole)

Based on study in normal subjects; 30% decrease in bioavailability of ketoconazole; monitor clinical status

Reboxetine
Possible reboxetine toxicity with ketoconazole (decreased metabolism; CYP3A4)
> BD Herman et al, Ketoconazole inhibits the clearance of the enantiomers of the antidepressant reboxetine in humans. Clin Pharmacol Ther, 66:374, 1999

Based on study in healthy subjects; monitor clinical status

Rifabutin
Uveitis with fluconazole or itraconazole; theoretically should also occur with ketoconazole (decreased rifabutin metabolism; CYP3A4)
> JD Fuller et al, Rifabutin prophylaxis and uveitis. N Engl J Med, 330:1315, 1994; CB Trapnell et al, Increased plasma rifabutin levels with concomitant fluconazole therapy in HIV-infected patients. Ann Intern Med, 14:573, 1996; A Lefort et al, Uveitis associated with rifabutin prophylaxis and itraconazole therapy. Ann Intern Med, 125:939, 1996

Single case reports with fluconazole (1994) and itraconazole (1996)

Rifampin
Decreased fluconazole, itraconazole and ketoconazole effect (increased metabolism)
> N Doble et al, Pharmacokinetic study of the interaction between rifampicin and ketoconazole. J Antimicrob Chemother, 21:633, 1988; RJ Coker et al, Interaction between fluconazole and rifampicin. BMJ, 301:818, 1990; G Apseloff et al, Induction of fluconazole metabolism by rifampin: *in vivo* study in humans. J Clin Pharmacol, 31:358, 1991; J Drayton et al, Coadministration of rifampin and itraconazole leads to undetectable levels of serum itraconazole. Clin Infect Dis, 18:266, 1994; DP Nicolau et al, Rifampin-fluconazole interaction in critically ill patients. Ann Pharmacother, 29:994, 1995; S Jaruratanasirikul and A Kleepkaew, Lack of effect of fluconazole on the pharmacokinetics of rifampicin in AIDS patients. J Antimicrob Chemother, 38:877, 1996; S Jaruratanasirikul and S. Sriwiriyajan, Effect of rifampicin on the pharmacokinetics of itraconazole in normal volunteers and AIDS patients. Eur J Clin Pharmacol, 54:155, 1998

Avoid concurrent use if possible; possible decreased rifampin effect with ketoconazole in some patients but not normal subjects; fluconazole may not affect rifampin pharmacokinetics in patients

ANTIFUNGALS, IMIDAZOLES AND TRIAZOLES, with: *(continued)*

Ritonavir
Possible ritonavir and itraconazole or ketoconazole toxicity (mutual decreased metabolism; CYP3A)
> AR MacKenzie-Wood et al, Itraconazole and HIV protease inhibitors: an important interaction. Med J Aust, 170:46, 1999; manufacturer's package insert (ritonavir)

Monitor clinical status

Saquinavir
Possible saquinavir toxicity (probably inhibition of P-glycoprotein; decreased metabolism; CYP3A4)
> CHW Koks et al, Itraconazole as an alternative for ritonavir liquid formulation when combined with saquinavir. AIDS, 14:89, 2000

Interaction used intentionally in 3 patients to increase saquinavir (Invirase – hard gelatin capsule formulation) plasma concentrations; monitor clinical status

Selective serotonin reuptake inhibitors (SSRIs)
Possible fluoxetine toxicity with itraconazole (possible decreased metabolism of fluoxetine metabolite)
> PN Black, Probable interaction between fluoxetine and itraconazole. Ann Pharmacother, 29:1048, 1995

Single case report (1995); monitor clinical status

Sibutramine
Possible sibutramine toxicity with itraconazole and ketoconazole (decreased metabolism)
> Manufacturer's package insert

Monitor clinical status

Sildenafil
Possible sildenafil toxicity (probably decreased metabolism)
> Manufacturer's package insert; JS Warrington et al, In vitro biotransformation of sildenafil (Viagra): indentification of human cytochromes and potential drug interactions. Drug Metab Dispos, 28:392, 2000

Theoretical; monitor clinical status; avoid the combination if possible; consider decreasing sildenafil dose

Sirolimus
Possible sirolimus toxicity with ketoconazole
> Manufacturer's package insert (sirolimus)

Avoid concurrent use

Sucralfate
Possible decreased ketoconazole effect (decreased absorption)
> PL Carver et al, *In vivo* interaction of ketoconazole and sucralfate in healthy volunteers. Antimicrob Agents Chemother, 38:326, 1994

Give at least 2 hours apart; based on studies in healthy men

Tacrolimus
Possible tacrolimus toxicity with fluconazole, itraconazole or ketoconazole (decreased metabolism; CYP3A; possibly decreased transport; P-glycoprotein)
> R Assan et al, FK506/Fluconazole interaction enhances FK506

(continued)

ANTIFUNGALS, IMIDAZOLES AND TRIAZOLES, with: *(continued)*
nephrotoxicity. Diabete Metab, 20:49, 1994; CL Osowski et al, Evaluation of the drug interaction between intravenous high-dose fluconazole and cyclosporine or tacrolimus in bone marrow transplant patients. Transplantation. 61:1268, 1996; LC Floren et al, Tacrolimus oral bioavailability doubles with coadministration of ketoconazole. Clin Pharmacol Ther, 62:41, 1997; A Dhawan et al, Tacrolimus (FK506) malabsorption: management with fluconazole coadministration. Transpl Int, 10:331, 1997; EM Billaud et al, Evidence for a pharmacokinetic interaction between itraconazole and tacrolimus in organ transplant patients. Br J Clin Pharmacol, 46:271, 1998; M Moreno et al, Clinical management of tacrolimus drug interactions in renal transplant patients. Transplant Proc, 31:2252, 1999; D Capone et al, Effects of itraconazole on tacrolimus blood concentrations in a renal transplant recipient. Ann Pharmacother, 33:1124, 1999; MO Macías et al, Tacrolimus-itraconazole interaction in a kidney transplant patient. Ann Pharmacother, 34:536, 2000

Monitor tacrolimus concentration; fluconazole has been used to increase subtherapeutic tacrolimus concentrations

Tacrolimus toxicity with clotrimazole (mechanism not established)
L Mieles et al, Interaction between FK506 and clotrimazole in a liver transplant recipient. Transplantation, 52:1086, 1991

Monitor tacrolimus concentration

Theophyllines
Possible decreased theophylline effect with ketoconazole (increased metabolism)
E Murphy et al, Ketoconazole – theophylline interaction. Ir Med J, 80:123, 1987

Monitor theophylline concentration; single case report with oral long-acting theophylline (1987)

Possible IV theophylline toxicity with ketoconazole (decreased metabolism)
JJ Heusner et al, Effect of chronically administered ketoconazole on the elimination of theophylline in man. Drug Intell Clin Pharm, 21:514, 1987

Questionable clinical significance; based on studies in healthy subjects, who showed a large individual variation

Possible theophylline toxicity with fluconazole (decreased metabolism)
H Konishi et al, Effect of fluconazole on theophylline disposition in humans. Eur J Clin Pharmacol, 46:309, 1994

Questionable clinical significance, based on study of normal subject

Verapamil
Possible verapamil toxicity (decreased metabolism; CYP3A4 and possibly P-glycoprotein transport)
R Sandström et al, The effect of ketoconazole on the jejunal permeability and CYP3A metabolism of (R/S)-verapamil in humans. Br J Clin Pharmacol, 48:180, 1999

ANTIFUNGALS, IMIDAZOLES AND TRIAZOLES, with: *(continued)*
Based on study in healthy subjects with ketoconazole; itraconazole and large doses of fluconazole likely to interact similarly; monitor clinical status

Vincristine

Severe neurotoxicity (probably decreased metabolism)

A Böhme et al, Unusual severe vincristine-induced neurotoxicity in four patients with all simultaneously receiving antifungal prophylaxis with itraconazole. Onkologie, 17(suppl 2):13, 1994; JA Murphy et al, Vincristine toxicity in five children with acute lymphoblastic leukaemia. Lancet, 346:443, 1995; A Böhme et al, Aggravation of vincristine-induced neurotoxicity by itraconazole in the treatment of adult ALL. Ann Hematol, 71:311, 1995; J Gillies et al, Severe vincristine toxicity in combination with itraconazole. Clin Lab Haematol, 20:123, 1998

Avoid concurrent use

Zidovudine

Possible zidovudine toxicity with fluconazole (decreased metabolism)

J Sahai et al, Effect of fluconazole on zidovudine pharmacokinetics in patients infected with human immunodeficiency virus. J Infect Dis, 169:1103, 1994; NH Brockmeyer et al, Pharmacokinetic interaction of fluconazole and zidovudine in HIV-positive patients. Eur J Med Res, 2:377, 1997

Monitor clinical status and zidovudine concentration; one study found only small increases in zidovudine plasma concentrations (1997)

Zolpidem

Possible zolpidem toxicity with ketoconazole (decreased metabolism; CYP3A)

DJ Greenblatt et al, Kinetic and dynamic interaction study of zolpidem with ketoconazole, itraconazole, and fluconazole. Clin Pharmacol Ther, 64:661, 1998

Based on study in healthy subjects; monitor clinical status; itraconazole and fluconazole had only small effect on zolpidem

ANTIFUNGALS, TERBINAFINE, with:

Anticoagulants, oral - See Anticoagulants, oral with Antifungals, terbinafine, page 61

Antidepressants, tricyclic - See Antidepressants, tricyclic with Antifungals, terbinafine, page 81

Cyclosporine

Possible decrease in cyclosporine effect (mechanism not established)

ACY Lo et al, The interaction of terbinafine and cyclosporine A in renal transplant patients. Br J Clin Pharmacol, 43:340, 1997

One of 4 patients who were given the combination required increased cyclosporine dosage

ANTIHISTAMINES, H$_1$-BLOCKERS: ASTEMIZOLE, TERFENADINE, with:

Acetaminophen - See Acetaminophen with Antihistamines, H$_1$-blockers: astemizole, terfenadine, page 7

Amprenavir - See Amprenavir with Antihistamines, H$_1$-blockers: astemizole, terfenadine, page 38

(continued)

ANTIHISTAMINES, H$_1$-BLOCKERS: ASTEMIZOLE, TERFENADINE, with: *(continued)*

Antifungals, imidazoles and triazoles - See Antifungals, imidazoles and triazoles with Antihistamines, H$_1$-blockers: astemizole, terfenadine, page 95

Beta-adrenergic blockers

Torsades de pointes with terfenadine or astemizole and sotalol (additive)
H Feroze et al, Torsades de pointes from terfenadine and sotalol given in combination. Pacing Clin Electrophysiol, 19:1519, 1996
Use antihistamine other than terfenadine or astemizole; single case report (1996); astemizole and terfenadine are no longer available

Carbamazepine

Carbamazepine toxicity with terfenadine (possible displacement from binding)
S Hirschfeld and P Jarosinski, Drug interaction of terfenadine and carbamazepine. Ann Intern Med, 118:907, 1993
Single case report (1993); monitor clinical status, and free carbamazepine concentration if available; terfenadine is no longer available

Delavirdine

Delavirdine decreases metabolism and may increase toxicity; high concentrations of astemizole or terfenadine may lead to dangerous cardiac arrhythmias
Manufacturer's package insert
Theoretical; manufacturer recommends avoiding concurrent use if possible; astemizole and terfenadine are no longer available

Efavirenz

Possible arrhythmias with astemizole (decreased metabolism)
Manufacturer's package insert (efavirenz)
Manufacturer recommends avoiding concurrent use; theoretical; astemizole is no longer available

Fluoroquinolones

Possible ventricular arrhythmia with sparfloxacin or grepafloxacin and astemizole or terfenadine (decreased antihistamine metabolism; also additive with grepafloxacin)
Manufacturer's package insert
Theoretical; manufacturer recommends avoiding concurrent use; astemizole and terfenadine are no longer available

Grapefruit juice

Possible increase in risk of ventricular arrhythmias with terfenadine or astemizole (decreased metabolism)
P Honig et al, Pharmacokinetics and cardiac effects of terfenadine in poor metabolizers receiving concomitant grapefruit juice. Clin Pharmacol Ther, 57:185, 1995; SE Rau et al, Grapefruit juice-terfenadine single-dose interaction: magnitude, mechanism, and relevance. Clin Pharmacol Ther, 61:401, 1997; CP Clifford et al, The cardiac effects of terfenadine after inhibition of its metabolism by grapefruit juice. Eur J Clin Pharmacol, 52:311, 1997; manufacturer's package insert
Based on studies with terfenadine in healthy subjects; monitor ECG; avoid concurrent use; astemizole and terfenadine are no longer available

ANTIHISTAMINES, H$_1$-BLOCKERS: ASTEMIZOLE, TERFENADINE, with: *(continued)*

Indinavir

Possible ventricular arrhythmia with astemizole or terfenadine (decreased antihistamine metabolism)

Manufacturer's package insert

Theoretical; manufacturer recommends avoiding concurrent use; astemizole and terfenadine are no longer available

Macrolide antibiotics

Arrhythmias with terfenadine or astemizole (decreased metabolism)

KE Biglin, Drug-induced torsades de pointes: a possible interaction of terfenadine and erythromycin. Ann Pharmacother, 28:282, 1994; PK Honig et al, Comparison of the effect of the macrolide antibiotics erythromycin, clarithromycin and azithromycin on terfenadine steady-state pharmacokinetics and electrocardiographic parameters. Drug Invest, 7:148, 1994; S Harris et al, Azithromycin and terfenadine: lack of drug interaction. Clin Pharmacol Ther, 58:310, 1995; MJ Goldberg et al, Effect of dirithromycin on human CYP3A *in vitro* and on pharmacokinetics and pharmacodynamics of terfenadine *in vivo*. J Clin Pharmacol, 36:1154, 1996; VS Watkins et al, Drug interactions of macrolides: emphasis on dirithromycin. Ann Pharmacother, 31:349, 1997; K Bachmann et al, A study of the interaction between dirithromycin and astemizole in healthy adults. Am J Ther, 4:73, 1997

Use antihistamine other than terfenadine or astemizole; azithromycin and dirithromycin do not appear to interact with terfenadine or astemizole; astemizole and terfenadine are no longer available

Nefazodone

Possible ventricular arrhythmias (decreased terfenadine and astemizole metabolism)

Manufacturer's package insert; astemizole and terfenadine are no longer available

Theoretical; manufacturer recommends avoiding concurrent use

Nelfinavir

Astemizole and terfenadine toxicity (decreased metabolism; CYP3A)

Manufacturer's package insert (nelfinavir)

Avoid concurrent use; astemizole and terfenadine are no longer available

Nifedipine

Possible nifedipine toxicity with terfenadine (mechanism not established)

HM Falkenberg, Possible interaction report. Can Pharm J, 121:294, 1988

Single case report (1988); terfenadine is no longer available

Quinine

Ventricular arrhythmia with astemizole (decreased astemizole metabolism)

Manufacturer's package insert (astemizole); ES Martin et al, Quinine may trigger torsades de pointes during astemizole therapy. Pacing Clin Electrophysiol, 20:2024, 1997

Avoid concurrent use; astemizole is no longer available

(continued)

ANTIHISTAMINES, H$_1$-BLOCKERS: ASTEMIZOLE, TERFENADINE, with: *(continued)*

Ritonavir
Possible ventricular arrhythmia with astemizole or terfenadine (decreased antihistamine metabolism)

Manufacturer's package insert (ritonavir)

Theoretical; listed as contraindicated in product information; astemizole and terfenadine are no longer available

Saquinavir
Possible ventricular arrhythmia with astemizole or terfenadine (decreased antihistamine metabolism)

K Jorga and NE Buss, Pharmacokinetic (PK) drug interaction with saquinavir soft gelatin capsule. Intersci Conf Antimicrob Agents Chemother, 39:20, 1999, abstract 339; N Buss, Saquinavir soft gel capsule (Fortovase): pharmacokinetics and drug interactions. Conf Retrovir Opportun Infect, 5:145, 1998, abs 354; Manufacturer's package insert

Product information states that concomitant use is not recommended; astemizole and terfenadine are no longer available

Selective serotonin reuptake inhibitors (SSRIs)
Possible arrhythmia with astemizole and fluoxetine, fluvoxamine, paroxetine or sertraline (mechanism not established); terfenadine may not interact with fluoxetine, paroxetine or sertraline.

Manufacturer's package insert (astemizole); RJ Marchiando and MD Cook, Probable terfenadine-fluoxetine-associated cardiac toxicity. Ann Pharmacother, 29:937, 1995; FDC Reports, Pharmaceutical Approvals Monthly, 2:23, April 1997; DE Martin et al, Paroxetine does not affect the cardiac safety and pharmacokinetics of terfenadine in healthy adult men. J Clin Psychopharmacol, 17:451, 1997; RF Bergstrom et al, Assessment of the potential for a pharmacokinetic interaction between fluoxetine and terfenadine. Clin Pharmacol Ther, 62:643, 1997

Avoid concurrent use; astemizole and terfenadine are no longer available

Troglitazone
Possible decreased terfenadine effect (increased metabolism; probably CYP3A4)

Manufacturer's package insert (troglitazone)

Avoid concurrent use; terfenadine is no longer available

Troleandomycin
Abnormal ECG with terfenadine and possibly astemizole (elevated concentrations due to decreased metabolism)

P Fournier et al, Une nouvelle cause de torsades de pointes: association terfénadine et troléandomycine. Ann Cardiol Angéiol, 42:249, 1993; manufacturer's package insert

Arrhythmias have occurred with elevated terfenadine concentrations; avoid concurrent use; astemizole and terfenadine are no longer available

Verapamil
Possible verapamil toxicity with terfenadine (mechanism not established)

HM Falkenberg, Possible interaction report. Can Pharm J, 121:294, 1988

ANTIHISTAMINES, H₁-BLOCKERS: ASTEMIZOLE, TERFENADINE, with: *(continued)*
Single case report (1988); terfenadine is no longer available

Zafirlukast
Possible decreased zafirlukast effect with terfenadine (increased metabolism; CYP3A4)

Manufacturer's package insert

Avoid concurrent use if zafirlukast concentration can not be monitored; terfenadine is no longer available

Zileuton
Possible astemizole or terfenadine toxicity (decreased metabolism)

Manufacturer's package insert; WM Awni et al, The pharmacokinetic and pharmacodynamic interaction between zileuton and terfenadine. Eur J Clin Pharmacol, 52:49, 1997

Study in 16 healthy subjects found increases in terfenadine serum levels but no changes in the ECG; avoid concurrent use; astemizone and terfenadine are no longer available

ANTIHISTAMINES, H₁-BLOCKERS: DIPHENHYDRAMINE, with:

Acetaminophen - See Acetaminophen with Antihistamines, H₁-blockers: diphenhydramine, page 8

Beta-adrenergic blockers
Possible metoprolol toxicity with diphenhydramine (decreased metabolism; CYP2D6)

BA Hamelin et al, Significant interaction between the nonprescription antihistamine diphenhydramine and the CYP2D6 substrate metoprolol in healthy men with high or low CYP2D6 activity. Clin Pharmacol Ther, 67:466, 2000

Based on study in healthy subjects; interaction occurred in subjects with high CYP2D6 activity (EMs) but not in those with low CYP2D6 activity (PMs)

Venlafaxine
Possible venlafaxine toxicity with diphenhydramine (decreased metabolism; CYP2D6)

E Lessard et al, Venlafaxine-diphenhydramine interaction in subjects with extensive or poor CYP2D6 activity. Clin Pharmacol Ther, 65:171, 1999

Based on study in healthy subjects; monitor clinical status

ANTIHISTAMINES, H₁-BLOCKERS: LORATADINE, with:

Antifungals, imidazoles and triazoles - See Antifungals, imidazoles and triazoles with Antihistamines, H₁-blockers: Loratadine, page 96

Antihistamines, H₂-blockers
Possible loratadine toxicity with cimetidine (probably decreased metabolism)

MD Brannan et al, Effects of various cytochrome P450 inhibitors on the metabolism of loratadine. Clin Pharmacol Ther, 57:193, 1995

Clinical significance not established; loratadine does not appear to cause ventricular arrhythmias as has been reported with terfenadine and astemizole

Macrolide antibiotics
Possible loratadine toxicity with erythromycin or clarithromycin (probably decreased metabolism)

MD Branna et al, Effects of various cytochrome P450 inhibitors on the

(continued)

ANTIHISTAMINES, H₁-BLOCKERS: LORATADINE, with: *(continued)*
    metabolism of loratadine. Clin Pharmacol Ther, 57:193, 1995; MD Brannan et al, Loratadine administered concomitantly with erythromycin: pharmacokinetic and electrocardiographic evaluations. Clin Pharmacol Ther, 58:269, 1995; RA Carr et al, Steady-state pharmacokinetics and electrocardiographic pharmacodynamics of clarithromycin and loratadine after individual or concomitant administration. Antimicrob Agents Chemother, 42:1176, 1998

Clinical significance not established; loratadine does not appear to cause ventricular arrhythmias as has been reported with terfenadine and astemizole

ANTIHISTAMINES, H₂-BLOCKERS, with:
  Alcohol - See Alcohol with Antihistamines, H₂-blockers, page 14
  Angiotensin-converting enzyme (ACE) inhibitors - See Angiotensin-converting enzyme (ACE) inhibitors with Antihistamines, H₂-blockers, page 43
  Antacids - See Antacids with Antihistamines, H₂-blockers, page 50
  Anticholinergics - See Anticholinergics with Antihistamines, H₂-blockers, page 58
  Anticoagulants, oral - See Anticoagulants, oral with Antihistamines, H₂-blockers, page 61
  Antidepressants, tricyclic - See Antidepressants, tricyclic with Antihistamines, H₂-blockers, page 81
  Antifungals, imidazoles and triazoles - See Antifungals, imidazoles and triazoles with Antihistamines, H₂-blockers, page 96
  Antihistamines, H₁-blockers: loratadine - See Antihistamines, H₁-blockers: loratadine with Antihistamines, H₂-blockers, page 113
  Barbiturates
    Possible decreased cimetidine effect (increased metabolism)
      A Somogyi et al, Influence of phenobarbital treatment on cimetidine kinetics. Eur J Clin Pharmacol, 19:343, 1981
    Small effect; significance not established
  Benzodiazepines
    Possible benzodiazepine toxicity with cimetidine (decreased metabolism)
      PV Desmond et al, Cimetidine impairs elimination of chlordiazepoxide *(Librium)* in man. Ann Intern Med, 93:266, 1980; DJ Greenblatt et al, Noninteraction of temazepam and cimetidine. J Pharm Sci, 73:399, 1984; DJ Greenblatt et al, Interaction of cimetidine with oxazepam, clorazepam, and flurazepam. J Clin Pharmacol, 24:187, 1984; S Pourbaix et al, Pharmacokinetic consequences of long term coadministration of cimetidine and triazolobenzodiazepines, alprazolam and triazolam, in healthy subjects. Int J Clin Pharmacol Ther Toxicol, 23:447, 1985; A Locniskar et al, Interaction of diazepam with famotidine and cimetidine, two H₂-receptor antagonists. J Clin Pharmacol, 26:299, 1986; H Friedman et al, Triazolam kinetics: interaction with cimetidine, propranolol, and the combination. J Clin Pharmacol, 28:228, 1988
    Monitor clinical status; oxazepam, lorazepam, and temazepam do not interact; famotidine, and possibly nizatidine, may be used instead of cimetidine

ANTIHISTAMINES, H$_2$-BLOCKERS, with: *(continued)*

Altered benzodiazepine effect with ranitidine (altered absorption; mechanism involving midazolam not established)

> JPH Fee et al, Cimetidine and ranitidine increase midazolam bioavailability. Clin Pharmacol Ther, 41:80, 1987; CM Wilson et al, Effect of pretreatment with ranitidine on the hypnotic action of single doses of midazolam, temazepam and zopiclone. Br J Anaesth, 58:483, 1986; U Klotz et al, Nocturnal doses of ranitidine and nizatidine do not affect the disposition of diazepam. J Clin Pharmacol, 27:210, 1987; RP Vanderveen et al, Effect of ranitidine on the disposition of orally and intravenously administered triazolam. Clin Pharm, 10:539, 1991

Monitor benzodiazepine effect or concentration; diazepam absorption was decreased; temazepam, nizatidine, and zopiclone may not interact

Beta-adrenergic blockers

Possible beta-blocker toxicity with high doses of cimetidine (decreased metabolism and decreased renal excretion in varying degrees for all stereoisomers)

> W Kirch et al, Interaction of cimetidine with metoprolol, propranolol, or atenolol. Lancet, 2:531, 1981; J Feely et al, Reduction of liver blood flow and propranolol metabolism by cimetidine. N Engl J Med, 304:692, 1981; E Rey et al, Effect of cimetidine on the pharmacokinetics of the new β-blocker betaxolol. Arzneimittelforschung, 37:952, 1987; RL Lalonde et al, Labetalol pharmacokinetics and pharmacodynamics: evidence of stereoselective disposition. Clin Pharmacol Ther, 48:509, 1990; AA Somogyi et al, Stereoselective inhibition of pindolol renal clearance by cimetidine in humans. Clin Pharmacol Ther, 51:379, 1992; W Kirch et al, Interaction of bisoprolol with cimetidine and rifampicin. Eur J Clin Pharmacol, 31:59, 1986; Y Ishii et al, Drug interaction between cimetidine and timolol ophthalmic solution: effect on heart rate and intraocular pressure in healthy Japanese volunteers. J Clin Pharmacol, 40:193, 2000

Monitor cardiac performance; may not occur with betaxolol or bisoprolol; may occur with ophthalmic timolol

Possible ophthalmoplegia with cimetidine (mechanism not established)

> GM Cunningham, Drug-induced internuclear ophthalmoplegia. Can Med Assoc J, 128:892, 1983

Single case report (1983)

Possible metoprolol toxicity with ranitidine (decreased metabolism)

> JG Kelly et al, Effects of ranitidine on the disposition of metoprolol. Br J Clin Pharmacol, 19:219, 1985

Clinical significance not established

Bupivacaine

Possible bupivacaine toxicity with cimetidine and ranitidine (decreased metabolism)

> DW Noble et al, Effects of H-2 antagonists on the elimination of bupivacaine. Br J Anaesth, 59:735, 1987; KK Pihlajamäki et al, Lack of effect of cimetidine on the pharmacokinetics of bupivacaine in healthy subjects. Br J Clin Pharmacol, 26:403, 1988; CM Wilson et al, Plasma bupivacaine con-

(continued)

ANTIHISTAMINES, H$_2$-BLOCKERS, with: *(continued)*
centrations associated with extradural anaesthesia for caesarean section: influence of pretreatment with ranitidine. Br J Anaesth, 58:1330P, 1986

Conflicting reports; monitor clinical status

Carbamazepine

Toxicity of carbamazepine with cimetidine (decreased metabolism)

MJ Dalton et al, Cimetidine and carbamazepine: a complex drug interaction. Epilepsia, 27:553, 1986

Experimental studies indicate that temporary increase in carbamazepine concentration (lasting about 7 days) can occur after starting cimetidine; ranitidine probably does not interact

Carmustine

Increased bone marrow depression with cimetidine (additive)

SA Klotz and BF Kay, Cimetidine and agranulocytosis. Ann Intern Med, 88:579, 1978; RG Selker et al, Bone-marrow depression with cimetidine plus carmustine. N Engl J Med, 299:834, 1978

Avoid concurrent use, if possible

Cephalosporins

Possible decreased cefpodoxime effect with famotidine (decreased absorption due to increased pH)

N Saathoff et al, Pharmacokinetics of cefpodoxime proxetil and interactions with an antacid and an H$_2$ receptor antagonist. Antimicrob Agents Chemother, 36:796, 1992

Monitor for decreased response to cefpodoxime

Chloramphenicol

Aplastic anemia with cimetidine (possibly additive or synergism)

BC West et al, Aplastic anemia associated with parenteral chloramphenicol: review of 10 cases, including the second case of possible increased risk with cimetidine. Rev Infect Dis, 10:1048, 1988

Two case reports (1981, 1988); avoid concurrent use

Chloroquine

Possible chloroquine toxicity with cimetidine (decreased metabolism)

El Ette et al, Chloroquine elimination in humans: effect of low-dose cimetidine. J Clin Pharmacol, 27:813, 1987

Study in healthy men; monitor for symptoms of toxicity

Clozapine

Clozapine toxicity with cimetidine (possibly decreased metabolism)

S Szymanski et al, A case report of cimetidine-induced clozapine toxicity. J Clin Psychiatry, 52:21, 1991

Single case report (1991); did not occur with ranitidine

Cyclosporine

Possible cyclosporine toxicity with famotidine (increased absorption)

H Reichenspurner et al, The influence of gastrointestinal agents on resorption and metabolism of cyclosporine after heart transplantation: experimental and clinical results. J Heart Lung Transplant, 12:1987, 1993; VT Tsang et al, Cyclosporin pharmacokinetics in heart-lung transplant recipients with cystic fibrosis. Eur J Clin Pharmacol, 46:261, 1994

ANTIHISTAMINES, H$_2$-BLOCKERS, with: *(continued)*
> *Monitor cyclosporine concentration; effect may occur with all drugs that increase gastric pH*

> **Delavirdine**
>> Possible decreased delavirdine effect (decreased absorption)
>>> Manufacturer's package insert
>>
>> *Theoretical; any agent that increases gastric pH may also interact; manufacturer recommends avoiding chronic concurrent use*

> **Digitoxin**
>> Possible digitoxin toxicity with cimetidine (decreased metabolism)
>>> LB Polish et al, Digitoxin-quinidine interaction: potentiation during administration of cimetidine. South Med J, 74:633, 1981
>>
>> *Monitor digitoxin concentration*

> **Digoxin**
>> Possible digoxin toxicity with cimetidine (mechanism not established)
>>> B Mouser et al, Effect of cimetidine on oral digoxin absorption. DICP, 24:286, 1990
>>
>> *Conflicting reports; clinical significance questionable; monitor digoxin concentration*

> **Diltiazem**
>> Possible diltiazem toxicity with cimetidine (decreased metabolism)
>>> LC Winship et al, The effect of ranitidine and cimetidine on single-dose diltiazem pharmacokinetics. Pharmacotherapy, 5:16, 1985
>>
>> *Monitor diltiazem concentration; ranitidine effect on diltiazem metabolism is small and probably not clinically significant*

> **Dofetilide**
>> Possible dofetilide toxicity with cimetidine (probably decreased renal excretion)
>>> S Abel et al, Effect of cimetidine and ranitidine on pharmacokinetics and pharmacodynamics of a single dose of dofetilide. Br J Clin Pharmacol, 49:64, 2000
>>
>> *Avoid concurrent use; based on study in healthy subjects; ranitidine did not interact*

> **Dolasetron**
>> Possible dolasetron toxicity with cimetidine (decreased metabolism)
>>> Manufacturer's package insert
>>
>> *Theoretical; monitor clinical status*

> **Encainide**
>> Possible encainide toxicity with cimetidine (probably decreased metabolism)
>>> Manufacturer's package insert
>>
>> *Monitor encainide concentration*

> **Epirubicin**
>> Possible increased epirubicin toxicity with cimetidine (mechanism not established)
>>> LS Murray et al, The effect of cimetidine on the pharmacokinetics of epirubicin in patients with advanced breast cancer: preliminary evidence of a potentially common drug interaction. Clin Oncol, 10:33, 1998

(continued)

ANTIHISTAMINES, H$_2$-BLOCKERS, with: *(continued)*
>   *Based on study of 8 patients; monitor clinical status; theoretically, famotidine, nizatidine and ranitidine may be less likely to interact*

Flecainide
>   Possible flecainide toxicity with cimetidine (decreased metabolism)
>>   TB Tjandra-Maga et al, Altered pharmacokinetics of oral flecainide by cimetidine. Br J Clin Pharmacol, 22:108, 1986
>   *Preliminary study in healthy volunteers; monitor flecainide concentration*

Fluoroquinolones
>   Possible decreased enoxacin effect with ranitidine (possibly decreased absorption); ciprofloxacin minimally affected by cimetidine; sparfloxacin and trovafloxacin may not be affected by cimetidine
>>   TH Grasela, Jr et al, Inhibition of enoxacin absorption by antacids or ranitidine. Antimicrob Agents Chemother, 33:615, 1989; ME Lebsack et al, Effect of gastric acidity on enoxacin absorption. Clin Pharmacol Ther, 52:252, 1992; manufacturer's package insert; RA Prince et al, Effect of cimetidine on ciprofloxacin pharmacokinetics. J Infect Dis Pharmacother, 3:85, 1999
>   *Avoid concurrent use; ciprofloxacin may not be affected 2 hours after ranitidine*

Fluorouracil
>   Possible fluorouracil toxicity with cimetidine (decreased metabolism)
>>   VJ Harvey et al, The influence of cimetidine on the pharmacokinetics of 5-fluorouracil. Br J Clin Pharmacol, 18:421, 1984; F de' Clari, Beschleunigtes Auftreten einer multifokalen Leukenzephalopathie unter Fluorouracil und Ranitidin. Dtsch Med Wochenschr, 118:1176, 1993
>   *Based on pharmacokinetic studies; effect may be delayed for several weeks after starting cimetidine; monitor serum concentration; single case report with ranitidine (1993)*

HMG-CoA reductase inhibitors
>   Possible fluvastatin toxicity (mechanism not established)
>>   Manufacturer's package insert
>   *Monitor fluvastatin concentration*

Hydroxyzine
>   Possible hydroxyzine toxicity with cimetidine (probably decreased metabolism)
>>   FER Simons et al, Effect of the H/d/s-22/s+2/u-antagonist cimetidine on the pharmacokinetics and pharmacodynamics of the H/d/s-21/s+2/u-antagonists hydroxyzine and cetirizine in patients with chronic urticaria. J Allergy Clin Immunol, 95:685, 1995
>   *Clinical significance not established*

Hypoglycemics, sulfonylurea
>   Increased hypoglycemic effect with glipizide or glyburide and cimetidine or ranitidine; other hypoglycemics may also interact (decreased metabolism)
>>   K Lee et al, Glyburide-induced hypoglycemia and ranitidine. Ann Intern Med, 107:261, 1987; EW Cate et al, Inhibition of tolbutamide elimination by cimetidine but not ranitidine. J Clin Pharmacol, 26:372, 1986; GI Adebayo and HAB Coker, Lack of efficacy of cimetidine and ranitidine as inhibitors of tolbutamide metabolism. Eur J Clin Pharmacol, 34:653, 1988; J Feely et al, Potentiation of the hypoglycaemic response to glipizide in diabetic patients

ANTIHISTAMINES, H$_2$-BLOCKERS, with: *(continued)*
> by histamine H$_2$-receptor antagonists. Br J Clin Pharmacol, 35:321, 1993

Monitor blood glucose; tolbutamide interacted in one single dose study, but not multiple dose studies

Decreased hypoglycemic effect has been reported with glibenclamide (mechanism not established)
> RT Kubacka et al, The paradoxical effect of cimetidine and ranitidine on glibenclamide pharmacokinetics and pharmacodynamics. Br J Clin Pharmacol, 23:743, 1987

Monitor blood glucose

Iron
Decreased iron effect with cimetidine (decreased absorption)
> R Esposito, Cimetidine and iron-deficiency anaemia. Lancet, 2:1132, 1977

Avoid concurrent use; treat ulcers with sucralfate taken at least 2 hours before or after iron

Lidocaine
Possible IV or epidural lidocaine toxicity with cimetidine (decreased metabolism)
> AB Knapp et al, The cimetidine-lidocaine interaction. Ann Intern Med, 98:174, 1983; PA Dailey et al, Lidocaine levels during cesarean section after pretreatment with ranitidine or cimetidine. Anesthesiology, 63:A444, 1985; K Kishikawa et al, Effects of famotidine and cimetidine on plasma levels of epidurally administered lignocaine. Anaesthesia, 45:719, 1990

Decrease infusion rate and monitor lidocaine concentration

Macrolide antibiotics
Reversible hearing loss (decreased erythromycin metabolism)
> N Mogford et al, Erythromycin deafness and cimetidine treatment. BMJ, 309:1620, 1994

Based on single case report (1994) and study in 6 healthy subjects

Metoclopramide
Decreased cimetidine effect (decreased absorption)
> N Barzaghi et al, Effects on cimetidine bioavailability of metoclopramide and antacids given two hours apart. Eur J Clin Pharmacol, 37:409, 1989

Cimetidine given at least 2 hours after metoclopramide or antacids was only slightly affected

Metronidazole
Possible IV metronidazole toxicity with cimetidine (decreased metabolism)
> R Gugler and JC Jensen, Interaction between cimetidine and metronidazole. N Engl J Med, 309:1518, 1983

Avoid concurrent use; may occur only after several days of cimetidine therapy

Miglitol
Possible decreased ranitidine effect (decreased bioavailability)
> Manufacturer's package insert (miglitol)

Monitor clinical status

(continued)

ANTIHISTAMINES, H$_2$-BLOCKERS, with: *(continued)*

Mirtazapine
Possible mirtazapine toxicity with cimetidine (probably decreased metabolism)
>JMA Sitsen et al, Concomitant use of mirtazapine and cimetidine: a drug-drug interaction study in healthy male subjects. Eur J Clin Pharmacol, 56:389, 2000

Based on study in healthy subjects; clinical importance not established; other H2- receptor antagonists theoretically would not interact; monitor clinical status

Moricizine
Possible moricizine toxicity with cimetidine (probably decreased metabolism)
>J Biollaz et al, Cimetidine inhibition of ethmozine metabolism. Clin Pharmacol Ther, 37:665, 1985

Monitor moricizine concentration; based on study in healthy men

Narcotics: meperidine and congeners
Severe narcotic toxicity with cimetidine (decreased metabolism)
>EM Sorkin and GS Ogawa, Cimetidine potentiation of narcotic action. Drug Intell Clin Pharm, 17:60, 1983; DRP Guay et al, Cimetidine alters pethidine disposition in man. Br J Clin Pharmacol, 18:907, 1984

Avoid concurrent use in dialysis patients and use cautiously in others; respiratory depression reversible with naloxone

Increased alfentanil effect with cimetidine but not ranitidine (decreased metabolism)
>J Kienlen et al, Pharmacokinetics of alfentanil in patients treated with either cimetidine or ranitidine. Drug Invest, 6:257, 1993

Based on pharmacokinetic study in ICU patients

Narcotics: methadone and congeners
Possible narcotic toxicity with cimetidine (probably decreased metabolism)
>EM Sorkin and GS Ogawa, Cimetidine potentiation of narcotic action. Drug Intell Clin Pharm, 17:60, 1983

Avoid concurrent use in dialysis patients and use cautiously in others; respiratory depression reversible with naloxone

Narcotics: morphine-like
Severe narcotic toxicity with cimetidine (probably decreased metabolism)
>A Fine and DN Churchill, Potentially lethal interaction of cimetidine and morphine. Can Med Assoc J, 124:1434, 1981

Avoid concurrent use in dialysis patients and use cautiously in others; respiratory depression reversible with naloxone

Mental confusion in patients on ranitidine with infusion of morphine and ranitidine (mechanism not established)
>M Martinez-Abad et al, Ranitidine-induced confusion with concomitant morphine. Drug Intell Clin Pharm, 22:914, 1988

Single case report (1988)

Decreased pain relief with ranitidine (increased metabolism)
>HJ McQuay et al, Oral morphine in cancer pain: influences on morphine and metabolite concentration. Clin Pharmacol Ther, 48:236, 1990

ANTIHISTAMINES, H$_2$-BLOCKERS, with: *(continued)*
Monitor pain relief

Possible morphine toxicity with ranitidine (accumulation of morphine and morphine-6-glucuronide)

> TA Aasmundstad and P Størset, Influence of ranitidine on the morphine-3-glucuronide to morphine-6-glucuronide ratio after oral administration of morphine in humans. Hum Exper Toxicol, 17:347, 1998

Monitor clinical status; based on study of normal male subjects

Neuromuscular blocking agents

Prolonged neuromuscular blockade with cimetidine and succinylcholine or vecuronium (probably decreased metabolism)

> G McCarthy et al, Effect of H$_2$-receptor antagonist pretreatment on vecuronium- and atracurium-induced neuromuscular block. Br J Anaesth, 66:713, 1991; DR Turner et al, Neuromuscular block by suxamethonium following treatment with histamine type 2 antagonists or metoclopramide. Br J Anaesth, 63:348, 1989; YJ Kao and DR Turner, Prolongation of succinylcholine block by metoclopramide. Anesthesiology, 70:905, 1989

Conflicting reports; some patients also received metoclopramide, which may have caused interaction

Resistance to neuromuscular blockade with ranitidine (mechanism not established)

> RS Katende and I Dimich, Resistance to nondepolarizing muscle relaxants in a patient treated with ranitidine. Mt Sinai J Med, 54:330, 1987; GE Woodworth et al, The effect of cimetidine and ranitidine on the duration of action of succinylcholine. Anesth Analg, 68:295, 1989

Not confirmed by study in 10 patients

Nifedipine

Possible nifedipine toxicity with cimetidine or ranitidine (decreased metabolism)

> JB Schwartz et al, Effect of cimetidine or ranitidine administration on nifedipine pharmacokinetics and pharmacodynamics. Clin Pharmacol Ther, 43:673, 1988; A Khan et al, The pharmacokinetics and pharmacodynamics of nifedipine at steady state during concomitant administration of cimetidine or high dose ranitidine. Br J Clin Pharmacol, 32:519, 1991

Monitor cardiovascular status; no interaction in normal subjects with ranitidine

Nisoldipine

Possible increased nisoldipine toxicity with cimetidine (decreased metabolism: CYP3A4)

> R Heinig, Clinical pharmacokinetics of nisoldipine coat-core. Clin Pharmacokinet, 35:191, 1998

Based on study in 12 healthy volunteers taking cimetidine 400 mg bid; no interaction with ranitidine; monitor clinical status

Nonsteroidal anti-inflammatory drugs

Possible piroxicam toxicity with cimetidine (decreased metabolism)

> P Milligan et al, The consequences of histamine H$_2$-receptor administration in patients with joint disorders receiving chronic piroxicam therapy. Br J

(continued)

ANTIHISTAMINES, H$_2$-BLOCKERS, with: *(continued)*
> Clin Pharmacol, 32:666P, 1991
> *Based on study in healthy men; clinical significance not established*

Possible salicylate toxicity with cimetidine or nizatidine (decreased metabolism)
> Manufacturer's package insert; W Khoury et al, The effect of cimetidine on aspirin absorption. Gastroenterology, 76:1169, 1979; Z Trnavska et al, The effect of cimetidine on the pharmacokinetics of salicylic acid. Drugs Exp Clin Res, 11:703, 1985
> *Monitor salicylate concentration*

Possible decreased naproxen effect with famotidine or ranitidine
> TB Vree et al, The effects of cimetidine, ranitidine and famotidine on the single-dose pharmacokinetics of naproxen and its metabolites in humans. Int J Clin Pharmacol, 31:597, 1993
> *Monitor clinical status*

Possible bromfenac toxicity with cimetidine (probably decreased metabolism)
> Manufacturer's package insert
> *Clinical significance not established*

Pentagastrin
Increased incidence of dizziness with cimetidine (mechanism not established)
> A Wade and D Wingate, Use of pentagastrin test as a combined teaching and research project for medical students. Lancet, 5:516, 1980
> *Warn patients*

Pentoxifylline
Possible pentoxifylline toxicity with cimetidine (decreased metabolism)
> VF Mauro et al, Alteration of pentoxifylline pharmacokinetics by cimetidine. J Clin Pharmacol, 28:649, 1988
> *Monitor pentoxifylline concentration*

Phenothiazines
Excessive sedation with chlorpromazine with cimetidine (probably decreased metabolism)
> A Byrne and B O'Shea, Adverse interaction between cimetidine and chlorpromazine in two cases of chronic schizophrenia. Br J Psychiatry, 155:413, 1989
> *Monitor phenothiazine concentration*

Phenytoin
Phenytoin toxicity with cimetidine (decreased metabolism)
> M Levine et al, Differential effect of cimetidine on serum concentrations of carbamazepine and phenytoin. Neurology, 35:562, 1985; NC Sambol et al, A comparison of the influence of famotidine and cimetidine on phenytoin elimination and hepatic blood flow. Br J Clin Pharmacol, 27:83, 1989; RG Karlstadt and RH Palmer, Unrecognized drug interaction with famotidine and nizatidine. Arch Intern Med, 151:810, 1991; CST Tse et al, Phenytoin concentration elevation subsequent to ranitidine administration. Ann Pharmacother, 27:1448, 1993; JA Rafi et al, Effect of over-the-counter cimetidine on phenytoin concentrations in patients with seizures. Ann Pharmacother,

ANTIHISTAMINES, H₂-BLOCKERS, with: *(continued)*
33:769, 1999

Monitor phenytoin concentration; effect of cimetidine at OTC doses probably minimal; case reports with famotidine (1991) and ranitidine (1988,1993)

Pramipexole

Possible pramipexole toxicity with cimetidine (probably decreased renal excretion)

Manufacturer's package insert

Avoid concurrent use

Praziquantel

Possible increased praziquantel toxicity (probably decreased metabolism)

WD Dachman et al, Cimetidine-induced rise in praziquantel levels in a patients with neurocysticercosis being treated with anticonvulsants. J Infect Dis, 169:689, 1994

Single case report of favorable use of interaction in a patient receiving anticonvulsants (1994); substantial increase in praziquantel levels; monitor clinical status

Probenecid

Possible famotidine toxicity (decreased renal excretion)

N Inotsume et al, The inhibitory effect of probenecid on renal excretion of famotidine in young, healthy volunteers. J Clin Pharmacol, 30:50, 1990

Avoid concurrent use, if possible; based on study in young, healthy men; other H₂-blockers may also interact

Procainamide

Procainamide toxicity with cimetidine (decreased renal excretion)

CD Christian, Jr et al, Cimetidine inhibits renal procainamide clearance. Clin Pharmacol Ther, 36:221, 1984; KA Rodvold et al, Interaction of steady state procainamide with H₂-receptor antagonists cimetidine and ranitidine. Ther Drug Monit, 9:378, 1987

Monitor procainamide concentration; also occurs with sustained-release oral procainamide

Possible procainamide toxicity or decreased effect with ranitidine (decreased absorption; decreased renal excretion)

KA Rodvold et al, Interaction of steady state procainamide with H₂-receptor antagonists cimetidine and ranitidine. Ther Drug Monit, 9:378, 1987; ML Rocci, Jr et al, Ranitidine-induced changes in the renal and hepatic clearances of procainamide are correlated. J Pharmacol Exp Ther, 248:923, 1989

Based on studies in healthy subjects; monitor procainamide concentration

Proguanil

Possible decreased proguanil effect due to decreased concentrations of active metabolite, cycloguanil with cimetidine (possible decreased metabolism)

JA Kolawole et al, Effects of cimetidine on the pharmacokinetics of proguanil in healthy subjects and in peptic ulcer patients. J Pharm Biomed Anal, 20:737, 1999

ANTIHISTAMINES, H₂-BLOCKERS, with: *(continued)*
Based on study in healthy subjects and peptic ulcer patients; clinical importance not established

Quinidine
Possible quinidine toxicity with cimetidine (mechanism not established)
> LB Polish et al, Digitoxin-quinidine interaction: potentiation during administration of cimetidine. South Med J, 74:633, 1981; BG Hardy et al, Effect of cimetidine on the pharmacokinetics and pharmacodynamics of quinidine. Am J Cardiol, 52:172, 1983

Monitor quinidine concentration

Cardiotoxicity with ranitidine (mechanism not established)
> A Iliopoulou et al, Quinidine-ranitidine adverse reaction. Eur Heart J, 7:360, 1986

Single, well-documented case report (1986)

Quinine
Possible quinine toxicity with cimetidine (decreased metabolism)
> S Wanwimolruk et al, Effects of cimetidine and ranitidine on the pharmacokinetics of quinine. Br J Clin Pharmacol, 22:346, 1986

Ranitidine does not interact

Selective serotonin reuptake inhibitors (SSRIs)
Possible paroxetine or citalopram toxicity with cimetidine (decreased metabolism)
> SJ Bannister et al, Evaluation of the potential for interactions of paroxetine with diazepam, cimetidine, warfarin, and digoxin. Acta Psychiatr Scand, 80 suppl 350:102, 1989; manufacturer's package insert; M Priskorn et al, Pharmacokinetic interaction study of citalopram and cimetidine in healthy subjects. Eur J Clin Pharmacol, 52:241, 1997

Clinical significance not established; monitor clinical status; based on studies in healthy subjects

Sildenafil
Possible sildenafil toxicity with cimetidine (probably decreased metabolism)
> Manufacturer's package insert

Theoretical, monitor clinical status

Sucralfate
Possible decreased cimetidine effect (possibly decreased absorption)
> Y Yoshida et al, Effects of concomitant drugs on the blood concentration of a histamine H₂ antagonist (the 3rd report); concomitant or time lag oral administration of cimetidine and sucralfate. Jpn J Gastroenterol, 84:1025, 1987; R D'Angio et al, Cimetidine absorption in humans during sucralfate coadministration. Br J Clin Pharmacol, 21:515, 1986; H Albin et al, Effect of sucralfate on the bioavailability of cimetidine. Eur J Clin Pharmacol, 30:493, 1986

Two studies failed to confirm initial report

Sympathomimetic amines
Possible dobutamine toxicity with cimetidine (possibly decreased metabolism)
> A Baraka et al, Cimetidine – dobutamine interaction? Anaesthesia, 47:965,

ANTIHISTAMINES, H$_2$-BLOCKERS, with: *(continued)*
    1992
> *Single case report; being treated with atenolol and cimetidine before operation; anesthetized with fentanyl, midazolam, and vecuronium*

Tacrine
> Possible tacrine toxicity with cimetidine (decreased metabolism)
>> Manufacturer's package insert
>
> *Monitor tacrine concentration*

Tamsulosin
> Possible tamsulosin toxicity with cimetidine (probably decreased metabolism)
>> Manufacturer's package insert
>
> *Based on study in healthy subjects; monitor clinical status*

Theophyllines
> Theophylline toxicity with cimetidine (decreased metabolism)
>> K Hsu et al, The influence of orally administered cimetidine and theophylline on the elimination of each drug in patients with chronic airways obstruction. Am Rev Respir Dis, 130:740, 1984; JA Gaska et al, Theophylline pharmacokinetics: effect of continuous versus intermittent cimetidine IV infusion. J Clin Pharmacol, 31:668, 1991; RL Davis et al, Effect of the addition of ciprofloxacin on theophylline pharmacokinetics in subjects inhibited by cimetidine. Ann Pharmacother, 26:11, 1992; IM Fraser et al, Effects of cimetidine and ranitidine on the pharmacokinetics of a chronotherapeutically formulated once-daily theophylline preparation *(Uniphyl)*. Clin Ther, 15:383, 1993; K Bachmann et al, Controlled study of the putative interaction between famotidine and theophylline in patients with chronic obstructive pulmonary disease. J Clin Pharmacol, 35:529, 1995; C-M Loi et al, Aging and drug interactions. III. Individual and combined effects of cimetidine and ciprofloxacin on theophylline metabolism in healthy male and female nonsmokers. J Pharmacol Exper Ther, 280:627, 1997; DE Nix et al, The effect of low-dose cimetidine (200 mg twice daily) on the pharmacokinetics of theophylline. J Clin Pharmacol, 39:855, 1999
>
> *Monitor theophylline concentration; two negative studies in healthy volunteers; concurrent ciprofloxacin may cause theophylline toxicity; effect small with nonprescription doses of cimetidine (400 mg/day)*
>
> Possible theophylline toxicity with famotidine (possibly decreased metabolism)
>> RG Karlstadt and RH Palmer, Unrecognized drug interaction with famotidine and nizatidine. Arch Intern Med, 151:810, 1991; K Bachmann et al, Controlled study of the putative interaction between famotidine and theophylline in patients with chronic obstructive pulmonary disease. J Clin Pharmacol, 35:529, 1995
>
> *Single case report (1991); conflicting results from two studies of single IV theophylline doses in patients with COPD*
>
> Possible theophylline toxicity with nizatidine (possibly decreased metabolism)
>> K Bachmann et al, Comparative investigation of the influence of nizatidine, ranitidine, and cimetidine on the steady-state pharmacokinetics of theophylline in COPD patients. J Clin Pharmacol, 32:476, 1992

(continued)

ANTIHISTAMINES, H$_2$-BLOCKERS, with: *(continued)*
Single case report (1991); 3 case reports of elevated theophylline concentration (1991); negative study with sustained-release theophylline in patients with COPD (1992)

Possible theophylline toxicity with ranitidine (possibly decreased metabolism)
> K Bachmann et al, Comparative investigation of the influence of nizatidine, ranitidine, and cimetidine on the steady-state pharmacokinetics of theophylline in COPD patients. J Clin Pharmacol, 32:476, 1992; IM Fraser et al, Effects of cimetidine and ranitidine on the pharmacokinetics of a chronotherapeutically formulated once-daily theophylline preparation *(Uniphyl)*. Clin Ther, 15:383, 1993; CG Wilson et al, Wirkung der Vorbehandlung mit Ranitidin auf Pharmakokinetik und Gastrointestinale passage eines Theophyllin Retard-Präparates. Arzneimittelforschung, 48:561, 1998

Probably occurs rarely; monitor theophylline concentration; several negative studies, suggesting the extent of interactions is likely to be modest

Ticlopidine
Possible increased ticlopidine toxicity (decreased clearance with cimetidine)
> Manufacturer's package insert

Monitor clinical status

Tocainide
Possible decreased tocainide effect with cimetidine (possibly decreased absorption)
> DS North et al, The effect of histamine-2 receptor antagonists on tocainide pharmacokinetics. J Clin Pharmacol, 28:640, 1988

Monitor tocainide concentration; ranitidine did not interact

Tolazoline
Decreased tolazoline effect with cimetidine (mechanism not established)
> C Roll and L Hanssler, Interaktion von Tolazolin und Cimetidin bei persistierender fetaler zirkulation des Neugeborenen. Monatsschr Kinderheilkd, 141:297, 1993; C-B Huang and S-C Huang, Caution with use of cimetidine in tolazoline induced upper gastrointestinal bleeding. Chang Gung Med J, 19:268, 1996

In two infants pulmonary hypertension, which responded to tolazoline, recurred after addition of cimetidine (1993; 1996)

Triptans
Possible zolmitriptan toxicity with cimetidine (probably decreased metabolism)
> Manufacturer's package insert (zolmitriptan)

Avoid concurrent use

Tyramine-rich foods and beverages
Severe headache and hypertension in patients on cimetidine after consuming beef extract and English cheddar (mechanism not established)
> MJJ Griffin and JS Morris, MAOI-like reaction associated with cimetidine. Drug Intell Clin Pharm, 21:219, 1987

Single case report (1987)

ANTIHISTAMINES, H$_2$-BLOCKERS, with: *(continued)*

Valproate
Possible valproate toxicity with cimetidine (decreased metabolism)
> LK Webster, Effect of cimetidine and ranitidine on carbamazepine and sodium valproate pharmacokinetics. Eur J Clin Pharmacol, 27:341, 1984

Based on studies in non-epileptic ulcer patients; avoid concurrent use; ranitidine did not interact

Venlafaxine
Possible increased venlafaxine toxicity with cimetidine (probably decreased metabolism)
> SM Troy et al, The influence of cimetidine on the disposition kinetics of the antidepressant venlafaxine. J Clin Pharmacol, 38:467, 1998

Based on study in healthy subjects; venlafaxine active metabolite not affected; clinical significance not established

Verapamil
Possible verapamil toxicity with cimetidine (decreased metabolism)
> C-M Loi et al, Effect of cimetidine on verapamil disposition. Clin Pharmacol Ther, 37:654, 1985; G Mikus et al, Interaction of verapamil and cimetidine: Stereochemical aspects of drug metabolism, drug disposition and drug action. J Pharmacol Exp Ther, 253:1042, 1990

Monitor cardiovascular status or verapamil concentration

Zaleplon
Possible increased zaleplon toxicity with cimetidine (decreased metabolism; CYP3A4)
> Manufacturer's package insert (zaleplon)

Based on study in healthy volunteers; zaleplon plasma concentration increased 85%; monitor clinical status

ANTISEPTICS, MERCURIAL, with:

Tetracyclines
Conjunctivitis (mechanism not established)
> TG Crook and JJ Freeman, Reactions induced by the concurrent use of thimerosal and tetracycline. Am J Optom Physiol Optics, 60:759, 1983

Occurs with use of contact lens cleaning solution containing thimerosal and systemic tetracyclines

ANTITRYPSIN, with:

Gemfibrozil
Possible decreased alpha 1-antitrypsin effect (mechanism not established)
> S Janciauskiene and S Eriksson, An interaction between gemfibrozil and alpha$_1$-antitrypsin. J Int Med, 236:357, 1994

Clinical significance not established

Aprobarbital, see Barbiturates

APROTININ, with:

Heparins
Heparin resistance (mechanism not established)
> AR Fisher et al, Heparin resistance after aprotinin. Lancet, 340:1230, 1992

Monitor PTT; based on a study in patients after coronary artery bypass surgery

ARBUTAMINE, with:
- **Anticholinergics** - See Anticholinergics with Arbutamine, page 58
- **Antidepressants, tricyclic** - See Antidepressants, tricyclic with Arbutamine, page 82
- **Beta-adrenergic blockers**
  Decreased arbutamine effect (antagonism)
  Manufacturer's package insert
  Withdraw beta-adrenergic blockers at least 48 hours before using arbutamine
- **Digoxin**
  Possible interference with interpretation of arbutamine heart rate response (antagonism)
  Manufacturer's package insert
  Avoid concurrent use
- **Flecainide**
  Possible increased risk of arrhythmias (additive)
  Manufacturer's package insert
  Avoid concurrent use
- **Lidocaine**
  Possible increased risk of arrhythmias (additive)
  Manufacturer's package insert
  Avoid concurrent use
- **Quinidine**
  Possible increased risk of arrhythmias (additive)
  Manufacturer's package insert
  Avoid concurrent use

Ardeparin, no documented interactions, see page 4, Criteria for Listing Interactions

ARTEMETHER, with:
- **Grapefruit juice**
  Possible artemether toxicity (possibly decreased metabolism; CYP3A4)
  MA van Agtmael et al, Grapefruit juice increases the bioavailability of artemether. Eur J Clin Pharmacol, 55:405, 1999
  Based on study in healthy subjects; monitor clinical status

ARTEMISININ, with:
- **Omeprazole**
  Possible decreased omeprazole effect (probably increased metabolism; CYP2C19)
  USH Svensson et al, Artemisinin induces omeprazole metabolism in human beings. Clin Pharmacol Ther, 64:160, 1998; K Mihara et al, Stereospecific analysis of omeprazole supports artemisinin as a potent inducer of CYP2C19. Fundam Clin Pharmacol, 13:671, 1999
  Based on study in healthy subjects; clinical significance not established

Ascorbic acid, see Vitamin C

Asparaginase, no documented interactions, see page 4, Criteria for Listing Interactions

Aspirin, see Nonsteroidal anti-inflammatory drugs

Astemizole, see Antihistamines, H_1-blockers: Astemizole, terfenadine

Atenolol, see Beta-adrenergic blockers

Atorvastatin, see HMG-CoA Reductase Inhibitors
ATOVAQUONE, with:
  Lopinavir/Ritonavir
    Possible decreased atovaquone effect (increased metabolism)
      Manufacturer's package insert (*Kaletra*)
    Atovaquone dosage may need to be increased; clinical significance unknown
  Metoclopramide
    Decreased atovaquone effect (decreased atovaquone bioavailability)
      Manufacturer's package insert (*Malarone*)
    Use another antiemetic
  Rifampin
    Decreased atovaquone effect (mechanism unknown)
      Manufacturer's package insert
    Atovaquone concentration decreased by 50%; monitor clinical status
  Tetracyclines
    Decreased atovaquone effect (mechanism unknown)
      Manufacturer's package insert (*Malarone*)
    Plasma concentration of atovaquone decreaed 40% with tetracycline; monitor clinical status
  Zidovudine
    Possible zidovudine toxicity (decreased metabolism)
      BL Lee et al, Atovaquone inhibits the glucuronidation and increases the plasma concentrations of zidovudine. Clin Pharmacol Ther, 59:14, 1996
    Monitor clinical status
Atracurium, see Neuromuscular blocking agents
Atropine, see Anticholinergics
AURANOFIN, with:
  Theophyllines
    Possible decreased theophylline effect (mechanism not established)
      AC Falcão et al, Theophylline pharmacokinetics with concomitant steroid and gold therapy. J Clin Pharm Ther, 25:191, 2000
    Based on population pharmacokinetic study; causal relationship not established; monitor theophylline serum concentrations
Avobenzone, no documented interactions, see page 4, Criteria for Listing Interactions
Azapropazone, see Nonsteroidal anti-inflammatory drugs
Azatadine, no documented interactions, see page 4, Criteria for Listing Interactions
AZATHIOPRINE, with:
  Alkylating agents - See Alkylating agents with Azathioprine, page 23
  Allopurinol - See Allopurinol with Azathioprine, page 25
  Angiotensin-converting enzyme (ACE) inhibitors - See Angiotensin-converting enzyme (ACE) inhibitors with Azathioprine, page 43
  Anticoagulants, oral - See Anticoagulants, oral with Azathioprine, page 62
  Isotretinoin
    Curling of head hair (mechanism not established)
      JW van der Pijl et al, Isotretinoin and azathioprine: a synergy that makes hair curl? Lancet, 348:622, 1996

(continued)

AZATHIOPRINE, with: *(continued)*
> *Three case reports (1996); patients taking several other drugs*

  Methotrexate
> Azathioprine toxicity (fever, muscle pain, rash) (mechanism not established)
>> R Blanco et al, Acute febrile toxic reaction in patients with refractory rheumatoid arthritis who are receiving combined therapy with methotrexate and azathioprine. Arthritis Rheum, 39:1016, 1996
>
> *In four of 43 patients treated for rheumatoid arthritis*

  Sulfonamides
> Possible azathioprine toxicity with sulfasalazine (decreased metabolism)
>> CL Szumlanski and RM Weinshilboum, Sulphasalazine inhibition of thiopurine methyltransferase: possible mechanism for interaction with 6-mercaptopurine and azathioprine. Br J Clin Pharmacol, 39:456, 1995;
>
> *Based on an in vitro study showing inhibition of thiopurine methyltransferase (TPMT) by sulfasalazine; patients with genetically reduced TPMT are reported to have more severe thiopurine toxicity*

  Trimethoprim
> Leucopenia (mechanism not established)
>> RR Bailey, Leukopenia due to a trimethoprim – azathioprine interaction. N Z Med J, 97:739, 1984
>
> *Report of 3 cases; monitor white blood count*

Azelaic acid, no documented interactions, see page 4, Criteria for Listing Interactions

Azelastine, no documented interactions, see page 4, Criteria for Listing Interactions

Azidothymidine, see Zidovudine

Azithromycin, see Macrolide antibiotics

Azlocillin, see Penicillins

AZT, see Zidovudine

Aztreonam, no documented interactions, see page 4, Criteria for Listing Interactions

Bacitracin, no documented interactions, see page 4, Criteria for Listing Interactions

BACLOFEN, with:
  Antidepressants, tricyclic - See Antidepressants, tricyclic with Baclofen, page 82

BARBITURATES, with:
  Acetaminophen - See Acetaminophen with Barbiturates, page 8
  Alcohol - See Alcohol with Barbiturates, page 14
  Anticoagulants, oral - See Anticoagulants, oral with Barbiturates, page 62
  Antidepressants, tricyclic - See Antidepressants, tricyclic with Barbiturates, page 82
  Antihistamines, H$_2$-blockers - See Antihistamines, H$_2$-blockers with Barbiturates, page 114

  Benzodiazepines
> Decreased clonazepam effect with phenobarbital (increased metabolism)
>> K-C Khoo et al, Influence of phenytoin and phenobarbital on the disposition of a single oral dose of clonazepam. Clin Pharmacol Ther, 28:368, 1980
>
> *Monitor clonazepam concentration*

BARBITURATES, with: *(continued)*
   Respiratory failure with clonazepam and amobarbital (mechanism not established)
   > WG Honer et al, Respiratory failure after clonazepam and amobarbital. Am J Psychiatry, 143:1495, 1986

   Single case report (1986)

Beta-adrenergic blockers
   Decreased beta-blocker effect (increased metabolism) except with sotalol and probably atenolol and nadolol (minimal hepatic metabolism)
   > K Haglund et al, Influence of pentobarbital on metoprolol plasma levels. Clin Pharmacol Ther, 26:326, 1979; P Collste et al, Influence of pentobarbital on effect and plasma levels of alprenolol and 4-hydroxy-alprenolol. Clin Pharmacol Ther, 25:423, 1979; EA Sotaniemi et al, Plasma clearance of propranolol and sotalol and hepatic drug-metabolizing enzyme activity. Clin Pharmacol Ther, 26:153, 1979; P Seideman et al, Decreased plasma concentrations and clinical effects of alprenolol during combined treatment with pentobarbitone in hypertension. Br J Clin Pharmacol, 23:267, 1987; A Hoffmann-Traeger et al, The influence of phenobarbital on the pharmacokinetics of propranolol in pregnancy. Biol Res Pregnancy, 8:57, 1987

   Avoid concurrent use unless barbiturate essential as anticonvulsant

Carbamazepine
   Difficulty in evaluating carbamazepine concentration (increased metabolism to the epoxide)
   > E Spina et al, Effect of phenobarbital on the pharmacokinetics of carbamazepine-10,11-epoxide, an active metabolite of carbamazepine. Ther Drug Monit, 13:109, 1991; H Liu and MR Delgado, Interactions of phenobarbital and phenytoin with carbamazepine and its metabolites' concentrations, concentration ratios, and level/dose ratios in epileptic children. Epilepsia, 36:249, 1995; S Sennoune et al, Steady state pharmacokinetics of carbamazepine-phenobarbital interaction in patients with epilepsy. Biopharm Drug Dispos, 17:155, 1996; D Divanodlou et al, Pharmacokinetic behaviour of carbamazepine and its main metabolite-10, 11 epoxide of carbamazepine in monotherapy or in combination with other anti-epileptic drugs. Eur J Neurol, 5:397, 1998

   Low or normal carbamazepine concentration may not be significant if epoxide is increased; however, relative antiepileptic potencies of the 2 compounds are unknown; if possible, monitor concentration of both carbamazepine and its epoxide; combination of phenytoin and phenobarbital may produce additive decrease in carbamazepine concentrations

Cephalosporins
   Rash in children with cefotaxime and high-dosage phenobarbital (mechanism not established)
   > S Harder et al, Unerwünschte arzneimittelreaktionen bei gleichzeitiger Gabe von hochdosiertem phenobarbital und betalaktam-antibiotika. Klin Pädiatr, 202:404, 1990

   Monitor clinical status

(continued)

BARBITURATES, with: *(continued)*
  Chloramphenicol
    Possible barbiturate toxicity (decreased metabolism); decreased chloramphenicol effect (increased metabolism)
      DA Powell et al, Interactions among chloramphenicol, phenytoin, and phenobarbital in a pediatric patient. J Pediatr, 98:1001, 1981; RA Bloxham et al, Chloramphenicol and phenobarbitone – a drug interaction. Arch Dis Child, 54:76, 1979; H Reiche and H-H Frey, Interactions between chloramphenicol and intravenous anesthetics. Anaesthesist, 30:504, 1981; K Krasinski et al, Pharmacologic interactions among chloramphenicol, phenytoin and phenobarbital. Pediatr Infect Dis, 1:232, 1982
    Monitor barbiturate and chloramphenicol concentrations in epileptics; avoid concurrent use in others; adjust barbiturate dosage when used as anesthetic in epileptics; monitor barbiturate and chloramphenicol concentrations in epileptics; avoid concurrent use in others; adjust barbiturate dosage when used as anesthetic in epileptics
  Clozapine
    Possible decreased clozapine effect (increased metabolism)
      WH Wilson, Do anticonvulsants hinder clozapine treatment? Biol Psychiatry, 37:132, 1995; G Facciolá et al, Inducing effect of phenobarbital on clozapine metabolism in patients with chronic schizophrenia. Ther Drug Monit, 20:628, 1998
    Based on preliminary retrospective study and study in 22 schizophrenic patients (1998)
  Contraceptives, implant
    Decreased contraceptive effect (increased metabolism)
      L Shane-McWhorter et al, Enhanced metabolism of levonorgestrel during phenobarbital treatment and resultant pregnancy. Pharmacotherapy, 18:1360, 1998
    Single case report (1998)
  Contraceptives, oral
    Decreased contraceptive effect (increased metabolism)
      DJ Back et al, The interaction of phenobarbital and other anticonvulsants with oral contraceptive steroid therapy. Contraception, 22:495, 1980; DJ Back et al, Evaluation of Committee on Safety of Medicines yellow card reports on oral contraceptive-drug interactions with anticonvulsants and antibiotics. Br J Clin Pharmacol, 25:527, 1988; L Shane-McWhorter et al, Enhanced metabolism of levonorgestrel during phenobarbital treatment and resultant pregnancy. Pharmacotherapy, 18:1360, 1998; MA Eldon et al, Gabapentin does not interact with a contraceptive regimen of norethindrone acetate and ethinyl estradiol. Neurology, 50:1146, 1998; RI Shader and JR Oesterheld, Contraceptive effectiveness: cytochromes and induction. J Clin Psychopharmacol, 20:119, 2000; K Wilbur and MHH Ensom, Pharmacokinetic drug interactions between oral contraceptives and second-generation anticonvulsants. Clin Pharmacokinet, 38:355, 2000

BARBITURATES, with: *(continued)*
Avoid concurrent use; use alternative contraceptive in epileptics; gabapentin does not appear to interact with an oral contraceptive containing norethindrone and ethinyl estradiol

Corticosteroids

Decreased corticosteroid effect (increased metabolism)

SM Brooks et al, Adverse effects of phenobarbital on corticosteroid metabolism in patients with bronchial asthma. N Engl J Med, 286:1125, 1972; SJ Wassner et al, The adverse effect of anticonvulsant therapy on renal allograft survival. J Pediatr, 88:134, 1976; MR Stjernholm and FH Katz, Effects of diphenylhydantoin, phenobarbital, and diazepam on the metabolism of methylprednisolone and its sodium succinate. J Clin Endocrinol Metab, 41:887, 1975; PM Brooks et al, Effects of enzyme induction on metabolism of prednisolone. Ann Rheum Dis, 35:339, 1976; VN Sehgal and G Srivastava, Corticosteroid-unresponsive pemphigus vulgaris following antiepileptic therapy. Int J Dermatol, 27:258, 1988

Monitor corticosteroid effect or concentration in epileptics; avoid concurrent use in others

Cyclosporine

Possible decreased cyclosporine effect (increased metabolism)

H Carstensen et al, Interaction between cyclosporin A and phenobarbitone. Br J Clin Pharmacol, 21:550, 1986; T Nishioka et al, Interaction between phenobarbital and ciclosporin following renal transplantation: a case report. Hinyokika Kiyo, 36:447, 1990

Two case reports (1986, 1990); monitor cyclosporine concentration

Delavirdine

Possible decreased delavirdine effect (increased metabolism)

Manufacturer's package insert

Based on preliminary data; monitor clinical status

Digitoxin

Decreased digitoxin effect (increased metabolism)

HM Solomon and WB Abrams, Interactions between digitoxin and other drugs in man. Am Heart J, 83:277, 1972

Use digoxin in epileptic patients

Felbamate

Barbiturate toxicity (mechanism not established)

BE Gidal and ML Zupanc, Potential pharmacokinetic interaction between felbamate and phenobarbital. Ann Pharmacother, 28:455, 1994

Single case report (1994); monitor barbiturate concentration

Guanfacine

Decreased antihypertensive effect; rebound hypertension on withdrawal of guanfacine (increased metabolism; increased guanfacine concentration on withdrawal)

JR Kiechel et al, Pharmacokinetic aspects of guanfacine withdrawal syndrome in a hypertensive patient with chronic renal failure. Eur J Clin Pharmacol, 25:463, 1983

(continued)

BARBITURATES, with: *(continued)*
Taper barbiturate before withdrawing guanfacine

Haloperidol

Decreased haloperidol effect; increased fluctuation of haloperidol effect with depot (IM) haloperidol decanoate (increased metabolism)

> M Linnoila et al, Effect of anticonvulsants on plasma haloperidol and thioridazine levels. Am J Psychiatry, 137:7, 1980; G Pupeschi et al, Do enzyme inducers modify haloperidol decanoate rate of release? Prog Neuro-Psychopharmacol Biol Psychiat, 18:1323, 1994; G Hirokane et al, Interindividual variation of plasma haloperidol concentrations and the impact of concomitant medications: the analysis of therapeutic drug monitoring data. Ther Drug Monit, 21:82, 1999

If barbiturate essential as an anticonvulsant, monitor clinical response and haloperidol concentration; with haloperidol decanoate, interval between injections may need to be reduced

Influenza vaccine

Possible barbiturate toxicity (decreased metabolism)

> MW Jann and GS Fidone, Effect of influenza vaccine on serum anticonvulsant concentrations. Clin Pharm, 5:817, 1986

Monitor barbiturate concentration

Lamotrigine

Decreased lamotrigine effect (probably increased metabolism)

> JA Armijo et al, Lamotrigine serum concentraion-to-dose ratio: influence of age and concomitant antiepileptic drugs and dosage implications. Ther Drug Monit, 21:182, 1999

Monitor lamotrigine serum concentrations and clinical status; lamotrigine dosage may need to be adjusted

Methsuximide

Possible toxicity of both drugs (decreased metabolism)

> B Rambeck, Pharmacological interactions of mesuximide with phenobarbital and phenytoin in hospitalized epileptic patients. Epilepsia, 20:147, 1979

Monitor methsuximide and barbiturate concentrations

Metronidazole

Decreased metronidazole effect with phenobarbital (probably increased metabolism)

> PB Mead et al, Possible alteration of metronidazole metabolism by phenobarbital. N Engl J Med, 306:1490, 1982; S Gupte, Phenobarbital and metabolism of metronidazole. N Engl J Med, 308:529, 1983

Double dose of metronidazole if phenobarbital essential as anticonvulsant

Montelukast

Possible decreased montelukast effect (increased metabolism; CYP450

> Manufacturer's package insert (montelukast)

Monitor clinical status

Narcotics: meperidine and congeners

Increased CNS depression with meperidine (increased meperidine metabolites)

> JE Stambaugh et al, A potentially toxic drug interaction between pethidine (meperidine) and phenobarbitone. Lancet, 1:398, 1977

BARBITURATES, with: *(continued)*
Avoid concurrent use, except for anesthesia

Narcotics: methadone and congeners
Methadone withdrawal symptoms (increased metabolism)
> S-J Liu and RIH Wang, Case report of barbiturate-induced enhancement of methadone metabolism and withdrawal syndrome. Am J Psychiatry, 141:1287, 1984

Avoid concurrent use, if possible; monitor epileptics taking methadone for withdrawal

Nelfinavir
Possible decreased nelfinavir effect (increased metabolism; CYP3A)
> Manufacturer's package insert (nelfinavir)

Clinical significance remains to be established

Nonsteroidal anti-inflammatory drugs
Increased thiopentone effect with aspirin (displacement from binding)
> JW Dundee et al, Aspirin and probenecid pretreatment influences the potency of thiopentone and the onset of action of midazolam. Eur J Anaesthesiol, 3:247, 1986

Adjust induction dose

Oxcarbazepine
Possible decreased oxcarbazepine effect (increased metabolism)
> Manufacturer's package insert (oxcarbazepine)

Concentration of active metabolite decreased 25%; monitor oxcarbazepine concentration

Phenothiazines
Decreased phenothiazine effect (increased metabolism)
> M Linnoila et al, Effect of anticonvulsants on plasma haloperidol and thioridazine levels. Am J Psychiatry, 137:7, 1980; S Loga et al, Interactions of orphenadrine and phenobarbitone with chlorpromazine: plasma concentrations and effects in man. Br J Clin Pharmacol, 2:197, 1975

Avoid concurrent use; monitor phenothiazine concentration if barbiturates required for treating epilepsy

Prazosin
Hypotension during epidural bupivacaine anesthesia (mechanism not established)
> CA Lydiatt et al, Severe hypotension during epidural anesthesia in a prazosin-treated patient. Anesth Analg, 76:1152, 1993

Single case report (1993); no response to phenylephrine; responded to epinephrine

Probenecid
Possible IV thiopental toxicity (displacement from binding)
> TJ McMurray et al, The influence of probenecid on the induction dose of thiopentone. Br J Clin Pharmacol, 17:224P, 1984; S Kaukinen et al, Prolongation of thiopentone anaesthesia by probenecid. Br J Anaesth, 52:603, 1980

Avoid concurrent use

(continued)

BARBITURATES, with: *(continued)*
Pyridoxine
Decreased barbiturate effect (possibly increased metabolism)
> O Hansson and M Sillanpaa, Pyridoxine and serum concentration of phenytoin and phenobarbitone. Lancet, 1:256, 1976

Monitor barbiturate concentration in epileptics; avoid concurrent use in others

Quinidine
Decreased quinidine effect (increased metabolism)
> JL Data et al, Interaction of quinidine with anticonvulsant drugs. N Engl J Med, 294:699, 1976; DJ Chapron et al, Apparent quinidine-induced digoxin toxicity after withdrawal of pentobarbital. A case of sequential drug interactions. Arch Intern Med, 139:363, 1979

Monitor quinidine concentration in epileptics; avoid concurrent use in others

Quinine
Possible phenobarbital toxicity (possible decreased metabolism)
> GJ Amabeoku et al, Pharmacokinetic interaction of single doses of quinine and carbamazepine, phenobarbitone and phenytoin in healthy volunteers. East Afr Med J, 70:90, 1993

Monitor phenobarbital concentration; based on studies in normal subjects

Reserpine
Hypotension during thiopental anesthesia (additive)
> CH Ziegler and JB Lovette, Operative complications after therapy with reserpine and reserpine compounds. JAMA, 176:916, 1961

Discontinue reserpine 2 weeks before thiopental anesthesia

Rifampin
Decreased barbiturate effect (increased metabolism)
> DD Breimer et al, Influence of rifampicin on drug metabolism: differences between hexobarbital and antipyrine. Clin Pharmacol Ther, 21:470, 1977; W Zilly et al, Stimulation of drug metabolism by rifampicin in patients with cirrhosis or cholestasis measured by increased hexobarbital and tolbutamide clearance. Eur J Clin Pharmacol, 11:287, 1977; DA Smith et al, Age-dependent stereoselective increase in the oral clearance of hexobarbitone isomers caused by rifampicin. Br J Clin Pharmacol, 32:735, 1991

Monitor barbiturate concentration if required as anticonvulsant

Sulfonamides
Increased thiopental effect (decreased albumin binding)
> SI Csogor and SF Kerek, Enhancement of thiopentone anaesthesia by sulphafurazole. Br J Anaesthesiol, 42:988, 1970; SI Csogor and J Papp, Competition between sulphonamides and thiopental for the binding sites of plasma proteins. Arzneimittelforschung, 20:1925, 1970

Monitor for possible dosage reduction

Sympathomimetic amines
Possible phenobarbital toxicity with methylphenidate (decreased metabolism)
> Manufacturer's package insert *(Ritalin)*

Monitor phenobarbital concentration; dosage adjustment may be necessary

BARBITURATES, with: *(continued)*
Teniposide
Possible decreased teniposide effect (increased metabolism)
> DK Baker et al, Increased teniposide clearance with concomitant anticonvulsant therapy. J Clin Oncol, 10:311, 1992; MV Relling et al, Adverse effect of anticonvulsants on efficacy of chemotherapy for acute lymphoblastic leukaemia. Lancet, 356:285, 2000

Evidence of reduced teniposide efficacy in children with acute lymphoblastic leukemia; monitor clinical status and teniposide concentration if available

Tetracyclines
Decreased doxycycline effect (increased metabolism)
> O Penttila et al, Interaction between doxycycline and some antiepileptic drugs. Br Med J, 2:470, 1974; PJ Neuvonen et al, Effect of antiepileptic drugs on the elimination of various tetracycline derivatives. Eur J Clin Pharmacol, 9:147, 1975

Avoid concurrent use; choose another antibiotic in epileptics

Theophyllines
Decreased theophylline effect (increased metabolism)
> KM Piafsky et al, Effect of phenobarbital on the disposition of intravenous theophylline. Clin Pharmacol Ther, 22:336, 1977; RA Landay et al, Effect of phenobarbital on theophylline disposition. J Allergy Clin Immunol, 62:27, 1978; CL Saccar et al, The effect of phenobarbital on theophylline disposition in children with asthma. J Allergy Clin Immunol, 75:716, 1985; RJ Kandrotas et al, Effect of phenobarbital administration on theophylline clearance in premature neonates. Ther Drug Monit, 12:139, 1990

Monitor theophylline concentration in epileptics; avoid concurrent use in others; individual response varies; interaction may not be clinically significant in neonates

Tiagabine
Decreased tiagabine effect (increased tiagabine metabolism)
> Manufacturer's package insert

Monitor clinical status

Valproate
Phenobarbital toxicity (decreased metabolism)
> IH Patel et al, Phenobarbital-valproic acid interaction. Clin Pharmacol Ther, 27:515, 1980; IM Kapetanovic et al, Mechanism of valproate-phenobarbital interaction in epileptic patients. Clin Pharmacol Ther, 29:480, 1981; I Bernus et al, Inhibition of phenobarbitone *N*-glucosidation by valproate. Br J Clin Pharmacol, 38:411, 1994; R O'Neil and C Brands, Coma induced by valproate in the presence of phenobarbital. J Gen Intern Med, 14 suppl 2:188, 1999

Monitor phenobarbital concentration if essential as anticonvulsant

Possible decreased valproate effect (increased metabolism)
> E Yukawa et al, Population-based investigation of valproic acid relative clearance using nonlinear mixed effects modeling: influence of drug-drug interaction and patient characteristics. J Clin Pharmacol, 37:1160, 1997

(continued)

BARBITURATES, with: *(continued)*
Monitor clinical status and valproate concentration

Verapamil

Possible decreased oral verapamil effect with phenobarbital (increased metabolism)

DR Rutledge et al, Effects of chronic phenobarbital on verapamil disposition in humans. J Pharmacol Exp Ther, 246:7, 1988

Monitor clinical status or verapamil concentration; based on study in healthy men

Zonisamide

Decreased zonisamide effect with phenobarbital (increased metabolism; CYP3A4)

Manufacturer's package insert (zonisamide)

Monitor zonisamide concentration and clinical status; zonisamide dosage may need to be adjusted

Basiliximab, no documented interactions, see page 4, Criteria for Listing Interactions

BCG, no documented interactions, see page 4, Criteria for Listing Interactions

Becaplermin, no documented interactions, see page 4, Criteria for Listing Interactions

Beclomethasone, see Corticosteroids

Bee venom, see Insect venom extracts

Belladonna alkaloids, see Anticholinergics

Benazepril, see Angiotensin-converting enzyme (ACE) inhibitors

Bendrofluazide, see Thiazide diuretics

Bendroflumethiazide, see Thiazide diuretics

BENTIROMIDE, with:

Methotrexate

Possible methotrexate toxicity (displacement from binding)

Manufacturer's package insert

Avoid concurrent use

BENZODIAZEPINES, with:

Acetaminophen - See Acetaminophen with Benzodiazepines, page 8

Alcohol - See Alcohol with Benzodiazepines, page 14

Amiodarone - See Amiodarone with Benzodiazepines, page 34

Amprenavir - See Amprenavir with Benzodiazepines, page 38

Antacids - See Antacids with Benzodiazepines, page 51

Antidepressants, tricyclic - See Antidepressants, tricyclic with Benzodiazepines, page 82

Antifungals, imidazoles and triazoles - See Antifungals, imidazoles and triazoles with Benzodiazepines, page 96

Antihistamines, H_2-blockers - See Antihistamines, H_2-blockers with Benzodiazepines, page 114

Barbiturates - See Barbiturates with Benzodiazepines, page 130

BENZODIAZEPINES, with: *(continued)*
 Beta-adrenergic blockers
  Possible diazepam or clorazepate toxicity with propranolol or metoprolol (decreased metabolism)
   G Hawksworth et al, Diazepam/beta-adrenoceptor antagonist interactions. Br J Clin Pharmacol, 17:69S, 1984; U Klotz and IW Reimann, Pharmacokinetic and pharmacodynamic interaction study of diazepam and metoprolol. Eur J Clin Pharmacol, 26:223, 1984; HR Ochs et al, Influence of propranolol coadministration or cigarette smoking on the kinetics of desmethyldiazepam following intravenous clorazepate. Klin Wochenschr, 64:1217, 1986; AK Scott et al, Effect of metoprolol on the pharmacokinetics of bromazepam and lorazepam. Br J Clin Pharmacol, 28:234P, 1989
  Avoid concurrent use or monitor diazepam or desmethyldiazepam (metabolite of clorazepate) concentration; may also occur with bromazepam and metoprolol (large individual variation); atenolol, triazolam, or lorazepam may not interact

  Reaction time may be prolonged with oxazepam and propranolol (decreased metabolism)
   J Sonne et al, Single dose pharmacokinetics and pharmacodynamics of oral oxazepam during concomitant administration of propranolol and labetalol. Br J Clin Pharmacol, 29:33, 1990
  Warn patients about driving

 Buprenorphine
  Increased CNS depression, especially in overdose (additive)
   M Reynaud et al, Six deaths linked to concomitant use of buprenorphine and benzodiazepines. Addiction, 93:1385, 1998
  Avoid concurrent use

 Caffeine
  Both increased and decreased lorazepam effects reported (mechanism not established); possibly also with diazepam and other benzodiazepines
   SE File et al, Interaction between effects of caffeine and lorazepam in performance tests and self-ratings. J Clin Psychopharmacol, 2:102, 1982; MM Ghoneim et al, Pharmacokinetic and pharmacodynamic interactions between caffeine and diazepam. J Clin Psychopharmacol, 6:75, 1986; AJ Mercer et al, The effect of lorazepam and caffeine, alone and in combination, on the electroencephalogram of healthy, caffeine withdrawn volunteers. Br J Pharmacol, 37:502P, 1994
  Avoid large amounts of caffeine (400 to 500 mg) in caffeine-containing beverages or over-the-counter medications

 Carbamazepine
  Decreased alprazolam and possibly clobazam or clonazepam effect (probably increased metabolism)
   GW Arana et al, Carbamazepine-induced reduction of plasma alprazolam concentrations: a clinical case report. J Clin Psychiatry, 49:448, 1988; JJ Muñoz et al, The effect of clobazam on steady state plasma concentrations of carbamazepine and its metabolites. Br J Clin Pharmacol, 29:763, 1990; P

(continued)

BENZODIAZEPINES, with: *(continued)*
>Genton et al, Carbamazepine intoxication with negative myoclonus after the addition of clobazam. Epilepsia, 39:1115, 1998; K Ikawa et al, Influence of concomitant anticonvulsants on serum concentrations of clonazepam in epileptic subjects: an age- and dose-effect linear regression model analysis. Pharm Pharmacol Commun, 5:307, 1999

Single case report with alprazolam (1988); monitor clinical status

>Possible carbamazepine toxicity with clobazam (possibly decreased metabolism)
>>P Genton et al, Carbamazepine intoxication with negative myoclonus after the addition of clobazam. Epilepsia, 39:1115, 1998

Single case report with positive re-challenge (1998)

Clozapine
>Respiratory arrest and syncope (mechanism not established)
>>N Sassim and R Grohmann, Adverse drug reactions with clozapine and simultaneous application of benzodiazepines. Pharmacopsychiatry, 21:306, 1988; A Klimke and E Klieser, Sudden death after intravenous application of lorazepam in a patient treated with clozapine. Am J Psychiatry, 151:5, 1994; I Faisal et al, Clozapine-benzodiazepine interactions. J Clin Psychiatry, 58:547, 1997; AJ Gelenberg, Clozapine plus benzodiazepines: hazardous? Biol Ther Psychiatry, 22:11, 1999; E Tupala et al, Transient syncope and ECG changes associated with the concurrent administration of clozapine and diazepam. J Clin Psychiatry, 60:619, 1999

Has been reported more frequently with clozapine alone than with combination; monitor respiratory status; may be more likely when clozapine is added to established benzodiazepine regimen

Contraceptives, oral
>Possible chlordiazepoxide or IV diazepam toxicity (mechanism not established)
>>DR Abernethy et al, Impairment of diazepam metabolism by low-dose estrogen-containing oral-contraceptive steroids. N Engl J Med, 306:791, 1982

Use with caution

>Variable psychomotor impairment with single doses of oral diazepam and possibly other benzodiazepines (mechanism not established)
>>EH Ellinwood, Jr et al, Effects of oral contraceptives on diazepam-induced psychomotor impairment. Clin Pharmacol Ther, 35:360, 1984; PD Kroboth et al, Pharmacodynamic evaluation of the benzodiazepine-oral contraceptive interaction. Clin Pharmacol Ther, 38:525, 1985

Greatest impairment during menstrual pause in oral contraceptive dosage; possibly not with multiple doses of diazepam since tolerance develops rapidly

>Decreased oral oxazepam, temazepam, or lorazepam effects (possibly increased metabolism)
>>DR Abernethy et al, Lorazepam and oxazepam kinetics in women on low-dose oral contraceptives. Clin Pharmacol Ther, 33:628, 1983; RV Patwardhan et al, Differential effects of oral contraceptive steroids on the metabolism of benzodiazepines. Hepatology, 3:248, 1983

BENZODIAZEPINES, with: *(continued)*
> *Increased lorazepam, oxazepam, or temazepam dosage may be required*

> Possible triazolam or alprazolam toxicity (decreased metabolism)
>> GP Stoehr et al, Effect of oral contraceptives on triazolam, temazepam, alprazolam, and lorazepam kinetics. Clin Pharmacol Ther, 36:683, 1984; JM Scavone et al, Alprazolam pharmacokinetics in women on low-dose oral contraceptives. J Clin Pharmacol, 28:454, 1988
>
> *Based on studies in healthy subjects; clinical significance not established*

> Midazolam may not interact to a clinically significant extent
>> AA Holazo et al, Effects of age, gender and oral contraceptives on intramuscular midazolam pharmacokinetics. J Clin Pharmacol, 28:1040, 1988; S Palovaara et al, Effect of an oral contraceptive preparation containing ethinylestradiol and gestodene on CYP3A4 activity as measured by midazolam l'-hydroxylation. Br J Clin Pharmacol, 50:333. 2000
>
> *Based on studies in healthy subjects*

Corticosteroids
> Possible decreased midazolam effect (probably increased metabolism; CYP3A4)
>> M Nakajima et al, Effects of chronic administration of glucocorticoid on midazolam pharmacokinetics in humans. Ther Drug Monit, 21:507, 1999
>
> *Based on study in 18 patients given IV midazolam; effect relatively small; theoretically oral midazolam would interact to a greater degree*

Delavirdine
> Delavirdine decreases metabolism and may increase toxicity
>> Manufacturer's package insert
>
> *Theoretical; manufacturer recommends avoiding concurrent use if possible*

Digoxin
> Possible digoxin toxicity with diazepam (decreased metabolism; decreased renal excretion)
>> JR Castillo-Ferrando et al, Digoxin levels and diazepam. Lancet, 2:368, 1980; G Tollefson et al, Alprazolam-related digoxin toxicity. Am J Psychiatry, 141:1612, 1984; HR Ochs et al, Effect of alprazolam on digoxin kinetics and creatinine clearance. Clin Pharmacol Ther, 38:595, 1985; H Guven et al, Age-related digoxin-alprazolam interaction. Clin Pharmacol Ther, 54:42, 1993
>
> *Monitor digoxin concentration; single case report in elderly woman with alprazolam (1984); studies of alprazolam in young healthy subjects show no interaction, but a study in patients taking 1 mg/day did show increased concentrations, especially in one patient over 65*

Diltiazem
> Marked increase in oral midazolam or triazolam sedative effects; modest increase in intravenous midazolam effects (decreased metabolism)
>> JT Backman et al, Dose of midazolam should be reduced during diltiazem and verapamil treatments. Br J Clin Pharmacol, 37:221, 1994; J Ahonen et al, Effect of diltiazem on midazolam and alfentanil disposition in patients undergoing coronary artery bypass grafting. Anesthesiology, 85:1246, 1996; K Kosuge et al, Enhanced effect of triazolam with diltiazem. Br J Clin

(continued)

BENZODIAZEPINES, with: *(continued)*
>Pharmacol, 43:367, 1997
>
>*Avoid oral midazolam or triazolam with diltiazem; parenteral midazolam interacts with diltiazem to a lesser degree*

Disulfiram
>Possible benzodiazepine toxicity (decreased metabolism)
>>SM MacLeod et al, Interaction of disulfiram with benzodiazepines. Clin Pharmacol Ther, 24:583, 1978; B Diquet et al, Lack of interaction between disulfiram and alprazolam in alcoholic patients. Eur J Clin Pharmacol, 38:157, 1990; M Hardman et al, Temazepam toxicity precipitated by disulfiram. Lancet, 344:1231, 1994
>
>*Alprazolam and oxazepam do not interact and may be used with disulfiram*

Efavirenz
>Possible prolonged sedation with oral midazolam or triazolam (decreased metabolism)
>>Manufacturer's package insert (efavirenz)
>
>*Oral preparation of midazolam not available in USA; manufacturer recommends avoiding concurrent use; effect on parenteral midazolam likely to be minimal; theoretical*

Fluoroquinolones
>Possible diazepam toxicity with ciprofloxacin (decreased metabolism)
>>F Kamali et al, The influence of steady-state ciprofloxacin on the pharmacokinetics and pharmacodynamics of a single dose of diazepam in healthy volunteers. Eur J Clin Pharmacol, 44:365, 1993
>
>*Monitor clinical status; based on a study of normal subjects given single doses of diazepam; clinical significance not established*

>Possible IV diazepam toxicity with ciprofloxacin (decreased metabolism)
>>F Kamali et al, The effect of ciprofloxacin on diazepam pharmacokinetics. Br J Clin Pharmacol, 35:78P, 1993
>
>*Based on study in 12 healthy men and women*

>No effect of ciprofloxacin on temazepam metabolism
>>F Kamali et al, The influence of ciprofloxacin on the pharmacokinetics and pharmacodynamics of a single dose of temazepam in the young and elderly. J Clin Pharmacol Ther, 19:105, 1994
>
>*Based on study in 12 healthy young men and 9 elderly patients*

Grapefruit juice
>Increased triazolam and oral midazolam effect; theoretically should also increase alprazolam and diazepam (decreased benzodiazepine metabolism)
>>SK Hukkinen et al, Plasma concentrations of triazolam are increased by concomitant ingestion of grapefruit juice. Clin Pharmacol Ther, 58:127, 1995; HHT Kupferschmidt et al, Interaction between grapefruit juice and midazolam in humans. Clin Pharmacol Ther, 58:20, 1995; JT Backman et al, Lack of correlation between in vitro and in vivo studies on the effects of tangeretin and tangerine juice on midazolam hydroxylation. Clin Pharmacol Ther, 67:382, 2000; JJ Lilja et al, Effect of grapefruit juice dose on grapefruit juice-triazolam interaction: repeated consumption prolongs

BENZODIAZEPINES, with: *(continued)*
>   triazolam half-life. Eur J Clin Pharmacol, 56:411, 2000
>
>   *Monitor clinical status; effect on triazolam larger with multiple doses of grapefruit juice; tangerine juice had minimal effect on midazolam pharmacokinetics*

Isoniazid
> Possible IV diazepam toxicity (decreased metabolism)
>> HR Ochs et al, Diazepam interaction with antituberculosis drugs. Clin Pharmacol Ther, 29:671, 1981; N Brockmeyer et al, The metabolism of diazepam following different enzyme inducing agents. Br J Clin Pharmacol, 19:544P, 1985
>
> *Decreased dosage may control seizures; but in combined antituberculosis therapy, suppression of diazepam effect by rifampin tends to predominate*
>
> Possible triazolam toxicity (decreased metabolism)
>> HR Ochs et al, Differential effect of isoniazid on triazolam oxidation and oxazepam conjugation. Br J Clin Pharmacol, 16:743, 1983
>
> *Oxazepam metabolism was not affected*

Kava
> Increased CNS depression (additive)
>> JC Almeida and EW Grimsley, Coma from the health food store: interaction between kava and alprazolam. Ann Intern Med, 125:940, 1996
>
> *Single case report; avoid concurrent use*

Levodopa
> Decreased levodopa effect (mechanism not established)
>> S Yosselson-Superstine and AG Lipman, Chlordiazepoxide interaction with levodopa. Ann Intern Med, 96:259, 1982; J Rafferty and J Williamson, Deterioration in Parkinson's disease caused by lorazepam. Br Med J, 287:1596, 1983
>
> *Avoid concurrent use, if possible*

Lithium
> Hypothermia with diazepam (mechanism not established)
>> GJ Naylor and A McHarg, Profound hypothermia on combined lithium carbonate and diazepam treatment. Br Med J, 2:22, 1977
>
> *Single case report (1977)*
>
> Neurotoxicity with clonazepam (mechanism not established)
>> D Koczerginski et al, Clonazepam and lithium – a toxic combination in the treatment of mania? Int Clin Psychopharmacol, 4:195, 1989
>
> *Monitor clinical status and lithium concentration*

Lopinavir/Ritonavir
> Increased midazolam toxicity including prolonged sedation and respiratory depression (decreased metabolism; CYP3A4)
>> Manufacturer's package insert (*Kaletra*)
>
> *Avoid concurrent use*

(continued)

BENZODIAZEPINES, with: *(continued)*
Loxapine
Hypotension, stupor and respiratory distress with lorazepam (possibly synergism)
>J Battaglia et al, Loxapine-lorazepam-induced hypotension and stupor. J Clin Psychopharmacol, 9:227, 1989; S Cohen and A Khan, Respiratory distress with use of lorazepam in mania. J Clin Psychopharmacol, 7:199, 1987

Several case reports; avoid concurrent use

Macrolide antibiotics
Possible triazolam or midazolam toxicity with erythromycin, clarithromycin or roxithromycin (decreased metabolism)
>JP Phillips et al, A pharmacokinetic drug interaction between erythromycin and triazolam. J Clin Psychopharmacol, 6:297, 1986; A Hiller et al, Unconsciousness associated with midazolam and erythromycin. Br J Anaesth, 65:826, 1990; K Aranko et al, Clinically important interaction between erythromycin and midazolam. Br J Clin Pharmacol, 33:217P, 1992; JT Backman et al, A pharmacokinetic interaction between roxithromycin and midazolam. Eur J Clin Pharmacol, 46:551, 1994; H Luurila et al, Lack of interaction of erythromycin with temazepam. Ther Drug Monit, 16:548, 1994; JT Backman et al, Azithromycin does not increase plasma concentrations of oral midazolam. Int J Clin Pharmacol Ther, 33:356, 1995; H Luurila et al, Interaction between erythromycin and nitrazepam in healthy volunteers. Pharmacol Toxicol, 76:255, 1995; H Luurila et al, Interaction between erythromycin and the benzodiazepines diazepam and flunitrazepam. Pharmacol Toxicol, 78:117, 1996; N Tokinaga et al, Hallucinations after a therapeutic dose of benzodiazepine hypnotics with co-administration of erythromycin. Psychiatry Clin Neurosci, 50:337, 1996; RA Yeates et al, Pharmacokinetic and pharmacodynamic interaction study between midazolam and the macrolide antibiotics, erythromycin, clarithromycin, and the azalide azithromycin. Int J Clin Pharmacol Ther, 35:577, 1997; JC Gorski et al, The contribution of intestinal and hepatic CYP3A to the interaction between midazolam and clarithromycin. Clin Pharmacol Ther, 64:133, 1998; DJ Greenblatt et al, Inhibition of triazolam clearance by macrolide antimicrobial agents: in vitro correlates and dynamic consequences. Clin Pharmacol Ther, 64:278, 1998

If alternative antibiotic cannot be used, monitor for excessive benzodiazepine effect; unconsciousness with oral midazolam (1990); parenteral midazolam much less affected than oral; clinical significance of interaction with roxithromycin not established; azithromycin may not interact with midazolam; erythromycin may not interact with temazepam or nitrazepam; significance of interaction with diazepam not established

Mirtazapine
Impaired motor function and cognition, and sedation (additive)
>Manufacturer's package insert

Avoid concurrent use

BENZODIAZEPINES, with: *(continued)*
   Monoamine oxidase inhibitors
   Phenelzine toxicity with nitrazepam (mechanism not established)
   > AL Harris and N McIntyre, Interaction of phenelzine and nitrazepam in a slow acetylator. Br J Clin Pharmacol, 12:254, 1981

   Single report (1981); significance not established

   Headache and flushing with clonazepam and phenelzine (mechanism not established)
   > JL Karagianis and H March, Flushing reaction associated with the interaction of phenelzine and clonazepam. Can J Psychiatry, 36:389, 1991; AB Eppel, Interaction between clonazepam and phenelzine. Can J Psychiatry, 35:647, 1990

   Two case reports of headache (1990,1991), one report of flushing (1991)

   Narcotics: meperidine and congeners
   Hypotension with alfentanil and midazolam; hypoxemia and apnea with midazolam and fentanyl (decreased sympathetic tone)
   > K Skarvan and W Schwinn, Hamodynamische interaktion zwischen midazolam und alfentanil bei koronarkranken. Anaesthesist, 35:17, 1986; PL Bailey et al, Frequent hypoxemia and apnea after sedation with midazolam and fentanyl. Anesthesiology, 73:826, 1990; P Burtin et al, Hypotension with midazolam and fentanyl in the newborn. Lancet, 337:1545, 1991

   Avoid concurrent use; reported in newborns with fentanyl

   Reversible neurological deficits in children with midazolam and fentanyl (mechanism not established)
   > I Bergman et al, Reversible neurologic abnormalities associated with prolonged intravenous midazolam and fentanyl administration. J Pediatr, 119:644, 1991; JP Zacny et al, Midazolam does not influence intravenous fentanyl-induced analgesia in healthy volunteers. Pharmacol Biochem Behav, 55:275, 1996

   Short-term use of midazolam and fentanyl in healthy adults did not cause unexpected adverse effects; monitor neurological status of children

   Narcotics: methadone and congeners
   Possible alprazolam toxicity with propoxyphene (probably decreased metabolism)
   > DR Abernethy et al, Interaction of propoxyphene with diazepam, alprazolam and lorazepam. Br J Clin Pharmacol, 19:51, 1985

   Avoid concurrent use; lorazepam and probably diazepam are not affected

   Nefazodone
   Possible alprazolam or triazolam toxicity (decreased metabolism)
   > PD Kroboth et al, Coadministration of nefazodone and benzodiazepines: I. Pharmacodynamic assessment. J Clin Psychopharmacol, 15:306, 1995; RH Barbhaiya et al, Coadministration of nefazodone and benzodiazepines: II. A pharmacokinetic interaction study with triazolam. J Clin Psychopharmacol, 15:320, 1995; DS Greene et al, Coadministration of nefazodone and benzodiazepines. III. A pharmacokinetic interaction study with alprazolam. J Clin Psychopharmacol, 15:399, 1995

(continued)

BENZODIAZEPINES, with: *(continued)*
> *Monitor alprazolam or triazolam concentration or clinical status; reduce alprazolam or triazolam dosage by 50%*

Nelfinavir
> Possible midazolam and triazolam toxicity (decreased metabolism; CYP3A)
>> Manufacturer's package insert (nelfinavir)
>
> *Theoretical; manufacturer recommends avoiding concurrent use*

Neuromuscular blocking agents
> Prolonged neuromuscular blocking effect of succinylcholine with diazepam (mechanism not established)
>> JJ Driessen et al, Benzodiazepines and neuromuscular blocking drugs in patients. Acta Anaesthesiol Scand, 30:642, 1986
>
> *Monitor neuromuscular status; effect may be less with atracurium or vecuronium*

Nonsteroidal anti-inflammatory drugs
> Possible delayed onset of action of naproxen with diazepam (delayed absorption)
>> BR Rao and D Rambhau, Influence of diazepam on the pharmacokinetic properties of orally administered naproxen. Drug Invest, 4:416, 1992
>
> *Based on a study in healthy men; clinical significance not established*
>
> Shortened induction with midazolam anesthesia after aspirin (displacement from binding)
>> JW Dundee et al, Aspirin and probenecid pretreatment influences the potency of thiopentone and the onset of action of midazolam. Eur J Anaesthesiol, 3:247, 1986
>
> *Monitor closely*

Olanzapine
> Increased orthostatic hypotensive effect of olanzapine with diazepam (mechanism not established)
>> Manufacturer's package insert (olanzpine)
>
> *Avoid concurrent use*

Omeprazole
> Possible diazepam, flurazepam, clorazepate and triazolam toxicity (decreased metabolism)
>> T Andersson et al, Effect of omeprazole treatment on diazepam plasma levels in slow versus normal rapid metabolizers of omeprazole. Clin Pharmacol Ther, 47:79, 1990; JF Martí-Massó et al, Ataxia following gastric bleeding due to omeprazole-benzodiazepine interaction. Ann Pharmacother, 26:429, 1992; Y Caraco et al, Interethnic difference in omeprazole's inhibition of diazepam metabolism. Clin Pharmacol Ther, 58:62, 1995; R Gugler et al, Lack of pharmacokinetic interaction of pantoprazole with diazepam in man. Br J Clin Pharmacol, 42:249, 1996; A Konrad, Protracted episode of reduced consciousness following co-medication with omeprazole and clorazepate. Clin Drug Invest, 19:307, 2000

BENZODIAZEPINES, with: *(continued)*
> *Monitor response to diazepam; based on studies of IV and oral diazepam in healthy men; may be limited to rapid omeprazole metabolizers; single case reports of ataxia, with triazolam and with flurazepam (1992); single possible case with clorazepate (2000); pantoprazole may not interact with diazepam*

Papaverine
> Prolonged erection after intracavernous injection of papaverine and IV diazepam (mechanism not established)
>> JA Vale et al, Papaverine, benzodiazepines, and prolonged erections. Lancet, 337:1552, 1991
>
> *Two case reports (1991)*

Phenytoin
> Decreased clonazepam, clobazam, and possibly oxazepam effect (increased metabolism)
>> K-C Khoo et al, Influence of phenytoin and phenobarbital on the disposition of a single oral dose of clonazepam. Clin Pharmacol Ther, 28:368, 1980; AK Scott et al, Oxazepam pharmacokinetics in patients with epilepsy treated long-term with phenytoin alone or in combination with phenobarbitone. Br J Clin Pharmacol, 16:441, 1983; IN Saavedra et al, Phenytoin/clonazepam interaction. Ther Drug Monit, 7:481, 1985
>
> *Monitor benzodiazepine effect or concentration*

> Variable effects of clonazepam on phenytoin concentration (mechanism not established)
>> IN Saavedra et al, Phenytoin/clonazepam interaction. Ther Drug Monit, 7:481, 1985; S Sennoune et al, Interactions between clobazam and standard antiepileptic drugs in patients with epilepsy. Ther Drug Monit, 14:269, 1992
>
> *Monitor phenytoin concentration; conflicting reports on direction of effect*

Probenecid
> Possible adinazolam, lorazepam or nitrazepam toxicity (decreased metabolism); could occur with other benzodiazepines
>> DR Abernethy et al, Probenecid impairment of acetaminophen and lorazepam clearance: direct inhibition of ether glucuronide formation. J Pharmacol Exp Ther, 234:345, 1985; NH Brockmeyer et al, Comparative effects of rifampin and/or probenecid on the pharmacokinetics of temazepam and nitrazepam. Int J Clin Pharmacol Ther Toxicol, 28:387, 1990; PL Golden et al, Effects of probenecid on the pharmacokinetics and pharmacodynamics of adinazolam in humans. Clin Pharmacol Ther, 56:133, 1994
>
> *Avoid concurrent use or reduce dose of benzodiazepine*

> Shortened induction with midazolam anesthesia (displacement from binding)
>> JW Dundee et al, Aspirin and probenecid pretreatment influences the potency of thiopentone and the onset of action of midazolam. Eur J Anaesthesiol, 3:247, 1986
>
> *Monitor closely*

(continued)

BENZODIAZEPINES, with: *(continued)*
  Propofol
    Possible excessive midazolam effect (probably decreased metabolism; CYP3A4)
      N Hamaoka et al, Propofol decreases the clearance of midazolam by inhibiting CYP3A4: an in vivo and in vitro study. Clin Pharmacol Ther, 66:110, 1999; H Seifert et al, Sedation with propofol plus midazolam versus propofol alone for interventional endoscopic proceures: a prospective, randomized study. Aliment Pharmacol Ther, 14:1207, 2000
    Based on study in 24 patients undergoing anesthesia induction; in another study of 239 patients undergoing endoscopy, addition of midazolam resulted in a modest reduction in propofol requirement; monitor for increased or prolonged midazolam effect
  Quinupristin/dalfopristin
    Possible midazolam toxicity (decreased metabolism; CYP3A4)
      Manufacturer's package insert (quinupristin/dalfopristin)
    Based on study in healthy volunteers; monitor clinical status
  Rifampin
    Possible decreased oral and IV diazepam, triazolam or nitrazepam effect and oral midazolam effect (increased metabolism)
      HR Ochs et al, Diazepam interaction with antituberculosis drugs. Clin Pharmacol Ther, 29:671, 1981; N Brockmeyer et al, The metabolism of diazepam following different enzyme inducing agents. Br J Clin Pharmacol, 19:544P, 1985; NH Brockmeyer et al, Comparative effects of rifampin and/or probenecid on the pharmacokinetics of temazepam and nitrazepam. Int J Clin Pharmacol Ther Toxicol, 28:387, 1990; K Villikka et al, Triazolam is ineffective in patients taking rifampin. Clin Pharmacol Ther, 61:8, 1997; JT Backman et al, The area under the plasma concentration-time curve for oral midazolam is 400-fold larger during treatment with itraconazole than with rifampicin
    Increased dosage of IV diazepam may be necessary to control seizures; in combined antituberculosis therapy with isoniazid, effect of rifampin predominates; triazolam and oral midazolam may be ineffective in patients on rifampin
  Ritonavir
    Possible toxicity of alprazolam, clorazepate, diazepam, estazolam, flurazepam, midazolam (oral), triazolam (decreased metabolism)
      RI Shader and DJ Greenblatt, Protease inhibitors and drug interactions—an alert. J Clin Psychopharmacol, 16:343, 1996; manufacturer's package insert (ritonavir); DJ Greenblatt et al, Alprazolam-ritonavir interaction: product labeling implications. Clin Pharmacol Ther, 67:157, 2000, abs PIII-60; DJ Greenblatt et al, Differential impairment of triazolam and zolpidem clearance by ritonavir. J Acquir Immune Defic Syndr, 24:129, 2000
    Alprazolam study in 8 healthy subjects; single case (1996) and pharmacokinetic study in healthy subjects with triazolam; listed as contraindicated in product information; may be less likely with long-term ritonavir use
  Saquinavir
    Prolongation of midazolam sedative effect (probably decreased metabolism; CYP3A4)
      C Merry et al, Saquinavir interaction with midazolam: pharmacokinetic

BENZODIAZEPINES, with: *(continued)*
considerations when prescribing protease inhibitors for patients with HIV disease. AIDS, 11:268, 1997; VJ Palkama et al, Effect of saquinavir on the pharmacokinetics and pharmacodynamics of oral and intravenous midazolam. Clin Pharmacol Ther, 66:33, 1999

Single case report (1997) and study in healthy subjects; effect large with oral midazolam; bolus doses of intravenous midazolam probably minimally affected; monitor clinical status

Selective serotonin reuptake inhibitors (SSRIs)
Possible increased impairment of skills related to driving with diazepam or alprazolam and fluoxetine (decreased metabolism)

L Lemberger et al, The effect of fluoxetine on the pharmacokinetics and psychomotor responses of diazepam. Clin Pharmacol Ther, 43:412, 1988; TA Lasher et al, Pharmacokinetic pharmacodynamic evaluation of the combined administration of alprazolam and fluoxetine. Psychopharmacology, 104:323, 1991; CE Wright et al, A pharmacokinetic evaluation of the combined administration of triazolam and fluoxetine. Pharmacotherapy, 12:103, 1992; DJ Greenblatt et al, Fluoxetine impairs clearance of alprazolam but not of clonazepam. Clin Pharmacol Ther, 52:479, 1992; J Cavanaugh et al, Lack of effect of fluoxetine on the pharmacokinetics and pharmacodynamics of estazolam. Clin Pharmacol Ther, 55:141, 1994; LA Dent and MW Orrock, Warfarin-fluoxetine and diazepam-fluoxetine interaction. Pharmacotherapy, 17:170, 1997; A Nolting and W Abramowitz, Lack of interaction between citalopram and the CYP3A4 substrate triazolam. Pharmacotherapy, 20:750, 2000; PC Hassan et al, Dose-response evaluation of the interaction between sertraline and alprazolam *in vivo*. J Clin Psychopharmacol, 20:150, 2000

Warn patients taking the combination of the risk of driving; triazolam, estazolam or clonazepam may not interact, but patients should still be warned; sertraline may not interact with diazepam or alprazolam; citalopram may not interact with triazolam

Possible alprazolam and bromazepam toxicity with fluvoxamine (decreased metabolism)

J Van Harten et al, Influence of multiple-dose administration of fluvoxamine on the pharmacokinetics of the benzodiazepines bromazepam and lorazepam: a randomised, cross-over study. Eur Neuropsychopharmacol, 2:381, 1992, abs P-122; JC Fleishaker and LK Hulst, A pharmacokinetic and pharmacodynamic evaluation of the combined administration of alprazolam and fluvoxamine. Eur J Clin Pharmacol, 46:35, 1994; E Perucca et al, Inhibition of diazepam metabolism by fluvoxamine: a pharmacokinetic study in normal volunteers. Clin Pharmacol Ther, 56:471, 1994; MJ Gardner et al, Effect of sertraline on the pharmacokinetics and protein binding of diazepam in healthy volunteers. Clin Pharmacokinet, 32 suppl 1:43, 1997

Based on studies in healthy volunteers; lorazepam may not interact

Serotonin syndrome with clonazepam and paroxetine (additive)

JG Rella and RS Hoffman, Possible serotonin syndrome from paroxetine

(continued)

BENZODIAZEPINES, with: *(continued)*
> and clonazepam. J Toxicol Clin Toxicol, 36:257, 1998; PL Bonate et al,
> Clonazepam and sertraline: absence of drug interaction in a multiple-dose
> study. J Clin Psychopharmacol, 20:19, 2000

Single case report (1998); sertraline does not appear to affect clonazepam pharmacokinetics when tested in healthy volunteer subjects

Theophyllines

Decreased diazepam, alprazolam or midazolam effect with aminophylline (possibly adenosine receptor blockade)
> JA Stirt, Aminophylline is a diazepam antagonist. Anesth Analg, 60:767, 1981; SB Arvidsson et al, Aminophylline antagonises diazepam sedation. Lancet, 2:1467, 1982; D Niemand et al, Adenosine in the inhibition of diazepam sedation by aminophylline. Acta Anaesthesiol Scand, 30:493, 1986; Y Tuncok et al, The effects of theophylline on serum alprazolam levels. Int J Clin Pharmacol Ther, 32:642, 1994; MF Bonfiglio et al, A pilot pharmacokinetic-pharmacodynamic study of benzodiazepine antagonism by flumazenil and aminophylline. Pharmacotherapy, 16:1166, 1996

Other benzodiazepines probably also affected; avoid concurrent use except as an antidote

Troleandomycin

Triazolam toxicity (decreased metabolism)
> D Warot et al, Troleandomycin-triazolam interaction in healthy volunteers: pharmacokinetic and psychometric evaluation. Eur J Clin Pharmacol, 32:389, 1987

Avoid concurrent use

Valproate

Possible IV diazepam toxicity (displacement from binding and decreased metabolism)
> S Dhillon and A Richens, Valproic acid and diazepam interaction *in vivo*. Br J Clin Pharmacol, 13:553, 1982

Use IV diazepam with caution

Clonazepam may precipitate absence status (mechanism not established); possible decrease in clonazepam effect
> WA Watson, Interaction between clonazepam and sodium valproate. N Engl J Med, 300:678, 1979; K Ikawa et al, Influence of concomitant anticonvulsants on serum concentrations of clonazepam in epileptic subjects: an age- and dose-effect linear regression model analysis. Pharm Pharmacol Commun, 5:307, 1999

Avoid concurrent use

Possible midazolam toxicity (displacement from binding)
> R Calvo et al, Effect of sodium valproate on midazolam distribution. J Pharm Pharmacol, 40:150, 1988

Monitor midazolam

Possible lorazepam toxicity (decreased metabolism - glucuronidation)
> GD Anderson et al, Lorazepam-valproate interaction: studies in normal subjects and isolated perfused rat liver. Epilepsia, 35:221, 1994; E Samara et al,

BENZODIAZEPINES, with: *(continued)*
>Pharmacokinetic-pharmacodynamic interaction between valproate and lorazepam. Clin Pharmacol Ther, 57:153, 1995; EE Samara et al, Effect of valproate on the pharmacokinetics and pharmacodynamics of lorazepam. J Clin Pharmacol, 37:442, 1997
>
>*Monitor clinical status; based on studies in healthy males*

Venlafaxine
>Possible decreased alprazolam effect (mechanism not established)
>>J Amchin et al, Effect of venlafaxine on the pharmacokinetics of alprazolam. Psychopharmacol Bull, 34:211, 1998
>
>*Based on study in healthy subjects; clinical significance not established*

Verapamil
>Marked increase in oral midazolam effects (decreased metabolism)
>>JT Backman et al, Dose of midazolam should be reduced during diltiazem and verapamil treatments. Br J Clin Pharmacol, 37:221, 1994
>
>*Avoid oral midazolam with verapamil; theoretically parenteral midazolam would interact with verapamil to a lesser degree*

Zidovudine
>Increased incidence of headache with oxazepam (mechanism not established)
>>L Mole et al, Pharmacokinetics of zidovudine alone and in combination with oxazepam in the HIV infected patient. J Acquir Immune Defic Syndr, 6:56, 1993
>
>*Discontinue oxazepam if headache occurs*

Benzonatate, no documented interactions, see page 4, Criteria for Listing Interactions

Benzphetamine, see Sympathomimetic amines

Benzthiazide, see Thiazide diuretics

Benztropine, see Anticholinergics

Benzyl benzoate, no documented interactions, see page 4, Criteria for Listing Interactions

BEPRIDIL, with:

Amprenavir - See Amprenavir with Bepridil, page 39

Digoxin
>Possible digoxin toxicity (mechanism not established)
>>GG Belz et al, Digoxin and bepridil: pharmacokinetic and pharmacodynamic interactions. Clin Pharmacol Ther, 39:65, 1986
>
>*Monitor digoxin concentration; based on study in healthy subjects*

Dofetilide
>Increased risk of arrhythmias (additive effect on QTc interval)
>>Manufacturer's package insert (dofetilide)
>
>*Avoid concurrent use*

Fluoroquinolones
>Possible arrhythmia with grepafloxacin and bepridil (possible additive effect on QTc interval)
>>Manufacturer's package insert
>
>*Theoretical; manufacturer recommends avoiding concurrent use*

(continued)

BEPRIDIL, with: *(continued)*
  Lopinavir/Ritonavir
    Possible bepridil toxicity (decreased metabolism
        Manufacturer's package insert (*Kaletra*)
    Theoretical; avoid combination if possible
  Ritonavir
    Possible bepridil toxicity (decreased metabolism)
        Manufacturer's package insert (ritonavir)
    Theoretical; listed as contraindicated in product information

BETA-ADRENERGIC BLOCKERS, with:
  Acetaminophen - See Acetaminophen with Beta-adrenergic blockers, page 8
  Alcohol - See Alcohol with Beta-adrenergic blockers, page 15
  Amiodarone - See Amiodarone with Beta-adrenergic blockers, page 34
  Anabolic and androgenic steroids - See Anabolic and androgenic steroids with Beta-adrenergic blockers, page 41
  Antacids - See Antacids with Beta-adrenergic blockers, page 51
  Anticholinesterases - See Anticholinesterases with Beta-adrenergic blockers, page 59
  Anticoagulants, oral - See Anticoagulants, oral with Beta-adrenergic blockers, page 62
  Antidepressants, tricyclic - See Antidepressants, tricyclic with Beta-adrenergic blockers, page 83
  Antihistamines, H_1-blockers: astemizole, terfenadine - See Antihistamines, H_1-blockers: astemizole, terfenadine with Beta-adrenergic blockers, page 110
  Antihistamines, H_1-blockers: diphenhydramine - See Antihistamines, H_1-blockers: diphenhydramine with Beta-adrenergic blockers, page 113
  Antihistamines, H_2-blockers - See Antihistamines, H_2-blockers with Beta-adrenergic blockers, page 115
  Arbutamine - See Arbutamine with Beta-adrenergic blockers, page 128
  Barbiturates - See Barbiturates with Beta-adrenergic blockers, page 131
  Benzodiazepines - See Benzodiazepines with Beta-adrenergic blockers, page 139
  Cholestyramine
    Possible decreased propranolol effect (decreased absorption)
        DM Hibbard et al, Effects of cholestyramine and colestipol on the plasma concentrations of propranolol. Br J Clin Pharmacol, 18:337, 1984
    Monitor blood pressure; based on studies in healthy volunteers
  Clonidine
    Hypertension (mechanism not established)
        GA Landis and SM Zimmet, Arterial thrombosis with combined clonidine hydrochloride and propranolol hydrochloride therapy. Arch Intern Med, 140:135, 1980; SE Warren et al, Clonidine and propranolol paradoxical hypertension. Arch Intern Med, 139:253, 1979; AJ Jounela and M Lilja, Interactions between beta-blockers and clonidine. Ann Clin Res, 16:181, 1984
    Stop beta-blocker several days before withdrawing clonidine; stop clonidine at least 3 days before switching to a beta-blocker

BETA-ADRENERGIC BLOCKERS, with: *(continued)*
> Hypotension (mechanism not established)
>> D Perks and GC Fisher, Esmolol and clonidine – a possible interaction. Anaesthesia, 47:533, 1992
>
> *Single case report with intravenous esmolol (1992)*

Cocaine
> Potentiation of cocaine-induced coronary vasoconstriction by propranolol (potentiation of alpha-adrenergic effect of cocaine)
>> RA Lange et al, Potentiation of cocaine-induced coronary vasoconstriction by beta-adrenergic blockade. Ann Intern Med, 112:897, 1990
>
> *Avoid concurrent use*

Colestipol
> Possible decreased propranolol effect (decreased absorption)
>> DM Hibbard et al, Effects of cholestyramine and colestipol on the plasma concentrations of propranolol. Br J Clin Pharmacol, 18:337, 1984
>
> *Monitor blood pressure; based on studies in healthy volunteers*

Contraceptives, oral
> Increased metoprolol and possibly propranolol effect (decreased metabolism)
>> MJ Kendall et al, Metoprolol pharmacokinetics and the oral contraceptive pill. Br J Clin Pharmacol, 14:120, 1982; DB Jack et al, Variability of beta-blocker pharmacokinetics in young volunteers. Eur J Clin Pharmacol, 23:37, 1982; MJ Kendall et al, Beta-adrenoceptor blocker pharmacokinetics and the oral contraceptive pill. Br J Clin Pharmacol, 17:87S, 1984
>
> *Monitor cardiovascular status*

Contrast media
> Increased incidence of anaphylaxis (mechanism not established)
>> DM Lang et al, Increased risk for anaphylactoid reaction from contrast media in patients on β-adrenergic blockers or with asthma. Ann Intern Med, 115:270, 1991
>
> *Measures to avoid the interaction, such as corticosteroids, antihistamines, and nonionic contrast media, require further study*

Cyclopropane
> Hypotension (additive)
>> NWB Craythorne and PE Huffington, Effects of propranolol on the cardiovascular response to cyclopropane and halothane. Anesthesiology, 27:580, 1966
>
> *Monitor blood pressure; based on animal study*

Cyclosporine
> Possible cyclosporine toxicity (mechanism not established)
>> M Kaijser et al, Elevation of cyclosporin A blood levels during carvedilol treatment in renal transplant patients. Clin Transplantation, 11:577, 1997
>
> *Based on study in 21 renal transplant patients; monitor cyclosporine concentration; large interpatient variability*

Debrisoquine
> Possible propranolol toxicity (decreased metabolism)
>> L Anthony et al, Multiple pathways of propranolol's metabolism are inhibited by debrisoquin. Clin Pharmacol Ther, 46:297, 1989

BETA-ADRENERGIC BLOCKERS, with: *(continued)*
Based on a study in healthy extensive debrisoquine metabolizers

Diazoxide
Severe hypotension (additive)
> Manufacturer's package insert

Avoid concurrent use within 6 hours

Digoxin
Possible increased digoxin toxicity with talinolol (increased absorption; P-glycoprotein)
> K Westphal et al, Oral bioavailability of digoxin is enhanced by talinolol: evidence for involvement of intestinal P-glycoprotein. Clin Pharmacol Ther, 68:6, 2000

Based on study in healthy subjects; monitor digoxin serum concentrations and clinical status

Diltiazem
Cardiac failure (additive effects on contractility and blockade of compensating reflexes; decreased beta-blocker metabolism); A-V conduction disturbances and sinus bradycardia (additive)
> WE Strauss et al, Combination therapy with diltiazem and propranolol: precipitation of congestive heart failure. Clin Cardiol, 8:363, 1985; P Rocha et al, Hemodynamic effects of intravenous diltiazem in patients treated chronically with propranolol. Am Heart J, 111:62, 1986; A Sagie et al, Symptomatic bradycardia induced by the combination of oral diltiazem and beta blockers. Clin Cardiol, 14:314, 1991; I Yust et al, Life-threatening bradycardic reactions due to beta blocker-diltiazem interactions. Isr J Med Sci, 28:292, 1992

Monitor cardiac status; angina patients with normal cardiac contractility and conduction may tolerate propranolol and diltiazem without adverse effects

Disopyramide
Cardiac failure with practolol (additive effects on contractility and blockade of compensating reflexes)
> AD Cumming and C Robertson, Interaction between disopyramide and practolol. Br Med J, 2:1264, 1979; J Bonde et al, Atenolol inhibits the elimination of disopyramide. Eur J Clin Pharmacol, 28:41, 1985

Monitor cardiac status

Heart block with metoprolol (possibly additive)
> A Pernat et al, Heart conduction disturbances and cardiovascular collapse after disopyramide and low-dose metoprolol in a patient with hypertrophic obstructive cardiomyopathy. J Electrocardiol, 30:341, 1997

Single case of severe hypotension and bradycardia with metoprolol (1997)

Dofetilide
Possible increased risk of arrhythmias with sotalol (additive effect on QTc interval)
> Manufacturer's package insert (dofetilide); P Ferraro et al, Dofetilide for atrial fibrillation. N Engl J Med, 342:289, 2000

BETA-ADRENERGIC BLOCKERS, with: *(continued)*
Extent of increased risk not established; avoid concurrent use until more data available

Dolasetron

Possible increase in dolasetron effect with atenolol (mechanism not established)

    Manufacturer's package insert

Intravenous atenolol reduced clearance of hydrodolasetron, active metabolite of dolasetron; clinical significance not established; monitor clinical status

Ergot alkaloids

Severe peripheral vasoconstriction; possible gangrene (synergism)

    JF Baumrucker, Drug interaction – propranolol and cafergot. N Engl J Med, 288:916, 1973; CP Venter et al, Severe peripheral ischaemia during concomitant use of beta-blockers and ergot alkaloids. Br Med J, 289:288, 1984

Avoid concurrent use

Ether

Hypotension (additive)

    L Jorfeldt et al, Propranolol in ether anesthesia. Acta Anaesthesiol Scand, 11:159, 1967

Monitor blood pressure

Fenoldopam

Hypotension

    VS Mathur et al, Anesth Analg, 86:S86, 1998; manufacturer's package insert

Monitor blood pressure

Flecainide

Decreased cardiac contractility with propranolol (additive); arrhythmias and cardiac arrest with sotalol

    JL Holtzman et al, The pharmacodynamic and pharmacokinetic interaction of flecainide acetate with propranolol: effects on cardiac function and drug clearance. Eur J Clin Pharmacol, 33:97, 1987; R Warren et al, Serious interactions of sotalol with amiodarone and flecainide. Med J Aust, 152:277, 1990

Monitor cardiovascular status; single report with sotalol (1990)

Fluoroquinolones

Possible metoprolol toxicity with ciprofloxacin (decreased metabolism)

    NM Waite et al, Disposition of the (+) and (–) isomers of metoprolol following ciprofloxacin treatment. Pharmacotherapy, 10:236, 1990, abs 33

Based on a study in healthy men

Possible ventricular arrhythmia with grepafloxacin and sotalol (possible additive effect on QTc interval)

    Manufacturer's package insert

Theoretical; manufacturer recommends avoiding concurrent use

Furosemide

Possible propranolol toxicity (mechanism not established)

    J Feely et al, Increased clearance of propranolol due to furosemide. Clin Res, 29:189A, 1981; M Chiariello et al, Effect of furosemide on plasma con-

(continued)

BETA-ADRENERGIC BLOCKERS, with: *(continued)*
centration and beta-blockade by propranolol. Clin Pharmacol Ther, 26:433, 1979

Monitor cardiovascular status

Gabapentin
Possible increased risk of dystonia with propranolol (mechanism not established)

E Palomeras et al, Dystonia in a patient treated with propranolol and gabapentin. Arch Neurol, 57:570, 2000

Single case report (2000); monitor clinical status

Haloperidol
Severe hypotension with propranolol (mechanism not established)

HE Alexander, Jr et al, Hypotension and cardiopulmonary arrest associated with concurrent haloperidol and propranolol therapy. JAMA, 252:87, 1984

Single case report (1984)

Halothane
Hypotension (additive)

L Jorfeldt et al, Cardiovascular effects of beta-receptor blocking drugs during halothane anaesthesia in man. Acta Anaesthesiol Scand, 14:35, 1970; JA Kaplan and RW Dunbar, Propranolol and surgical anesthesia. Anesth Analg, 55:1, 1976; JM Hunter, Synergism between halothane and labetalol. Anaesthesia, 34:257, 1979

Monitor blood pressure

Hydralazine
Possible propranolol or metoprolol toxicity (mechanism not established)

DB Jack et al, The effect of hydralazine on the pharmacokinetics of three different beta adrenoceptor antagonists: metoprolol, nadolol, and acebutolol. Biopharm Drug Dispos, 3:47, 1982; DW Schneck and JE Vary, Mechanism by which hydralazine increases propranolol bioavailability. Clin Pharmacol Ther, 33:447, 1984; AJ McLean et al, Stable oral availability of atenolol coadministered with hydralazine. Drugs, 25 suppl 2:131, 1983; S Lindeberg et al, The effect of hydralazine on steady-state plasma concentrations of metoprolol in pregnant hypertensive women. Eur J Clin Pharmacol, 35:131, 1988

Monitor cardiovascular status; atenolol may not interact

Hydroxychloroquine
Possible metoprolol toxicity (probably decreased metabolism; CYP2D6)

M Somer et al, Influence of hydroxychloroquine on the bioavailability of oral metoprolol. Br J Clin Pharmacol, 49:549, 2000

Based on study in healthy subjects; clinical importance not established; monitor clinical status

Hypoglycemics, sulfonylurea
Decreased hypoglycemic effect (possibly decreased insulin release); after sulfonylurea overdose, prolonged hypoglycemia and decreased glycogenolysis (blocked beta effects of epinephrine); beta-receptor blockade masks tachycardia and tremor during hypoglycemia

PD Hansten, Beta-blocking agents and antidiabetic drugs. Drug Intell Clin

BETA-ADRENERGIC BLOCKERS, with: *(continued)*

Pharm, 14:46, 1980; R Zaman et al, The effect of acebutolol and propranolol on the hypoglycaemic action of glibenclamide. Br J Clin Pharmacol, 13:507, 1982; SP Deacon et al, Acebutolol, atenolol, and propranolol and metabolic responses to acute hypoglycaemia in diabetics. Br Med J, 2:1255, 1977; AJ Sinclair et al, Betaxolol and glucose-insulin relationships: studies in normal subjects taking glibenclamide or metformin. Br J Clin Pharmacol, 30:699, 1990

Monitor blood glucose; selective beta-blockers are less likely to interact; warn patient about absence of hypoglycemic symptoms

Insulin

With overdose, prolonged hypoglycemia and decreased glycogenolysis (blocked beta effects of epinephrine); beta-receptor blockade masks tachycardia and tremor during hypoglycemia

PD Hansten, Beta-blocking agents and antidiabetic drugs. Drug Intell Clin Pharm, 14:46, 1980; M Thamer et al, Association between antihypertensive drug use and hypoglycemia: a case-control study of diabeic users of insulin or sulfonylureas. Clin Ther, 21:1387, 1999

Monitor blood glucose and warn patient about absence of hypoglycemic symptoms; epidemiologic study suggests that beta-adrenergic blockers do not increase the risk of hypoglycemia in diabetics

Isradipine

Possible propranolol toxicity (possibly decreased metabolism)

AMM Shepherd et al, Pharmacokinetic interaction between isradipine and propranolol. Clin Pharmacol Ther, 43:194, 1988, abs IVB-1

Monitor propranolol concentration; based on study in 17 healthy men

Lidocaine

Lidocaine toxicity with propranolol, metoprolol, and possibly others (decreased metabolism)

DW Schneck et al, Effects of nadolol and propranolol on plasma lidocaine clearance. Clin Pharmacol Ther, 36:584, 1984; KA Conrad et al, Lidocaine elimination: effects of metoprolol and of propranolol. Clin Pharmacol Ther, 33:133, 1983; L Jordo et al, Pharmacokinetics of lidocaine in healthy individuals pretreated with multiple doses of metoprolol. Int J Clin Pharmacol Ther Toxicol, 22:312, 1984; NDS Bax et al, The impairment of lignocaine clearance by propranolol – major contribution from enzyme inhibition. Br J Clin Pharmacol, 19:597, 1985

Monitor lidocaine concentration; metoprolol had no effect after single IV doses of lidocaine in young, healthy subjects

Lithium

Bradycardia with propranolol (possibly synergism)

D Becker, Lithium and propranolol: possible synergism? J Clin Psychiatry, 50:473, 1989

Single case report (1989)

Maprotiline

Maprotiline toxicity with propranolol (decreased metabolism)

G Tollefson and T Lesar, Effect of propranolol on maprotiline clearance. Am

(continued)

BETA-ADRENERGIC BLOCKERS, with: *(continued)*
> J Psychiatry, 141:148, 1984; J Saiz-Ruiz and L Moral, Delirium induced by association of propranolol and maprotiline. J Clin Psychopharmacol, 8:77, 1988

Two case reports (1984, 1988)

Mefloquine
Increased risk of ECG abnormalities or cardiac arrest (mechanism not established)
> Manufacturer's package insert

Avoid concurrent use

Methyldopa
Hypertensive reaction (unopposed alpha-adrenergic stimulation)
> AS Nies and DG Shand, Hypertensive response to propranolol in a patient treated with methyldopa – a proposed mechanism. Clin Pharmacol Ther, 14:823, 1973

Avoid concurrent use

Metoclopramide
Increased hypotensive effect with labetolol (probably additive)
> M Blanco et al, Metoclopramide enhances labetalol-induced antihypertensive effect during handgrip in hypertensive patients. Am J Ther, 5:221, 1998

Based on study in hypertensive patients; monitor blood pressure and clinical status

Miglitol
Possible decreased propranolol effect (decreased bioavailability)
> Manufacturer's package insert (miglitol)

Monitor clinical status

Monoamine oxidase inhibitors
Bradycardia with phenelzine and nadolol or metoprolol (additive)
> A Reggev and BR Vollhardt, Bradycardia induced by an interaction between phenelzine and beta blockers. Psychosomatics, 30:106, 1989

In 2 patients over 60 years old (1989); monitor cardiovascular status

Narcotics: meperidine and congeners
Narcotic toxicity (mechanism not established)
> WM Davis and NS Hatoum, Possible toxic interaction of propranolol and narcotic analgesics. Drug Intell Clin Pharm, 15:290, 1981; DL Roerig et al, Effect of propranolol on the first pass uptake of fentanyl in the human and rat lung. Anesthesiology, 71:62, 1989

Data in 3 animal species and one study during human anesthesia with fentanyl; use concurrently with caution

Neuromuscular blocking agents
Bradycardia (possibly additive)
> B Yate and SM Mostafa, Drug interaction? Anaesthesia, 39:728, 1984; GL Glynne, Drug interaction? Anaesthesia, 39:293, 1984

Reported in 3 patients, one with atenolol and 2 with timolol eye drops

BETA-ADRENERGIC BLOCKERS, with: *(continued)*
>Both prolongation and reversal of neuromuscular blockade have been reported with tubocurarine (mechanism not established)
>>MS Rozen and FM Whan, Prolonged curarization associated with propranolol. Med J Aust, 1:467, 1972; YS Varma et al, Comparative effect of propranolol, oxprenolol and pindolol on neuromuscular blocking action of d-tubocurarine in man. Indian J Med Res, 61:1382, 1973
>
>*Monitor neuromuscular status*

Nicardipine
>Possible nicardipine toxicity with propranolol (decreased metabolism)
>>P Rocha et al, Kinetics and hemodynamic effects of intravenous nicardipine modified by previous propranolol oral treatment. Cardiovasc Drugs Ther, 4:1525, 1990; I Vercruysse et al, Increase in plasma propranolol caused by nicardipine is dependent on the delivery rate of propranolol. Eur J Clin Pharmacol, 49:121, 1995
>
>*Monitor clinical status*

Nifedipine
>Cardiac failure (additive adverse effects on contractility and blockade of compensating reflexes)
>
>A-V conduction disturbances and sinus bradycardia (additive)
>>U Elkayam et al, Effects of nifedipine on hemodynamics and cardiac function in patients with normal left ventricular ejection fraction already treated with propranolol. Am J Cardiol, 58:536, 1986; MJ Kendall et al, Lack of a pharmacokinetic interaction between nifedipine and the beta-adrenoceptor blockers metoprolol and atenolol. Br J Clin Pharmacol, 18:331, 1984; D Gangji et al, Study of the influence of nifedipine on the pharmacokinetics and pharmacodynamics of propranolol, metoprolol and atenolol. Br J Clin Pharmacol, 17:29S, 1984
>
>*Monitor cardiac status*

Nisoldipine
>Increased hypotensive effect (additive)
>>TA Shaw-Stiffel et al, Pharmacokinetic and pharmacodynamic interactions during multiple-dose administration of nisoldipine and propranolol. Clin Pharmacol Ther, 55:661, 1994; HL Elliott et al, The interactions between nisoldipine and two β-adrenoceptor antagonists—atenolol and propranolol. Br J Clin Pharmacol, 32:379, 1991; MAH Levine et al, Pharmacokinetic and pharmacodynamic interactions between nisoldipine and propranolol. Clin Pharmacol Ther, 43:39, 1988
>
>*Monitor blood pressure*

Nonsteroidal anti-inflammatory drugs
>Decreased antihypertensive effect (possibly prostaglandin synthesis inhibition)
>>J Watkins et al, Attenuation of hypotensive effect of propranolol and thiazide diuretics by indomethacin. Br Med J, 281:702, 1980; A Salvetti et al, The influence of indomethacin and sulindac on some pharmacological actions of atenolol in hypertensive patients. Br J Clin Pharmacol, 17:108S, 1984; DL Ebel et al, Effect of sulindac, piroxicam and placebo on the

(continued)

BETA-ADRENERGIC BLOCKERS, with: *(continued)*
> hypotensive effect of propranolol in patients with mild to moderate essential hypertension. Adv Ther, 2:131, 1985; J Webster, Interactions of NSAIDs with diuretics and beta-blockers; mechanisms and clinical implications. Drugs, 30:32, 1985; KL Radack et al, Ibuprofen interferes with the efficacy of antihypertensive drugs. Ann Intern Med, 107:628, 1987; AA Schuna et al, Lack of interaction between sulindac or naproxen and propranolol in hypertensive patients. J Clin Pharmacol, 29:524, 1989; MA Abate et al, Effect of naproxen and sulindac on blood pressure response to atenolol. DICP, 24:810, 1990; A Schoenfeld et al, Antagonism of antihypertensive drug therapy in pregnancy by indomethacin? Am J Obstet Gynecol, 161:1204, 1989; MA Abate et al, Interaction of indomethacin and sulindac with labetalol. Br J Clin Pharmacol, 31:363, 1991; A Halabi et al, Double-blind study on the interaction of oxaprozin with metoprolol in hypertensives. Cardiovasc Drugs Ther, 3:441, 1989

Monitor blood pressure; naproxen or oxaprozin may not interact; sulindac may interact only with labetalol

Penicillins
> Possible decreased atenolol effect with ampicillin (decreased absorption)
>> M Schafer-Korting et al, Atenolol interaction with aspirin, allopurinol, and ampicillin. Clin Pharmacol Ther, 33:283, 1983; AJ McLean et al, Dose-dependence of atenolol-ampicillin interaction. Br J Clin Pharmacol, 18:969, 1984

Despite large decrease in bioavailability, blood pressure remained under control, but exercise tachycardia increased; not studied in patients with angina; monitor clinical status

Phenothiazines
> Possible toxicity of both chlorpromazine and propranolol; possible thioridazine toxicity with propranolol or pindolol (decreased metabolism)
>> RE Vestal et al, Inhibition of propranolol metabolism by chlorpromazine. Clin Pharmacol Ther, 25:19, 1979; FA Miller and D Rampling, Adverse effects of combined propranolol and chlorpromazine therapy. Am J Psychiatry, 139:1198, 1982; RM Greendyke and DR Kanter, Plasma propranolol levels and their effect on plasma thioridazine and haloperidol concentrations. J Clin Psychopharmacol, 7:178, 1987; Manufacturer's package insert (thioridazine)

Manufacturer (thioridazine) states that concurrent use with propranolol or pindolol is contraindicated; with other combinations monitor clinical status

Prazosin
> Increased hypotensive effect of first dose of prazosin (mechanism not established)
>> P Seideman et al, Prazosin first dose phenomenon during combined treatment with a beta-adrenoceptor blocker in hypertensive patients. Br J Clin Pharmacol, 13:865, 1982; HL Elliott et al, Immediate cardiovascular responses to oral prazosin-effects of concurrent beta-blockers. Clin Pharmacol Ther, 29:303, 1981

BETA-ADRENERGIC BLOCKERS, with: *(continued)*
Use small initial dose and take at bedtime
Propafenone
Metoprolol neurological and cardiovascular toxicity (probably decreased metabolism)
> F Wagner et al, Drug interaction between propafenone and metoprolol. Br J Clin Pharmacol, 24:213, 1987

Monitor clinical status

Quinidine
Bradycardia with ophthalmic timolol (probably decreased timolol metabolism)
> Y Dinai et al, Bradycardia induced by interaction between quinidine and ophthalmic timolol. Ann Intern Med, 103:890, 1985; TI Edeki et al, Pharmacogenetic explanation for excessive β-blockade following timolol eye drops. JAMA, 274:1611, 1995

Selective beta-blockers may be preferable; effect accentuated in extensive metabolizers; monitor cardiac rhythm

Possible metoprolol toxicity (decreased metabolism)
> T Leemann et al, Single-dose quinidine treatment inhibits metoprolol oxidation in extensive metabolizers. Eur J Clin Pharmacol, 29:739, 1986; SL Bramer and A Suri, Inhibition of CYP2D6 by quinidine and its effects on the metabolism of cilostazol. Clin Pharmacokinet, 37 suppl 2:41, 1999

Monitor metoprolol concentration or cardiac status; based on studies in healthy subjects; genetic variability in response

Orthostatic hypotension with propranolol (mechanism not established)
> NR Loon et al, Orthostatic hypotension due to quinidine and propranolol. Am J Med, 81:1101, 1986; M Yasuhara et al, Alteration of propranolol pharmacokinetics and pharmacodynamics by quinidine in man. J Pharmacobio-Dyn, 13:681, 1990

Single case report (1986); study in healthy men found elevated plasma propranolol concentrations

Rifampin
Decreased beta-blockade (increased metabolism)
> RJ Herman et al, Induction of propranolol metabolism by rifampicin. Br J Clin Pharmacol, 16:565, 1983

Increased beta-blocker dosage may be required

Possible increased beta-blockade with metoprolol (decreased metabolism)
> PN Bennett et al, Effect of rifampicin on metoprolol and antipyrine kinetics. Br J Clin Pharmacol, 13:387, 1982

Monitor cardiovascular status

Selective serotonin reuptake inhibitors (SSRIs)
Heart block with fluoxetine and propranolol (possible decreased metabolism)
> WM Drake and GD Gordon, Heart block in a patient on propranolol and fluoxetine. Lancet, 343:425, 1994

Single case report (1994); poor documentation

BETA-ADRENERGIC BLOCKERS, with: *(continued)*
Bradycardia with metoprolol, fluoxetine, paroxetine, or citalopram (probably decreased metoprolol metabolism)
> T Walley et al, Interaction of metoprolol and fluoxetine. Lancet, 341:967, 1993; manufacturer's package insert (citalopram); A Hemeryck et al, Paroxetine affects metoprolol pharmacokinetics and pharmacodynamics in healthy volunteers. Clin Pharmacol Ther, 67:283, 2000

Single case report with fluoxetine (1993); citalopram doubled plasma metoprolol concentrations; paroxetine produced several-fold increase in metoprolol concentrations; sotalol did not interact with fluoxetine

Possible portosystemic encephalopathy (possibly decreased metabolism; CYP2D6)
> TJM van der Cammen et al, Stopping the pills. Lancet, 354:564, 1999

Single case report in a patient with hereditary hemorrhagic telangiectasia upon initiation of fluoxetine (1999); monitor clinical status, especially those with underlying liver disease

Sulfinpyrazone
Decreased hypotensive effect of oxprenolol (mechanism not established)
> LA Ferrara et al, Interference by sulphinpyrazone with the antihypertensive effects of oxprenolol. Eur J Clin Pharmacol, 29:717, 1986

Monitor blood pressure

Sympathomimetic amines
Decreased antihypertensive effect (pharmacological antagonism); hypertensive reactions with nonselective beta-blockers (unopposed alpha-adrenergic stimulation)
> DA Richards et al, Circulatory effects of noradrenaline and adrenaline before and after labetalol. Br J Clin Pharmacol, 7:371, 1979; CLA van Herwaarden et al, Effects of adrenaline during treatment with propranolol and metoprolol. Br Med J, 2:1029, 1977; I Goldberg et al, Timolol and epinephrine: a clinical study of ocular interactions. Arch Ophthalmol, 98:484, 1980; E Cass et al, Hazards of phenylephrine topical medication in persons taking propranolol. Can Med Assoc J, 120:1261, 1979; GD Alexander, Dangers of propranolol withdrawal prior to local anesthesia with epinephrine. Arch Otolaryngol, 111:280, 1985; TV Whelan, Propranolol, epinephrine, and accelerated hypertension during hemodialysis. Ann Intern Med, 106:327, 1987; H Houben et al, Effect of low-dose epinephrine infusion on hemodynamics after selective and nonselective beta-blockade in hypertension. Clin Pharmacol Ther, 31:685, 1982; M Sugimura et al, An echocardiographic study of interactions between pindolol and epinephrine contained in a local anesthetic solution. Anesth Prog, 42:29, 1995; ZJ Koscielniak-Nielsen, An unusual toxic reaction to axillary block by mepivacaine with adrenaline. Acta Anaesthesiol Scand, 42:868, 1998

Avoid concurrent use, if possible; discontinuing beta-blockers before surgery usually not recommended; use local anesthetics without epinephrine where possible

BETA-ADRENERGIC BLOCKERS, with: *(continued)*
> Decreased antianaphylactic effect of epinephrine (beta-blockade)
>> BR Newman and LK Schultz, Epinephrine-resistant anaphylaxis in a patient taking propranolol hydrochloride. Ann Allergy, 47:35, 1981; RL Jacobs et al, Potentiated anaphylaxis in patients with drug-induced beta-adrenergic blockade. J Allergy Clin Immunol, 68:125, 1981
>
> *Increased epinephrine dosage may be required in anaphylaxis*
>
> **Sympathomimetic bronchodilators**
>
> Decreased bronchodilator effect (antagonism)
>> J Wunderlich et al, Beta-adrenoceptor blockers and terbutaline in patients with chronic obstructive lung disease. Chest, 78:714, 1980; APM Greefhorst and CLA van Herwaarden, Ventilatory and haemodynamic effects of terbutaline infusion during beta$_1$-selective blockade with metoprolol and acebutolol in asthmatic patients. Eur J Clin Pharmacol, 23:203, 1982; JB Warren et al, Effect of penbutolol and propranolol on normal airway response to salbutamol. Clin Pharmacol Ther, 36:47, 1984
>
> *Avoid beta-blockers in asthmatics*
>
> **Theophyllines**
>
> Theophylline toxicity with propranolol and in smokers with metoprolol (decreased theophylline metabolism)
>> KA Conrad and DW Nyman, Effects of metoprolol and propranolol on theophylline elimination. Clin Pharmacol Ther, 28:463, 1980; JO Miners et al, Selectivity and dose-dependency of the inhibitory effect of propranolol on theophylline metabolism in man. Br J Clin Pharmacol, 20:219, 1985; SJ Warrington et al, Bisoprolol: studies of potential interactions with theophylline and warfarin in healthy volunteers. J Cardiovasc Pharmacol, 16 suppl 5:S164, 1990
>
> *Avoid beta-blockers in asthmatics; bisoprolol may not interact*
>
> **Thiazide diuretics**
>
> Increased hyperglycemic effect of thiazides in type II diabetics with propranolol (mechanism not established)
>> A Dornhorst et al, Aggravation by propranolol of hyperglycaemic effect of hydrochlorothiazide in type II diabetics without alteration of insulin secretion. Lancet, 1:123, 1985
>
> *Avoid concurrent use*
>
> Cardiac arrhythmias (mechanism not established)
>> O Odugbesan et al, Hazards of combined beta-blocker/diuretic tablets. Lancet, 1:1221, 1985; AJ Williams, JC Rodger et al, AR Scott, Hazards of combined beta-blocker/diuretic. Lancet, 1:1395, 1985; JK McKibbin et al, Sotalol, hypokalaemia, syncope, and torsade de pointes. Br Heart J, 51:157, 1984
>
> *Observed in patients with diuretic-induced hypokalemia given beta-blockers; monitor serum potassium concentration and cardiac rhythm*
>
> **Thyroid hormones**
>
> Decreased T$_3$ effect (increased metabolism)
>> J Feely et al, Propranolol, triiodothyronine, reverse triiodothyronine and thyroid disease. Clin Endocrinol, 10:531, 1979

(continued)

BETA-ADRENERGIC BLOCKERS, with: *(continued)*
- *Monitor thyroid status*

Tobacco, smoking
Decreased propranolol effect (increased metabolism)
> K Fox et al, Interaction between cigarettes and propranolol in treatment of angina pectoris. Br Med J, 281:191, 1980

Avoid concurrent use; not known whether interaction occurs with other beta-adrenergic blockers

Tocainide
Increased adverse psychiatric effects (mechanism not established)
> M Rubino and E Jackson, Severe paranoia with concomitant tocainide and propranolol therapy. Clin Pharm, 1:177, 1982

Single case report (1982)

Triptans
Possible rizatriptan or zolmitriptan toxicity with propranolol (decreased metabolism)
> Manufacturer's package insert; RW Peck et al, The interaction between propranolol and the novel antimigraine agent zolmitriptan (311C90). Br J Clin Pharmacol, 44:595, 1997; P Rolan, Potential drug interactions with the the novel antimigraine compound zolmitriptan (Zomig(tm), 311C90). Cephalalgia, 17 suppl:18:21, 1997

Based on studies in healthy subjects; monitor clinical status; rizatriptan dose should be limited to 5 mg when propranolol is also taken

Verapamil
Cardiac failure, A-V conduction disturbances and sinus bradycardia (probable decreased metabolism)
> J Zatuchni, Bradycardia and hypotension after propranolol HCl and verapamil. Heart Lung, 14:94, 1985; SG Carruthers et al, Synergistic adverse hemodynamic interaction between oral verapamil and propranolol. Clin Pharmacol Ther, 46:469, 1989; DL Johnston et al, Clinical and hemodynamic evaluation of propranolol in combination with verapamil, nifedipine and diltiazem in exertional angina pectoris: a placebo-controlled double-blind, randomized, crossover study. Am J Cardiol, 55:680, 1985; AJ McLean et al, Clearance-based oral drug interaction between verapamil and metoprolol and comparison with atenolol. Am J Cardiol, 55:1628, 1985; M Misra et al, Sinus arrest caused by atenolol – verapamil combination. Clin Cardiol, 10:365, 1987; AC Keech et al, Extent and pharmacokinetic mechanisms of oral atenolol-verapamil interaction in man. Eur J Clin Pharmacol, 35:363, 1988; Nl Sinclair and JL Benzie, Timolol eye drops and verapamil – a dangerous combination. Med J Aust, 1:548, 1983; SD Pringle and CJ MacEwen, Severe bradycardia due to interaction of timolol eye drops and verapamil. Br Med J, 294:155, 1987; BE Bleske et al, Evaluation of dosage-release formulations on inhibition of drug clearance: effect of sustained- and immediate-release verapamil on propranolol pharmacokinetic parameters. Ther Drug Monit, 16:216, 1994; Ul Schwarz et al, Unexpected effect of verapamil on oral bioavailability of the β-blocker talinolol in humans. Clin Pharmacol Ther, 65:283, 1999

BETA-ADRENERGIC BLOCKERS, with: *(continued)*
> Monitor cardiac status; may be less likely with nifedipine; timolol (ophthalmic) may also affect cardiovascular status

Vitamin C
> Possible decreased propranolol effect (probably increased first-pass metabolism)
>> JP Gonzalez et al, Influence of vitamin C on the absorption and first pass metabolism of propranolol. Eur J Clin Pharmacol, 48:295, 1995
>
> *Based on study in healthy men and women; clinical significance not established*

Zileuton
> Possible propranolol toxicity (decreased metabolism)
>> Manufacturer's package insert (zileuton)
>
> *Monitor propranolol concentration or clinical status*

Betaine, no documented interactions, see page 4, Criteria for Listing Interactions

Betamethasone, see Corticosteroids

Betaxolol, see Beta-adrenergic blockers

Bethanechol chloride, no documented interactions, see page 4, Criteria for Listing Interactions

BETHANIDINE, with:

Antidepressants, tricyclic - See Antidepressants, tricyclic with Bethanidine, page 83

Phenothiazines
> Decreased antihypertensive effect (blockade of uptake at target site)
>> WE Fann et al, Chlorpromazine reversal of the antihypertensive action of guanethidine. Lancet, 2:436, 1971; DS Janowsky et al, Guanethidine antagonism by antipsychotic drugs. J Tenn Med Assoc, 65:620, 1972
>
> *Avoid concurrent use; based on similarity to guanethidine*

Sympathomimetic amines
> Decreased antihypertensive effect (inhibition of norepinephrine uptake by neurons)
>> JR Misage and RH McDonald, Jr, Antagonism of hypotensive action of bethanidine by "common cold" remedy. Br Med J, 4:347, 1970
>
> *Avoid concurrent use*

BEXAROTENE, with:

Gemfibrozil
> Possible bexarotene toxicity (decreased metabolism; CYP3A4)
>> Manufacturer's package insert (bexarotene)
>
> *Avoid concurrent use*

Bicalutamide, no documented interactions, see page 4, Criteria for Listing Interactions

Bicarbonate of soda, see Antacids

Biperiden, no documented interactions, see page 4, Criteria for Listing Interactions

Bishydroxycoumarin, see Anticoagulants, oral

BISMUTH SUBSALICYLATE, with:
Tetracyclines
Decreased tetracycline effect (decreased absorption)
> KS Albert et al, Decreased tetracycline bioavailability caused by a bismuth subsalicylate antidiarrheal mixture. J Pharm Sci, 68:586, 1979; CD Ericsson et al, Influence of subsalicylate bismuth on absorption of doxycycline. JAMA, 247:2266, 1982; DP Healy et al, Reduced tetracycline bioavailability caused by magnesium aluminum silicate or in liquid formulations of bismuth subsalicylate. Ann Pharmacother, 31:1460, 1997

Effect may be due to magnesium-aluminum silicate suspending agent rather than bismuth subsalicylate; give tetracyclines at least 2 hours before or 6 hours after bismuth subsalicylate

BITOLTEROL, with:
Entacapone
Possible tachycardia and hypertension (decreased metabolism; COMT)
> Manufacturer's package insert (entacapone)

Avoid concurrent use

BLEOMYCIN, with:
Colony Stimulating Factors
Possible increased risk of pulmonary toxicity (mechanism not established)
> B Philippe et al, Pulmonary toxicity of chemotherapy and GM-CSF. Respir Med, 88:715, 1994; LY Dirix et al, Pulmonary toxicity and bleomycin. Lancet, 344:56, 1994; Y Bastion et al, Possible toxicity with the association of G-CSF and bleomycin. Lancet, 343:1221, 1994

Monitor pulmonary function

Oxygen
Pneumonitis (additive toxicity)
> RJ Cersosimo et al, Bleomycin pneumonitis potentiated by oxygen administration. Drug Intell Clin Pharm, 19:921, 1985; TS Ingrassia, III et al, Oxygen-exacerbated bleomycin pulmonary toxicity. Mayo Clin Proc, 66:173, 1991

Use oxygen at minimum effective concentration in patients who have received bleomycin

BLOOD TRANSFUSION, with:
Angiotensin-converting enzyme (ACE) inhibitors - See Angiotensin-converting enzyme (ACE) inhibitors with Blood transfusion, page 43
Methotrexate
Methotrexate toxicity (accumulation in red blood cells)
> AKL Yap et al, Methotrexate toxicity coincident with packed red cell transfusions. Lancet, 2:641, 1986

Avoid concurrent use, if possible

Bran, see Oat bran

BRETYLIUM, with:
Sympathomimetic amines
Possible hypertensive reaction (inhibition of norepinephrine uptake by neurons)
> MD Day, Effect of sympathomimetic amines on the blocking action of

BRETYLIUM, with: *(continued)*
> guanethidine, bretylium and xylocholine. Br J Pharmacol, 18:421, 1962; MO Day and MJ Rand, Antagonism of guanethidine and bretylium by various agents. Lancet, 2:1282, 1962

Based on animal studies; monitor blood pressure

BRIMONIDINE, with:

Antidepressants, tricyclic - See Antidepressants, tricyclic with Brimonidine, page 83

Monoamine oxidase inhibitors

Possible cardiovascular toxicity (mechanism not established)
> Manufacturer's package insert

Avoid concurrent use

Brinzolamide, no documented interactions, see page 4, Criteria for Listing Interactions

Bromazepam, see Benzodiazepines

Bromfenac, see Nonsteroidal anti-inflammatory drugs

BROMOCRIPTINE, with:

Alcohol - See Alcohol with Bromocriptine, page 15

Macrolide antibiotics

Possible bromocriptine toxicity with erythromycin (mechanism not established)
> MV Nelson et al, Pharmacokinetic evaluation of erythromycin and caffeine administered with bromocriptine. Clin Pharmacol Ther, 47:694, 1990

Monitor bromocriptine concentration or clinical status; based on study in healthy men

Phenothiazines

Decreased bromocriptine effect with thioridazine (antagonism)
> RJ Robbins et al, Interactions between thioridazine and bromocriptine in a patient with a prolactin-secreting pituitary adenoma. Am J Med, 76:921, 1984

Single report (1984); thioridazine, a dopamine antagonist, blocked bromocriptine suppression of prolactin-secreting pituitary adenoma

Sympathomimetic amines

Cardiac arrhythmias (mechanism not established)

In one patient who received capsules containing isometheptene, a sympathomimetic amine, acetaminophen and dichloralphenazone, a sedative (1991)

Seizures (mechanism not established)
> K Kulig et al, Bromocriptine-associated headache: possible life-threatening sympathomimetic interaction. Obstet Gynecol, 78:941, 1991

In one patient who received capsules containing phenylpropanolamine and guaifenesin (1991)

Postpartum hypertension (mechanism not established)
> JCN Chan et al, Postpartum hypertension, bromocriptine and phenylpropanolamine. Drug Invest, 8:254, 1994

In one patient who received phenylpropanolamine (1994)

Brompheniramine, no documented interactions, see page 4, Criteria for Listing Interactions

Budesonide, see Corticosteroids
BUMETANIDE, with:
   Aminoglycoside antibiotics - See Aminoglycoside antibiotics with Bumetanide, page 30
   Nonsteroidal anti-inflammatory drugs
      Decreased diuretic effect with indomethacin or sulindac (inhibition of prostaglandin synthesis)
         S Ahmad, Indomethacin-bumetanide interaction: an alert. Am J Cardiol, 54:246, 1984; MH Skinner et al, Sulindac inhibits bumetanide-induced sodium and water excretion. Clin Pharmacol Ther, 42:542, 1987
      Monitor diuretic effect
   Probenecid
      Possible decreased bumetanide effect (blocked access to site of action)
         MT Velasquez et al, Effect of probenecid on the natriuresis and renin release induced by bumetanide in man. J Clin Pharmacol, 21:657, 1981
      Monitor diuretic effect

BUPIVACAINE, with:
   Angiotensin-converting enzyme (ACE) inhibitors - See Angiotensin-converting enzyme (ACE) inhibitors with Bupivacaine, page 43
   Antifungals, imidazoles and triazoles - See Antifungals, imidazoles and triazoles with Bupivacaine, page 97
   Antihistamines, H_2-blockers - See Antihistamines, H_2-blockers with Bupivacaine, page 115
   Lidocaine
      Possible lidocaine toxicity (displacement from binding)
         DL Goolkasian et al, Displacement of lidocaine from serum a_1-acid glycoprotein binding sites by basic drugs. Eur J Clin Pharmacol, 25:413, 1983
      Monitor lidocaine concentration
   Mepivacaine
      Mepivacaine toxicity (displacement from binding)
         CT Hartrick et al, Compounding of bupivacaine and mepivacaine for regional anesthesia. A safe practice? Reg Anesth, 9:94, 1984; CT Hartrick et al, Influence of bupivacaine on mepivacaine protein binding. Clin Pharmacol Ther, 36:546, 1984
      Avoid concurrent use; single case report (1984); supported by in vitro studies
   Narcotics: morphine-like
      Possible respiratory depression (mechanism not established)
         CY Piquet et al, Respiratory depression following administration of intrathecal bupivacaine to an opioid-dependent patient. Ann Pharmacother, 32:653, 1998
      Report of two patients, one fatal (1998)
   Prazosin
      Hypotension during epidural bupivacaine anesthesia (mechanism not established)
         CA Lydiatt et al, Severe hypotension during epidural anesthesia in a prazosin-treated patient. Anesth Analg, 76:1152, 1993

BUPIVACAINE, with: *(continued)*
   Single case report (1993); no response to phenylephrine; responded to epinephrine
   Verapamil
      Severe hypotension and bradycardia (mechanism not established)
         C Collier, Verapamil and epidural bupivacaine. Anaesth Intensive Care, 13:101, 1985
      With bupivacaine for epidural block; lidocaine may not interact

BUPRENORPHINE, with:
   Benzodiazepines - See Benzodiazepines with Buprenorphine, page 139

BUPROPION, with:
   Amantadine - See Amantadine with Bupropion, page 27
   Antidepressants, tricyclic - See Antidepressants, tricyclic with Bupropion, page 83
   Carbamazepine
      Decreased bupropion effect (probably increased metabolism)
         AP Popli et al, Bupropion and anticonvulsant drug interactions. Ann Clin Psychiatry, 7:99, 1995; TA Ketter et al, Carbamazepine but not valproate induces bupropion metabolism. J Clin Psychopharmacol, 15:327, 1995
      Monitor clinical status
   Corticosteroids
      Increased seizure risk with system steroids (additive)
         Manufacturer's package insert
      Use only with caution; monitor clinical status
   Guanfacine
      Seizures (mechanism not established)
         P Tilton, Bupropion and guanfacine. J Am Acad Child Adolesc Psychiatry, 37:682, 1998
      Single case report (1998); causal relationship not established
   Levodopa
      Possible increase in adverse effects (mechanism not established)
         Manufacturer's package insert
      Monitor clinical status; the manufacturer recommends small initial doses of bupropion and gradual increases
   Monoamine oxidase inhibitors
      Possible seizures (mechanism not established)
         Manufacturer's package insert; RS Kent, Bupropion clarification. J Clin Psychiatry, 60:196, 1999
      Avoid concurrent use; MAOI should be stopped at least 14 days before starting bupropion
   Phenothiazines
      Increased seizure risk (additive)
         Manufacturer's package insert
      Use only with caution; monitor clinical status
   Ritonavir
      Possible bupropion toxicity (decreased metabolism)
         Manufacturer's package insert (ritonavir)

(continued)

BUPROPION, with: *(continued)*
Theoretical considerations; listed as contraindicated in product information

Selective serotonin reuptake inhibitors (SSRIs)

Catatonia when bupropion given right after fluoxetine (mechanism not established)

SH Preskorn, Should bupropion dosage be adjusted based upon therapeutic drug monitoring? Psychopharmacol Bull, 27:637, 1991

Single case report (1991)

Anxiety and panic with fluoxetine (mechanism not established)

SJ Young, Panic associated with combining fluoxetine and bupropion. J Clin Psychiatry, 57:177, 1996

Single case report confirmed by rechallenge (1996)

Theophyllines

Increased seizures risk (additive)

Manufacturer's package insert

Use only with caution; monitor clinical status

Zolpidem

Hallucinations (additive)

CJ Elko et al, Zolpidem-associated hallucinations and serotonin reuptake inhibition: a possible interaction. Clin Toxicol, 36:195, 1998

Single case report (1998)

BUSPIRONE, with:

Antifungals, imidazoles and triazoles - See Antifungals, imidazoles and triazoles with Buspirone, page 97

Diltiazem

Possible buspirone toxicity (probably decreased first-pass metabolism of buspirone; CYP3A4)

TS Lamberg et al, Effects of verapamil and diltiazem on the pharmacokinetics and pharmacodynamics of buspirone. Clin Pharmacol Ther, 63:640, 1998

Based on study in healthy subjects; monitor clinical status

Grapefruit juice

Possible buspirone toxicity (decreased metabolism)

JJ Lilja et al, Grapefruit juice substantially increases plasma concentrations of buspirone. Clin Pharmacol Ther, 64:655, 1998

Based on study in healthy subjects; avoid concurrent use

Macrolide antibiotics

Possible buspirone toxicity with erythromycin (decreased metabolism)

KT Kivistö et al, Buspirone concentrations are greatly increased by erythromycin and itraconazole. Eur J Clin Pharmacol, 52:A134, 1997

Avoid concurrent use; based on study in healthy subjects; clarithromycin likely to produce similar effect, but azithromycin would not interact

Monoamine oxidase inhibitors

Hypertension (mechanism not established)

Manufacturer's package insert

BUSPIRONE, with: *(continued)*
  Avoid concurrent use
  Rifampin
    Decreased buspirone effect (increased metabolism; probable CYP3A4)
      TS Lamberg et al, Concentrations and effects of buspirone are considerably reduced by rifampicin. Br J Clin Pharmacol, 45:381, 1998; KT Kivistö et al, Interactions of buspirone with itraconazole and rifampicin: effects on the pharmacokinetics of the active 1-(2-pyriminidyl)-piperazine metabolite of buspirone. Pharmacol Toxicol, 84:94, 1999
    Avoid concurrent use; based on study in healthy subjects
  Selective serotonin reuptake inhibitors (SSRIs)
    Loss of anxiolytic effect of buspirone (mechanism not established)
      P Fischer et al, Weak antidepressant response after buspirone augmentation of serotonin reuptake inhibitors in refractory severe depression. Int Clin Psychopharmacol, 13:83, 1998
    Buspirone did not provide much benefit to 10 refractory depressive patients on various SSRIs (1998)

    Seizure with fluoxetine (mechanism not established)
      TA Grady et al, Seizure associated with fluoxetine and adjuvant buspirone therapy. J Clin Psychopharmacol, 12:70, 1992
    Single case report (1992)

    Possible buspirone toxicity with fluvoxamine (probably decreased metabolism)
      IM Anderson et al, The effect of chronic fluvoxamine on hormonal and psychological responses to buspirone in normal volunteers. Pschopharmacology, 128:74, 1996; TS Lamberg et al, The effect of fluvoxamine on the pharmacokinetics and pharmacodynamics of buspirone. Eur J Clin Pharmacol, 54:761, 1998
    Based on studies in healthy subjects; clinical significance not established

    Serotonin syndrome (mechanism not established)
      M Baetz and D Malcolm, Serotonin syndrome from fluvoxamine and buspirone. Can J Psychiatry, 40:428, 1995; GH Manos, Possible serotonin syndrome associated with buspirone added to fluoxetine. Ann Pharmacother, 34:871, 2000
    Single case reports with fluvoxamine (1995) and fluoxetine (2000)
  Trazodone
    Serotonin syndrome (additive)
      RJ Goldberg and M Huk, Serotonin syndrome from trazodone and buspirone. Psychosomatics, 33:235, 1992
    Single case report (1992)
  Verapamil
    Possible buspirone toxicity (probably decreased first-pass metabolism of buspirone; CYP3A4)
      TS Lamberg et al, Effects of verapamil and diltiazem on the pharmacokinetics and pharmacodynamics of buspirone. Clin Pharmacol Ther, 63:640, 1998

(continued)

BUSPIRONE, with: *(continued)*
  Based on study in healthy subjects; monitor clinical status
Busulfan, see Alkylating agents
Butabarbital, see Barbiturates
Butalbital, see Barbiturates
Butaperazine, see Phenothiazines
Butenafine, no documented interactions, see page 4, Criteria for Listing Interactions
Butoconazole, no documented interactions, see page 4, Criteria for Listing Interactions
Butorphanol, no documented interactions, see page 4, Criteria for Listing Interactions

CABERGOLINE, with:
  Haloperidol
    Decreased effect of both drugs (antagonism)
      Manufacturer's package insert
    Avoid concurrent use
  Metoclopramide
    Decreased effect of both drugs (antagonism)
      Manufacturer's package insert
    Avoid concurrent use
  Phenothiazines
    Decreased effect of both drugs (antagonism)
      Manufacturer's package insert
    Avoid concurrent use

CAFFEINE, with:
  Alcohol - See Alcohol with Caffeine, page 16
  Antifungals, imidazoles and triazoles - See Antifungals, imidazoles and triazoles with Caffeine, page 98
  Benzodiazepines - See Benzodiazepines with Caffeine, page 139
  Carbamazepine
    Decreased caffeine effect (increased metabolism)
      AC Parker et al, Induction of CYP1A2 activity by carbamazepine in children using the caffeine breath test. Br J Clin Pharmacol, 45:176, 1998
    Based on study in 5 children

    Possible decreased carbamazepine effect (decreased absorption)
      J Vaz et al, Influence of caffeine on pharmacokinetic profile of sodium valproate and carbamazepine in normal volunteers. Indian J Exp Biol, 36:112, 1998
    Monitor carbamazepine concentration and clinical status; avoid large fluctuations in caffeine intake

  Clozapine
    Possible exacerbation of schizophrenia (mechanism not established)
      JL Vainer and G Chouinard, Interaction between caffeine and clozapine. J Clin Psychopharmacol, 14:284, 1994; L Bertilsson et al, Clozapine disposition covaries with CYP1A2 activity determined by a caffeine test. Br J Clin Pharmacol, 38:471, 1994; S Hägg et al, Effect of caffeine on clozapine phar-

CAFFEINE, with: *(continued)*
macokinetics in healthy volunteers. Br J Clin Pharmacol, 49:59, 2000

Based on a single case report (1994) and pharmacokinetic study in healthy subjects; monitor clinical status

Contraceptives, oral

Possible caffeine toxicity (decreased metabolism)

EC Rietveld et al, Rapid onset of an increase in caffeine residence time in young women due to oral contraceptive steroids. Eur J Clin Pharmacol, 26:371, 1984; RV Patwardhan et al, Impaired elimination of caffeine by oral contraceptive steroids. J Lab Clin Med, 95:603, 1980; A Balogh et al, Influence of ethinylestradiol-containing combination oral contraceptives with gestodene or levonorgestrel on caffeine elimination. Eur J Clin Pharmacol, 48:161, 1995

Possibly significant with large doses of caffeine, especially with prolonged use

Dipyridamole

Decreased dipyridamole effect (caffeine blockade of adenosine receptors)

P Smits et al, Dose-dependent inhibition of the hemodynamic response to dipyridamole by caffeine. Clin Pharmacol Ther, 50:529, 1991; P Smits et al, Caffeine reduces dipyridamole-induced myocardial ischemia. J Nucl Med, 30:1723, 1989

Single case report (1989); confirmed by study in healthy volunteers; avoid concurrent use

Disulfiram

Possible caffeine toxicity (decreased metabolism)

CA Beach et al, Inhibition of elimination of caffeine by disulfiram in normal subjects and recovering alcoholics. Clin Pharmacol Ther, 39:265, 1986

Greatest effect observed in recovering alcoholics; avoid concurrent use during early rehabilitation of alcoholics

Fluoroquinolones

Possible caffeine toxicity with enoxacin, ciprofloxacin, grepafloxacin and pefloxacin; may be less likely with norfloxacin and trovafloxacin; does not occur with ofloxacin, levofloxacin, lomefloxacin, sparfloxacin or temafloxacin (decreased metabolism; CYP1A2)

G Barnett et al, Pharmacokinetic determination of relative potency of quinolone inhibition of caffeine disposition. Eur J Clin Pharmacol, 39:63, 1990; G Mahr et al, Effects of temafloxacin and ciprofloxacin on the pharmacokinetics of caffeine. Clin Pharmacokinet, 22 suppl 1:90, 1992; DP Healy et al, Lack of interaction between lomefloxacin and caffeine in normal volunteers. Antimicrob Agents Chemother, 35:660, 1991; manufacturer's package inserts; M Kinzig-Schippers et al, Interaction of pefloxacin and enoxacin with the human cytochrome P450 enzyme CYP1A2. Clin Pharmacol Ther, 65:262, 1999; JA Carrillo and J Benitez, Clinically significant pharmacokinetic interactions between dietary caffeine and medications. Clin Pharmacokinet, 39:127, 2000

Avoid large caffeine intake

(continued)

CAFFEINE, with: *(continued)*

Iron
Decreased iron effect (decreased absorption)
> TA Morck et al, Inhibition of food iron absorption by coffee. Am J Clin Nutr, 37:416, 1983

Give at least 2 hours apart

Lithium
Possible decreased lithium effect (probably increased renal excretion)
> JW Jefferson, Lithium tremor and caffeine intake: two cases of drinking less and shaking more. J Clin Psychiatry, 49:72, 1998; R Mester et al, Caffeine withdrawal increases lithium blood levels. Biol Psychiatry, 37:348, 1995

Monitor lithium concentration

Nicotine gum
Possible increased blood pressure and heart rate after IV caffeine causing blood levels similar to 2 cups of coffee and nicotine gum (additive)
> P Smits et al, The cardiovascular interaction between caffeine and nicotine in humans. Clin Pharmacol Ther, 54:194, 1993

Warn patients and monitor cardiovascular status

Selective serotonin reuptake inhibitors (SSRIs)
Possible caffeine toxicity with fluvoxamine (decreased metabolism; probably CYP1A2)
> U Jeppesen et al, Dose-dependent inhibition of CYP1A2, CYP2C19 and CYP2D6 by citalopram, fluoxetine, fluvoxamine and paroxetine. Eur J Clin Pharmacol, 51:73, 1996; U Jeppesen et al, A fluvoxamine-caffeine interaction study. Pharmacogenetics, 6:213, 1996; O Spigset, Are adverse drug reactions attributed to fluvoxamine caused by concomitant intake of caffeine? Eur J Clin Pharmacol, 54:665, 1998; BB Rasmussen et al, Fluvoxamine is a potent inhibitor of the metabolism of caffeine *in vitro*. Pharmacol Toxicol, 83:240, 1998

Based on studies in healthy subjects; effect not seen with other SSRIs tested (citalopram, fluoxetine, paroxetine); in vitro studies show fluvoxamine is a potent inhibit of CYP1A2

Sympathomimetic amines
Acute increase in blood pressure with phenylpropanolamine (mechanism not established)
> NJ Brown et al, A pharmacodynamic interaction between caffeine and phenylpropanolamine. Clin Pharmacol Ther, 50:363, 1991

Avoid concurrent use

Theophyllines
Toxicity of both drugs in patients with liver disease (decreased metabolism)
> SA Iverson et al, Unsuspected caffeine toxicity complicating theophylline therapy. Hum Toxicol, 3:509, 1984; JHG Jonkman et al, The influence of caffeine on the steady-state pharmacokinetics of theophylline. Clin Pharmacol Ther, 49:248, 1991; J Sato et al, Influence of usual intake of dietary caffeine on single-dose kinetics of theophylline in healthy human subjects. Eur J Clin Pharmacol, 44:295, 1993

CAFFEINE, with: *(continued)*

Monitor methylxanthine as well as theophylline concentration in patients with liver disease; large amounts of caffeine (equivalent to 6 to 10 cups of coffee) may cause the interaction in healthy men

Verapamil

Possible caffeine toxicity (decreased metabolism)

S Nawoot et al, Inhibition of caffeine elimination by verapamil. Clin Pharmacol Ther, 43:148, 1988

Monitor cardiovascular status; based on studies in healthy men

Calcifediol, see Vitamin D

Calciferol, see Vitamin D

Calcipotriene, no documented interactions, see page 4, Criteria for Listing Interactions

CALCITONIN, with:

Lithium

Possible decreased lithium effect (increased renal excretion)

G Passiu et al, Calcitonin decreases lithium plasma levels in man. Preliminary report. Int J Clin Pharm Res, 18:179, 1998

Based on study of four patients; monitor lithium concentration and clinical status

Calcitriol, no documented interactions, see page 4, Criteria for Listing Interactions

CALCIUM, with:

Fluoride

Decreased fluoride effect (decreased absorption)

H Spencer et al, Effect of aluminum hydroxide on fluoride metabolism. Clin Pharmacol Ther, 28:529, 1980; D Briançon et al, Comparative study of fluoride bioavailability following the administration of sodium fluoride alone and in combination with different calcium salts. J Bone Mineral Res, 5 suppl 1:S71, 1990; J-P Devogelaer et al, Bioavailability of enteric-coated sodium fluoride tablets as affected by the administration of calcium supplements at different time intervals. J Bone Mineral Res, 5 suppl 1:S75, 1990

Avoid concurrent use or give as far apart as possible; enteric-coated fluoride and calcium solutions may not interact

Risedronate

Decreased risedronate effect (decreased absorption)

Manufacturer's package insert (risedronate)

Calcium supplements should be taken at a different time of the day

Thyroid hormones

Possible decreased levothyroxine effect with calcium carbonate (decreased absorption)

CR Schneyer, Calcium carbonate and reduction of levothyroxine efficacy. JAMA, 279:750, 1998; LE Butner et al, Calcium carbonate – induced hypothroidism. Ann Intern Med, 132:595, 2000; N Singh et al, Effect of calcium carbonate on the absorption of levothyroxine. JAMA, 283:2822, 2000; LE Butner et al, Calcium carbonate-induced hypothyroidism. Ann Intern Med, 132:595, 2000

(continued)

CALCIUM, with: *(continued)*
Based on several case reports and study in 20 patients; monitor T4 or TSH concentrations; calcium and levothyroxine should be taken at least 4 hours apart

Zinc

Possible decreased zinc effect (decreased absorption)

V Argiratos and S Samman, The effect of calcium carbonate and calcium citrate on the absorption of zinc in healthy female subjects. Eur J Clin Nutr, 48:198, 1994

Avoid concurrent use

Calcium disodium edetate, no documented interactions, see page 4, Criteria for Listing Interactions

Calusterone, see Anabolic and androgenic steroids

Candesartan, no documented interactions, see page 4, Criteria for Listing Interactions

Capecitabine, see Fluorouracil

Capreomycin, no documented interactions, see page 4, Criteria for Listing Interactions

CAPSAICIN, with:

Angiotensin-converting enzyme (ACE) inhibitors - See Angiotensin-converting enzyme (ACE) inhibitors with Capsaicin, page 43

Captopril, see Angiotensin-converting enzyme (ACE) inhibitors

Carbachol, no documented interactions, see page 4, Criteria for Listing Interactions

CARBAMAZEPINE, with:

Anabolic and androgenic steroids - See Anabolic and androgenic steroids with Carbamazepine, page 41

Anticoagulants, oral - See Anticoagulants, oral with Carbamazepine, page 62

Antidepressants, tricyclic - See Antidepressants, tricyclic with Carbamazepine, page 83

Antifungals, imidazoles and triazoles - See Antifungals, imidazoles and triazoles with Carbamazepine, page 98

Antihistamines, H$_1$-blockers: astemizole, terfenadine - See Antihistamines, H$_1$-blockers: astemizole, terfenadine with Carbamazepine, page 110

Antihistamines, H$_2$-blockers - See Antihistamines, H$_2$-blockers with Carbamazepine, page 116

Barbiturates - See Barbiturates with Carbamazepine, page 131

Benzodiazepines - See Benzodiazepines with Carbamazepine, page 139

Bupropion - See Bupropion with Carbamazepine, page 169

Caffeine - See Caffeine with Carbamazepine, page 172

Cisplatin

Decreased carbamazepine effect (decreased absorption)

C Neef and I de Voogd-van der Straaten, An interaction between cytostatic and anticonvulsant drugs. Clin Pharmacol Ther, 43:372, 1988

Single well-documented case report (1988); monitor carbamazepine concentration

Clozapine

Neuroleptic malignant syndrome (mechanism not established)

T Müller et al, Neuroleptic malignant syndrome after clozapine plus carba-

CARBAMAZEPINE, with: *(continued)*

mazepine. Lancet, 2:1500, 1988

Single case report (1988) in patient who received clozapine shortly after lithium was stopped; syndrome has been reported with clozapine or lithium alone

Bone marrow suppression

SL Gerson et al, Polypharmacy in fatal clozapine-associated agranulocytosis. Lancet, 338:262, 1991; U Junghan et al, Increased risk of hematological side-effects in psychiatric patients treated with clozapine and carbamazepin? Pharmacopsychiat, 26:262, 1993

Single case report of agranulocytosis with pancytopenia (1991); retrospective study found incidence of granulocytopenia with concurrent carbamazepine and clozapine not significantly increased; avoid concurrent use or monitor white cell count

Possibly decreased clozapine effect (possibly increased metabolism)

V Raitasuo et al, Carbamazepine and plasma levels of clozapine. Am J Psychiatry, 150:169, 1993; M Jerling et al, Fluvoxamine inhibition and carbamazepine induction of the metabolism of clozapine: evidence from a therapeutic drug monitoring service. Ther Drug Monit, 16:368, 1994; WH Wilson, Do anticonvulsants hinder clozapine treatment? Biol Psychiatry, 37:132, 1995

Two case reports (1993), data from therapeutic drug monitoring service, and a retrospective review of 88 patients

Contraceptives, oral

Decreased contraceptive effect (increased metabolism)

DJ Rapport and JR Calabrese, Interactions between carbamazepine and birth control pills. Psychosomatics, 30:462, 1989; DJ Back et al, Evaluation of Committee on Safety of Medicines yellow card reports on oral contraceptive-drug interactions with anticonvulsants and antibiotics. Br J Clin Pharmacol, 25:527, 1988; MA Eldon et al, Gabapentin does not interact with a contraceptive regimen of norethindrone acetate and ethinyl estradiol. Neurology, 50:1146, 1998

Use alternative contraceptive; gabapentin does not appear to interact with an oral contraceptive containing norethindrone and ethinyl estradiol

Corticosteroids

Decreased corticosteroid effect (probably increased metabolism)

A Olivesi, Modified elimination of prednisolone in epileptic patients on carbamazepine monotherapy, and in women using low-dose oral contraceptives. Biomed Pharmacother, 40:301, 1986; J Kobberling and A v zur Muhlen, The influence of diphenylhydantoin and carbamazepine on the circadian rhythm of free urinary corticoids and on the suppressibility of the basal and the "impulsive" activity by dexamethasone. Acta Endocrinol, 72:308, 1973; MR Privitera et al, Interference by carbamazepine with the dexamethasone suppression test. Biol Psychiatry, 17:611, 1982

Monitor corticosteroid effect

(continued)

CARBAMAZEPINE, with: *(continued)*
  Cyclosporine
    Decreased cyclosporine effect (increased metabolism)
      G Hillebrand et al, Valproate for epilepsy in renal transplant recipients receiving cyclosporine. Transplantation, 43:915, 1987; OMV Schofield et al, Cyclosporin A in psoriasis: interaction with carbamazepine. Br J Dermatol, 122:425, 1990; J Soto Alvarez et al, Effect of carbamazepine on ciclosporin blood level. Nephron, 58:235, 1991
    Use alternative anticonvulsant, if possible; valproate does not interact
  Delavirdine
    Possible decreased delavirdine effect (increased metabolism)
      Manufacturer's package insert
    Based on preliminary data; monitor clinical status
  Diltiazem
    Neurotoxicity (probably decreased carbamazepine metabolism; CYP3A4)
      MJ Brodie and GJA Macphee, Carbamazepine neurotoxicity precipitated by diltiazem. Br Med J, 292:1170, 1986; E Maoz et al, Carbamazepine neurotoxic reaction after administration of diltiazem. Arch Intern Med, 152:2503, 1992; PH Silverstone and L Birkett, Diltiazem as augmentation therapy in patients with treatment-resistant bipolar disorder: a retrospective study. J Psychiatry Neurosci, 25:276, 2000
    Avoid concurrent use if possible; if combination used, monitor carbamazepine levels and adjust carbamazepine dose as needed; combination used to advantage in several patients with resistant bipolar disorder
  Etretinate
    Decreased effect of etretinate in erythroderma (mechanism not established)
      KN Mohammed, Unresponsiveness to etretinate during anticonvulsant therapy. Dermatology, 185:79, 1992
    Single case report (1992)
  Felbamate
    Possible decreased carbamazepine effect (increased metabolism); possible carbamazepine toxicity (decreased epoxide metabolism)
      ML Wagner et al, Effect of felbamate on carbamazepine and its major metabolites. Clin Pharmacol Ther, 53:536, 1993
    Monitor carbamazepine and carbamazepine epoxide concentration; clinical significance not established
  Furosemide
    Hyponatremia (mechanism not established)
      R Yassa et al, Carbamazepine, diuretics, and hyponatremia: a possible interaction. J Clin Psychiatry, 48:281, 1987
    Single case report (1987); monitor sodium concentration
  Grapefruit juice
    Possible carbamazepine toxicity (decreased metabolism; CYP3A4)
      SK Garg et al, Effect of grapefruit juice on carbamazepine bioavailability in patients with epilepsy. Clin Pharmacol Ther, 64:286, 1998
    Based on study in epileptic patients; monitor carbamazepine concentration

CARBAMAZEPINE, with: *(continued)*
- **Haloperidol**

    Decreased haloperidol effect; increased fluctuation of haloperidol effect with depot (IM) haloperidol decanoate (increased metabolism)

    > EM Kahn et al, Change in haloperidol level due to carbamazepine – a complicating factor in combined medication for schizophrenia. J Clin Psychopharmacol, 10:54, 1990; J Brayley and P Yellowlees, An interaction between haloperidol and carbamazepine in a patient with cerebral palsy. Aust N Z J Psychiatry, 21:605, 1987; G Pupeschi et al, Do enzyme inducers modify haloperidol decanoate rate of release? Prog Neuro-Psychopharmacol Biol Psychiat, 18:1323, 1994; K Iwahashi et al, The drug—drug interaction effects of haloperidol on plasma carbamazepine levels. Clin Neuropharmacol, 18:233, 1995; K Nisijima et al, Addition of carbamazepine to long-term treatment with neuroleptics may induce neuroleptic malignant syndrome. Biol Psychiatry, 44:930, 1998; G Hirokane et al, Interindividual variation of plasma haloperidol concentrations and the impact of concomitant medications: the analysis of therapeutic drug monitoring data. Ther Drug Monit, 21:82, 1999; B Hesslinger et al, Effects of carbamazepine and valproate on haloperidol plasma levels and on psychopathologic outcome in schizophrenic patients. J Clin Psychopharmacol, 19:310, 1999

    Monitor clinical status and haloperidol concentration; single case report of neurotoxicity (1987) and neuroleptic malignant syndrome (1998); with haloperidol decanoate, interval between injections may need to be reduced

- **Indinavir**

    Decreased indinavir effect (increased metabolism)

    > PWH Hugen et al, Carbamazepine-indinavir interaction causes antiretroviral therapy failure. Ann Pharmacother, 34:465, 2000

    Single case report (2000); avoid concurrent use or monitor for reduced indinavir effect

- **Influenza vaccine**

    Possible carbamazepine toxicity (decreased metabolism)

    > MW Jann and GS Fidone, Effect of influenza vaccine on serum anticonvulsant concentrations. Clin Pharm, 5:817, 1986

    Monitor carbamazepine concentration

- **Isoniazid**

    Toxicity of both drugs (altered metabolism)

    > SH Block, Carbamazepine-isoniazid interaction. Pediatrics, 69:494, 1982; JM Wright et al, Isoniazid-induced carbamazepine toxicity and vice versa: a double drug interaction. N Engl J Med, 307:1325, 1982; FE Berkowitz et al, Acute liver failure caused by isoniazid in a child receiving carbamazepine. Int J Tuberc Lung Dis, 2:603, 1998

    Avoid concurrent use, if possible; monitor liver function if combination used

- **Isotretinoin**

    Possible altered carbamazepine bioavailability and/or metabolism (mechanism not established)

    > JR Marsden, Effect of isotretinoin on carbamazepine pharmacokinetics. Br J Dermatol, 119:403, 1988

(continued)

CARBAMAZEPINE, with: *(continued)*
Single case report (1988); clinical significance not established

Lamotrigine

Carbamazepine toxicity (decreased metabolism of carbamazepine epoxide)

T Warner et al, Lamotrigine-induced carbamazepine toxicity: an interaction with carbamazepine-10,11-epoxide. Epilepsy Res, 11:147, 1992; FMC Besag et al, Carbamazepine toxicity with lamotrigine: pharmacokinetic or pharmacodynamic interaction? Epilepsia, 39:183, 1998

Monitor clinical status; serum carbamazepine measurements alone may not predict toxicity

Decreased lamotrigine effect (probably increased metabolism)

TW May et al, Influence of oxcarbazepine and methsuximide on lamotrigine concentrations in epileptic patients with and without valproic acid comedication: results of a retrospective study. Ther Drug Monit, 21:175, 1999; Y Böttiger et al, Lamotrigine drug interactions in a TDM material. Ther Drug Monit, 21:171, 1999; JA Armijo et al, Lamotrigine serum concentration-to-dose ratio: influence of age and concomitant antiepileptic drugs and dosage implications. Ther Drug Monit, 21:182, 1999

Monitor lamotrigine serum concentrations and clinical status; lamotrigine dosage may need to be adjusted

Lithium

Neurotoxicity and sinus node dysfunction (possibly synergism)

S Shukla et al, Lithium-carbamazepine neurotoxicity and risk factors. Am J Psychiatry, 141:1604, 1984; KG Kramlinger and RM Post, Addition of lithium carbonate to carbamazepine: hematological and thyroid effects. Am J Psychiatry, 147:615, 1990; TL Steckler, Lithium- and carbamazepine-associated sinus node dysfunction: nine-year experience in a psychiatric hospital. J Clin Psychopharmacol, 14:336, 1994; M-U Manto et al, Cerebellar ataxia in upper limbs triggered by addition of carbamazepine to lithium treatment. Acta Neurol Belg, 96:316, 1996

Monitor neurological and cardiac status; patients with hypothyroidism may be especially susceptible to neurotoxicity

Loxapine

Neuroleptic malignant syndrome on withdrawal of carbamazepine (possibly reversal of increased metabolism)

GA Keepers, Neuroleptic malignant syndrome associated with withdrawal from carbamazepine. Am J Psychiatry, 147:1687, 1990

Single case report (1990)

Macrolide antibiotics

Carbamazepine toxicity with clarithromycin (decreased metabolism; CYP3A4)

F Albani et al, Clarithromycin-carbamazepine interaction: a case report. Epilepsia, 34:161, 1993; WO Tatum, IV and MA Gonzalez, Carbamazepine toxicity in an epileptic induced by clarithromycin. Hosp Pharm, 29:45, 1994; DC Metz and HD Getz, *Helicobacter pylori* gastritis therapy with omeprazole and clarithromycin increases serum carbamazepine levels. Dig Dis Sci, 40:912, 1995; NK O'Connor and J Fris, Clarithromycin-carbamazepine

CARBAMAZEPINE, with: *(continued)*
>   interaction in a clinical setting. J Am Board Fam Pract, 7:489, 1994; GC Ibáñez et al, Toxicidad de carbamacepina inducida por eritromicina y claritromicina, un problema frencuente. Farm Clin, 13:698, 1996; N Yasui et al, Carbamazepine toxicity induced by clarithromycin coadministration in psychiatric patients. Int Clin Psychopharmacol, 12:225, 1997; S Alegre-Herrera et al, Interacción claitromicina-carbamazepina: sintomas neurológicos e hiponatremia. An Med Interna, 15:48, 1998
>   *Avoid concurrent use; azithromycin unlikely to interact*
>
>   Possible reduction in clarithromycin effect (mechanism not established)
>   C Sungur, Acute rheumatic fever despite clarithromycin treatment of beta-hemolytic streptococcal tonsillitis. Ann Pharmacother, 28:1197, 1994
>   *Based on single case report (1994); causal relationship not established*
>
>   Carbamazepine toxicity with erythromycin (decreased metabolism)
>   YY Wong et al, Effect of erythromycin on carbamazepine kinetics. Clin Pharmacol Ther, 33:460, 1983; E Carrcenco et al, Carbamazepine toxicity induced by concurrent erythromycin therapy. Arch Neurol, 42:187, 1985; KJ Goulden et al, Severe carbamazepine intoxication after coadministration of erythromycin. J Pediatr, 109:135, 1986; N Barzaghi et al, Inhibition by erythromycin of the conversion of carbamazepine to its active 10,11-epoxide metabolite. Br J Clin Pharmacol, 24:836, 1987; AJ Macnab et al, Heart block secondary to erythromycin-induced carbamazepine toxicity. Pediatrics, 80:951, 1987; RA Mitsch, Carbamazepine toxicity precipitated by intravenous erythromycin. DICP, 23:878, 1989; CE Stafstrom et al, Erythromycin-induced carbamazepine toxicity: a continuing problem. Arch Pediatr Adolesc Med, 149:99, 1995; GC Ibáñez et al, Toxicidad de carbamacepina inducida por eritromicina y claritromicina, un problema frencuente. Farm Clin, 13:698, 1996
>   *Avoid concurrent use; azithromycin unlikely to interact*
>
> **Metoclopramide**
>   Neurotoxicity (mechanism not established)
>   R Sandyk, Carbamazepine and metoclopramide interaction: possible neurotoxicity. Br Med J, 288:830, 1984
>   *Single case report (1984)*
>
> **Metronidazole**
>   Possible carbamazepine toxicity (possibly decreased metabolism)
>   BD Patterson, Possible interaction between metronidazole and carbamazepine. Ann Pharmacother, 28:1303, 1994
>   *Single case report (1994)*
>
> **Mianserin**
>   Possible decreased mianserin effect (increased metabolism)
>   E Leinonen et al, Effects of carbamazepine on serum antidepressant concentrations in psychiatric patients. J Clin Psychopharmacol, 11:313, 1991; CB Eap et al, Effects of carbamazepine coadministration on plasma concentrations of the enantiomers of mianserin and of its metabolites. Ther Drug Monit, 21:166, 1999

(continued)

CARBAMAZEPINE, with: *(continued)*
> *Based on studies in depressed patients; monitor mianserin concentration and clinical status*

Monoamine oxidase inhibitors
Possible decreased carbamazepine effect with tranylcypromine (mechanism not established)
> NE Barklage et al, Do monoamine oxidase inhibitors alter carbamazepine blood levels? J Clin Psychiatry, 53:258, 1992

Report of several cases (1992); monitor carbamazepine concentration

Narcotics: methadone and congeners
Carbamazepine toxicity with propoxyphene and dextropropoxyphene (decreased metabolism; CYP3A)
> M Dam and J Christiansen, Interaction of propoxyphene with carbamazepine. Lancet, 2:509, 1977; YL Yu et al, Interaction between carbamazepine and dextropropoxyphene. Postgrad Med J, 62:231, 1986; S Allen, Cerebellar dysfunction following dextropropoxyphene-induced carbamazepine toxicity. Postgrad Med J, 70:764, 1994; L Bergendal et al, The clinical relevance of the interaction between carbamazepine and dextropropoxyphene in elderly patients in Gothenburg, Sweden. Eur J Clin Pharmacol, 53:203, 1997

Avoid concurrent use

Methadone withdrawal symptoms (probably increased metabolism)
> J Bell et al, The use of serum methadone levels in patients receiving methadone maintenance. Clin Pharmacol Ther, 43:623, 1988

Single case report (1988); monitor methadone concentration

Narcotics: tramadol
Decreased tramadol effect (increased metabolism)
> Manufacturer's package insert

Monitor clinical status; as much as a two fold increase in dosage may be required

Nefazodone
Possible carbamazepine toxicity and decreased nefazodone effect (decreased metabolism; enzyme induction)
> C Laroudie et al, Carbamazepine-nefazodone interaction in healthy subjects. J Clin Psychopharmacol, 20:46, 2000

Based on study in healthy subjects; monitor clinical status

Nelfinavir
Possible decreased nelfinavir effect (increased metabolism; CYP3A)
> Manufacturer's package insert (nelfinavir)

Clinical significance remains to be established

Neuromuscular blocking agents
Accelerated recovery from neuromuscular blockade (possible increased metabolism)
> R Tempelhoff et al, Resistance to atracurium-induced neuromuscular blockade in patients with intractable seizure disorders treated with anticonvulsants. Anesth Analg, 71:665, 1990; F Varin et al, Carbamazepine induced changes on vecuronium pharmacokinetics in anesthetized patients. Clin

CARBAMAZEPINE, with: *(continued)*
> Pharmacol Ther, 55:143, 1994; Soriano et al, Pharmacokinetics and pharmacodynamics of vecuronium in children on anticonvulsant drugs. Anesthesiology, 83, suppl 3A:167, 1995; manufacturer's package insert for doxacurium; A Spacek et al, Rocuronium-induced neuromuscular block is affected by chronic carbamazepine therapy. Anesthesiology, 90:109, 1999

Monitor neuromuscular status

Nicardipine
> Reduced nicardipine effect (possibly by increased metabolism; CYP3A4)
>> P Laria et al, Une nouvelle cause d'hypertension artérielle résistante: la coprescription avec des traitements anticomitiaux. Arch Mal Coeur Vaiss, 92:1005, 1999
>
> *Single case report (1999); monitor blood pressure*

Olanzapine
> Possible decreased olanzapine effect (increased metabolism; CYP1A2)
>> RA Lucas et al, A pharmacokinetic interaction between carbamazepine and olanzapine: observations on possible mechanism. Eur J Clin Pharmacol, 54:639, 1998; OV Olesen and K Linnet, Olanzapine serum concentrations in psychiatric patients given standard doses: the influence of comedication. Ther Drug Monit, 21:87, 1999; RW Licht et al, Olanzapine serum concentrations lowered by concomitant treatment with carbamazepine. J Clin Psychopharmacol, 20:110, 2000
>
> *Monitor clinical status; adjust olanzapine dose as needed*

Omeprazole
> Possible carbamazepine toxicity (possible decreased metabolism)
>> MUR Naidu et al, Effect of multiple dose omeprazole on the pharmacokinetics of carbamazepine. Drug Invest, 7:8, 1994
>
> *Based on study in 7 patients with duodenal ulcer; clinical significance not established*
>
> Possible decreased omeprazole effect (increased metabolism; CYP3A)
>> L Bertilsson et al, Carbamazepine treatment induces the CYP3A4 catalysed sulphoxidation of omeprazole, but has no or less effect on hydroxylation via CYP2C19. Br J Clin Pharmacol, 44:186, 1997
>
> *Based on study in 5 patients; clinical significance not established*

Oxcarbazepine
> Possible decreased oxcarbazepine effect (possible increased metabolism)
>> Manufacturer's package insert (oxcarbazepine)
>
> *Active metabolite decreased 40%; monitor oxcarbazepine concentrations*

Phenothiazines
> Possible decreased perphenazine effect (possible increased metabolism)
>> GL Ellenor and AB Kodsi, Drug interaction: case report of carbamazepine versus valproic acid with perphenazine. ASHP Midyear Clinical Meeting, 28:P-169(D), 1993
>
> *Single case report (1993)*

CARBAMAZEPINE, with: *(continued)*
  Phenytoin
    Decreased carbamazepine effect (increased metabolism); altered phenytoin effect (mechanism not established)
      E Perucca and A Richens, Reversal by phenytoin of carbamazepine-induced water intoxication: a pharmacokinetic interaction. J Neurol Neurosurg Psychiatry, 43:540, 1980; DJ Chapron et al, Unmasking the significant enzyme-inducing effects of phenytoin on serum carbamazepine concentrations during phenytoin withdrawal. Ann Pharmacother, 27:708, 1993; JJ Zielinski and D Haidukewych, Dual effects of carbamazepine – phenytoin interaction. Ther Drug Monit, 9:21, 1987; H Liu and MR Delgado, Interactions of phenobarbital and phenytoin with carbamazepine and its metabolites' concentrations, concentration ratios, and level/dose ratios in epileptic children. Epilepsia, 36:249, 1995; D Divanoglou et al, Pharmacokinetic behaviour of carbamazepine and its main metabolite-10,11 epoxide of carbamazepine in monotherapy or in combination with other anti-epileptic drugs. Eur J Neurol, 5:397, 1998
    Monitor carbamazepine and phenytoin concentrations; both increased and decreased concentrations have been reported; combination of phenytoin and phenobarbital may produce additive decrease in carbamazepine concentrations
  Praziquantel
    Decreased praziquantel effect (increased metabolism)
      PRM Bittencourt et al, Phenytoin and carbamazepine decrease oral bioavailability of praziquantel. Neurology, 42:492, 1992
    Monitor for decreased response to praziquantel
  Primidone
    Decreased primidone effect and increased phenobarbital effect (increased conversion of primidone to phenobarbital)
      JC Cloyd et al, Primidone kinetics: effects of concurrent drugs and duration of therapy. Clin Pharmacol Ther, 29:402, 1981
    Monitor primidone and phenobarbital concentrations

    Decreased carbamazepine effect (increased metabolism)
      D Battino et al, Plasma levels of primidone and its metabolite phenobarbital: effect of age and associated therapy. Ther Drug Monit, 5:73, 1983; P Benetello and M Furlanut, Primidone – carbamazepine interaction: clinical consequences. Int J Clin Pharm Res, 7:165, 1987
    Monitor carbamazepine and carbamazepine epoxide concentrations
  Quinine
    Possible carbamazepine toxicity (possible decreased metabolism)
      GJ Amabeoku et al, Pharmacokinetic interaction of single doses of quinine and carbamazepine, phenobarbitone and phenytoin in healthy volunteers. East Afr Med J, 70:90, 1993
    Monitor carbamazepine concentration; based on studies in normal subjects
  Ritonavir
    Possible carbamazepine toxicity (decreased metabolism; CYP3A4)
      Y Kato et al, Potential interaction between ritonavir and carbamazepine.

CARBAMAZEPINE, with: *(continued)*
    Pharmacotherapy, 20:851, 2000
    Single case report (2000); monitor carbamazepine serum concentration and clinical status
Selective serotonin reuptake inhibitors (SSRIs)
Carbamazepine toxicity with fluoxetine or fluvoxamine (decreased metabolism), or sertraline (mechanism not established)
    SR Grimsley et al, Pharmacodynamics and pharmacokinetics of fluoxetine/carbamazepine interaction. Clin Pharmacol Ther, 49:135, 1991 abs PI-48; HBPE Gernaat et al, Fluoxetine and parkinsonism in patients taking carbamazepine. Am J Psychiatry, 148:1604, 1991; BE Gidal et al, Evaluation of the effect of fluoxetine on the formation of carbamazepine epoxide. Ther Drug Monit, 15:405, 1993; E Spina et al, Carbamazepine coadministration with fluoxetine or fluvoxamine. Ther Drug Monit, 15:247, 1993; C Debruille et al, Carbamazepine/fluvoxamine interaction: about two observations. J Pharm Clin, 13:128, 1994; manufacturer's package insert (citalopram)
Fluoxetine interaction well documented; report of 6 cases with fluvoxamine (1991, 1992, 1994); one report of 8 epileptic patients on fluoxetine and 7 on fluvoxamine found no interaction; monitor carbamazepine concentration (preferably of epoxide metabolite); citalopram may not interact

Toxic serotonin syndrome - shivering, agitation, incoordination, restless legs, diaphoresis, hyperreflexia (mechanism not established)
    SM Dursun et al, Toxic serotonin syndrome after fluoxetine plus carbamazepine. Lancet, 342:442, 1993; L Vercueil et al, Surdosage en carbamazépine après administration d'un comprimé de sertraline: relation au syndrome sérotoninergique? Therapie, 53:499, 1998; T Apelland et al, Serotonergt syndrom med dødelig utgang utløst av selektiv serotonin-reopptakshemmer. Tidsskr Nor Laegeforen, 119:647, 1999
Single case reports with fluoxetine (1993), sertraline (1998), and paroxetine, but patient was also taking two other drugs (1999)

Possible decreased sertraline effect (probably increased metabolism; CYP3A4)
    A Khan et al, Lack of sertraline efficacy probably due to an interaction with carbamazepine. J Clin Psychiatry, 61:526, 2000
Two case reports (2000); monitor clinical status
Stiripentol
Possible carbamazepine toxicity (decreased metabolism)
    A Tran et al, Effect of stiripentol on carbamazepine plasma concentration and metabolism in epileptic children. Eur J Clin Pharmacol, 50:497, 1996
Based on study of 16 children with epilepsy; monitor carbamazepine concentration and clinical status
Sympathomimetic amines
Decreased methylphenidate effect (increased metabolism; CYP2D6)
    JL Schaller and D Behar, Carbamazepine and methylphenidate in ADHD. J Am Acad Child Adolesc Psychiatry, 38:112, 1999; D Behar et al, Extreme reduction of methylphenidate levels by carbamazepine. J Am Acad Child

(continued)

CARBAMAZEPINE, with: *(continued)*
>Adolesc Psychiatry, 37:1128, 1998; V Gross-Tsur, Carbamazepine and methylphenidate. J Am Acad Child Adolesc Psychiatry, 38:6, 1999
>
>*Two case reports (1998, 1999); monitor clinical status; may necessitate substantial increase in methylphenidate dose; effect may not be seen in every patient*

Teniposide
>Possible decreased teniposide effect (mechanism not established)
>>MV Relling et al, Adverse effect of anticonvulsants on efficacy of chemotherapy for acute lymphoblastic leukaemia. Lancet, 356:285, 2000
>
>*Evidence of reduced teniposide efficacy in children with acute lymphoblastic leukemia; monitor clinical status*

Tetracyclines
>Decreased doxycycline effect (increased metabolism)
>>O Penttila et al, Interaction between doxycycline and some antiepileptic drugs. Br Med J, 2:470, 1974; PJ Neuvonen et al, Effect of antiepileptic drugs on the elimination of various tetracycline derivatives. Eur J Clin Pharmacol, 9:147, 1975
>
>*Choose another antibiotic*

Theophyllines
>Decreased effect of both theophylline and carbamazepine (increased theophylline metabolism; reduced carbamazepine bioavailability)
>>KR Rosenberry et al, Reduced theophylline half-life induced by carbamazepine therapy. J Pediatr, 102:472, 1983; EA Mitchell et al, Interaction between carbamazepine and theophylline. N Z Med J, 99:69, 1986; C Kulkarni et al, Aminophylline alters pharmacokinetics of carbamazepine but not that of sodium valproate — a single dose pharmacokinetic study in human volunteers. Indian J Physiol Pharmacol, 39:122, 1995
>
>*Monitor carbamazepine and theophylline concentration*

Thiazide diuretics
>Hyponatremia (mechanism not established)
>>R Yassa et al, Carbamazepine, diuretics, and hyponatremia: a possible interaction. J Clin Psychiatry, 48:281, 1987
>
>*Single case report (1987); monitor sodium concentration*

Tiagabine
>Decreased tiagabine effect (increased tiagabine metabolism)
>>Manufacturer's package insert
>
>*Based on patient studies; monitor clinical status*

Ticlopidine
>Carbamazepine toxicity (probably decreased metabolism; CYP3A4)
>>RIG Brown and TG Cooper, Ticlopidine-carbamazepine interaction in a coronary stent patient. Can J Cardiol, 13:853, 1997
>
>*Single case report with positive rechallenge (1997)*

Topiramate
>Possible decreased topiramate effect (mechanism not established)
>>Manufacturer's package insert (topiramate)
>
>*Monitor topiramate concentration*

CARBAMAZEPINE, with: *(continued)*
- **Trazodone**

    Possible carbamazepine toxicity (mechanism not established)

    > AS Romero et al, Interaction between trazodone and carbamazepine. Ann Pharmacother, 33:1370, 1999

    Single case report (1999); monitor carbamazepine levels and clinical status

- **Troleandomycin**

    Carbamazepine toxicity (decreased metabolism)

    > C Dravet et al, Interaction between carbamazepine and triacetyloleandomycin. Lancet, 1:810, 1977; E Mesdjian et al, Carbamazepine intoxication due to triacetyloleandomycin administration in epileptic patients. Epilepsia, 21:489, 1980

    Choose another antibiotic

- **Valproate**

    Decreased valproate effect and possible increased toxicity (increased metabolism and formation of toxic metabolite)

    > SK Panesar et al, The effect of carbamazepine on valproic acid disposition in adult volunteers. Br J Clin Pharmacol, 27:323, 1989; PJW McKee et al, variability and clinical relevance of the interaction between sodium valproate and carbamazepine in epileptic patients. Epilepsy Res, 11:193, 1992; E Yukawa et al, Population-based investigation of valproic acid relative clearance using nonlinear mixed effects modeling: influence of drug-drug interaction and patient characteristics. J Clin Pharmacol, 37:1160, 1997

    Monitor valproate concentration and clinical status; one study in patients failed to confirm

    Psychosis (mechanism not established)

    > RJW McKee et al, Acute psychosis with carbamazepine and sodium valproate. Lancet, 1:167, 1989

    Single patient with both drugs within target range (1989)

    Carbamazepine toxicity (decreased metabolism of carbamazepine epoxide) and protein binding displacement

    > DK Robbins et al, Inhibition of epoxide hydrolase by valproic acid in epileptic patients receiving carbamazepine. Br J Clin Pharmacol, 29:759, 1990; B Rambeck et al, Valproic acid-induced carbamazepine-10,11-epoxide toxicity in children and adolescents. Eur Neurol, 30:79, 1990; F Pisani et al, Interaction of carbamazepine-10,11-epoxide, an active metabolite of carbamazepine, with valproate: a pharmacokinetic study. Epilepsia, 31:339, 1990; H Liu and MR Delgado, The influence of polytherapy on the relationships between serum carbamazepine and its metabolites in epileptic children. Epilepsy Res, 17:257, 1994; H Liu et al, Interactions of valproic acid with carbamazepine and its metabolites' concentrations, concentration ratios, and level/dose ratios in epileptic children. Clin Neuropharmacol, 18:1, 1995; DA Svinarov and CE Pippenger, Valproic acid-carbamazepine interaction: is valproic acid a selective inhibitor of epoxide hydrolase? Ther Drug Monit, 17:217, 1995

(continued)

CARBAMAZEPINE, with: *(continued)*
    Monitor carbamazepine and carbamazepine epoxide concentrations

  Possible increased risk of osteomalacia (mechanism not established)
    Y Karaaslan et al, Osteomalacia associated with carbamazepine/valproate. Ann Pharmacother, 34:264, 2000
  Based on single case report (2000); monitor for evidence of osteomalacia

Valpromide
Carbamazepine toxicity (increased epoxide metabolite concentrations)
    JWA Meijer et al, Possible hazard of valpromide-carbamazepine combination therapy in epilepsy. Lancet, 1:802, 1984; F Pisani et al, Sodium valproate and valpromide: differential interactions with carbamazepine in epileptic patients. Epilepsia, 27:548, 1986; BM Kerr et al, Inhibition of human liver microsomal epoxide hydrolase by valproate and valpromide: in vitro/in vivo correlation. Clin Pharmacol Ther, 46:82, 1989
Avoid concurrent use

Verapamil
Carbamazepine toxicity (decreased metabolism)
    GJA Macphee et al, Verapamil potentiates carbamazepine neurotoxicity: a clinically important inhibitory interaction. Lancet, 1:700, 1986; WA Price and LR DiMarzio, Verapamil-carbamazepine neurotoxicity. J Clin Psychiatry, 49:80, 1988; B Beattie et al, Verapamil-induced carbamazepine neurotoxicity; a report of two cases. Eur Neurol, 28:104, 1988
Avoid concurrent use

Vincristine
Decreased vincristine effect (enzyme induction; CYP3A4)
    K Villikka et al, Cytochrome P450-inducing antiepileptics increase the clearance of vincristine in patients with brain tumors. Clin Pharmacol Ther, 66:589, 1999
Based on study in patients with brain tumors; monitor clinical status

Zonisamide
Decreased zonisamide effect (increased metabolism; CYP3A4)
    Manufacturer's package insert (zonisamide)
Monitor zonisamide concentration and clinical status; zonisamide dosage may need to be adjusted

Carbenicillin, see Penicillins

Carbidopa-Levodopa, see Levodopa

Carbonates, see Antacids

CARBONIC ANHYDRASE INHIBITORS, with:

Cyclosporine
Possible cyclosporine toxicity with acetazolamide (mechanism not established)
    KF Tabbara et al, Interaction between acetazolamide and cyclosporine. Arch Ophthalmol, 116:832, 1998
Three case reports (1998); monitor cyclosporine concentration

Lithium
Lithium toxicity (probably decreased renal excretion)
    C Gay et al, Intoxication au lithium. L'Encephale, 11:261, 1985

CARBONIC ANHYDRASE INHIBITORS, with: *(continued)*
One case report (1985); reported with most other diuretics; monitor lithium concentration

Nonsteroidal anti-inflammatory drugs

Adverse effects of either aspirin or both drugs (mechanism not established)
> CJ Anderson et al, Toxicity of combined therapy with carbonic anhydrase inhibitors and aspirin. Am J Ophthalmol, 86:516, 1978; RA Cowan et al, Metabolic acidosis induced by carbonic anhydrase inhibitors and salicylates in patients with normal renal function. Br Med J, 289:347, 1984; KR Sweeney et al, Toxic interaction between acetazolamide and salicylate: case reports and a pharmacokinetic explanation. Clin Pharmacol Ther, 40:518, 1986

Avoid concurrent use; other NSAIDs may not interact

Quinidine

Possible quinidine toxicity (decreased renal excretion due to alkaline urine)
> RE Gerhardt et al, Quinidine excretion in aciduria and alkaluria. Ann Intern Med, 71:927, 1969

Avoid concurrent use

Sympathomimetic amines

Pseudoephedrine toxicity (decreased renal excretion due to alkaline urine)
> RG Kuntzman et al, The influence of urinary pH on the plasma half-life of pseudoephedrine in man and dog and a sensitive assay for its determination in human plasma. Clin Pharmacol Ther, 12:62, 1971; DC Brater et al, Renal excretion of pseudoephedrine. Clin Pharmacol Ther, 28:690, 1980

Avoid concurrent use

Topiramate

Possible renal calculus (additive increase in urinary pH; topiramate is a carbonic anhydrase inhibitor)
> Manufacturer's package insert (topiramate)

Theoretical; manufacturer recommends avoiding concurrent use

CARBOPLATIN, with:

Phenytoin

Decreased phenytoin effect (mechanism not established)
> ASM Dofferhoff and HH Berendsen, Decreased phenytoin level after carboplatin treatment. Am J Med, 89:247, 1990

Single case report (1990); monitor phenytoin concentration; also occurs with cisplatin

Cardiotech, no documented interactions, see page 4, Criteria for Listing Interactions
Carisoprodol, no documented interactions, see page 4, Criteria for Listing Interactions

CARMUSTINE, with:

Antihistamines, H_2-blockers - See Antihistamines, H_2-blockers with Carmustine, page 116

Carphenazine, see Phenothiazines
Carteolol, see Beta-adrenergic blockers
Carvedilol, see Beta-adrenergic blockers
Cefaclor, see Cephalosporins
Cefadroxil, see Cephalosporins

Cefazolin, see Cephalosporins
Cefdinir, see Cephalosporins
Cefepime, see Cephalosporins
Cefixime, see Cephalosporins
Cefmetazole, see Cephalosporins
Cefonicid, see Cephalosporins
Cefoperazone, see Cephalosporins
Ceforanide, see Cephalosporins
Cefotaxime, see Cephalosporins
Cefotetan, see Cephalosporins
Cefoxitin, see Cephalosporins
Cefpodoxime, see Cephalosporins
Cefprozil, see Cephalosporins
Ceftibuten, see Cephalosporins
Ceftizoxime, see Cephalosporins
Ceftriaxone, see Cephalosporins
Cefuroxime, see Cephalosporins
Cefuroxime axetil, see Cephalosporins
Celecoxib, see COX-2 inhibitors
Cephalexin, see Cephalosporins
Cephaloglycin, see Cephalosporins
Cephaloridine, see Cephalosporins
CEPHALOSPORINS, with:

  Alcohol - See Alcohol with Cephalosporins, page 16

  Aminoglycoside antibiotics - See Aminoglycoside antibiotics with Cephalosporins, page 30

  Antacids - See Antacids with Cephalosporins, page 51

  Anticoagulants, oral - See Anticoagulants, oral with Cephalosporins, page 63

  Antihistamines, H_2-blockers - See Antihistamines, H_2-blockers with Cephalosporins, page 116

  Barbiturates - See Barbiturates with Cephalosporins, page 131

  Contraceptives, oral

    Decreased contraceptive effect (mechanism not established)

      DJ Back et al, Evaluation of Committee on Safety of Medicines yellow card reports on oral contraceptive-drug interactions with anticonvulsants and antibiotics. Br J Clin Pharmacol, 25:527, 1988

    Two case reports (1988)

  Cyclosporine

    Possible cyclosporine toxicity with ceftriaxone (mechanism not established)

      J Soto Alvarez et al, Interaction between ciclosporin and ceftriaxone. Nephron, 59:681, 1991

    Two case reports (1991); monitor cyclosporine concentration

  Ethacrynic acid

    Cephaloridine nephrotoxicity (mechanism not established)

      MG Dodds and RD Foord, Enhancement by potent diuretics of renal tubular necrosis induced by cephaloridine. Br J Pharmacol, 40:227, 1970; GL Mandell, Cephaloridine. Ann Intern Med, 79:561, 1973; DH Lawson et al, The

CEPHALOSPORINS, with: *(continued)*
>nephrotoxicity of cephaloridine. Postgrad Med J, 46 suppl:36, 1970
>
>*Monitor renal function*

Furosemide
>Possible ceftazidime toxicity (delayed renal elimination)
>>G Chrysos et al, Pharmacokinetic interactions of ceftaziadime and frusemide. J Chemother, 7 suppl 4:107, 1995
>
>*Based on study in healthy subjects; clinical significance not established; give at least 6 hours apart*

Heparins
>Possible increased bleeding risk with moxalactam (additive)
>>Anonymous, Moxalactam boxed warning about bleeding problems. FDA Drug Bull, 13:16, 1983; package insert
>
>*Avoid concurrent use of more than 20,000 U/day of heparin with moxalactam*

Iron
>Decreased cefdinir effect (decreased absorption)
>>Manufacturer's package insert (cefdinir)
>
>*Give at least 2 hours apart*

Methyldopa
>Pustular eruption with cephradine or cefazolin (mechanism not established)
>>D Stough et al, Pustular eruptions following administration of cefazolin: a possible interaction with methyldopa. J Am Acad Dermatol, 16:1051, 1987
>
>*Single case report (1987) with each of these cephalosporins and methyldopa*

Nonsteroidal anti-inflammatory drugs
>Possible increased bleeding risk with moxalactam and aspirin (additive)
>>Anonymous, Moxalactam boxed warning about bleeding problems. FDA Drug Bull, 13:16, 1983
>
>*Avoid concurrent use*

Penicillins
>Possible cefotaxime toxicity with azlocillin or mezlocillin in patients with renal impairment (decreased excretion)
>>D Kampf et al, Kinetic interactions between azlocillin, cefotaxime, and cefotaxime metabolites in normal and impaired renal function. Clin Pharmacol Ther, 35:214, 1984; LC Rodondi et al, Influence of coadministration on the pharmacokinetics of mezlocillin and cefotaxime in healthy volunteers and in patients with renal failure. Clin Pharmacol Ther, 45:527, 1989
>
>*Decrease cefotaxime dosage if GFR less than 40 ml/min*

Pentoxifylline
>Serum sickness with cefoxitin (mechanism not established)
>>AP Panwalker et al, Serum sickness associated with cefoxitin and pentoxifylline therapy. Drug Intell Clin Pharm, 20:953, 1986
>
>*Single case report (1986)*

Verapamil
>Verapamil toxicity with ceftriaxone (mechanism not established)
>>K Kishore et al, Acute verapamil toxicity in a patient with chronic toxicity: possible interaction with ceftriaxone and clindamycin. Ann Pharmacother,

(continued)

CEPHALOSPORINS, with: *(continued)*
27:877, 1993
Single case report; patient was also receiving clindamycin (1993)

Cephalothin, see Cephalosporins

Cephapirin, see Cephalosporins

Cephradine, see Cephalosporins

Cerivastatin, see HMG-CoA Reductase Inhibitors

Cetirizine, no documented interactions, see page 4, Criteria for Listing Interactions

Cevimeline, no documented interactions, see page 4, Criteria for Listing Interactions

Chewing tobacco, see Tobacco, smokeless

CHLORAL HYDRATE, with:

Alcohol - See Alcohol with Chloral hydrate, page 16

Anticoagulants, oral - See Anticoagulants, oral with Chloral hydrate, page 63

Furosemide

Vasomotor instability (mechanism not established)

M Malach and N Berman, Furosemide and chloral hydrate: adverse drug interaction. JAMA, 232:638, 1975; RP Dean et al, Interaction of chloral hydrate and intravenous furosemide in a child. Clin Pharm, 10:385, 1991

Avoid concurrent use

Selective serotonin reuptake inhibitors (SSRIs)

Prolonged drowsiness with fluoxetine (mechanism not established)

S Devarajan, Interaction of fluoxetine and chloral hydrate. Can J Psychiatry, 37:590, 1992

Single case report (1992)

CHLORAMBUCIL, with:

Cyclosporine

Inability to maintain therapeutic concentrations of cyclosporine (mechanism not established)

G Emilia and C Messora, Interaction between cyclosporin and chlorambucil. Eur J Haematol, 51:179, 1993

Single case report (1993) of a woman with chronic lymphocytic leukemia treated with cyclosporine for autoimmune hemolytic anemia

CHLORAMPHENICOL, with:

Anticoagulants, oral - See Anticoagulants, oral with Chloramphenicol, page 63

Antihistamines, H$_2$-blockers - See Antihistamines, H$_2$-blockers with Chloramphenicol, page 116

Barbiturates - See Barbiturates with Chloramphenicol, page 132

Cyclosporine

Possible cyclosporine toxicity (mechanism not established)

LL Bui and DD Huang, Possible interaction between cyclosporine and chloramphenicol. Ann Pharmacother, 33:252, 1999

Single case report (1999)

Etomidate

Prolonged anesthesia (decreased metabolism)

H Reiche and H-H Frey, Interactions between chloramphenicol and intravenous anesthetics. Anaesthesist, 30:504, 1981

CHLORAMPHENICOL, with: *(continued)*
Adjust anesthetic dosage

Hypoglycemics, sulfonylurea
Increased hypoglycemic effect of chlorpropamide or tolbutamide (mechanism not established)
> B Petitpierre et al, Behaviour of chlorpropamide in renal insufficiency and under the effect of associated drug therapy. Int J Clin Pharmacol Ther Toxicol, 6:120, 1972; E Brunova et al, Interaction of tolbutamide and chloramphenicol in diabetic patients. Int J Clin Pharmacol, 15:7, 1977

Monitor blood glucose

Phenytoin
Phenytoin toxicity (decreased metabolism)
> JO Rose et al, Intoxication caused by interaction of chloramphenicol and phenytoin. JAMA, 237:2630, 1977; FM Vincent et al, Chloramphenicol-induced phenytoin intoxication. Ann Neurol, 3:469, 1978

Choose another antibiotic, if possible; otherwise, monitor chloramphenicol and phenytoin concentrations

Possible chloramphenicol toxicity (mechanism not established)
> K Krasinski et al, Pharmacologic interactions among chloramphenicol, phenytoin and phenobarbital. Pediatr Infect Dis, 1:232, 1982

Choose another antibiotic, if possible; otherwise, monitor chloramphenicol and phenytoin concentrations

Rifampin
Decreased chloramphenicol effect (increased metabolism)
> CG Prober, Effect of rifampin on chloramphenicol levels. N Engl J Med, 312:788, 1985; HW Kelly et al, Interaction of chloramphenicol and rifampin. J Pediatr, 112:817, 1988

Avoid concurrent use

Tacrolimus
Possible tacrolimus toxicity (probably decreased metabolism; CYP3A)
> SL Schulman et al, Interaction between tacrolimus and chloramphenicol in a renal transplant recipient. Transplantation, 65:1397, 1998; DJ Taber et al, Drug-drug interaction between chloramphenicol and tacrolimus in a liver transplant recipient. Transplant Proc, 32:660, 2000

Two case reports (1998, 2000); monitor tacrolimus concentration and clinical status

Chlordiazepoxide, see Benzodiazepines

Chlorhexidine, no documented interactions, see page 4, Criteria for Listing Interactions

CHLORMETHIAZOLE, with:
Alcohol - See Alcohol with Chlormethiazole, page 16

Chlorodeoxyadenosine, no documented interactions, see page 4, Criteria for Listing Interactions

CHLOROQUINE, with:
Acetaminophen - See Acetaminophen with Chloroquine, page 8

(continued)

CHLOROQUINE, with: *(continued)*

Antihistamines, H$_2$-blockers - See Antihistamines, H$_2$-blockers with Chloroquine, page 116

Cyclosporine

Possible cyclosporine toxicity (possibly decreased metabolism)

MRN Nampoory et al, Drug interaction of chloroquine with ciclosporin. Nephron, 62:108, 1992; P Finielz et al, Interaction between cyclosporin and chloroquine. Nephron, 65:333, 1993; J Guiserix and A Aizel, Interactions ciclosporine-chloroquine. La Presse Médicale, 14:1214, 1996

Three case reports (1992, 1993, 1996); monitor cyclosporine concentration

Kaolin or Kaolin-pectin

Possible decreased chloroquine effect (decreased absorption)

JC McElnay et al, *In vitro* experiments on chloroquine and pyrimethamine absorption in the presence of antacid constituents or kaolin. J Trop Med Hyg, 85:153, 1982; JC McElnay et al, The effect of magnesium trisilicate and kaolin on the *in vivo* absorption of chloroquine. J Trop Med Hyg, 85:159, 1982

Give at least 4 hours apart

Mefloquine

Increased risk of convulsions (mechanism not established)

Manufacturer's package insert

Avoid concurrent use

Methotrexate

Possible reduction in methotrexate effect (possible decreased absorption)

P Seideman et al, Chloroquine reduces the bioavailability of methotrexate in patients with rheumatoid arthritis. Arthritis Rheum, 37:830, 1994

Based on study in patients with rheumatoid arthritis given drugs simultaneously; effect of separating doses not studied

Metronidazole

Dystonic reactions (mechanism not established)

JI Achumba et al, Chloroquine-induced acute dystonic reactions in the presence of metronidazole. Drug Intell Clin Pharm, 22:308, 1988

Single case report (1988)

Penicillamine

Possible penicillamine toxicity (mechanism not established)

P Seideman and B Lindström, Pharmacokinetic interactions of penicillamine in rheumatoid arthritis. J Rheumatol, 16:473, 1989

Monitor penicillamine concentration or for clinical signs of toxicity

Phenothiazines

Possible chlorpromazine toxicity (decreased metabolism)

ROA Makanjuola et al, Effects of antimalarial agents on plasma levels of chlorpromazine and its metabolites in schizophrenic patients. Trop Geographic Med, 40:31, 1988

Monitor chlorpromazine concentration

Praziquantel

Possible decreased praziquantel effect (mechanism not established)

CM Masimirembwa et al, The effect of chloroquine on the pharmacokine-

CHLOROQUINE, with: *(continued)*
>tics and metabolism of praziquantel in rats and in humans. Biopharm Drug Dispos, 15:33, 1994
>
>*Of 8 patients studied, 4 had subtherapeutic praziquantel concentrations*

Promethazine
Possible chloroquine toxicity (probably decreased metabolism)
>AO Ehiemua et al, Effect of promethazine on the metabolism of chloroquine. Eur J Drug Metab Pharmacokinet, 13:15, 1988

Monitor for symptoms of toxicity

Rabies vaccine
Decreased antibody response to human diploid rabies vaccine (mechanism not established)
>DN Taylor et al, Chloroquine prophylaxis associated with a poor antibody response to human diploid cell rabies vaccine. Lancet, 1:1405, 1984; M Pappaioanou et al, Antibody response to preexposure human diploid-cell rabies vaccine given concurrently with chloroquine. N Engl J Med, 314:280, 1986

Some patients were also taking Fansidar; avoid concurrent use

Thyroid hormones
Possible reduction in thyroxine effect (possibly increased metabolism)
>Y Munera et al, Interaction of thyroxine sodium with antimalarial drugs. BMJ, 314:1593, 1997

Single case report (1997)

Chlorothiazide, see Thiazide diuretics

Chlorpheniramine, no documented interactions, see page 4, Criteria for Listing Interactions

Chlorpromazine, see Phenothiazines

Chlorpropamide, see Hypoglycemics, sulfonylurea

Chlorprothixene, see Phenothiazines

Chlorthalidone, see Thiazide diuretics

CHLORZOXAZONE, with:

Disulfiram
Possible chlorzoxazone toxicity (decreased metabolism)
>ED Kharasch et al, Single-dose disulfiram inhibition of chlorzoxazone metabolism: A clinical probe for P450 2E1. Clin Pharmacol Ther, 56:643, 1993

Based on a study of normal males

CHOLESTYRAMINE, with:

Acetaminophen - See Acetaminophen with Cholestyramine, page 8

Amiodarone - See Amiodarone with Cholestyramine, page 34

Anticoagulants, oral - See Anticoagulants, oral with Cholestyramine, page 63

Antidepressants, tricyclic - See Antidepressants, tricyclic with Cholestyramine, page 84

Beta-adrenergic blockers - See Beta-adrenergic blockers with Cholestyramine, page 152

Corticosteroids
Possible decreased effect of hydrocortisone (decreased absorption)
>V Audetat et al, Beeintrachtigt cholestyramin die biologische verfugbarkeit

CHOLESTYRAMINE, with: *(continued)*
> von prednisolon? Schweiz Med Wochenschr, 107:527, 1977; C Johansson et al, Interaction by cholestyramine on the uptake of hydrocortisone in the gastrointestinal tract. Acta Med Scand, 204:509, 1978

Monitor corticosteroid concentration; does not occur with prednisolone

Digitoxin
Decreased digitoxin effect (binding in intestine)
> DD Brown et al, A steady-state evaluation of the effects of propantheline bromide and cholestyramine on the bioavailability of digoxin when administered as tablets or capsules. J Clin Pharmacol, 25:360, 1985

Give digitoxin 1½ hours before cholestyramine and monitor digitoxin concentration

Digoxin
Decreased digoxin effect (binding in intestine)
> DD Brown et al, A steady-state evaluation of the effects of propantheline bromide and cholestyramine on the bioavailability of digoxin when administered as tablets or capsules. J Clin Pharmacol, 25:360, 1985

Give digoxin 1½ hours before cholestyramine and monitor digoxin concentration; solution-containing capsules preferable to tablets

Fenofibrate
Possible reduced fenofibrate effect (decreased absorption)
> Manufacturer's package insert (fenofibrate)

Give fenofibrate at least 1 hour before or 4 to 6 hours after cholestyramine

Furosemide
Decreased diuretic effect (decreased absorption)
> PJ Neuvonen et al, Effects of resins and activated charcoal on the absorption of digoxin, carbamazepine and frusemide. Br J Clin Pharmacol, 25:229, 1988

Give at least 6 hours apart

HMG-CoA reductase inhibitors
Decreased cerivastatin, fluvastatin or pravastatin effect (decreased absorption)
> W Mück et al, Int J Clin Pharmacol Ther, 35:250, 1997; manufacturer's package insert

Give statin 1 hour before or 4 hours after cholestyramine; may occur with other statins

Hypoglycemics, sulfonylurea
Decreased glipizide effect (decreased absorption)
> KT Kivistö and PJ Neuvonen, The effect of cholestyramine and activated charcoal on glipizide absorption. Br J Clin Pharmacol, 30:733, 1990

Give at least 2 hours apart; based on study in healthy men

Leflunomide
Decreased leflunomide effect (decreased absorption)
> Manufacturer's package insert

Giving leflunomide at least 2 hours before or 6 hours after cholestyramine may reduce (but not eliminate) effect, due to enterohepatic cycling of leflunomide; interaction useful in case of leflunomide overdose

CHOLESTYRAMINE, with: *(continued)*
Metronidazole
Possible decreased metronidazole effect (decreased absorption)
> AM Molokhia and S Al-Rahman, Effect of concomitant oral administration of some adsorbing drugs on the bioavailability of metronidazole. Drug Devel Indust Pharm, 13:1229, 1987

Based on studies in 5 healthy volunteers; monitor metronidazole concentration or clinical status

Mycophenolate mofetil
Possible decreased mycophenolate effect (decreased absorption)
> Manufacturer's package insert

Monitor mycophenolate concentration

Narcotics: meperidine and congeners
Possible decreased loperamide effect (decreased absorption)
> TY Ti et al, Probable interaction of loperamide and cholestyramine. Can Med Assoc J, 119:607, 1978

Give drugs as far apart as possible

Nicotinic acid
Possible decreased niacin effect (possible decreased absorption)
> Manufacturer's package insert *(Niaspan)*

Based on in vitro study; separate doses by 4 to 6 hours, or as much as possible; colestipol may interact to a greater extent

Nonsteroidal anti-inflammatory drugs
Possible decreased naproxen effect (delayed absorption)
> MV Calvo and A Dominguez-Gil, Interaction of naproxen with cholestyramine. Biopharm Drug Dispos, 5:33, 1984

Monitor clinical status; give naproxen 2 hours before or 6 hours after cholestyramine; based on study in 8 healthy volunteers

Possible decreased ibuprofen effect (decreased rate and extent of absorption)
> A Mohamed et al, The effect of colestipol and cholestyramine on ibuprofen bioavailability in man. Bispharm Drug Dispos, 15:463, 1994

Based on study in healthy subjects; give ibuprofen 2 hours before or 6 hours after cholestyramine; colestipol did not interact

Possible decreased diclofenac effect (decreased rate and extent of absorption)
> SR Al-Balla et al, The effects of cholestyramine and colestipol on the absorption of diclofenac in man. J Clin Pharmacol Ther, 32:441, 1994

Based on study in healthy subjects; give diclofenac 2 hours before or 6 hours after cholestyramine

Possible decreased meloxicam effect (decreased absorption)
> Manufacturer's package insert (meloxicam)

Meloxicam clearance increased by 50%; monitor clinical status

Raloxifene
Reduction in raloxifene effect (decreased absorption and interference with enterohepatic cycling)
> Manufacturer's package insert

(continued)

CHOLESTYRAMINE, with: *(continued)*
> *Avoid concurrent use; colestipol may have similar effect; separating doses may not completely avoid interaction*

Spironolactone
Hyperchloremic acidosis (decreased renal chloride clearance)
> WM Clouston and HM Lloyd, Cholestyramine induced hyperchloremic metabolic acidosis. Aust N Z J Med, 15:271, 1985; ER Eaves and MG Korman, Cholestyramine induced hyperchloremic metabolic acidosis. Aust N Z J Med, 14:670, 1984; P Zapater and D Alba, Acidosis and extreme hyperkalemia associated with cholestyramine and spironolactone. Ann Pharmacother, 29:1991, 1995

Reported in patients with cirrhosis; avoid concurrent use in such patients

Thiazide diuretics
Decreased thiazide effect (decreased absorption)
> DB Hunninghake et al, The effect of cholestyramine and colestipol on the absorption of hydrochlorothiazide. Int J Clin Pharmacol Ther Toxicol, 20:151, 1982; DB Hunninghake and DM Hibbard, Influence of time intervals for cholestyramine dosing on the absorption of hydrochlorothiazide. Clin Pharmacol Ther, 39:329, 1986

Give drugs as far apart as possible

Thyroid hormones
Decreased thyroid effect (binding in intestine)
> RC Northcutt et al, The influence of cholestyramine on thyroxine absorption. JAMA, 208:1857, 1969; SM Harmon and CF Seifert, Levothyroxine-cholestyramine interaction reemphasized. Ann Intern Med, 115:658, 1991

Give drugs at least 5 hours apart

Troglitazone
Possible decreased troglitazone effect (decreased absorption)
> Manufacturer's package insert (troglitazone)

Avoid concurrent use; troglitazone is no longer available

Ursodiol
Possible decreased ursodiol effect (decreased absorption)
> Manufacturer's package insert

Give at least 2 hours apart

Valproate
Decreased valproate effect (decreased absorption)
> AT Pennell et al, Cholestyramine decreases valproic acid serum concentrations. J Clin Pharmacol, 32:755, 1992, abs 55

Give at least 3 hours apart; based on study in 6 healthy volunteers

Choline magnesium trisalicylate, see Nonsteroidal anti-inflammatory drugs
Ciclopirox, no documented interactions, see page 4, Criteria for Listing Interactions
Cidofovir, no documented interactions, see page 4, Criteria for Listing Interactions
CILOSTAZOL, with:

Diltiazem
Possible cilostazol toxicity (decreased metabolism; CYP3A4)
> Manufacturer's package insert (cilostazol)

CILOSTAZOL, with: *(continued)*
> *Manufacturer recommends decreasing dose of cilostazol to 50 mg bid*

HMG-COA reductase inhibitors
Possible lovastatin toxicity (mechanism not established)
> SL Bramer et al, Effect of multiple cilostazol doses on single dose lovastatin pharmacokinetics in healthy volunteers. Clin Pharmacokinet, 37 suppl 2:69, 1999

Based on study in healthy subjects; effect modest; monitor clinical status

Macrolide antibiotics
Possible cilostazol toxicity (decreased metabolism)
> A Suri et al, Effects of CYP3A inhibition on the metabolism of cilostazol. Clin Pharmacokinet, 37 suppl 2:61, 1999; manufacturer's package insert (cilostazol)

Manufacturer recommends decreasing dose of cilostazol to 50 mg bid; other macrolide antibiotics such as clarithromycin and troleandomycin will probably interact, but theoretically azithromycin and dirithromycin would not

Omeprazole
Possible cilostazol toxicity (decreased metabolism; omeprazole inhibits CYP2C19)
> A Suri and SL Bramer, Effect of omeprazole on the metabolism of cilostazol. Clin Pharmacokinet, 37 suppl 2:53, 1999; manufacturer's package insert (cilostazol)

Manufacturer recommends decreasing dose of cilostazol to 50 mg bid

Cimetidine, see Antihistamines, H_2-blockers
Ciprofloxacin, see Fluoroquinolones
CISAPRIDE, with:

Alcohol - See Alcohol with Cisapride, page 16
Amprenavir - See Amprenavir with Cisapride, page 39
Anticoagulants, oral - See Anticoagulants, oral with Cisapride, page 63
Antifungals, imidazoles and triazoles - See Antifungals, imidazoles and triazoles with Cisapride, page 98

Delavirdine
Delavirdine decreases metabolism and may increase toxicity; high concentrations of cisapride may lead to dangerous cardiac arrhythmias
> Manufacturer's package insert

Theoretical; manufacturer recommends avoiding concurrent use if possible; cisapride is no longer marketed in the USA

Dofetilide
Increased risk of arrhythmias (additive effect on QTc interval)
> Manufacturer's package insert (dofetilide)

Avoid concurrent use; cisapride is no longer marketed in the USA

Efavirenz
Possible cisapride-induced arrhythmias (decreased metabolism)
> Manufacturer's package insert (efavirenz)

Manufacturer recommends avoiding concurrent use; theoretical; cisapride is no longer marketed in the USA

(continued)

CISAPRIDE, with: *(continued)*
  Fluoroquinolones
    Possible ventricular arrhythmia with grepafloxacin (possible additive effect on QTc interval; CYP3A4)
      Manufacturer's package insert
    Theoretical; manufacturer recommends avoiding concurrent use; cisapride is no longer marketed in the USA
  Grapefruit juice
    Possible cisapride toxicity (decreased metabolism; CYP3A4)
      Manufacturer's package insert (cisapride); AS Gross et al, Influence of grapefruit juice on cisapride pharmacokinetics. Clin Pharmacol Ther, 65:395, 1999; KT Kivistö et al, Repeated consumption of grapefruit juice considerably increases plasma concentrations of cisapride. Clin Pharmacol Ther, 66:448, 1999
    Based on studies in healthy subjects; avoid concurrent use; cisapride is no longer marketed in the USA
  Indinavir
    Possible ventricular arrhythmia (decreased cisapride metabolism; CYP3A4)
      Manufacturer's package insert
    Theoretical; avoid concurrent use; cisapride is no longer marketed in the USA
  Lopinavir/Ritonavir
    Increased cisapride toxicity, including cardiac arrhythmias
      Manufacturer's package insert (*Kaletra*)
    Avoid concurrent use; cisapride is no longer marketed in the USA
  Macrolide antibiotics
    Ventricular arrhythmias with clarithromycin or erythromycin (probably decreased metabolism, CYP3A4; possible synergism)
      IR Jenkins and J Gibson, Cisapride, erythromycin and arrhythmia. Anaesth Intensive Care, 24:728, 1996; MA Sekkarie, Torsades de pointes in two chronic renal failure patients treated with cisapride and clarithromycin. Am J Kidney Dis, 30:437, 1997; VS Gray, Syncopal episodes associated with cisapride and concurrent drugs. Ann Pharmacother, 32:648, 1998; AD van Haarst et al, The influence of cisapride and clarithromycin on QT intervals in healthy volunteers. Clin Pharmacol Ther, 64:542, 1998; R Trinkle, Comment: syncopal episodes associated with cisapride. Ann Pharmacother, 33:251, 1999
    Several case reports; avoid concurrent use; cisapride is no longer marketed in the USA
  Nefazodone
    Possible ventricular arrhythmia (decreased cisapride metabolism)
      Manufacturer's package insert
    Theoretical; manufacturer recommends avoiding concurrent use; cisapride is no longer marketed in the USA
  Nelfinavir
    Possible cisapride toxicity (decreased metabolism; CYP3A)
      Manufacturer's package insert (nelfinavir)

CISAPRIDE, with: *(continued)*
Avoid concurrent use; cisapride is no longer marketed in the USA

Nifedipine
Possible hypotension (increased gastrointestinal motility)
> C Satoh et al, Influence of cisapride on the pharmacokinetics and antihypertensive effect of sustained-release nifedipine. Intern Med, 35:941, 1996

Based on study in 20 hypertensive patients; monitor blood pressure; cisapride is no longer marketed in the USA

Ritonavir
Possible ventricular arrhythmias (decreased metabolism)
> Manufacturer's package insert (ritonavir)

Theoretical; listed as contraindicated in product information; cisapride is no longer marketed in the USA

Saquinavir
Possible ventricular arrhythmia (saquinavir decreases metabolism)
> Manufacturer's package insert

Theoretical; manufacturer recommends avoiding concurrent use if possible; cisapride is no longer marketed in the USA

Selective serotonin reuptake inhibitors (SSRIs)
Possible ventricular arrhythmias (possible decreased metabolism, CYP3A4)
> R Trinkle, Comment: syncopal episodes associated with cisapride. Ann Pharmacother, 33:251, 1999

Single case report (1999); cisapride is no longer marketed in the USA

Troleandomycin
Possible ventricular arrhythmias (probably decreased metabolism)
> Manufacturer's package insert

Based on cases reported to the manufacturer and in vitro study of human hepatic microsomes; avoid concurrent use; cisapride is no longer marketed in the USA

CISPLATIN, with:

Aminoglycoside antibiotics - See Aminoglycoside antibiotics with Cisplatin, page 30
Carbamazepine - See Carbamazepine with Cisplatin, page 176

Ifosfamide
Increased hearing loss (mechanism not established)
> WH Meyer et al, Ifosfamide and exacerbation of cisplatin-induced hearing loss. Lancet, 341:754, 1993

Monitor hearing

Lithium
Reduced lithium effect (probably due to sodium loading with cisplatin)
> JH Beijnen et al, Lithium pharmacokinetics during cisplatin-based chemotherapy: a case report. Cancer Chemother Pharmacol, 33:523, 1994

Case report of a 33-year-old man who also received bleomycin and etoposide (1994); clinical significance not established

Methotrexate
Methotrexate toxicity (decreased renal clearance)
> WR Crom et al, The effect of prior cisplatin therapy on the pharmacokinetics of high-dose methotrexate. J Clin Oncol, 2:655, 1984; N Haim et al,

CISPLATIN, with: *(continued)*
> Methotrexate-related deaths in patients previously treated with cis-diamminedichloride platinum. Cancer Chemother Pharmacol, 13:223, 1984

Monitor methotrexate concentration, especially in patients who have previously received more than 360 mg per square meter of cisplatin (cumulative dose)

Ondansetron
Possible small alteration in cisplatin effect (mechanism not established)
> PJ Cagnoni et al, Modification of the pharmacokinetics of high-dose cyclophosphamide and cisplatin by antiemetics. Bone Marrow Transplant, 24:1, 1999

Based on study in patients undergoing bone marrow transplant; clinical importance not established

Paclitaxel
Possible taxol neurotoxicity (mechanism not established)
> G Cavaletti et al, Peripheral neurotoxicity of taxol in patients previously treated with cisplatin. Cancer, 75:1141, 1995

Based on study in 22 patients given taxol for a relapse of cisplatin-treated ovarian cancer

Phenytoin
Decreased phenytoin effect (increased metabolism)
> C Neef and I de Voogd-van der Straaten, An interaction between cytostatic and anticonvulsant drugs. Clin Pharmacol Ther, 43:372, 1988; SA Grossman et al, Decreased phenytoin levels in patients receiving chemotherapy. Am J Med, 87:505, 1989

Single well-documented case report (1988); monitor phenytoin concentration; also reported in many patients receiving cisplatin alone or with carmustine; also occurs with carboplatin

Valproate
Decreased valproate effect (decreased absorption)
> C Neef and I de Voogd-van der Straaten, An interaction between cytostatic and anticonvulsant drugs. Clin Pharmacol Ther, 43:372, 1988

Single well-documented case report (1988); monitor valproate concentration

Citalopram, see Selective serotonin reuptake inhibitors (SSRIs)

CITRATES, with:
  Antacids - See Antacids with Citrates, page 51

Citric acid, see Citrates

Clarithromycin, see Macrolide antibiotics

Clemastine, no documented interactions, see page 4, Criteria for Listing Interactions

CLINDAMYCIN, with:
Cyclosporine
Possible decreased cyclosporine effect (mechanism not established)
> R Thurnheer et al, Possible interaction between clindamycin and cyclosporin. BMJ, 319:163, 1999

CLINDAMYCIN, with: *(continued)*
> *Two case reports with positive dechallenge (1999); monitor cyclosporine concentrations during clindamycin therapy*

Neuromuscular blocking agents
Increased neuromuscular blockade (additive)
> D Avery and R Finn, Succinylcholine-prolonged apnea associated with clindamycin and abnormal liver function tests. Dis Nerv Syst, 38:473, 1977; LD Becker and RD Miller, Clindamycin enhances a nondepolarizing neuromuscular blockade. Anesthesiology, 45:84, 1976

Monitor neuromuscular status when blocking agents must be given

Verapamil
Verapamil toxicity (mechanism not established)
> K Kishore et al, Acute verapamil toxicity in a patient with chronic toxicity: possible interaction with ceftriaxone and clindamycin. Ann Pharmacother, 27:877, 1993

Single case report; patient was also receiving ceftriaxone (1993)

Clobazam, see Benzodiazepines
Clobetasol, no documented interactions, see page 4, Criteria for Listing Interactions
Clobetasol propionate, no documented interactions, see page 4, Criteria for Listing Interactions
Clocortolone, no documented interactions, see page 4, Criteria for Listing Interactions

CLOFAZIMINE, with:

Phenytoin
Decreased phenytoin effect (mechanism not established)
> LA Cone et al, Drug interactions in patients with AIDS. Clin Infect Dis, 15:1066, 1992

Single case report (1992)

CLOFIBRATE, with:

Anticoagulants, oral - See Anticoagulants, oral with Clofibrate, page 64

Contraceptives, oral
Possible decreased clofibrate effect (increased metabolism)
> JO Miners et al, Gender and oral contraceptive steroids as determinants of drug glucuronidation: effects on clofibric acid elimination. Br J Clin Pharmacol, 18:240, 1984

Monitor blood lipids or chlorphenoxyisobutyric acid concentration

Hypoglycemics, sulfonylurea
Increased hypoglycemic effect (mechanism not established)
> J-C Daubresse et al, Clofibrate and diabetes control in patients treated with oral hypoglycemic agents. Br J Clin Pharmacol, 7:599, 1979

Monitor blood glucose

Phenformin
Increased hypoglycemic effect (mechanism not established)
> J-C Daubresse et al, Clofibrate and diabetes control in patients treated with oral hypoglycemic agents. Br J Clin Pharmacol, 7:599, 1979

Monitor blood glucose

(continued)

CLOFIBRATE, with: *(continued)*
Probenecid
Clofibrate toxicity (possibly decreased metabolism)
> JR Veenendaal et al, Probenecid-clofibrate interaction. Clin Pharmacol Ther, 29:351, 1981

Avoid concurrent use, if possible

Probucol
Decreased HDL-cholesterol concentration (mechanism not established)
> J Davignon et al, Severe hypoalphalipoproteinemia induced by a combination of probucol and clofibrate. Adv Exp Med Biol, 201:111, 1986; S Yokoyama et al, A little more information about aggravation of probucol-induced HDL-reduction by clofibrate. Atherosclerosis, 70:179, 1988

Avoid concurrent use

Rifampin
Possible decreased clofibrate effect (increased metabolism)
> G Houin and J-P Tillement, Clofibrate and enzymatic induction in man. Int J Clin Pharmacol, 16:150, 1978

Monitor blood lipids or chlorphenoxyisobutyric acid concentration

Thiazide diuretics
Severe hyponatremia (mechanism not established)
> J Soler-Bel et al, Hiponatremia intensa por clofibrato y diurético tiacídico. Med Clin (Barc), 91:438, 1988

Single case report (1988)

Clomipramine, see Antidepressants, tricyclic
Clonazepam, see Benzodiazepines

CLONIDINE, with:
Antidepressants, tricyclic - See Antidepressants, tricyclic with Clonidine, page 84
Beta-adrenergic blockers - See Beta-adrenergic blockers with Clonidine, page 152

Insulin
Decreased insulin effect (mechanism not established)
> A Mimouni-Bloch and M Mimouni, Clonidine-induced hyperglycemia in a young diabetic girl. Ann Pharmacother, 27:980, 1993

Single case report (1993); 9½ year old girl 6 months after onset of diabetes, who required low doses of insulin ("honeymoon period")

Levodopa
Decreased levodopa effect (mechanism not established)
> I Shoulson and TN Chase, Clonidine and the anti-parkinsonian response to L-dopa or piribedil. Neuropharmacology, 15:25, 1976

Use alternative antihypertensive drug

Mirtazapine
Possible decreased antihypertensive effect of clonidine (probably antagonism)
> RA Abo-Zena et al, Hypertensive urgency induced by an interaction of mirtazapine and clonidine. Pharmacotherapy, 20:476, 2000

Single case report involving a patient on hemodialysis (2000); monitor blood pressure and clinical status

CLONIDINE, with: *(continued)*

Naloxone

Decreased clonidine effect (possibly due to blockade of clonidine effect by release of CNS endogenous opioid)

C Farsang et al, Reversal by naloxone of the antihypertensive action of clonidine: involvement of the sympathetic nervous system. Circulation, 69:461, 1984

Only about half of patients affected; monitor blood pressure and clinical status

Propofol

Possible propofol toxicity (mechanism not established)

J Guglielminotti et al, Effects of premedication on dose requirements for propofol: comparison of clonidine and hydroxyzine. Br J Anaesth, 80:733, 1998

Based on study in 28 patients undergoing surgery; decrease propofol dose as indicated

Sympathomimetic amines

ECG abnormalities and sudden death in children taking methylphenidate and clonidine (mechanism not established)

JM Swanson et al, Clonidine in the treatment of ADHD: questions about safety and efficacy. J Child Adoles Phychopharmacol, 5:301, 1995; RR Fenichel, Combining methylphenidate and clonidine: the role of post-marketing surveillance. J Child Adoles Psychopharmacol, 5:155, 1995; F Levy, Clonidine: adverse responses. J Paediatr Child Health, 34:501, 1998

Cause and effect not established; monitor clinical status

Tolazoline

Decreased antihypertensive effect (mechanism not established)

P Merguet et al, Experimental study of the circulatory effects of 2-(2,6-dichlorophenylamine)-2-imidazoline hydrochloride in man. Pharmacol Clin, 1:30, 1968

Avoid concurrent use

Verapamil

A-V Block (possible synergy)

R Jaffe et al, Adverse interaction between clonidine and verapamil. Ann Pharmacother, 28:881, 1994

Two cases (1994)

CLOPIDOGREL, with:

Anticoagulants, oral - See Anticoagulants, oral with Clopidogrel, page 64

Nonsteroidal anti-inflammatory drugs

Gastrointestinal blood loss (possibly additive)

Manufacturer's package insert (clopidogrel); A Van Hecken et al, Effect of clopidogrel on naproxen-induced gastrointestinal blood loss in healthy volunteers. Drug Metab Drug Interact, 14:193, 1998; JD Easton, Clinical aspects of the use of clopidogrel, a new antiplatelet agent. Semin Thromb Hemost, 25 suppl 2:77, 1999

(continued)

CLOPIDOGREL, with: *(continued)*
>*Based on study in healthy subjects with naproxen (1998) and aspirin (1999); monitor hemoglobin and hematocrit*

Clorazepate, see Benzodiazepines

CLOZAPINE, with:

Antidepressants, tricyclic - See Antidepressants, tricyclic with Clozapine, page 84

Antihistamines, H$_2$-blockers - See Antihistamines, H$_2$-blockers with Clozapine, page 116

Barbiturates - See Barbiturates with Clozapine, page 132

Benzodiazepines - See Benzodiazepines with Clozapine, page 140

Caffeine - See Caffeine with Clozapine, page 172

Carbamazepine - See Carbamazepine with Clozapine, page 176

Cocaine
>Hypotension and syncope (mechanism not established)
>>FA Hameedi et al, Near syncope associated with concomitant clozapine and cocaine use. J Clin Psychiatry, 57:371, 1996
>
>*Single case report (1996)*

Fluoroquinolones
>Possible clozapine toxicity with ciprofloxacin (probably decreased metabolism; CYP1A2)
>>JS Markowitz et al, Fluoroquinolone inhibition of clozapine metabolism. Am J Psychiatry, 153:881, 1997; AAB Joos et al, Pharmacokinetic interaction of clozapine and rifampicin in a forensic patient with an atypical mycobacterial infection. J Clin Psychopharmacol, 18:83, 1998; JL Karagianis et al, Clozapine-associated neuroleptic malignant syndrome: two new cases and a review of the literature. Ann Pharmacother, 33:623, 1999
>
>*Three case reports (1997, 1998, 1999); toxicity occurred in two; enoxacin likely to interact but little or no interaction would be expected with other fluoroquinolones*

Haloperidol
>Possible haloperidol toxicity (possibly decreased metabolism)
>>SA Allen, Effect of chlorpromazine and clozapine on plasma concentrations of haloperidol in a patient with schizophrenia. J Clin Pharmacol, 40:1296, 2000
>
>*Single case report (2000); causal relationship not established; monitor clinical status*

Interferon
>Agranulocytosis (probably additive)
>>RM Hoffmann et al, Interferon-α-induced agranulocytosis in a patient on long-term clozapine therapy. J Hepatology, 29:170, 1998
>
>*Single case report (1998)*

Lithium
>CNS toxicity (mechanism not established)
>>LM Blake et al, Reversible neurologic symptoms with clozapine and lithium. J Clin Psychopharmacol, 12:297, 1992; B Hellwig et al, Tapering off clozapine in a clozapine-lithium co-medication may cause an acute organic psychosis: a case report. Pharmacopsychiatry, 28:187, 1995

CLOZAPINE, with: *(continued)*
> *Monitor clinical status and maintain lithium concentration below 0.5 mEq/L; toxicity may occur when clozapine is tapered and lithium continued*

Macrolide antibiotics

Possible clozapine toxicity with erythromycin (decreased metabolism); erythromycin inhibits CYP1A2 and CYP3A4

> LG Funderburg et al, Seizure following addition of erythromycin to clozapine treatment. Am J Psychiatry, 151:12, 1994; L Glassner et al, Erythromycin-induced clozapine toxic reaction. Arch Intern Med, 156:675, 1996; S Hägg et al, Absence of interaction between erythromycin and a single dose of clozapine. Eur J Clin Pharmacol, 55:221, 1999; SI Usiskin et al, Retreatment with clozapine after erythromycin-induced neutropenia. Am J Psychiatry, 157:1021, 2000

Single case report of seizures (1994); single case report of neurotoxicity (1996); single case report of neutropenia (2000); negative study in healthy subjects did not involve sufficient duration of erythromycin treatment (1999)

Phenothiazines

Possible clozapine toxicity with perphenazine (mechanism not established)

> C Cooke and J de Leon, Adding other antipsychotics to clozapine. J Clin Psychiatry, 60:710, 1999

Single case report (1999); monitor clinical status

Phenytoin

Decreased clozapine effect (increased metabolism)

> DD Miller, Effect of phenytoin on plasma clozapine concentrations in two patients. J Clin Psychiatry, 52:23, 1991

Two cases (1991)

Rifampin

Reduced clozapine effect (increased metabolism; CYP1A2, 3A)

> AAB Joos et al, Pharmacokinetic interaction of clozapine and rifampicin in a forensic patient with an atypical mycobacterial infection. J Clin Psychopharmacol, 18:83, 1998

Single case report of marked decrease in clozapine concentrations (1998)

Risperidone

Possible clozapine toxicity (mechanism not established)

> SC Tyson et al, Pharmacokinetic interaction between risperidone and clozapine. Am J Psychiatry, 152:9, 1995; SA Chong et al, Atrial ectopics with clozapine-risperidone combination. J Clin Psychopharmacol, 17:130, 1997

Two case reports (1995, 1997); monitor clinical status and clozapine concentrations

Ritonavir

Possible clozapine toxicity (decreased metabolism)

> Manufacturer's package insert (ritonavir)

Theoretical; listed as contraindicated in product information

Selective serotonin reuptake inhibitors (SSRIs)

Clozapine toxicity with fluvoxamine, and possibly sertraline, fluoxetine, citalopram or paroxetine (decreased metabolism; CYP1A2; CYP2C19; CYP2D6)

> H Weigmann et al, Interactions of fluvoxamine with the metabolism of

(continued)

CLOZAPINE, with: *(continued)*
clozapine. Pharmacopsychiatry, 26:209, 1993; F Centorrino et al, Serum concentrations of clozapine and its major metabolites: effects of cotreatment with fluoxetine or valproate. Am J Psychiatry, 151:1, 1994; M Jerling et al, Fluvoxamine inhibition and carbamazepine induction of the metabolism of clozapine: evidence from a therapeutic drug monitoring service. Ther Drug Monit, 16:368, 1994; F Centorrino et al, Serum levels of clozapine and norclozapine in patients treated with selective serotonin reuptake inhibitors. Am J Psychiatry, 153:820, 1996; HJ Koponen et al, Fluvoxamine increases the clozapine serum levels significantly. Eur Neuropsychopharmacol, 6:69, 1996; JS Markowitz et al, Fluvoxamine–clozapine dose-dependent interaction. Can J Psychiatry, 41:670, 1996; A Szegedi et al, Improved efficacy and fewer side effects under clozapine treatment after addition of fluvoxamine. J Clin Psychopharmacol, 15:141, 1995; SA Chong et al, Worsening of psychosis with clozapine and selective serotonin reuptake inhibitor combination: two case reports. J Clin Psychopharmacol, 17:68, 1997; NR Pinninti and J De Leon, Interaction of sertraline with clozapine. J Clin Psychopharmacol, 17:119, 1997; TP George et al, Leukopenia associated with addition of paroxetine to clozapine. J Clin Psychiatry, 59:31, 1998; AAB Joos et al, Dose-dependent pharmacokinetic interaction of clozapine and paroxetine in an extensive metabolizer. Pharmacopsychiatria, 30:266, 1997; SE Purdon and M Snaterse, Selective serotonin reuptake inhibitor modulation of clozapine effects on cognition in schizophrenia. Can J Psychiatry, 43:84, 1998; KE Ferslew et al, A fatal drug interaction between clozapine and fluoxetine. J Forensic Sci, 43:1082, 1998; F-J Kuo et al, Extrapyramidal symptoms after addition of fluvoxamine to clozapine. J Clin Psychopharmacol, 18:483, 1998; D Taylor et al, Co-administration of citalopram and clozapine: effect on plasma clozapine levels. Int Clin Psychopharmacol, 13:19, 1998; W-H Chang et al, In-vitro and in-vivo evaluation of the drug-drug interaction between fluvoxamine and clozapine. Psychopharmacology, 145:91, 1999; OV Olesen and K Linnet, Fluvoxamine-clozapine drug interaction: inhibition *in vitro* of five cytochrome P450 isoforms involved in clozapine metabolism. J Clin Psychopharmacol, 20:35, 2000; M Heeringa et al, Elevated plasma levels of clozapine after concomitant use of fluvoxamine. Pharm World Sci, 21:243, 1999; A Szegedi et al, Addition of low-dose fluvoxamine to low-dose clozapine monotherapy in schizophrenia: drug monitoring and tolerability data from a prospective clinical trial. Pharmacopsychiatry, 32:148, 1999; CP Borba and DC Henderson, Citalopram and clozapine: potential drug interaction. J Clin Psychiatry, 61:301, 2000; D Hinze-Selch et al, Effect of coadministration of clozapine and fluvoxamine versus clozapine monotherapy on blood cell counts, plasma levels of cytokines and body weight. Psychopharmacology, 149:163, 2000

CLOZAPINE, with: *(continued)*

Marked increases in clozapine levels (5 to 10 fold) with fluvoxamine; monitor clozapine concentration and WBC count; single case reports with paroxetine (1997) and citalopram (2000); fluvoxamine or fluoxetine have been used with clozapine to improve efficacy in a number of cases; fatality with fluoxetine (1998) but a causal relationship was not established

Possible increased toxicity of fluoxetine when discontinued (mechanism not established)

> M-L Lu et al, Selective serotonin reuptake inhibitor syndrome: precipitated by concomitant clozapine? J Clin Psychopharmacol, 19:386, 1999

Single case report with fluoxetine (1999); clinical importance not established

Tobacco, smoking

Decreased clozapine effect (increased metabolism)

> H Wetzel et al, Pharmacokinetic interactions of clozapine with selective serotonin reuptake inhibitors: differential effects of fluvoxamine and paroxetine in a prospective study. J Clin Psychopharmacol, 18:2, 1998; LK Oyewumi, Smoking cessation and clozapine side effects. Can J Psychiatry, 43:748, 1998; E Skogh et al, Could discontinuing smoking be hazardous for patients administered clozapine medication? A Case report. Ther Drug Monit, 21:580, 1999

Smokers may have higher dosage requirements for clozapine; watch for clozapine toxicity if patient stops smoking

Valproate

Possible decreased clozapine effect (mechanism not established)

> P Finley and D Warner, Potential impact of valproic acid therapy on clozapine disposition. Biol Psychiatry, 36:487, 1994; LP Longo and C Salzman, Valproic acid effects on serum concentrations of clozapine and norclozapine. Am J Psychiatry, 152:4, 1995; G Facciolá et al, Small effects of valproic acid on the plasma concentrations of clozapine and its major metabolites in patients with schizophrenic or affective disorders. Ther Drug Monit, 21:341, 1999

Monitor clozapine concentration; one study found slight increases in clozapine concentrations after valproate; another study found clozapine plus valproate to be efficacious and well tolerated

Possible hepatotoxicity (mechanism not established)

> WC Wirshing et al, Hepatic encephalopathy associated with combined clozapine and divalproex sodium treatment. J Clin Psychopharmacol, 17:120, 1997

Single case report of hepatic encephalopathy (1997); causal relationship not established.

COCAINE, with:

Beta-adrenergic blockers - See Beta-adrenergic blockers with Cocaine, page 153
Clozapine - See Clozapine with Cocaine, page 206
Disulfiram

Possible cocaine toxicity (probably decreased metabolism)

> EF McCance-Katz et al, Disulfiram effects on acute cocaine administration.

(continued)

COCAINE, with: *(continued)*
>   Drug Alcohol Depend, 52:27, 1998
>
> *Increased cardiovascular effects of intranasal cocaine, especially heart rate; avoid concurrent use*

Nonsteroidal anti-inflammatory drugs
> Fetal renal failure and gastrointestinal hemorrhage with cocaine and indomethacin (possibly additive)
>
>   SJ Carlan et al, Cocaine and indomethacin: fetal anuria, neonatal edema, and gastrointestinal bleeding. Obstet Gynecol, 78:501, 1991
>
> *Single case report (1991)*

Propofol
> Convulsions after topical cocaine and propofol general anesthesia (mechanism not established)
>
>   BJ Hendley, Convulsions after cocaine and propofol. Anaesthesia, 45:788, 199
>
> *Single case report (1990)*

Sympathomimetic amines
> Ventricular arrhythmias with topical cocaine plus epinephrine or phenylephrine in nasal surgery (possible additive effects)
>
>   KEA Nicholson and JEG Rogers, Cocaine and adrenaline paste: a fatal combination? BMJ, 311:250, 1995; M Ashchi et al, Cardiac complication from use of cocaine and phenylephrine in nasal septoplasty. Arch Otolaryngol Head Neck Surg, 121:681, 1995
>
> *Avoid concurrent use*
>
> Possible increased risk of ischemic brain lesions with combined cocaine-amphetamine abuse (probably additive)
>
>   M Strupp et al, Combined amphetamine and cocaine abuse caused mesencephalic ischemia in a 16-year-old boy – due to vasospasm? Eur Neurol, 43:181, 2000
>
> *Single case report (2000); avoid concurrent use*

Codeine, see Narcotics: morphine-like

COLCHICINE, with:

Cyclosporine
> Cyclosporine toxicity (mechanism not established)
>
>   R Menta et al, Reversible acute cyclosporin nephrotoxicity induced by colchicine administration. Nephrol Dialysis Transplant, 2:380, 1987; A Yussim et al, Gastrointestinal, hepatorenal, and neuromuscular toxicity caused by cyclosporine-colchicine interaction in renal transplantation. Transplant Proc, 26:2825, 1994
>
> *Single case report (1987), and a study of 4 renal transplant patients*
>
> Possible colchicine-induced myopathy (mechanism not established)
>
>   BI Lee et al, Acute myopathy induced by colchicine in a cyclosporine-treated renal transplant recipient. J Korean Med Sci, 12:160, 1997; JT Jagose and RR Bailey, Muscle weakness due to colchicine in a renal transplant recipient. NZ Med J, 110:34, 1997
>
> *Two case reports (1997)*

COLCHICINE, with: *(continued)*
Macrolide antibiotics
Colchicine toxicity with erythromycin (mechanism not established)
> Y Caraco et al, Acute colchicine intoxication – possible role of erythromycin administration. J Rheumatol, 19:494, 1992

Single case report (1992)

COLESEVELAM, with:
Verapamil
Decreased verapamil effect (possibly decreased absorption)
> Manufacturer's package insert (colesevelam)

Plasma concentration of sustained-release verpamil decreased in one study; clinical significance unknown

COLESTIPOL, with:
Beta-adrenergic blockers - See Beta-adrenergic blockers with Colestipol, page 153
Digoxin
Possible decreased digoxin effect (decreased absorption)
> RJ van Bever et al, The effect of colestipol on digitoxin plasma levels. Arzneimittelforschung, 26:1891, 1976; VW Payne et al, Use of colestipol in a patient with digoxin intoxication. Drug Intell Clin Pharm, 15:902, 1981

Based on analogy with cholestyramine and reversal of digoxin toxicity with colestipol; may not be clinically significant with usual doses of colestipol for hypercholesterolemia; digitoxin may not interact

Fenofibrate
Possible reduced fenofibrate effect (decreased absorption)
> Manufacturer's package insert (fenofibrate)

Give fenofibrate at least 1 hour before or 4 to 6 hours after colestipol

Furosemide
Decreased diuretic effect (decreased absorption)
> PJ Neuvonen et al, Effects of resins and activated charcoal on the absorption of digoxin, carbamazepine and frusemide. Br J Clin Pharmacol, 25:229, 1988

Give at least 6 hours apart

Gemfibrozil
Decreased gemfibrozil effect (decreased absorption)
> SC Forland et al, Apparent reduced absorption of gemfibrozil when given with colestipol. J Clin Pharmacol, 30:29, 1990

Give at least 2 hours apart

HMG-CoA reductase inhibitors
Decreased pravastatin effect (decreased absorption)
> Manufacturer's package insert

Give 1 hour before colestipol; may occur with other statins

Mycophenolate mofetil
Possible decreased mycophenolate effect (decreased absorption)
> Manufacturer's package insert

Monitor mycophenolate concentration

(continued)

COLESTIPOL, with: *(continued)*
  Nicotinic acid
   Possible decreased niacin effect (possible decreased absorption)
     Manufacturer's package insert *(Niaspan)*
   Based on in vitro study; separate doses by 4 to 6 hours, or as much as possible; cholestyramine may interact to lesser extent
  Nonsteroidal anti-inflammatory drugs
   Possible decreased diclofenac effect (decreased rate and extent of absorption)
     SR Al-Balla et al, The effects of cholestyramine and colestipol and the absorption of diclofenac in man. Int J Clin Pharmacol ther, 32:441, 1994
   Based on a study in healthy subjects; give diclofenac 2 hours before or 6 hours after colestipol
  Thiazide diuretics
   Decreased thiazide effect (decreased absorption)
     RE Kauffman and DL Azarnoff, Effect of colestipol on gastrointestinal absorption of chlorothiazide in man. Clin Pharmacol Ther, 14:886, 1973
   Give drugs as far apart as possible
  Ursodiol
   Possible decreased ursodiol effect (decreased absorption)
     Manufacturer's package insert
   Give at least 2 hours apart
Colistimethate, see Polymyxins
COLONY STIMULATING FACTORS, with:
  Bleomycin - See Bleomycin with Colony Stimulating Factors, page 166
CONTRACEPTIVES, IMPLANT, with:
  Barbiturates - See Barbiturates with Contraceptives, implant, page 132
  Phenytoin
   Decreased contraceptive effect (probably increased metabolism)
     V Odlind and S-E Olsson, Enhanced metabolism of levonorgestrel during phenytoin treatment in a woman with Norplant implants. Contraception, 33:257, 1986; M Haukkamaa, Contraception by Norplant subdermal capsules is not reliable in epileptic patients on anticonvulsant treatment. Contraception, 33:559, 1986
   Use alternative contraceptive
CONTRACEPTIVES, ORAL, with:
  Acetaminophen - See Acetaminophen with Contraceptives, oral, page 8
  Alcohol - See Alcohol with Contraceptives, oral, page 16
  Anticoagulants, oral - See Anticoagulants, oral with Contraceptives, oral, page 64
  Antidepressants, tricyclic - See Antidepressants, tricyclic with Contraceptives, oral, page 84
  Antifungals, Griseofulvin - See Antifungals, Griseofulvin with Contraceptives, oral, page 95
  Antifungals, imidazoles and triazoles - See Antifungals, imidazoles and triazoles with Contraceptives, oral, page 98
  Barbiturates - See Barbiturates with Contraceptives, oral, page 132
  Benzodiazepines - See Benzodiazepines with Contraceptives, oral, page 140

CONTRACEPTIVES, ORAL, with: *(continued)*

Beta-adrenergic blockers - See Beta-adrenergic blockers with Contraceptives, oral, page 153

Caffeine - See Caffeine with Contraceptives, oral, page 173

Carbamazepine - See Carbamazepine with Contraceptives, oral, page 177

Cephalosporins - See Cephalosporins with Contraceptives, oral, page 190

Clofibrate - See Clofibrate with Contraceptives, oral, page 203

Corticosteroids

Possible corticosteroid toxicity with prednisolone (probably decreased metabolism)

> UF Legler and LZ Benet, Marked alterations in dose-dependent prednisolone kinetics in women taking oral contraceptives. Clin Pharmacol Ther, 39:425, 1986; UF Legler, Lack of impairment of fluocortolone disposition in oral contraceptive users. Eur J Clin Pharmacol, 35:101, 1988; J Seidegård et al, Effect of an oral contraceptive on the plasma levels of budesonide and prednisolone and the influence on plasma cortisol. Clin Pharmacol Ther, 67:373, 2000

Clinical significance not established; budesonide and fluocortolone may be less likely to interact

Cyclosporine

Hepatotoxicity (mechanism not established)

> G Deray et al, Oral contraceptive interaction with cyclosporin. Lancet, 1:158, 1987

Single case report (1987)

Efavirenz

Possible decreased contraceptive effect (mechanism not established)

> Manufacturer's package insert (efavirenz); AS Joshi et al, Lack of a pharmacokinetic interaction between efavirenz (DMP266) and ethinyl estradiol in healthy female volunteers. Conf Retrovir Opportun Infect, 5:144, 1998, abstract 348

In one study in healthy volunteers there was no effect on estrogen concentrations

Ethosuximide

Decreased contraceptive effect (mechanism not established)

> DJ Back et al, Evaluation of Committee on Safety of Medicines yellow card reports on oral contraceptive-drug interactions with anticonvulsants and antibiotics. Br J Clin Pharmacol, 25:527, 1988

Four case reports; use alternative contraceptive

Felbamate

Possible decreased oral contraceptive effect (possible increased estrogen metabolism)

> V Saano et al, Effects of felbamate on the pharmacokinetics of a low-dose combination oral contraceptive. Clin Pharmacol Ther, 58:523, 1995

Effect greater on gestodene than ethinyl estradiol; use alternate contraceptive method

(continued)

CONTRACEPTIVES, ORAL, with: *(continued)*

Guanethidine

Decreased guanethidine effect (mechanism not established)

TM Clezy, Oral contraceptives and hypertension: the effect of guanethidine. Med J Aust, 1:638, 1970

Avoid concurrent use

Hypoglycemics, sulfonylurea

Possible decreased hypoglycemic effect (mechanism not established)

WN Spellacy, A review of carbohydrate metabolism and the oral contraceptives. Am J Obstet Gynecol, 104:448, 1969

Monitor blood glucose

Lopinavir/Ritonavir

Possible decreased contraceptive effect (mechanism not established)

Manufacturer's package insert (*Kaletra*)

Use alternative contraceptive

Macrolide antibiotics

Possible decreased contraceptive effect with erythromycin (mechanism not established)

DJ Back et al, Evaluation of Committee on Safety of Medicines yellow card reports on oral contraceptive-drug interactions with anticonvulsants and antibiotics. Br J Clin Pharmacol, 25:527, 1988;

Singe case report (1988); theoretically, erythromycin and clarithromycin would inhibit the CYP3A4 metabolism of estrogens, thus decreasing the likelihood of reduced contraceptive effect

Possible decreased contraceptive effect with dirithromycin (mechanism not established)

VS Watkins et al, Drug interactions of macrolides: emphasis on dirithromycin. Ann Pharmacother, 31:349, 1997

Based on study in healthy women; consider adding alternative contraceptive

Methyldopa

Decreased antihypertensive effect (mechanism not established)

TM Clezy, Oral contraceptives and hypertension: the effect of guanethidine. Med J Aust, 1:638, 1970

Avoid concurrent use

Metronidazole

Decreased contraceptive effect (mechanism not established)

DJ Back et al, Evaluation of Committee on Safety of Medicines yellow card reports on oral contraceptive-drug interactions with anticonvulsants and antibiotics. Br J Clin Pharmacol, 25:527, 1988

Three case reports

Monoamine oxidase inhibitors

Possible selegiline toxicity (probably decreased metabolism)

K Laine et al, Dose linearity study of selegiline pharmacokinetics after oral administration: evidence for strong drug interaction with female sex steroids.

CONTRACEPTIVES, ORAL, with: *(continued)*
Marked increase in selegiline concentrations; based on study in healthy women; avoid concurrent use

Narcotics: morphine-like

Possible decreased morphine effect (increased metabolism)
> KJR Watson et al, The oral contraceptive pill increases morphine clearance but does not increase hepatic blood flow. Gastroenterology, 90:1779, 1986

Monitor clinical status; based on study in healthy women

Nelfinavir

Possible decreased contraceptive effect (increased metabolism; CYP3A)
> Manufacturer's package insert (nelfinavir)

Use alternate contraceptive method

Nevirapine

Possible decreased contraceptive effect (increased metabolism; CYP3A)
> Manufacturer's package insert (nevirapine)

Theoretical; use alternate contraceptive method

Oxcarbazepine

Decreased contraceptive effect (increased metabolism; CYP3A)
> C Fattore et al, Induction of ethinylestradiol and levonorgestrel metabolism by oxcarbazepine in healthy women. Epilepsia, 40:783, 1999; PK Jensen et al, Possible interaction between oxcarbazepine and an oral contraceptive. Epilepsia, 33:1149, 1992; K Wilbur and MHH Ensom, Pharmacokinetic drug interactions between oral contraceptives and second-generation anticonvulsants. Clin Pharmacokinet, 38:355, 2000

In one study breakthrough bleeding was reported; use alternative or additional contraceptive method

Penicillamine

Macromastia and gingival hyperplasia (mechanism not established)
> BI Rose et al, Macromastia in a woman treated with penicillamine and oral contraceptives; a case report. J Reprod Med, 35:43, 1990

Single case report (1990)

Penicillins

Decreased contraceptive effect with ampicillin, oxacillin, or penicillin V (probably decreased enterohepatic circulation of estrogen)
> DJ Back et al, The effects of ampicillin on oral contraceptive steroids in women. Br J Clin Pharmacol, 14:43, 1982; TJ Silber, Apparent oral contraceptive failure associated with antibiotic administration. J Adolesc Health Care, 4:287, 1983; SK Vong and THHG Koh, Contraceptive failure caused by antibiotics. Br J Pharmaceutical Pract, 11:248, 1989; DJ Back et al, Evaluation of Committee on Safety of Medicines yellow card reports on oral contraceptive-drug interactions with anticonvulsants and antibiotics. Br J Clin Pharmacol, 25:527, 1988; E Weisberg, Interactions between oral contraceptives and antifungals/antibacterials: is contraceptive failure the result? Clin Pharmacokinet, 36:309, 1999; KE Burroughs and ML Chambliss, Antibiotics and oral contraceptive failure. Arch Fam Med, 9:81: 2000

(continued)

CONTRACEPTIVES, ORAL, with: *(continued)*
Low (probably <1%) but unpredictable incidence; consider adding other contraceptive methods (i.e. barrier) or abstinence during the course of antibiotic therapy

Phenytoin
Decreased contraceptive effect (increased metabolism)
   CB Coulam and JF Annegers, Do anticonvulsants reduce the efficacy of oral contraceptives? Epilepsia, 20:519, 1979; DJ Back et al, Evaluation of Committee on Safety of Medicines yellow card reports on oral contraceptive-drug interactions with anticonvulsants and antibiotics. Br J Clin Pharmacol, 25:527, 1988; P Crawford et al, The interaction of phenytoin and carbamazepine with combined oral contraceptive steroids. Br J Clin Pharmacol, 30:892, 1990; MA Eldon et al, Gabapentin does not interact with a contraceptive regimen of norethindrone acetate and ethinyl estradiol. Neurology, 50:1146, 1998

Use alternative contraceptive; gabapentin does not appear to interact with an oral contraceptive containing norethindrone and ethinyl estradiol

Possible phenytoin toxicity (possibly decreased metabolism)
   EA DeLeacy et al, Effects of subject's sex, and intake of tobacco, alcohol, and oral contraceptives on plasma phenytoin levels. Br J Clin Pharmacol, 8:33, 1979

Monitor phenytoin concentration

Primidone
Decreased contraceptive effect (increased metabolism)
   CB Coulam and JF Annegers, Do anticonvulsants reduce the efficacy of oral contraceptives? Epilepsia, 20:519, 1979; DJ Back et al, Evaluation of Committee on Safety of Medicines yellow card reports on oral contraceptive-drug interactions with anticonvulsants and antibiotics. Br J Clin Pharmacol, 25:527, 1988

Use alternative contraceptive

Rifabutin
Possible decreased contraceptive effect (increased metabolism)
   M LeBel et al, Effects of rifabutin and rifampicin on the pharmacokinetics of ethinylestradiol and norethindrone. J Clin Pharmacol, 38:1042, 1998; P Barditch-Crovo et al, The effects of rifampin and rifabutin on the pharmacokinetics and pharmacodynamics of a combination oral contraceptive. Clin Pharmacol Ther, 65:428, 1999

Reduced serum concentrations of both ethinyl estradiol and norethindrone in healthy women; use alternative contraceptive

Rifampin
Decreased contraceptive effect (increased metabolism)
   Editor, Rifampicin, "pill" do not go well together. JAMA, 227:608, 1974; DJ Back et al, The effect of rifampicin on norethisterone pharmacokinetics. Eur J Clin Pharmacol, 15:193, 1979; JL Skolnick et al, Rifampin, oral contraceptives, and pregnancy. JAMA, 236:1382, 1976; M LeBel et al, Effects of rifabutin and rifampicin on the pharmacokinetics of ethinylestradiol and

CONTRACEPTIVES, ORAL, with: *(continued)*

norethindrone. J Clin Pharmacol, 38:1042, 1998; E Weisberg, Interactions between oral contraceptives and antifungals/antibacterials: is contraceptive failure the result? Clin Pharmacokinet, 36:309, 1999; From the Clinical Effectiveness Committee, Use of rifampicin and contraceptive steroids. Br J Fam Plann, 24:169, 1999; P Barditch-Crovo et al, The effects of rifampin and rifabutin on the pharmacokinetics and pharmacodynamics of a combination oral contraceptive. Clin Pharmacol Ther, 65:428, 1999

Use alternative contraceptive; reduced serum concentrations of both ethinyl estradiol and norethindrone in healthy women; rifampicin appears to have a greater inducing effect than rifabutin

Ritonavir

Possible decreased contraceptive effect of ethinyl estradiol (probably increased metabolism)

Manufacturer's package insert (ritonavir); D Ouellet et al, Effect of ritonavir on the pharmacokinetics of ethinyl oestradiol in healthy female volunteers. Br J Clin Pharmacol, 46:111, 1998

Use alternative contraceptive

Saint John's wort

Possible increased risk of pregnancy (probably enzyme induction [CYP3A4], and transport CP-glycoprotein)

Q-Y Yue et al, Safety of St John's wort. Lancet, 355:576, 2000; RI Shader and DJ Greenblatt, More on oral contraceptives, drug interactions, herbal medicines, and hormone replacement therapy. J Clin Psychopharmacol, 20:397, 2000

Based on several case reports of menstrual irregularities (2000); causal relationship not established; avoid concurrent use or add additional contraception

Tetracyclines

Decreased contraceptive effect (mechanism not established)

JF Bacon and GM Shenfield, Pregnancy attributable to interaction between tetracycline and oral contraceptives. Br Med J, 280:293, 1980; JL Neely et al, The effect of doxycycline on serum levels of ethinyl estradiol, norethindrone, and endogenous progesterone. Obstet Gynecol, 77:416, 1991; AA Murphy et al, The effect of tetracycline on levels of oral contraceptives. Am J Obstet Gynecol, 164:28, 1991; DJ Back et al, Evaluation of Committee on Safety of Medicines yellow card reports on oral contraceptive-drug interactions with anticonvulsants and antibiotics. Br J Clin Pharmacol, 25:527, 1988

Use alternative contraceptive; one study in 7 women reports no change in contraceptive steroid concentrations after 24 hours or 5-10 days of 500 mg q6h of tetracycline

Theophyllines

Possible theophylline toxicity (decreased metabolism)

KM Tornatore et al, Effect of chronic oral contraceptive steroids on theophylline disposition. Eur J Clin Pharmacol, 23:129, 1982; RK Roberts et al, Oral contraceptive steroids impair the elimination of theophylline. J Lab Clin Med, 101:821, 1983; MJ Gardner et al, Effects of tobacco smoking and

CONTRACEPTIVES, ORAL, with: *(continued)*

oral contraceptive use on theophylline disposition. Br J Clin Pharmacol, 16:271, 1983

Monitor theophylline concentration; opposing effects of contraceptives and smoking, which increases metabolism, tend to offset each other

Tizanidine

Tizanidine toxicity (probably decreased metabolism)

Manufacturer's package insert

Start with reduced doses of tizanidine; monitor clinical status

Topiramate

Possible decreased contraceptive effect (mechanism not established)

Manufacturer's package insert (topiramate)

Use alternate contraceptive

Trimethoprim

Decreased contraceptive effect (mechanism not established)

DJ Back et al, Evaluation of Committee on Safety of Medicines yellow card reports on oral contraceptive-drug interactions with anticonvulsants and antibiotics. Br J Clin Pharmacol, 25:527, 1988

Two case reports (1988); use alternative contraceptive

Trimethoprim-sulfamethoxazole

Decreased contraceptive effect (mechanism not established)

DJ Back et al, Evaluation of Committee on Safety of Medicines yellow card reports on oral contraceptive-drug interactions with anticonvulsants and antibiotics. Br J Clin Pharmacol, 25:527, 1988

Five case reports; use alternative contraceptive; also reported with trimethoprim alone

Troglitazone

Possible decreased contraceptive effect (increased metabolism of both estrogen and progestin; probably CYP3A4)

Manufacturer's package insert (troglitazone); C-M Loi et al, Effect of troglitazone on the pharmacokinetics of an oral contraceptive agent. J Clin Pharmacol, 39:410, 1999

Use alternate contraceptive; troglitazone is no longer available

Troleandomycin

Jaundice (additive)

J-P Miguet et al, Jaundice from troleandomycin and oral contraceptives. Ann Intern Med, 92:434, 1980

Avoid concurrent use

Vitamin C

Increased serum concentration and possible adverse effects of estrogens with 1 gram/day of vitamin C (decreased metabolism)

DJ Back et al, Interaction of ethinyloestradiol with ascorbic acid in man. Br Med J, 282:1516, 1981; MH Briggs, Megadose vitamin C and metabolic effects of the pill. Br Med J, 283:1547, 1981; JC Morris et al, Interaction of ethinyloestradiol with ascorbic acid in man. Br Med J, 283:503, 1981

Decrease vitamin C to 100 mg/day

CONTRAST MEDIA, with:
  Amiodarone - See Amiodarone with Contrast media, page 34
  Beta-adrenergic blockers - See Beta-adrenergic blockers with Contrast media, page 153
  Interleukin-2
    "Recall" of rIL-2 toxicity after intravenous injection of iohexol or diatrizoate or other ionic contrast media (mechanism not established)
      AS Abi-Aad et al, Metastatic renal cell cancer: interleukin-2 toxicity induced by contrast agent injection. J Immunother, 10:292, 1991; AA Zukiwski et al, Increased incidence of hypersensitivity to iodine-containing radiographic contrast media after interleukin-2 administration. Cancer, 65:1521, 1990; RK Oldham et al, Contrast medium "recalls" interleukin-2 toxicity. J Clin Oncol, 8:942, 1990
    Patients who have had reactions following rIL-2 have renewed symptoms; antihistamines and steroids have been suggested for prophylaxis, but there are no reports of effectiveness
  Metformin
    Lactic acidosis (decreased renal function)
      Manufacturer's package insert; CL Kay and NS Curry, Intravascular injection of iodinated contrast media. Clinical Radiol, 52:403, 1997; MJ Duddy, Metformin and contrast: the risk. Clin Radio, 53:310, 1998; P Rasuli and I Hammond, Metformin and contrast media: where is the conflict? Can Assoc Radiol J, 49:161, 1998; MM McCartney et al, Metformin and contrast media — a dangerous combination? Clin Radiol, 54:29, 1999
    Manufacturer recommends discontinuing metformin for 48 hours after contrast media and resuming when renal function is restored; lactic acidosis is unlikely if patient has normal renal function

CORTICOSTEROIDS, with:
  Alkylating agents - See Alkylating agents with Corticosteroids, page 23
  Aminoglutethimide - See Aminoglutethimide with Corticosteroids, page 29
  Antacids - See Antacids with Corticosteroids, page 51
  Anticoagulants, oral - See Anticoagulants, oral with Corticosteroids, page 64
  Antifungals, imidazoles and triazoles - See Antifungals, imidazoles and triazoles with Corticosteroids, page 99
  Barbiturates - See Barbiturates with Corticosteroids, page 133
  Benzodiazepines - See Benzodiazepines with Corticosteroids, page 141
  Bupropion - See Bupropion with Corticosteroids, page 169
  Carbamazepine - See Carbamazepine with Corticosteroids, page 177
  Cholestyramine - See Cholestyramine with Corticosteroids, page 195
  Contraceptives, oral - See Contraceptives, oral with Corticosteroids, page 213
  Cyclosporine
    Toxicity of low doses of corticosteroids (decreased metabolism)
      E Langhoff et al, Inhibition of prednisolone metabolism by cyclosporine in kidney-transplanted patients. Transplantation, 39:107, 1985; S Durrant et al, Cyclosporin A, methylprednisolone, and convulsions. Lancet, 2:829, 1982; L Öst, Impairment of prednisolone metabolism by cyclosporine treatment in renal graft recipients. Transplantation, 44:533, 1987

(continued)

CORTICOSTEROIDS, with: *(continued)*
> *Monitor corticosteroid effect or concentration*

Possible cyclosporine toxicity with high doses of corticosteroids (possibly decreased metabolism)
> G Klintmalm and J Sawe, High dose methylprednisolone increases plasma cyclosporin levels in renal transplant recipients. Lancet, 1:731, 1984; CS Ubhi et al, Interaction of intravenous methylprednisolone with oral cyclosporin. Nephrol Dial Transplant, 5:376, 1990; Y Hatta et al, Microangiopathic hemolytic anemia in a graft-versus-host disease patient treated with cyclosporine A and prednisolone. Intern Med, 31:434, 1992

Monitor cyclosporine concentration; clinically significant elevations appear to occur only rarely; single case of microangiopathic hemolytic anemia in graft vs host disease (1992)

Diltiazem
Possible methylprednisolone toxicity (probably decreased metabolism [CYP3A4] and inhibition of P-glycoprotein)
> T Varis et al, Diltiazem and mibefradil increase the plasma concentrations and greatly enhance the adrenal-suppressant effect of oral methylprednisolone. Clin Pharmacol Ther, 67:215, 2000

Based on study in healthy subjects; monitor clinical status; greater potential for suppression of adrenal function

Estrogens
Possible corticosteroid toxicity (mechanism not established)
> UF Legler and LZ Benet, Marked alterations in dose-dependent prednisolone kinetics in women taking oral contraceptives. Clin Pharmacol Ther, 39:425, 1986; LE Gustavson et al, Impairment of prednisolone disposition in women taking oral contraceptives or conjugated estrogens. J Clin Endocrinol Metab, 62:234, 1986; UF Legler, Lack of impairment of fluocortolone disposition in oral contraceptive users. Eur J Clin Pharmacol, 35:101, 1988

Clinical significance not established

Ethacrynic acid
Increased potassium loss and risk of gastric hemorrhage (additive)
> Manufacturer's package insert; H Jick and J Porter, Drug-induced gastrointestinal bleeding. Lancet, 2:87, 1978; M Weintraub, Recording events in clinical trials. Br Med J, 1:581, 1978

Avoid concurrent use

Furosemide
Increased potassium loss (additive)
> GW Thorn, Clinical considerations in the use of corticosteroids. N Engl J Med, 274:775, 1966

Monitor potassium concentration

Macrolide antibiotics
Possible toxicity of methylprednisolone with erythromycin or clarithromycin (decreased excretion)
> CF LaForce et al, Inhibition of methylprednisolone elimination in the presence of erythromycin therapy. J Allergy Clin Immunol, 72:34, 1983; DA Fost

CORTICOSTEROIDS, with: *(continued)*
> et al, Inhibition of methylprednisolone elimination in the presence of clarithromycin therapy. J Allergy Clin Immunol, 103:1031, 1999

Does not occur with prednisone or prednisolone

Methotrexate
> Disseminated herpes zoster (mechanism not established)
>> DJ Anderson and EN Janoff, Herpes zoster infection in a patient on methotrexate given prednisone to prevent post-herpetic neuralgia. Ann Intern Med, 107:783, 1987
>
> *Single case report (1987)*
>
> Possible methotrexate toxicity (mechanism not established)
>> P Lafforgue et al, Is there an interaction between low doses of corticosteroids and methotrexate in patients with rheumatoid arthritis? J Rheumatol, 20:263, 1993
>
> *Based on a study in patients with rheumatoid arthritis; clinical significance not established*
>
> Possible increased risk of bladder carcinoma (mechanism not established)
>> RJ Millard and S McCredie, Bladder cancer in patients on low-dose methotrexate and corticosteroids. Lancet, 343:1222, 1994
>
> *Based on two case reports (1994)*
>
> Hepatotoxicity (mechanism not established)
>> JEA Wolff et al, Dexamethasone increases hepatotoxicity of MTX in children with brain tumors. Anticancer Res, 18:2895, 1998
>
> *Based on study in children with brain tumors; dexamethasone is not necessary to prevent cerebral edema during methotrexate treatment*

Metronidazole
> Decreased metronidazole effect (increased metabolism)
>> O Eradiri et al, Interaction of metronidazole with phenobarbital, cimetidine, prednisone, and sulfasalazine in Crohn's disease. Biopharm Drug Dispos, 9:219, 1988
>
> *Monitor metronidazole concentration*

Montelukast
> Possible increased risk of edema (mechanism not established)
>> M Geller, Marked peripheral edema associated with montelukast and prednisone. Ann Intern Med, 132:924, 2000
>
> *Single case report (2000); causal relationship not established; monitor clinical status*

Neuromuscular blocking agents
> Decreased pancuronium or vecuronium effect (mechanism not established)
>> MJ Laflin, Interaction of pancuronium and corticosteroids. Anesthesiology, 47:471, 1977; EF Meyers, Partial recovery from pancuronium neuromuscular blockade following hydrocortisone administration. Anesthesiology, 46:148, 1979; AE Schwartz et al, Acute steroid therapy does not alter nondepolarizing muscle relaxant effects in humans. Anesthesiology, 65:326, 1986; SM Parr et al, Betamethasone-induced resistance to vecuronium: a potential problem in neurosurgery? Anaesth

CORTICOSTEROIDS, with: *(continued)*
>> Intensive Care, 19:103, 1991
> *Monitor clinical status*

> Myopathy with pancuronium or vecuronium and chronic corticosteroids (mechanism not established)
>> JL Vasquez et al, Myopathie aiguë compliquant une curarisation et une corticothérapie prolongées pour état de mal asthmatique. Presse Med, 21:1433, 1992; JL Gooch, AAEM case report #29: prolonged paralysis after neuromuscular blockade. Muscle Nerve, 18:937, 1995; JR Fischer and RK Baer, Acute myopathy associated with combined use of corticosteroids and neuromuscular blocking agents. Ann Pharmacother, 30:1437, 1996
> *Numerous case reports; avoid concurrent use if possible*

Nonsteroidal anti-inflammatory drugs
> Decreased salicylate effect (mechanism not established)
>> JR Klinenberg and F Miller, Effect of corticosteroids on blood salicylate concentration. JAMA, 194:601, 1965; GG Graham et al, Patterns of plasma concentrations and urinary excretion of salicylate in rheumatoid arthritis. Clin Pharmacol Ther, 22:410, 1977; J Edelman et al, The effect of intra-articular steroids on plasma salicylate concentrations. Br J Clin Pharmacol, 21:301, 1986
> *Monitor salicylate concentration; also occurs with intra-articular steroids*

Omeprazole
> Decreased prednisone effect (mechanism not established)
>> P Joly et al, Possible interaction prednisone-oméprazole dans la pemphigoïde bulleuse. Gastroenterol Clin Biol, 14:682, 1990; O Chosidow et al, Pemphigoïde bulleuse secondairement corticorésistante; rôle inhibiteur de l'oméprazole sur le métabolisme des corticoïdes? Ann Dermatol Venereol, 118:45, 1991
> *Monitor clinical status; well documented report of a single case (1990)*

Paclitaxel
> Possible increased risk of skin necrosis with fluorometholone (mechanism not established)
>> A Aboolian et al, Skin necrosis in the presence of paclitaxel and fluorometholone. Support Care Cancer, 7:158, 1999
> *Single case report with fluorometholone eye drops (1999)*

Phenytoin
> Decreased corticosteroid effect (increased metabolism)
>> FM Vincent, Phenytoin/dexamethasone interaction. Lancet, 1:1360, 1978; EE Werk, Jr et al, Interference in the effect of dexamethasone by diphenylhydantoin. N Engl J Med, 281:32, 1969; J McLelland and W Jack, Phenytoin/dexamethasone interaction: a clinical problem. Lancet, 2:1096, 1978; SJ Wassner et al, Allograft survival in patients receiving anticonvulsant medications. Clin Nephrol, 8:293, 1977; U Keilholz and GP Guthrie, Jr, Case report: adverse effect of phenytoin on mineralocorticoid replacement with fludrocortisone in adrenal insufficiency. Am J Med Sci, 291:280, 1986; M Bartoszek et al, Prednisolone and methylprednisolone kinetics in

CORTICOSTEROIDS, with: *(continued)*
>children receiving anticonvulsant therapy. Clin Pharmacol Ther, 42:424, 1987

Monitor corticosteroid effect or concentration; increased corticosteroid dosage may be necessary both for therapy and in a suppression test

Possible toxicity of parenteral phenytoin with IV dexamethasone (possibly decreased metabolism)
>LA Lawson et al, Phenytoin-dexamethasone interaction: a previously unreported observation. Surg Neurol, 16:23, 1981; DD Wong et al, Phenytoin-dexamethasone: a possible drug-drug interaction. JAMA, 254:2062, 1985

Monitor phenytoin concentration

Decreased phenytoin effect (increased metabolism)
>PF Jarosinski et al, Altered phenytoin clearance during intensive chemotherapy for acute lymphoblastic leukemia. J Pediatr, 112:996, 1988; TE Lackner, Interaction of dexamethasone with phenytoin. Pharmacotherapy, 11:344, 1991

Two well-studied cases (1988,1991); monitor phenytoin concentration

Possible increased risk of phenytoin hypersensitivity syndrome with dexamethasone (mechanism not established)
>U Tröger et al, A very early onset of respiratory failure due to phenytoin-associated hypersensitivity syndrome and concomitant glucocorticoid administration. Intensive Care Med 2000; 26:258

Single case report (2000); causal relationship not established; monitor clinical status

Praziquantel
>Decreased praziquantel effect with dexamethasone (mechanism not established)
>>ML Vazquez et al, Plasma levels of praziquantel decrease when dexamethasone is given simultaneously. Neurology, 37:1561, 1987
>
>*Based on study of 8 patients with neurocysticercosis; avoid use of dexamethasone as preventive treatment of praziquantel adverse effects; may result in lower praziquantel levels*

Primidone
>Decreased corticosteroid effect (probably increased metabolism)
>>MC Young and IA Hughes, Loss of therapeutic control in congenital adrenal hyperplasia due to interaction between dexamethasone and primidone. Acta Paediatr Scand, 80:120, 1991; KW Hancock and MJ Levell, Primidone/dexamethasone interaction. Lancet, 2:97, 1978
>
>*In 2 patients with congenital adrenal hyperplasia (1978,1991)*

Rifampin
>Marked decrease in corticosteroid effect (increased metabolism)
>>KH Lee et al, Time course of the changes in prednisolone pharmacokinetics after co-administration or discontinuation of rifampin. Eur J Clin Pharmacol, 45:287, 1993; F Carrie et al, Rifampin-induced nonresponsiveness of giant cell arteritis to prednisone treatment. Arch Intern Med, 154:1521, 1994; EJ Schenkel, Severe exacerbation of asthma secondary to rifampin in

CORTICOSTEROIDS, with: *(continued)*
    a steroid-dependent asthmatic. J Allergy Clin Immunol, 95:314, 1995
Avoid concurrent use, if possible; if combination is used, substantial increase in corticosteroid dosage may be needed

Ritonavir

Possible adrenal suppression with nasal fluticasone (decreased metabolism)
    F Chen et al, Severe adrenal suppression in a patient treated with ritonavir and nasal fluticasone. AIDS, 12:S56, 1998; ME Hillebrand-Haverkort et al, Ritonavir-induced Cushing's syndrome in a patient treated with nasal fluticasone. AIDS, 13:1803, 1999

Two case reports (1998, 1999)

Sympathomimetic amines

Decreased dexamethasone effect with ephedrine (mechanism not established)
    SM Brooks et al, The effects of ephedrine and theophylline on dexamethasone metabolism in bronchial asthma. J Clin Pharmacol, 17:308, 1977

Use another bronchodilator

Possible cardiopulmonary toxicity with ritodrine (mechanism not established)
    L Spatling et al, Effect of ritodrine and betamethasone on metabolism, respiration, and circulation. Am J Perinatol, 3:41, 1986; HR Elliott et al, Pulmonary oedema associated with ritodrine infusion and betamethasone administration in premature labor. Br Med J, 2:799, 1978

Avoid concurrent use, if possible

Sympathomimetic bronchodilators

Hypokalemia with prednisone and fenoterol or albuterol (probably additive)
    DR Taylor et al, Interaction between corticosteroid and β-agonist drugs; biochemical and cardiovascular effects in normal subjects. Chest, 102:519, 1992; DR Taylor and RJ Hancox, Interactions between corticosteroids and [beta] agonists. Thorax, 55:595, 2000

Based on study in healthy subjects; combination frequently used without undue adverse effects; monitor potassium concentration

Theophyllines

Theophylline toxicity (mechanism not established)
    DC Leavengood et al, The effect of corticosteroids on theophylline metabolism. Ann Allergy, 50:249, 1983; N Buchanan et al, Asthma a possible interaction between hydrocortisone and theophylline. S Afr Med J, 56:1147, 1979; EN Squire, Jr and HS Nelson, Corticosteroids and theophylline clearance. N Engl Regional Allergy Proc, 8:113, 1987; RJ Fergusson et al, Effect of prednisolone on theophylline pharmacokinetics in patients with chronic airflow obstruction. Thorax, 42:195, 1987

Conflicting reports; monitor theophylline concentration

Thiazide diuretics

Increased potassium loss (additive)
    GW Thorn, Clinical considerations in the use of corticosteroids. N Engl J Med, 274:775, 1966

Monitor potassium concentration

CORTICOSTEROIDS, with: *(continued)*
Troleandomycin
Methylprednisolone toxicity (decreased metabolism)
> SJ Szefler et al, Dose- and time-related effect of troleandomycin on methylprednisolone elimination. Clin Pharmacol Ther, 32:166, 1982; R Lantner et al, Fatal varicella in a corticosteroid-dependent asthmatic receiving troleandomycin. Allergy Proc, 11:83, 1990

Avoid concurrent use

Vitamin D
Lack of vitamin D effect (mechanism not established)
> P Vardi et al, Hypocalcaemia induced by glucocorticoids in a child with hypoparathyroidism treated with 1-a-hydroxyvitamin D_3. Eur J Pediatr, 144:280, 1985

Report in a child with hypoparathyroidism; parathyroid replacement may be necessary; dihydrotachysterol might be tried

CORTICOTROPIN, with:
Valproate
Marked hyfibrinogenemia
> K Tokuda et al, Three cases of hypofibrinogenemia induced by chemotherapy with a combination of synthetic ACTH and valproic acid. No to Hattatsu, 26:50, 1994

Report of 3 epileptic children given synthetic corticotropin and valproate (1994)

COX-2 INHIBITORS, with:
Angiotensin-converting enzyme (ACE) inhibitors - See Angiotensin-converting enzyme (ACE) inhibitors with COX-2 inhibitors, page 43

Antacids - See Antacids with COX-2 inhibitors, page 52

Anticoagulants, oral - See Anticoagulants, oral with COX-2 inhibitors, page 64

Antifungals, imidazoles and triazoles - See Antifungals, imidazoles and triazoles with COX-2 inhibitors, page 99

Furosemide
Decreased diuretic and antihypertensive effect (inhibition of renal prostaglandin synthesis)
> Manufacturer's package insert

Monitor blood pressure and diuretic effect

Lithium
Lithium toxicity (decreased renal excretion)
> Manufacturer's package inserts (celecoxib and rofecoxib)

Monitor lithium concentration

Methotrexate
Methotrexate toxicity (decreased renal excretion)
> Manufacturer's package insert (rofecoxib)

Monitor methotrexate toxicity

Nonsteroidal anti-inflammatory drugs
Increased gastric toxicity (additive)
> Manufacturer's package insert

(continued)

COX-2 INHIBITORS, with: *(continued)*

In endoscopic studies more patients taking both aspirin and COX-2 inhibitors developed ulcers; monitor clinical status; avoid concurrent use of multiple NSAIDs

Rifampin

Decreased rofecoxib effect (increased metabolism)

Manufacturer's package insert (rofecoxib)

Manufacturer recommends beginning rofecoxib treatment of osteoarthritis with 25 mg when co-administered with rifampin

Thiazide diuretics

Decreased diuretic and antihypertensive effect (inhibition of renal prostaglandin synthesis)

Manufacturer's package insert

Monitor blood pressure and diuretic effect

Cromolyn sodium, no documented interactions, see page 4, Criteria for Listing Interactions

Cyanocobalamin, no documented interactions, see page 4, Criteria for Listing Interactions

CYCLOBENZAPRINE, with:

Alcohol - See Alcohol with Cyclobenzaprine, page 17

Droperidol

Torsade de pointes (possible additive QT interval prolongation)

EL Michalets et al, Torsade de pointes resulting from the addition of droperidol to an existing cytochrome P450 drug interaction. Ann Pharmacother, 32:761, 1998

Single case report (1998); patient also receiving fluoxetine; causal relationship not established

Selective serotonin reuptake inhibitors (SSRIs)

Torsade de pointes with fluoxetine (possible decreased cyclobenzaprine metabolism)

EL Michalets et al, Torsade de pointes resulting from the addition of droperidol to an existing cytochrome P450 drug interaction. Ann Pharmacother, 32:761, 1998

Single case report (1998); patient also receiving droperidol; causal relationship not established

Cyclophosphamide, see Alkylating agents

CYCLOPROPANE, with:

Angiotensin-converting enzyme (ACE) inhibitors - See Angiotensin-converting enzyme (ACE) inhibitors with Cyclopropane, page 44

Beta-adrenergic blockers - See Beta-adrenergic blockers with Cyclopropane, page 153

Reserpine

Probable hypotension (additive)

CS Coakley et al, Circulatory responses during anesthesia of patients on rauwolfia therapy. JAMA, 161:1143, 1958; RL Katz et al, Anesthesia, surgery and rauwolfia. Anesthesiology, 25:142, 1964

CYCLOPROPANE, with: *(continued)*
   Monitor blood pressure
  Spironolactone
    Hypotension (additive)
      Manufacturer's package insert
   Monitor blood pressure
  Sympathomimetic amines
    Cardiac arrhythmias (mechanism not established)
      RS Matteo et al, The injection of epinephrine during general anesthesia with halogenated hydrocarbons and cyclopropane in man. Anesthesiology, 24:327, 1963
   Monitor cardiac rhythm

CYCLOSERINE, with:
  Alcohol - See Alcohol with Cycloserine, page 17
  Isoniazid
    CNS effects, dizziness, drowsiness (mechanism not established)
      MJ Mattila et al, Serum levels, urinary excretion, and side-effects of cycloserine in the presence of isoniazid and p-aminosalicylic acid. Scand J Respir Dis, 50:291, 1969; VMK Venho and R Koskinen, The effect of pyrazinamide, rifampicin and cycloserine on the blood levels and urinary excretion of isoniazid. Ann Clin Res, 3:277, 1971
   Monitor frequently and warn about impaired driving ability

CYCLOSPORINE, with:
  Alcohol - See Alcohol with Cyclosporine, page 17
  Alkylating agents - See Alkylating agents with Cyclosporine, page 23
  Allopurinol - See Allopurinol with Cyclosporine, page 25
  Aminoglycoside antibiotics - See Aminoglycoside antibiotics with Cyclosporine, page 30
  Amiodarone - See Amiodarone with Cyclosporine, page 34
  Amlodipine - See Amlodipine with Cyclosporine, page 37
  Anabolic and androgenic steroids - See Anabolic and androgenic steroids with Cyclosporine, page 41
  Angiotensin-converting enzyme (ACE) inhibitors - See Angiotensin-converting enzyme (ACE) inhibitors with Cyclosporine, page 44
  Antacids - See Antacids with Cyclosporine, page 52
  Anticoagulants, oral - See Anticoagulants, oral with Cyclosporine, page 64
  Antifungals, Amphotericin B - See Antifungals, Amphotericin B with Cyclosporine, page 94
  Antifungals, Griseofulvin - See Antifungals, Griseofulvin with Cyclosporine, page 95
  Antifungals, imidazoles and triazoles - See Antifungals, imidazoles and triazoles with Cyclosporine, page 99
  Antifungals, terbinafine - See Antifungals, terbinafine with Cyclosporine, page 109
  Antihistamines, H$_2$-blockers - See Antihistamines, H$_2$-blockers with Cyclosporine, page 116

(continued)

CYCLOSPORINE, with: *(continued)*
  Barbiturates - See Barbiturates with Cyclosporine, page 133
  Beta-adrenergic blockers - See Beta-adrenergic blockers with Cyclosporine, page 153
  Carbamazepine - See Carbamazepine with Cyclosporine, page 178
  Carbonic anhydrase inhibitors - See Carbonic anhydrase inhibitors with Cyclosporine, page 188
  Cephalosporins - See Cephalosporins with Cyclosporine, page 190
  Chlorambucil - See Chlorambucil with Cyclosporine, page 192
  Chloramphenicol - See Chloramphenicol with Cyclosporine, page 192
  Chloroquine - See Chloroquine with Cyclosporine, page 194
  Clindamycin - See Clindamycin with Cyclosporine, page 202
  Colchicine - See Colchicine with Cyclosporine, page 210
  Contraceptives, oral - See Contraceptives, oral with Cyclosporine, page 213
  Corticosteroids - See Corticosteroids with Cyclosporine, page 219
  Digoxin
    Digoxin toxicity (decreased clearance); inhibition of transport (P-glycoprotein)
      P Dorian et al, Digoxin-cyclosporine interaction: severe digitalis toxicity after cyclosporine treatment. Clin Invest Med, 11:108, 1988; I Robieux et al, The effects of cardiac transplantation and cyclosporine therapy on digoxin pharmacokinetics. J Clin Pharmacol, 32:338, 1992
    Monitor digoxin concentration
  Diltiazem
    Cyclosporine toxicity (decreased metabolism; CYP3A4 inhibition of transport; p-glycoprotein)
      JM Pochet and Y Pirson, Cyclosporin – diltiazem interaction. Lancet, 1:979, 1986; JM Grino et al, Influence of diltiazem on cyclosporin clearance. Lancet, 1:1387, 1986; K Kohlhaw et al, Effect of the calcium channel blocker diltiazem on cyclosporine A blood levels and dose requirements. Transplant Proc, 20 suppl 2:572, 1988; K Wagner et al, Prevention of posttransplant acute tubular necrosis by the calcium antagonist diltiazem: a prospective randomized study. Am J Nephrol, 7:287, 1987; K Wagner et al, Interaction of cyclosporin and calcium antagonists. Transplant Proc, 21:1453, 1989; K Wagner et al, Interaction of calcium blockers and cyclosporine. Transplant Proc, 20 suppl 2:561, 1988; GR Bailie and G Eisele, Cyclosporine-associated arthralgia. Clin Nephrol, 33:256, 1990; RC Bourge et al, Diltiazem-cyclosporine interaction in cardiac transplant recipients: impact on cyclosporine dose and medication costs. Am J Med, 90:402, 1991; CE Cook, Nontherapeutic cyclosporine levels: sustained-release diltiazem products are not the same. Transplantation, 57:1687, 1994; IS Sketris et al, Effect of calcium-channel blockers on cyclosporine clearance and use in renal transplant patients. Ann Pharmacother, 28:1227, 1994; TE Jones et al, Formulation of diltiazem affects cyclosporin-sparing activity. Eur J Clin Pharmacol, 52:55, 1997; TE Jones et al, Diltiazem-cyclosporin pharmacokinetic interaction — dose-response relationship. Br J Clin Pharmacol, 44:499, 1997; AJ McLachlan and SE Tett, Effect of metabolic inhibitors on cyclosporine pharmacokinetics using a population approach. Ther Drug Monit, 20:390, 1998;

CYCLOSPORINE, with: *(continued)*

A Foradori et al, Modification of the pharmacokinetics of cyclosporine A and metabolites by the concomitant use of Neoral and diltiazem or ketoconazole in stable adult kidney transplants. Transplant Proc, 30:1685, 1998; JG Preuner et al, First-pass metabolism of cyclosporine A in human intestine: inhibition by diltiazem. Transplant Proc, 30:2545, 1998; TT Jiang et al, Cyclosporine-induced encephalopathy predisposed by diltiazem in a patient with aplastic anemia. Ann Pharmacother, 33:750, 1999; A Asberg et al, Pharmacokinetic interactions between microemulsion formulated cyclosporine A and diltiazem in renal transplant recipients. Eur J Clin Pharmacol, 55:383, 1999

Although there are 2 case reports of deterioration in renal function, there are reports of a series of more than 40 patients in whom diltiazem appeared to improve renal function despite increased cyclosporine concentrations; in a small controlled trial the incidence of rejection was similar with and without diltiazem; in one patient the interaction was associated with severe arthralgia (1990) and encephalopathy in another (1999); studies in cardiac and renal transplant patients indicate that the combination can be used safely with decreased cyclosporine dosage; effect can be seen with as little as 10 mg/day of diltiazem; sustained-release preparations of diltiazem may differ and the same preparation should always be prescribed; interaction occurs with both the microemulsion formulation and old formulation of cyclosporine

Disopyramide

Renal toxicity (mechanism not established)

G Nanni et al, Effect of disopyramide in a cyclosporine-treated patient. Transplantation, 45:257, 1988

Single case report (1988); cyclosporine concentration did not change

Doxorubicin

Doxorubicin toxicity (probable decreased metabolism)

SR Raber et al, Effects of cyclosporin on pharmacokinetics and pharmacodynamics of doxorubicin. Clin Pharmacol Ther, 55:189, 1994

Avoid concurrent use

Etoposide

Etoposide toxicity with high-dose cyclosporine (mechanism not established)

BL Lum et al, Alteration of etoposide pharmacokinetics and pharmacodynamics by cyclosporine in a phase I trial to modulate multidrug resistance. J Clin Oncol, 10:1635, 1992; G Bisogno et al, High-dose cyclosporin with etoposide—toxicity and pharmacokinetic interaction in children with solid tumours. Br J Cancer, 77:2304, 1998

Monitor clinical status and etoposide concentration

Felodipine

Possible felodipine toxicity (decreased metabolism)

JK Madsen et al, Pharmacokinetic interaction between cyclosporine and the dihydropyridine calcium antagonist felodipine. Eur J Clin Pharmacol, 50:203, 1996; K Yeleswaram, Comment on "Pharmacokinetic interaction between cyclosporine and the dihydropyridine calcium antagonist felodipine." Eur J Clin Pharmacol, 2:159, 1997; JK Madsen et al, Comment on

CYCLOSPORINE, with: *(continued)*
> "Pharmacokinetic interaction between cyclosporine and the dihydropyridine calcium antagonist felodipine." Eur J Clin Pharmacol, 52:161, 1997; A Yildiz et al, Interaction between cyclosporine A and verapamil, felodipine, and isradipine. Nephron, 81:117, 1999

Based on several studies in healthy subjects; felodipine does not appear to affect cyclosporine serum concentrations

Fluoroquinolones

Possible cyclosporine toxicity with ciprofloxacin or norfloxacin (possibly decreased metabolism)
> RA Elston and J Taylor, Possible interaction of ciprofloxacin with cyclosporin A. J Antimicrob Chemother, 21:679, 1988; DJ Thomson et al, Norfloxacin-cyclosporine interaction. Transplantation, 46:312, 1988; CK Avent et al, Synergistic nephrotoxicity due to ciprofloxacin and cyclosporine. Am J Med, 85:452, 1988; KKC Tan et al, Co-administration of ciprofloxacin and cyclosporin: lack of evidence for a pharmacokinetic interaction. Br J Clin Pharmacol, 28:185, 1989; M Nasir et al, Interaction between ciclosporin and ciprofloxacin. Nephron, 57:245, 1991; A Wynckel et al, Traitement des légionelloses par ofloxacine chez le transplanté rénal; absence d'interférence avec la ciclosporine A. Pressé Méd, 20:291, 1991; BA Ryerson et al, "Effect of enoxacin on cyclosporine pharmacokinetics in healthy subjects." In *Program and Abstracts of the 31st Interscience Conference on Antimicrobial Agents and Chemotherapy, Chicago IL, Sept 29-Oct 2, 1991*, page 198, abs 597. Am Soc Microbiol:Washington DC, 1991; RA McLellan et al, Norfloxacin interferes with cyclosporine disposition in pediatric patients undergoing renal transplantation. Clin Pharmacol Ther, 58:322, 1995; DR Doose et al, Levofloxacin does not alter cyclosporine disposition. J Clin Pharmacol, 38:90, 1998; manufacturer's package insert

Monitor renal status; concentration of both drugs may remain within normal range; adjustment of cyclosporine dosage may avoid nephrotoxicity; effectiveness of decreased cyclosporine dosage in avoiding rejection has not been established; levofloxacin, ofloxacin or enoxacin may not interact

Possible increased rejection rates in renal transplant patients with ciprofloxacin (possible decreased cyclosporine immunosuppressive effect)
> RE Wrishko et al, Investigation of a possible interaction between ciprofloxacin and cyclosporine in renal transplant patients. Transplantation, 64:996, 1997

Based on retrospective case-control study

Furosemide

Gout (additive hyperuricemia)
> DJ Tiller et al, Gout and hyperuricaemia in patients on cyclosporin and diuretics. Lancet, 1:453, 1985

Avoid concurrent use, if possible

CYCLOSPORINE, with: *(continued)*
  Grapefruit juice
    Possible cyclosporine toxicity (decreased first-pass metabolism; possible inhibition of P-glycoprotein)
      AAMJ Hollander et al, The effect of grapefruit juice on cyclosporine and prednisone metabolism in transplant patients. Clin Pharmacol Ther, 57:318, 1995; LL Ioannides-Demos et al, Dosing implications of a clinical interaction between grapefruit juice and cyclosporine and metabolite concentrations in patients with autoimmune diseases. J Rheumatol, 24:49, 1997; LJ Brunner et al, Interaction between cyclosporine and grapefruit juice requires long-term ingestion in stable renal transplant recipients. Pharmacotherapy, 18:23, 1998; Y-M Ku et al, Effect of grapefruit juice on the pharmacokinetics of microemulsion cyclosporine and its metabolite in healthy volunteers: does the formulation difference matter? J Clin Pharmacol, 38:959, 1998; DJ Edwards et al, 6',7'-Dihydroxybergamottin in grapefruit juice and Seville orange juice: effects on cyclosporine, disposition, enterocyte CYP3A4, and P-glycoprotein. Clin Pharmacol Ther, 65:237, 1999
    Based on studies in healthy subjects and in patients with kidney transplants and autoimmune diseases; occurs with both conventional cyclosporine formulation and microemulsion; monitor cyclosporine concentration
  HMG-CoA reductase inhibitors
    Rhabdomyolysis with lovastatin, simvastatin, atorvastatin and possibly cerivastatin (probably decreased metabolism; CYP3A4)
      CL Corpier et al, Rhabdomyolysis and renal injury with lovastatin use; report of two cases in cardiac transplant recipients. JAMA, 260:239, 1988; C East et al, Rhabdomyolysis in patients receiving lovastatin after cardiac transplantation. N Engl J Med, 318:47, 1988; DJ Norman et al, Myolysis and acute renal failure in a heart-transplant recipient receiving lovastatin. N Engl J Med, 109:46, 1988; DSJ Alejandro et al, Myoglobinuric acute renal failure in a cardiac transplant patient taking lovastatin and cyclosporine. J Am Soc Nephrol, 5:153, 1994; PKT Li et al, The interaction of fluvastatin and cyclosporin A in renal transplant patients. Int J Clin Pharmacol Ther, 33:246, 1995; RB Goldberg and D Roth, A preliminary report of the safety and efficacy of fluvastatin for hypercholesterolemia in renal transplant patients receiving cyclosporine. Am J Cardiol, 76:107A, 1995; H Holdaas et al, Effect of fluvastatin for safely lowering atherogenic lipids in renal transplant patients receiving cyclosporine. Am J Cardiol, 76:102A, 1995; G Blaison et al, Rhabdomyolyse causée par la simvastatine chez un transplanté cardiaque sous ciclosporine. Rev Med Interne, 13:61, 1992; M Arnadottir et al, Plasma concentration profiles of simvastatin 3-hydroxy-3-methylglutaryl-coenzyme A reductase inhibitory activity in kidney transplant recipients with and without ciclosporin. Nephron, 65:410, 1993; U Christians, Combination of pravastatin and cyclosporin in transplant patients. Clin Pharmacokinet, 32:173, 1997; W Mück et al, Increase in cerivastatin systemic exposure after single and multiple dosing in cyclosporine-treated kidney transplant recipients. Clin Pharmacol Ther, 65:251, 1999; XU Feng et al, Delay of metabolism rate of ciclosporin by simvastatin in 7

CYCLOSPORINE, with: *(continued)*
>Chinese healthy men. Acta Pharmacologica Sinica, 19:443, 1998; D Capone et al, Effects of simvastatin and pravastatin on hyperlipidemia and cyclosporin blood levels in renal transplant recipients. Am J Nephrol, 19:411, 1999; L Gullestad et al, Interaction between lovastatin and cyclosporine A after heart and kidney transplantation. Transplant Proc, 31:2163, 1999; HC Maltz et al, Rhabdomyolysis associated with concomitant use of atorvastatin and cyclosporine. Ann Pharmacother, 33:1176, 1999; A Jardine and H Holdaas, Fluvastatin in combination with cyclosporin in renal transplant recipients: a review of clinical and safety experience. J Clin Pharm Ther, 24:397, 1999; ML Rodriguez et al, Cerivastatin-induced rhabdomyolysis. Ann Intern Med, 132:598, 2000; E Cohen et al, Cyclosporin drug-interaction-induced rhabdomyolysis. A report of two cases in lung transplant recipients. Transplantation, 70:119, 2000

Several case reports; hepatotoxicity due to cyclosporine may have been primary; monitor cyclosporine and creatinine phosphokinase (CPK) concentrations and for signs of rhabdomyolysis (muscle pain, weakness or dark urine); 3 to 5 fold increase in cerivastatin concentration in 12 renal transplant patients, but no myopathy; fluvastatin and pravastatin appear less likely to interact

Possible increased risk of cyclosporine toxicity (mechanism not established)
>J Lill et al, Cyclosporine-drug interactions and the influence of patient age. Am J Health Syst Pharm, 57:1579, 2000

Possible increased risk of cyclosporine toxicity (mechanism not established)

Hypoglycemics, sulfonylurea
Possible cyclosporine toxicity with glipizide or glyburide (mechanism not established)
>PD Chidester and DJ Connito, Interaction between glipizide and cyclosporine: report of two cases. Transplant Proc, 25:2136, 1993; SI Islam et al, Possible interaction between cyclosporine and glibenclamide in posttransplant diabetic patients. Ther Drug Monit, 18:624, 1996; S Sagedal et al, Glipizide treatment of post-transplant diabetes does not interfere with cyclosporine pharmacokinetics in renal allograft recipients. Clin Transplant, 12:553, 1998

Monitor cyclosporine concentration; two cases with glipizide (1993); six cases with glyburide (1996); no effect of glipizide on cyclosporine pharmacokinetics in one study of 11 renal transplant patients

Idarubicin
Possible idarubicin toxicity (probably decreased metabolism; CYP3A4)
>F Pea et al, Multidrug resistance modulation in vivo: the effect of cyclosporin A alone or with dexverapamil on idarubicin pharmacokinetics in acute leukemia. Eur J Clin Pharmacol, 55:361, 1999

Based on study of patients with leukemia; monitor clinical status

Imipenem
CNS disturbances and seizures (mechanism not established)
>J Zazgornik et al, Potentiation of neurotoxic side effects by coadministration of imipenem to cyclosporine therapy in a kidney transplant

CYCLOSPORINE, with: *(continued)*

recipient – synergism of side effects or drug interaction? Clin Nephrol, 26:265, 1986; C Bösmüller et al, Increased risk of central nervous system toxicity in patients treated with ciclosporin and imipenem/cilastatin. Nephron, 58:362, 1991

Avoid concurrent use in patients with decreased renal function

Lipids, intravenous preparations

Possible cyclosporine toxicity (decreased binding due to altered serum lipoprotein composition)

N De Klippel et al, Cyclosporin leukoencephalopathy induced by intravenous lipid solution. Lancet, 339:1114, 1992

Single case with leukoencephalopathy (1992); patient received Intralipid; leukoencephalopathy has been reported with cyclosporine alone

Losartan

Possible increased cyclosporine toxicity (mechanism not established)

J Lill et al, Cyclosporine-drug interactions and the influence of patient age. Am J Health Syst Pharm, 57:1579, 2000

Based on population-based pharmacokinetic study; causal relationship not established; monitor clinical status

Macrolide antibiotics

Cyclosporine toxicity with erythromycin or clarithromycin (probably decreased presystemic metabolism; CYP3A4)

LM Gersema et al, Suspected drug interaction between cyclosporine and clarithromycin. J Heart Lung Transplant, 13:343, 1994; SK Gupta et al, Cyclosporin-erythromycin interaction in renal transplant patients. Br J Clin Pharmacol, 27:475, 1989; E Zylber-Katz, Multiple drug interactions with cyclosporine in a heart transplant patient. Ann Pharmacother, 29:127, 1995; D Ljutic and Z Rumboldt, Possible interaction between azithromycin and cyclosporin: a case report. Nephron, 70:130, 1995; E Gómez et al, Interaction between azithromycin and cyclosporin? Nephron, 73:724, 1996; VS Watkins et al, Drug interactions of macrolides: emphasis on dirithromycin. Ann Pharmacother, 31:349, 1997; S Treille et al, Kidney graft dysfunction after drug interaction between clarithromycin and cyclosporin. Nephrol Dial Transplant. 11:1192, 1996; ST Spicer et al, The mechanism of cyclosporine toxicity induced by clarithromycin. Br J Clin Pharmacol, 43:194, 1997; B Sádaba et al, Concurrent clarithromycin and cyclosporin A treatment. J antimicrob Chemother, 42:393, 1998

Avoid concurrent use of cyclosporine with erythromycin or clarithromycin; single case report with azithromycin (1995), but most evidence suggests no interaction with cyclosporine; dirithromycin may produce small increases in cyclosporine serum concentrations

Methotrexate

Toxicity of both drugs (decreased elimination)

AV Powles et al, Cyclosporin toxicity. Lancet, 335:610, 1990; MJ Korstanje et al, Cyclosporine and methotrexate: a dangerous combination. J Am Acad Dermatol, 23:320, 1990; M Baraldi et al, Cyclosporine A pharmacokinetics in rheumatoid arthritis patients after 6 months of methotrexate

CYCLOSPORINE, with: *(continued)*
> therapy. Pharmacol Res, 40:483, 1999

Although concurrent use has been discouraged, some have recommended cautious use of the combination in patients with severe rheumatoid arthritis

Metoclopramide

Possible cyclosporine toxicity (increased absorption)
> NK Wadhwa et al, The effect of oral metoclopramide on the absorption of cyclosporine. Transplantation, 43:211, 1987; NK Wadhwa et al, The effect of oral metoclopramide on the absorption of cyclosporine. Transplant Proc, 19:1730, 1987

Combined use might be an advantage if safe dosage is used

Metronidazole

Possible cyclosporine toxicity (probably decreased metabolism; CYP3A4)
> E Zylber-Katz et al, Cyclosporine interactions with metronidazole and cimetidine. Drug Intell Clin Pharm, 22:504, 1988; F Vincent et al, Insuffisance rénale aiguë chez un transplanté rénal traité par cyclosporine A et métronidazole. Therapie, 49:155, 1994; F Vincent et al, Insuffisance rénale aiguë chez un transplanté rénal traité par cyclosporine A et métronidazole. Therapie, 49:155, 1994; K Herzig and DW Johnson, Marked elevation of blood cyclosporin and tacrolimus levels due to concurrent metronidazole therapy. Nephrol Dial Transplant, 14:521, 1999

Four case reports (1988, 1994, 1999)

Mifepristone

Possible cyclosporine toxicity (mechanism not established)
> VS DeVore et al, Drug interaction between mifepristone and cyclosporine. ASHP Midyear Clinical Meeting, 33:P-94D, 1998

Single preliminary case report (1998); monitor cyclosporine concentrations

Minoxidil

Severe hypertrichosis (possibly additive)
> MS Sever et al, Limited use of minoxidil in renal transplant recipients because of the additive side-effects of cyclosporine on hypertrichosis. Transplantation, 50:536, 1990

Report in 6 patients (1990)

Modafinil

Decreased cyclosporine effect (increased metabolism)
> Manufacturer's package insert (modafinil)

Single case reported by manufacturer (1998)

Muromonab-CD3

Possible cyclosporine toxicity (probably decreased metabolism)
> D Vrahnos et al, Cyclosporine (CSA) levels during OKT3 treatment of acute renal allograft rejection. Pharmacotherapy, 11:278, 1991, abs 95; EM Vasquez and R Pollak, OKT3 therapy increases cyclosporine blood levels. Clin Transplant, 11:38, 1997

Monitor cyclosporine concentration

Mycophenolate mofetil

Possible decreased mycophenolate mofetil (mechanism not established)
> PJH Smak Gregoor et al, Effect of cyclosporine on mycophenolic acid

CYCLOSPORINE, with: *(continued)*
> trough levels in kidney transplant recipients. Transplantation, 68:1603, 1999
>
> *Based on study in transplant patients; plasma levels of the active metabolite mycophenolic acid (MPA) increased in subjects who discontinued concomitant cyclosporine; monitor clinical status*

Nefazodone
> Possible cyclosporine toxicity (decreased metabolism; CYP3A4)
>> KM Helms-Smith and SL Curtis, Apparent interaction between nefazodone and cyclosporine. Ann Intern Med, 125:424, 1996; JP Vella and MH Sayegh, Interactions between cyclosporine and newer antidepressant medications. Am J Kidney Dis, 31:320, 1998; DH Wright et al, Nefazodone and cyclosporine drug-drug interaction. J Heart Lung Transplant, 18:913, 1999; DH Wright et al, Nefazodone and cyclosporine drug-drug interaction. J Heart Lung Transplant, 18:913, 1999
>
> *Four case reports (1996, 1998, 1999); monitor cyclosporine concentrations and clinical status*

Neuromuscular blocking agents
> Prolonged neuromuscular blockade (mechanism not established)
>> E Crosby and JA Robblee, Cyclosporine[sic]-pancuronium interaction in a patient with a renal allograft. Can J Anaesth, 35:300, 1988; GG Wood, Cyclosporine-vecuronium interaction. Can J Anaesth, 36:358, 1989; JY Lepage et al, Interaction cyclosporine atracurium et vecuronium. Ann Fr Anesth Reanim, 8 suppl:R135, 1989; A Sidi et al, Prolonged neuromuscular blockade and ventilatory failure after renal transplantation and cyclosporine. Can J Anaesth, 37:543, 1990; P Ganjoo and P Tewari, Oral cyclosporine-vecuronium interaction. Can J Anaesth, 41:1017, 1994
>
> *Several case reports*

Nicardipine
> Renal toxicity (decreased cyclosporine metabolism)
>> M Cantarovich et al, Confirmation of the interaction between cyclosporine and the calcium channel blocker nicardipine in renal transplant patients. Clin Nephrol, 28:190, 1987; B Bourbigot et al, Nicardipine increases cyclosporin blood levels. Lancet, 1:1447, 1986; M Kessler et al, Influence of nicardipine on renal function and plasma cyclosporin in renal transplant patients. Eur J Clin Pharmacol, 36:637, 1989
>
> *Monitor cyclosporine concentration*

Nifedipine
> Possible nifedipine toxicity (decreased metabolism)
>> JP McFadden et al, Cyclosporin decreases nifedipine metabolism. BMJ, 299:1224, 1989
>
> *Monitor clinical status; 2 case reports of paresthesias, rash (1989)*

Nonsteroidal anti-inflammatory drugs
> Nephrotoxicity or hypertension with diclofenac, mefenamic acid, or sulindac (mechanism not established)
>> G Deray et al, Enhancement of cyclosporine A nephrotoxicity by diclofenac. Clin Nephrol, 27:213, 1987; KP Harris et al, Nonsteroidal antiinflammatory drugs and cyclosporine; a potentially serious adverse interaction.

(continued)

CYCLOSPORINE, with: *(continued)*
> Transplantation, 46:598, 1988; GP Sesin et al, Sulindac-induced elevation of serum cyclosporine concentration. Clin Pharm, 8:445, 1989; JP Branthwaite and A Nicholls, Cyclosporin and diclofenac interaction in rheumatoid arthritis. Lancet, 337:252, 1991; JWM Agar, Cyclosporin A and mefenamic acid in a renal transplant patient. Aust N Z J Med, 21:784, 1991; JM Kovarik et al, Diclofenac combined with cyclosporine in treatment refractory rheumatoid arthritis: longitudinal safety assessment and evidence of a pharmacokinetic/dynamic interaction. J Rheumatol, 23:2033, 1996; A Constantopoulos, Colitis induced by interaction of cyclosporine A and non-steroidal anti-inflammatory drugs. Pediatr Int, 41:184, 1999

Several case reports with sulindac or diclofenac; single case report with mefenamic acid (1991); monitor renal function and blood pressure (cyclosporine concentration may not change); one case of colitis with cyclosporine and indomethacin (1999); use conservative doses of diclofenac initially (diclofenac concentrations may increase)

Possible diclofenac toxicity (possibly decreased metabolism)
> JM Kovarik et al, Cyclosporine and nonsteroidal antiinflammatory drugs: exploring potential drug interactions and their implications for the treatment of rheumatoid arthritis. J Clin Pharmacol, 37:336, 1997

Based on study in healthy subjects; monitor clinical status

Omeprazole
Possible cyclosporine toxicity (increased absorption)
> H Reichenspurner et al, The influence of gastrointestinal agents on resorption and metabolism of cyclosporine after heart transplantation: experimental and clinical results. J Heart Lung Transplant, 12:1987, 1993; L Schouler et al, Omeprazole-cyclosporin interaction. Am J Gastroenterol, 86:1097, 1991; I Blohmé et al, A study of the interaction between omeprazole and cyclosporine in renal transplant patients. Br J Clin Pharmacol, 35:156, 1993; T Lorf et al, The effect of pantoprazole on tacrolimus and cyclosporin A blood concentration in transplant recipients. Eur J Clin Pharmacol, 56:439, 2000

Monitor cyclosporine concentration; pantoprazole may not interact; study in 10 male transplant patients failed to confirm

Orlistat
Decreased cyclosporine effect (probably decreased absorption)
> H Nägele et al, Effect of orlistat on blood cyclosporin concentration in an obese heart transplant patient. Eur J Clin Pharmacol, 55:667, 1999; E Colman and M Fossler, Reduction in blood cyclosporine concentrations by orlistat. N Engl J Med, 342:1141, 2000

Several case reports; marked reduction in cyclosporine serum concentrations; avoid concurrent use

Penicillins
Decreased cyclosporine effect with nafcillin (probably increased metabolism)
> SA Veremis et al, Subtherapeutic cyclosporine concentrations during nafcillin therapy. Transplantation, 43:913, 1987

CYCLOSPORINE, with: *(continued)*
Single, well-documented case report (1987)

Cyclosporine toxicity with nafcillin and ticarcillin (mechanism not established)
C Lambert et al, Interaction ciclosporine-ticarcilline chez un transplanté rénal. Pressé Méd, 18:230, 1989; F Jahansouz et al, Potentiation of cyclosporine nephrotoxicity by nafcillin in lung transplant recipients. Transplantation, 55:1045, 1993
Avoid concurrent use

Phenytoin
Decreased cyclosporine effect (mechanism not established)
DJ Freeman et al, Evaluation of cyclosporin-phenytoin interaction with observations on cyclosporin metabolites. Br J Clin Pharmacol, 18:887, 1984; M Rowland and SK Gupta, Cyclosporin – phenytoin interaction: re-evaluation using metabolite data. Br J Clin Pharmacol, 24:329, 1987
Monitor cyclosporine concentration

Polyethylene glycol and electrolytes
Decreased cyclosporine effect (possibly decreased absorption)
T Santa et al, Decreased cyclosporine absorption after treatment with *GoLytely* lavage solution in a kidney transplant patient. Ann Pharmacother, 28:963, 1994
Single case report (1994); monitor cyclosporine concentration

Probucol
Decreased cyclosporine effect (possibly decreased absorption)
C Gallego et al, Interaction between probucol and cyclosporine in renal transplant patients. Ann Pharmacother, 28:940, 1994
Monitor cyclosporine concentration

Progestins
Cyclosporine toxicity with norethindrone or oral contraceptives (decreased metabolism)
WB Ross et al, Cyclosporin interaction with danazol and norethisterone. Lancet, 1:330, 1986; G Deray et al, Oral contraceptive interaction with cyclosporin. Lancet, 1:158, 1987
Monitor cyclosporine concentration

Propafenone
Cyclosporine toxicity (mechanism not established)
CH Spes et al, Ciclosporin-propafenone interaction. Klin Wochenschr, 68:872, 1990
Single well-documented case report (1990)

Pyrazinamide
Decreased cyclosporine effect (possibly increased metabolism)
LA Jiménez del Cerro and FR Hernández, Effect of pyrazinamide on ciclosporin levels. Nephron, 62:113, 1992
Single case report (1992); effect appeared to be additive to that of isoniazid and rifampin

Acute myopathy (possibly additive)
J Fernández-Solà et al, Acute toxic myopathy due to pyrazinamide in a

CYCLOSPORINE, with: *(continued)*
>patient with renal transplantation and cyclosporine therapy. Nephrol Dial Transplant, 11:1850, 1996

Single case report (1996)

Quinine
>Possible alteration in cyclosporine effect (mechanism not established)
>>HW Tan and SL Ch'ng, Drug interaction between cyclosporine A and quinine in a renal transplant patient with malaria. Singapore Med J, 32:189, 1991; J Lill et al, Cyclosporine-drug interactions and the influence of patient age. Am J Health Syst Pharm, 57:1579, 2000

Single case report of decreased cyclosporine effect (1991); population-based pharmacokinetic study suggested increased cyclosporine effect; monitor clinical status

Quinupristin/dalfopristin
>Possible cyclosporine toxicity (decreased metabolism; CYP3A4)
>>Manufacturer's package insert (quinupristin/dalfopristin)

Monitor cyclosporine concentrations

Rifampin
>Decreased cyclosporine effect (increased intestinal and hepatic metabolism; CYP3A4)
>>E Renoult et al, Effect of topical rifamycin SV treatment on cyclosporin A blood levels in a renal transplant recipient. Eur J Clin Pharmacol, 40:433, 1991; MF Hebert et al, Bioavailability of cyclosporine with concomitant rifampin administration is markedly less than predicted by hepatic enzyme induction. Clin Pharmacol Ther, 52:453, 1992; E Zylber-Katz, Multiple drug interactions with cyclosporine in a heart transplant patient. Ann Pharmacother, 29:127, 1995; D Capone et al, Drug interaction between cyclosporine and two antimicrobial agents, josamycin and rifampicin, in organ-transplanted patients. Int J Clin Pharm Res, 16:73, 1996; YH Kim et al, Effects of rifampin on cyclosporine disposition in kidney recipients with tuberculosis. Transplant Proc, 30:3570, 1998; VL Freitag et al, Effect of short-term rifampin on stable cyclosporine concentrations. Ann Pharmacother, 33:871, 1999

Avoid concurrent use, if possible; cyclosporine dose may have to be increased by 2.5 to 3 fold; single case report with topical rifampin precursor rifamycin SV (1991); even 2 to 4 doses of rifampin can result in subtherapeutic cyclosporine concentrations

Saint John's wort
>Decreased cyclosporine effect (possibly increased metabolism; possibly increased transport; P-glycoprotein)
>>F Ruschitzka et al, Acute heart transplant rejection due to Saint John's wort. Lancet, 355:548, 2000; T Breidenbach et al, Drug interaction of St John's wort with ciclosporin. Lancet, 355:1912, 2000; GW Barone et al, Drug interaction between St. John's wort and cyclosporine. Ann Pharmacother, 34:1013, 2000; T Breidenbach et al, Profound drop of cyclosporin A whole blood trough levels caused by St. John's wort (Hypericum perforatum). Transplantation, 69:2229, 2000

CYCLOSPORINE, with: *(continued)*
> *Three case reports with positive dechallenge; additional 45 cases subsequently reported; avoid combination*

Saquinavir
> Probable cyclosporine and saquinavir toxicity (probably mutual inhibition of metabolism; CYP3A4)
>> K Brinkman et al, Pharmacokinetic interaction between saquinavir and cyclosporine. Ann Intern Med, 129:914, 1998
>
> *Monitor cyclosporine concentration and clinical status; theoretical interaction confirmed by single case*

Selective serotonin reuptake inhibitors (SSRIs)
> Possible cyclosporine toxicity with fluvoxamine or fluoxetine (probably decreased metabolism; CYP3A4)
>> RC Horton and RS Bonser, Interaction between cyclosporine and fluoxetine. BMJ, 311:422, 1995; JS Markowitz et al, Lack of antidepressant-cyclosporine pharmacokinetic interactions. J Clin Psychopharmacol, 18:91, 1998; JP Vella and MH Sayegh, Interactions between cyclosporine and newer antidepressant medications. Am J Kidney Dis, 31:320, 1998
>
> *Single case report with fluoxetine (1995) and fluvoxamine (1998); several patients have taken SSRIs, including fluoxetine, and cyclosporine concurrently without adverse effects (1998)*

Sirolimus
> Possible sirolimus toxicity with microemulsion formulation of cyclosporine (decreased metabolism; CYP3A4; possible decreased p-glycoprotein transport)
>> B Kaplan et al, The effects of relative timing of sirolimus and cyclosporine microemulsion formulation coadministration on the pharmacokinetics of each agent. Clin Pharmacol Ther, 63:48, 1998
>
> *In one study in 24 transplant recipients, concomitant administration of the microemulsion formulation of cyclosporine increased sirolimus concentrations; sirolimus and the microemulsion formulation of cyclosporine should be given 4 hours apart*
>
> Possible sirolimus toxicity with cyclosporine oral solution (decreased metabolism; CYP3A4; decreased P-glycoprotein transport)
>> Manufacturer's package insert (sirolimus)
>
> *In one study in 150 psoriasis patients, sirolimus trough concentrations increased 67% to 86%; monitor sirolimus concentrations*

Sulfonamides
> Decreased cyclosporine effect with sulfasalazine, sulfamethazine or sulfadiazine (possibly increased metabolism)
>> DK Jones et al, Serious interaction between cyclosporin A and sulphadimidine. Br Med J, 292:728, 1986; CH Spes et al, Sulfadiazine therapy for toxoplasmosis in heart transplant recipients decreases cyclosporine concentration. Clin Invest, 70:752, 1992; D Du Cheyron et al, Effect of sulfasalazine on cyclosporin blood concentration. Eur J Clin Pharmacol, 55:227, 1999
>
> *Monitor cyclosporine concentration*

(continued)

CYCLOSPORINE, with: *(continued)*

Tacrolimus

Possible cyclosporine toxicity (mechanism not established)

U Christians et al, Interactions of FK 506 and cyclosporine metabolism. Transplant Proc, 23:2794, 1991; TE Starzl et al, FK 506 for liver, kidney, and pancreas transplantation. Lancet, 2:1000, 1989

Avoid concurrent use

Thiazide diuretics

Gout or renal toxicity (additive hyperuricemia; mechanism of renal toxicity not established)

DJ Tiller et al, Gout and hyperuricaemia in patients on cyclosporin and diuretics. Lancet, 1:453, 1985; G Deray et al, Enhancement of cyclosporin nephrotoxicity by diuretic therapy. Clin Nephrol, 32:47, 1989

Avoid concurrent use, if possible

Ticlopidine

Decreased cyclosporine effect (probably increased metabolism)

B Birmelé et al, Interaction of cyclosporin and ticlopidine. Nephrol Dial Transplant, 6:150, 1991; P Boissonnat et al, A drug interaction study between ticlopidine and cyclosporin in heart transplant recipients. Eur J Clin Pharmacol, 53:45, 1997

Single case report (1991); in some transplant patients half normal doses of ticlopidine can inhibit platelet aggregation without interacting

Trimethoprim

Nephrotoxicity (synergism)

JF Thompson et al, Nephrotoxicity of trimethoprim and cotrimoxazole in renal allograft recipients treated with cyclosporine. Transplantation, 36:204, 1983; O Ringden et al, Nephrotoxicity by co-trimoxazole and cyclosporin in transplanted patients. Lancet, 1:1016, 1984

Avoid concurrent use

Troglitazone

Decreased cyclosporine effect (probable increase in metabolism; CYP3A)

B Kaplan et al, Potential interaction of troglitazone and cyclosporine. Transplantation, 65:1399, 1998; SJ Burgess et al, Effect of troglitazone on cyclosporine whole blood levels. Transplantation, 66:272, 1998; MH Park et al, Troglitazone, a new antidiabeic agent, decreases cyclosporine level. J Heart Lung Transplant, 17:1139, 1998; RP Frantz and TT Nguyen, Rezulin (troglitazone) greatly increases cyclosporine metabolism. J Heart Lung Transplant, 17:1037, 1998

Several case reports and review of 18 transplant patients; monitor cyclosporine concentration; troglitazone is no longer available

Verapamil

Possible cyclosporine toxicity (decreased metabolism or absorption)

RL Howard et al, The effect of calcium channel blockers on the cyclosporine dose requirement in renal transplant recipients. Renal Failure, 12:89, 1990; KL Tortorice et al, The effects of calcium channel blockers on cyclosporine and its metabolites in renal transplant recipients. Ther Drug Monit, 12:321, 1990; IS Sketris et al, Effect of calcium-channel blockers on

CYCLOSPORINE, with: *(continued)*
    cyclosporine clearance and use in renal transplant patients. Ann Pharmacother, 28:1227, 1994; C Bagnis and G Deray, Intérêt des antagonistes calciques dans la prise en charge thérapeutique des patients hypertendus traités par ciclosporine. Arch Mal Coeur Vaiss, 91:411, 1998; A Yildiz et al, Interaction between cyclosporine A and verapamil, felodipine, and isradipine. Nephron, 81:117, 1999

Monitor cyclosporine concentration; combination has been used safely to reduce cyclosporine dosage and to treat cyclosporine-induced hypertension; effect not seen with felodipine or isradipine

Vincristine
Neurotoxicity (mechanism not established)
    Y Bertrand et al, Cyclosporin A used to reverse drug resistance increases vincristine neurotoxicity. Am J Hematol, 40:158, 1992

Single case report (1992); occurred during treatment of leukemia (ALL), only when cyclosporine was added to a regimen containing vincristine

Cyclothiazide, see Thiazide diuretics

CYPROHEPTADINE, with:
  Antidepressants, tricyclic - See Antidepressants, tricyclic with Cyproheptadine, page 84

Monoamine oxidase inhibitors
Hallucinations with cyproheptadine and phenelzine (mechanism not established)
    DA Kahn, Possible toxic interaction between cyproheptadine and phenelzine. Am J Psychiatry, 144:1242, 1987

Single case report (1987)

Selective serotonin reuptake inhibitors (SSRIs)
Decreased antidepressant effect with cyproheptadine and fluoxetine or paroxetine (mechanism not established)
    RJ Katz and M Rosenthal, Adverse interaction of cyproheptadine with serotonergic antidepressants. J Clin Psychiatry, 55:314, 1994; RC Christensen, Adverse interaction of paroxetine and cyproheptadine. J Clin Psychiatry, 56:9, 1995; F Boon, Cyproheptadine and SSRIs. J Am Acad Child Adolesc Psychiatry, 38:112, 1999

Monitor antidepressant effect; theoretically would occur with any SSRI

Cysteamine, no documented interactions, see page 4, Criteria for Listing Interactions

CYTARABINE, with:
  Alcohol - See Alcohol with Cytarabine, page 17

DACARBAZINE, with:
Levodopa
Decreased levodopa effect (mechanism not established)
    M Merello et al, Impaired levodopa response in Parkinson's disease during melanoma therapy. Clin Neuropharmacol, 15:69, 1992

Single case report (1992)

Daclizumab, no documented interactions, see page 4, Criteria for Listing Interactions

Dactinomycin, no documented interactions, see page 4, Criteria for Listing Interactions

Dalfopristin/quinupristin, see Quinupristin/dalfopristin

Dalteparin, no documented interactions, see page 4, Criteria for Listing Interactions

Danaparoid, no documented interactions, see page 4, Criteria for Listing Interactions

Danazol, see Anabolic and androgenic steroids

DANTROLENE, with:

Metoclopramide
Possible dantrolene toxicity (increased absorption)
> JL Segal and SR Brunnemann, Comparative bioavailability of oral dantrolene in patients with spinal cord injury (SCI). J Clin Pharmacol, 29:835, 1989, abs 15

Monitor clinical status or dantrolene concentration

Verapamil
Myocardial depression and hyperkalemia (synergism)
> AS Rubin and AD Zablocki, Hyperkalemia, verapamil, and dantrolene. Anesthesiology, 66:246, 1987

Occurred with IV dantrolene given to prevent malignant hyperthermia; avoid concurrent use, if possible; nifedipine may not interact; diltiazem interacts in swine

DAPSONE, with:

Didanosine
Decreased dapsone effect (decreased absorption – dapsone requires low pH; didanosine buffered at pH 7-8)
> CE Metroka et al, Failure of prophylaxis with dapsone in patients taking dideoxyinosine. N Engl J Med, 325:737, 1991; J Sahai et al, Effects of the antacids in didanosine tablets on dapsone pharmacokinetics. Ann Intern Med, 123:584, 1995

Failure of prophylaxis for pneumocystis pneumonia in HIV patients; drugs should be given at least 2 hours apart; interaction not confirmed in subsequent study (1995)

Primaquine
Possible increased risk of methemoglobinemia (additive)
> DD Sin and SD Shafran, Dapsone- and primaquine-induced methemoglobinemia in HIV-infected individuals. J Acquir Immune Defic Syndr Hum Retrovirol, 12:477, 1996

Based on observations in HIV-positive patients

Pyrimethamine
Agranulocytosis (mechanism not established)
> Manufacturer's package insert

Avoid concurrent use

Rifampin
Possible decreased dapsone effect (increased metabolism)
> FAJM Pieters et al, Influence of once-monthly rifampicin and daily clofazimine on the pharmacokinetics of dapsone in leprosy patients in Nigeria. Eur J Clin Pharmacol, 34:73, 1988; UP Jorde et al, SM Borcherding and TH

DAPSONE, with: *(continued)*

Self, Significance of drug interactions with rifampin in *Pneumocystis carinii* pneumonia prophylaxis. Arch Intern Med, 152:2348, 1992

Current practice in leprosy is to give rifampin only once a month, which does not affect dapsone metabolism; important in Pneumocystis carinii prophylaxis and treatment

Trimethoprim

Dapsone toxicity, methemoglobinemia (probably decreased metabolism)

BL Lee et al, Dapsone, trimethoprim, and sulfamethoxazole plasma levels during treatment of Pneumocystis pneumonia in patients with the acquired immunodeficiency syndrome (AIDS). Ann Intern Med, 110:606, 1989

In patients with AIDS; monitoring methemoglobin appears more sensitive than dapsone concentration; trimethoprim concentration increased, but clinical significance has not been established

Trimethoprim-sulfamethoxazole

Dapsone toxicity and methemoglobinemia, with trimethoprim alone (probably decreased metabolism)

BL Lee et al, Dapsone, trimethoprim, and sulfamethoxazole plasma levels during treatment of Pneumocystis pneumonia in patients with the acquired immunodeficiency syndrome (AIDS). Ann Intern Med, 110:606, 1989

In patients with AIDS; monitoring methemoglobin appears more sensitive than dapsone concentration; trimethoprim concentration increased, but clinical significance has not been established

Daunorubicin, no documented interactions, see page 4, Criteria for Listing Interactions

DdC, see Zalcitabine

DdI, see Didanosine

DEBRISOQUINE, with:

Antidepressants, tricyclic - See Antidepressants, tricyclic with Debrisoquine, page 85

Beta-adrenergic blockers - See Beta-adrenergic blockers with Debrisoquine, page 153

Insulin

Hypotension with short-acting insulin (possibly additive)

L Hume, Potentiation of hypotensive effect of debrisoquine by insulin. Diabetic Med, 2:390, 1985

Single case report (1985)

Phenothiazines

Possible debrisoquine toxicity (decreased metabolism)

E Spina et al, Debrisoquine oxidation phenotype during neuroleptic monotherapy. Eur J Clin Pharmacol, 41:467, 1991

Monitor debrisoquine concentration or clinical status

Sympathomimetic amines

Decreased antihypertensive effect and possible hypertension with phenylephrine (release of norepinephrine and blockade of reuptake of amines by neurons)

W Allum et al, Interaction between debrisoquine and phenylephrine in

(continued)

DEBRISOQUINE, with: *(continued)*
>man. Br J Clin Pharmacol, 1:51, 1974; Br J Pharmacol, 47:675P, 1973; J Aminu et al, Interaction between debrisoquine and phenylephrine. Lancet, 2:935, 1970
>
>*Avoid concurrent use*

Decamethonium, see Neuromuscular blocking agents

Deet, no documented interactions, see page 4, Criteria for Listing Interactions

Dehydroepiandrosterone, no documented interactions, see page 4, Criteria for Listing Interactions

DELAVIRDINE, with:

Antacids - See Antacids with Delavirdine, page 52

Antifungals, imidazoles and triazoles - See Antifungals, imidazoles and triazoles with Delavirdine, page 100

Antihistamines, H$_1$-blockers: astemizole, terfenadine - See Antihistamines, H$_1$-blockers: astemizole, terfenadine with Delavirdine, page 110

Antihistamines, H$_2$-blockers - See Antihistamines, H$_2$-blockers with Delavirdine, page 117

Barbiturates - See Barbiturates with Delavirdine, page 133

Benzodiazepines - See Benzodiazepines with Delavirdine, page 141

Carbamazepine - See Carbamazepine with Delavirdine, page 178

Cisapride - See Cisapride with Delavirdine, page 199

Didanosine
>Decreased absorption of both drugs
>>Manufacturer's package insert
>
>*Give at least 1 hour apart*

Indinavir
>Possible indinavir toxicity (decreased metabolism)
>>JJ Ferry et al, Pharmacokinetic drug-drug interaction study of delavirdine and indinavir in healthy volunteers. J Acquir Immune Defic Syndr Hum Retrovirol, 18:252, 1998
>
>*Based on study in healthy subjects; monitor clinical status*

Lopinavir/Ritonavir
>Increased lopinavir toxicity (decreased metabolism)
>>Manufacturer's package insert (*Kaletra*)
>
>*Doses of the combination may need to be adjusted*

Macrolide antibiotics
>Possible increased delavirdine or clarithromycin toxicity (decreases each others metabolism)
>>Manufacturer's package insert
>
>*Theoretical; monitor clinical status*

Nelfinavir
>Possible nelfinavir toxicity (decreased metabolism); decreased delavirdine effect (mechanism unknown); neutropenia has occurred
>>Manufacturer's package insert and information received from the manufacturer
>
>*Monitor clinical status and neutrophil counts*

DELAVIRDINE, with: *(continued)*
Paclitaxel
Possible paclitaxel toxicity (probably decreased metabolism; CYP3A4)
> JD Schwartz et al, Potential interaction of antiretroviral therapy with paclitaxel in patients with AIDS-related Kaposi's sarcoma. AIDS, 13:283, 1999

Two case reports (1999); patients also received saquinavir and fluconazole

Phenytoin
Possible decreased delavirdine effect (increased metabolism)
> Manufacturer's package insert

Based on preliminary data; monitor clinical status

Rifabutin
Possible decreased delavirdine effect (probably increased metabolism)
> MT Borin et al, Pharmacokinetic study of the interaction between rifabutin and delavirdine mesylate in HIV-1 infected patients. Antiviral Res, 35:53, 1997

Based on study in 12 HIV+ patients; monitor delavirdine concentration

Rifampin
Decreased delavirdine effect (increased metabolism)
> Manufacturer's package insert

Avoid concurrent use

Ritonavir
Possible ritonavir toxicity (decreased metabolism)
> GD Morse et al, Ritonavir (RIT) pharmacokinetics (PK) during combination therapy with delavirdine (DLV). Conf Retrovir Opportun Infect, 5:143, 1998, abstract 343

In one study ritonavir concentration increased 70%; dose of ritonavir may need to be lowered

Saquinavir
Possible saquinavir toxicity (decreased metabolism); may cause hepatotoxicity
> Manufacturer's package insert

Monitor clinical status

Selective serotonin reuptake inhibitors (SSRIs)
Possible delavirdine toxicity (probably decreased metabolism)
> Manufacturer's package insert

Based on population pharmacokinetic data; monitor clinical status

Demeclocycline, see Tetracyclines

Deoxyribonuclease, no documented interactions, see page 4, Criteria for Listing Interactions

DES, see Estrogens

DESFLURANE, with:
Sympathomimetic amines
Possible increased risk of cardiac ischemia with dopamine or dobutamine (mechanism not established)
> CL Moir, Cardiac ischemia and desflurane. Can J Anaesth, 46:810, 1999; JM Murray and SR Luncy, Fatal cardiac ischaemia associated with prolonged desflurane anaesthesia and administration of exogenous catecholamines. Can J Anaesth, 45:1200, 1998

DESFLURANE, with: *(continued)*
> *Four fatal cases of cardiac ischemia in study of 21 patients undergoing head and neck surgery (1998); more study needed to establish causal relationship*

Desipramine, see Antidepressants, tricyclic

Desonide, no documented interactions, see page 4, Criteria for Listing Interactions

Desoximetasone, no documented interactions, see page 4, Criteria for Listing Interactions

Dexamethasone, see Corticosteroids

Dexchlorpheniramine maleate, no documented interactions, see page 4, Criteria for Listing Interactions

Dexrazoxane, no documented interactions, see page 4, Criteria for Listing Interactions

DEXTRAN SULFATE, with:
   Angiotensin-converting enzyme (ACE) inhibitors - See Angiotensin-converting enzyme (ACE) inhibitors with Dextran sulfate, page 44

Dextroamphetamine, see Sympathomimetic amines

Dextromethorphan, see Narcotics: dextromethorphan

DEXTROTHYROXINE, with:
   Anticoagulants, oral - See Anticoagulants, oral with Dextrothyroxine, page 65

Dezocine, no documented interactions, see page 4, Criteria for Listing Interactions

Diatrizoate meglumine, see Contrast media

Diazepam, see Benzodiazepines

DIAZOXIDE, with:
   Anticoagulants, oral - See Anticoagulants, oral with Diazoxide, page 65
   Beta-adrenergic blockers - See Beta-adrenergic blockers with Diazoxide, page 154
   Hydralazine
     Severe hypotension (additive)
       WL Henrich et al, Hypotensive sequelae of diazoxide and hydralazine therapy. JAMA, 237:264, 1977
     Avoid concurrent use within 6 hours
   Methyldopa
     Severe hypotension (additive)
       Manufacturer's package insert
     Avoid concurrent use within 6 hours
   Minoxidil
     Severe hypotension (additive)
       Manufacturer's package insert
     Avoid concurrent use within 6 hours
   Nitrates
     Severe hypotension (additive)
       Manufacturer's package insert
     Avoid concurrent use within 6 hours
   Nonsteroidal anti-inflammatory drugs
     Decreased hypotensive effect of diazoxide by tenoxicam (possibly inhibition prostaglandins)
       DK Sommers et al, The countering of diazoxide-induced vasodilatation by tenoxicam in normal volunteers. Eur J Clin Pharmacol, 46:569, 1994

DIAZOXIDE, with: *(continued)*
Based on study in 10 healthy subjects

Phenothiazines

Hyperglycemia with chlorpromazine (mechanism not established)
> A Aynsley-Green and R Illig, Enhancement by chlorpromazine of hyperglycaemic action of diazoxide. Lancet, 2:658, 1975

Single case report in patient also receiving bendroflumethiazide (1975); monitor blood glucose

Phenytoin

Decreased anticonvulsant effect (mechanism not established)
> TF Roe et al, Drug interaction: diazoxide and diphenylhydantoin. J Pediatr, 87:480, 1975

Monitor phenytoin concentration

Possible decreased hyperglycemic effect of diazoxide (possibly increased metabolism)
> DJ Petro et al, Diazoxide-diphenylhydantoin interaction. J Pediatr, 89:331, 1975

Monitor blood glucose

Prazosin

Severe hypotension (additive)
> Manufacturer's package insert

Avoid concurrent use within 6 hours

Reserpine

Severe hypotension (additive)
> Manufacturer's package insert

Avoid concurrent use within 6 hours

Thiazide diuretics

Increased hyperglycemic and hyperuricemic effect (mechanism not established)
> Manufacturer's package insert; HS Seltzer and EW Allen, Hyperglycemia and inhibition of insulin secretion during administration of diazoxide and trichlormethiazide in man. Diabetes, 19:19, 1969

Monitor blood glucose and uric acid

Dibenamine, see Alpha-adrenergic blockers

Dichloralphenazone, no documented interactions, see page 4, Criteria for Listing Interactions

Dichlorphenamide, see Carbonic anhydrase inhibitors

Diclofenac, see Nonsteroidal anti-inflammatory drugs

Dicloxacillin, see Penicillins

Dicumarol, see Anticoagulants, oral

Dicyclomine, see Anticholinergics

DIDANOSINE, with:

Amprenavir - See Amprenavir with Didanosine, page 39

Antifungals, imidazoles and triazoles - See Antifungals, imidazoles and triazoles with Didanosine, page 100

Dapsone - See Dapsone with Didanosine, page 242

DIDANOSINE, with: *(continued)*

Delavirdine - See Delavirdine with Didanosine, page 244

Fluoroquinolones

Decreased ciprofloxacin effect; other fluoroquinolones probably also interact (decreased absorption)

> J Sahai et al, Cations in the didanosine tablet reduce ciprofloxacin bioavailability. Clin Pharmacol Ther, 53:292, 1993; J Sahai, Avoiding the ciprofloxacin-didanosine interaction. Ann Intern Med, 123:394, 1995; CA Knuff and RH Barbhaiya, A multiple-dose pharmacokinetic interaction study between didanosine (Videx®) and ciprofloxacin (Cipro®) in male subjects seropositive for HIV but asymptomatic. Biopharm Drug Dispos, 18:65, 1997

Avoid concurrent use or give ciprofloxacin 2 hours before or 6 hours after didanosine; didanosine is acid labile and chewable tablets contain aluminum and magnesium buffers that bind ciprofloxacin; based on studies in 12 healthy volunteers and 16 HIV positive men

Ganciclovir

Possible didanosine toxicity (mechanism not established)

> CB Trapnell et al, Altered didanosine pharmacokinetics with concomitant oral ganciclovir. Clin Pharmacol Ther, 55:193, 1994; PJ Cimoch et al, Pharmacokinetics of oral ganciclovir alone and in combination with zidovudine, didanosine, and probenecid in HIV-infected subjects. J Acquir Immune Defic Syndr Hum Retrovirol, 17:227, 1998; D Jung et al, Effect of high-dose oral ganciclovir on didanosine disposition in human immunodeficiency virus (HIV)-positive patients. J Clin Pharmacol, 38:1057, 1998

Monitor clinical status

Possible decreased ganciclovir effect (mechanism not established)

> PJ Cimoch et al, Pharmacokinetics of oral ganciclovir alone and in combination with zidovudine, didanosine, and probenecid in HIV-infected subjects. J Acquir Immune Defic Syndr Hum Retrovirol, 17:227, 1998; D Jung et al, Effect of high-dose oral ganciclovir on didanosine disposition in human immunodeficiency virus (HIV)-positive patients. J Clin Pharmacol, 38:1057, 1998

Monitor clinical status; didanosine had no effect on serum ganciclovir concentrations in one study of 9 patients (1998)

Hydroxyurea

Possible increased risk of peripheral neuropathy (mechanism not established)

> JA Cepeda and D Wilks, Excess peripheral neuropathy in patients treated with hydroxyurea plus didanosine and stavudine for HIV infection. AIDS, 14:332, 2000

Patients also on stavudine; causal relationship not established; monitor clinical status

Indinavir

Possible decreased indinavir effect (decreased absorption)

> Manufacturer's package insert (indinavir)

DIDANOSINE, with: *(continued)*
> *Indinavir requires acid pH and didanosine formulated with buffer; give one hour apart on an empty stomach*

> **Narcotics: methadone and congeners**
>> Possible decreased didanosine effect (probably decreased bioavailability)
>>> PM Rainey et al, Interaction of methadone with didanosine and stavudine. J Acquir Immune Defic Syndr, 24:241, 2000
>> *Based on study in HIV(+) patients using didanosine tablets; monitor clinical status and adjust didanosine dosage as needed*

> **Ritonavir**
>> Gout (possible additive effect)
>>> DL Mehlhaff and DS Stein, Gout secondary to ritonavir and didanosine. AIDS, 10:1744, 1996
>> *Single case report (1996); monitor uric acid concentration*

> **Stavudine**
>> Increased risk of pancreatitis
>>> Manufacturer's package insert
>> *Monitor for clinical and laboratory sign of pancreatitis*

> **Zalcitabine**
>> Aggravation of neuropathy (possibly synergism)
>>> SF LeLacheur and GL Simon, Exacerbation of dideoxycytidine-induced neuropathy with dideoxyinosine. J Acquir Immune Defic Syndr, 4:538, 1991
>> *Single case report (1991)*

> **Zidovudine**
>> Possible zidovudine toxicity (possibly decreased metabolism)
>>> M Barry et al, Pharmacokinetics of zidovudine and dideoxyinosine alone and in combination in patients with the acquired immunodeficiency syndrome. Br J Clin Pharmacol, 37:421, 1994; D Gibb et al, Pharmacokinetics of zidovudine and dideoxyinosine alone and in combination in children with HIV infection. Br J Clin Pharmacol, 39:527, 1995; GD Morse et al, Pharmacokinetics of zidovudine and didanosine during combination therapy. Antiviral Res, 27:419, 1995
>> *Monitor zidovudine response; clinical significance not established; study in HIV-positive children found the drugs could be used safely together*

Dideoxycytidine, see Zalcitabine

Dideoxyinosine, see Didanosine

Dienestrol, see Estrogens

Diethylpropion, see Sympathomimetic amines

Diethylstilbestrol, see Estrogens

Diflunisal, see Nonsteroidal anti-inflammatory drugs

DIGITOXIN, with:
> **Aminoglutethimide** - See Aminoglutethimide with Digitoxin, page 29
> **Antifungals, Amphotericin B** - See Antifungals, Amphotericin B with Digitoxin, page 94
> **Antihistamines, H$_2$-blockers** - See Antihistamines, H$_2$-blockers with Digitoxin, page 117

(continued)

DIGITOXIN, with: *(continued)*

Barbiturates - See Barbiturates with Digitoxin, page 133

Cholestyramine - See Cholestyramine with Digitoxin, page 196

Diltiazem

Possible digitoxin toxicity (mechanism not established)

> J Kuhlmann, Effects of verapamil, diltiazem, and nifedipine on plasma levels and renal excretion of digitoxin. Clin Pharmacol Ther, 38:667, 1985

Monitor digitoxin concentration; not observed with nifedipine

Ethacrynic acid

Digitoxin toxicity (potassium and magnesium depletion)

> DC Brater and HF Morrelli, Digoxin toxicity in patients with normokalemic potassium depletion. Clin Pharmacol Ther, 22:21, 1977; E Steiness and KH Olesen, Cardiac arrhythmias induced by hypokalaemia and potassium loss during maintenance digoxin therapy. Br Heart J, 38:167, 1976

Monitor potassium and magnesium concentrations

Furosemide

Digitoxin toxicity (potassium and magnesium depletion)

> FJ Ascione, Digitalis glycosides with potassium-depleting diuretics. Drug Ther (Hosp), 7:5, 1977

Monitor potassium and magnesium concentrations

Macrolide antibiotics

Possible digitoxin toxicity with azithromycin (mechanism not established)

> F Thalhammer et al, Azithromycin-related toxic effects of digitoxin. Br J Clin Pharmacol, 45:91, 1998

Two case reports (1998); monitor digitoxin serum concentration and clinical status

Neuromuscular blocking agents

Increased incidence of arrhythmias (mechanism not established)

> EG Dowdy and LW Fabian, Ventricular arrhythmias induced by succinylcholine in digitalized patients: a preliminary report. Anesth Analg, 42:501, 1963; RS Bartolone and TLK Rao, Dysrhythmias following muscle relaxant administration in patients receiving digitalis. Anesthesiology, 58:567, 1983

Fewer arrhythmias with succinylcholine than with pancuronium; treat resulting arrhythmias with tubocurarine

Quinidine

Possible digitoxin toxicity (mechanism not established)

> J Kuhlmann et al, Effects of quinidine on pharmacokinetics and pharmacodynamics of digitoxin achieving steady-state conditions. Clin Pharmacol Ther, 39:288, 1986

Monitor digitoxin concentration

Rifampin

Decreased digitoxin effect (increased metabolism)

> G Boman et al, Acute cardiac failure during treatment with digitoxin – an interaction with rifampicin. Br J Clin Pharmacol, 10:89, 1980; DM Poor et al, Interaction of rifampin and digitoxin. Arch Intern Med, 143:599, 1983

Monitor digitoxin concentration

DIGITOXIN, with: *(continued)*

Tamoxifen

Possible digitoxin toxicity (mechanism not established)

M Middeke et al, Interaction between tamoxifen and digitoxin? Klin Wochenschr, 64:1211, 1986

Monitor digitoxin concentration

Thiazide diuretics

Digitoxin toxicity (potassium and magnesium depletion)

FJ Ascione, Digitalis glycosides with potassium-depleting diuretics. Drug Ther (Hosp), 7:5, 1977

Monitor potassium and magnesium concentrations

Verapamil

Possible digitoxin toxicity (mechanism not established)

J Kuhlmann, Effects of verapamil, diltiazem, and nifedipine on plasma levels and renal excretion of digitoxin. Clin Pharmacol Ther, 38:667, 1985; J Kuhlmann, Effects of quinidine, verapamil and nifedipine on the pharmacokinetics and pharmacodynamics of digitoxin during steady state conditions. Arzneimittelforschung, 37:545, 1987

Monitor digitoxin concentration; not observed with nifedipine

DIGOXIN, with:

Acarbose - See Acarbose with Digoxin, page 6

Adenosine - See Adenosine with Digoxin, page 11

Alkylating agents - See Alkylating agents with Digoxin, page 23

Aminoglycoside antibiotics - See Aminoglycoside antibiotics with Digoxin, page 30

Amiodarone - See Amiodarone with Digoxin, page 34

Antacids - See Antacids with Digoxin, page 52

Anticholinergics - See Anticholinergics with Digoxin, page 58

Antifungals, Amphotericin B - See Antifungals, Amphotericin B with Digoxin, page 94

Antifungals, imidazoles and triazoles - See Antifungals, imidazoles and triazoles with Digoxin, page 101

Antihistamines, H_2-blockers - See Antihistamines, H_2-blockers with Digoxin, page 117

Arbutamine - See Arbutamine with Digoxin, page 128

Benzodiazepines - See Benzodiazepines with Digoxin, page 141

Bepridil - See Bepridil with Digoxin, page 151

Beta-adrenergic blockers - See Beta-adrenergic blockers with Digoxin, page 154

Cholestyramine - See Cholestyramine with Digoxin, page 196

Colestipol - See Colestipol with Digoxin, page 211

Cyclosporine - See Cyclosporine with Digoxin, page 228

Diltiazem

Digoxin toxicity (decreased renal excretion)

WN Jones et al, Digoxin-diltiazem interaction: a pharmacokinetic evaluation. Eur J Clin Pharmacol, 31:351, 1986; M Andrejak et al, Diltiazem increases steady state digoxin serum levels in patients with cardiac disease. J Clin Pharmacol, 27:967, 1987

(continued)

DIGOXIN, with: *(continued)*
>   *Monitor clinical status and digoxin concentration; possibly increased digoxin concentration in studies of healthy volunteers*
>
> **Ethacrynic acid**
>   Digoxin toxicity (potassium and magnesium depletion)
> > FJ Ascione, Digitalis glycosides with potassium-depleting diuretics. Drug Ther (Hosp), 7:5, 1977
>
>   *Monitor potassium and magnesium concentrations*
>
> **Felodipine**
>   Possible digoxin toxicity (mechanism not established)
> > PHJM Dunselman et al, Digoxin-felodipine interaction in patients with congestive heart failure. Eur J Clin Pharmacol, 35:461, 1988
>
>   *Monitor digoxin concentration*
>
> **Flecainide**
>   Possible digoxin toxicity (possibly decreased metabolism)
> > CE Weeks et al, The effect of flecainide acetate, a new antiarrhythmic, on plasma digoxin levels. J Clin Pharmacol, 26:27, 1986
>
>   *Small effect; might be clinically significant at upper end of digoxin dosage range*
>
> **Fluoroquinolones**
>   Possible digoxin toxicity with gatifloxacin
> > Manufacturer's package insert (gatifloxacin)
>
>   *In one study in 3 of 11 healthy volunteers, digoxin concentrations increased significantly; monitor clinical status and digoxin concentration*
>
> **Furosemide**
>   Digoxin toxicity (potassium and magnesium depletion)
> > FJ Ascione, Digitalis glycosides with potassium-depleting diuretics. Drug Ther (Hosp), 7:5, 1977
>
>   *Monitor potassium and magnesium concentrations*
>
> **Ginseng**
>   Digoxin toxicity with Siberian ginseng (mechanism not established)
> > S McRae, Elevated serum digoxin levels in a patient taking digoxin and Siberian ginseng. Can Med Assoc J, 155:293, 1996
>
>   *Single well-documented case (1996); Siberian ginseng differs chemically from the Chinese variety*
>
> **HMG-CoA reductase inhibitors**
>   Possible modest decrease in digoxin effect with atorvastatin (mechanism not established)
> > RA Boyd et al, Atorvastatin coadministration may increase digoxin concentrations by inhibition of intestinal P-glycoprotein-mediated secretion. J Clin Pharmacol, 40:91, 2000
>
>   *Based on study in healthy subjects; effect relatively small; monitor clinical status*
>
> **Hydralazine**
>   Decreased digoxin effect with IV hydralazine (increased renal excretion)
> > JJ Cogan et al, Acute vasodilator therapy increases renal clearance of digoxin in patients with congestive heart failure. Circulation, 64:973, 1981

DIGOXIN, with: *(continued)*
  Monitor digoxin concentration
  Hydroxychloroquine
    Possible digoxin toxicity (mechanism not established)
      I Leden, Digoxin-hydroxychloroquine interaction? Acta Med Scand, 211:411, 1982
    Monitor digoxin concentration
  Hypoglycemics, sulfonylurea
    Possible digoxin toxicity (mechanism not established)
      G Pogatsa et al, Effect of various hypoglycaemic sulphonylureas on the cardiotoxicity of glycosides. Eur J Clin Pharmacol, 28:367, 1985
    Monitor digoxin concentration
  Isradipine
    Possible digoxin toxicity (possibly decreased metabolism)
      SM Rodin et al, Comparative effects of verapamil and isradipine on steady-state digoxin kinetics. Clin Pharmacol Ther, 43:668, 1988; BF Johnson et al, The comparative effects of verapamil and a new dihydropyridine calcium channel blocker on digoxin pharmacokinetics. Clin Pharmacol Ther, 42:66, 1987
    Clinical significance not established; based on studies in healthy men
  Kaolin or Kaolin-pectin
    Decreased digoxin effect (decreased absorption)
      MD Allen et al, Effect of magnesium-aluminum hydroxide and kaolin-pectin on absorption of digoxin from tablets and capsules. J Clin Pharmacol, 21:26, 1981
    Use digoxin capsules rather than tablets and monitor digoxin concentration
  Macrolide antibiotics
    Digoxin toxicity with clarithromycin and erythromycin (probable decreased hepatic and renal excretion; P-glycoprotein); possible decreased bacterial gut metabolism (less likely)
      J Lindenbaum et al, Inactivation of digoxin by the gut flora: reversal by antibiotic therapy. N Engl J Med, 305:789, 1981; SR Midoneck and OR Etingin, Clarithromycin-related toxic effects of digoxin. N Engl J Med, 333:1505, 1995; BA Brown et al, Clarithromycin-associated digoxin toxicity in the elderly. Clin Infect Dis, 24:92, 1997; JJ Nawarskas et al, Digoxin toxicity secondary to clarithromycin therapy. Ann Pharmacother, 31:864, 1997; S Nordt et al, Clarithromycin-induced digoxin poisoning. J Toxicol Clin Toxicol, 35:501, 1997; S Trivedi et al, Ann Intern Med, 128:604, 1998; H Wakasugi et al, Effect of clarithromycin on renal excretion of digoxin: interaction with P-glycoprotein. Clin Pharmacol Ther, 64:123, 1998; LL Lilley and R Guanci, A dangerous combination. Am J Nurs, 98:10, 1998; SR Letwin et al, Digoxin toxicity associated with clarithromycin-a "re-reminder". Can J Hosp Pharm, 51:273, 1998; MJ Gooderham et al, Concomitant digoxin toxicity and warfarin interaction in a patient receiving clarithromycin. Ann Pharmacother, 33:796, 1999; AP Ten Eick et al, Possible drug interaction between digoxin and azithromycin in a young child. Clin Drug Invest, 20:61, 2000

(continued)

DIGOXIN, with: *(continued)*
Monitor digoxin concentration and clinical status, or consider using an alternate non-macrolide antibiotic; single case report with azithromycin (2000)

Methyldopa

Sinus bradycardia (additive)

JC Davis et al, Sinus node dysfunction caused by methyldopa and digoxin. JAMA, 245:1241, 1981

Monitor heart rate

Metoclopramide

Possible decreased effect of digoxin tablets (decreased absorption)

BF Johnson et al, Effect of metoclopramide on digoxin absorption from tablets and capsules. Clin Pharmacol Ther, 36:724, 1984

Use digoxin capsules, which contain solution

Midodrine

Increased risk of bradycardia, AV block or arrhythmia (mechanism not established)

Manufacturer's package insert

Monitor cardiovascular status

Miglitol

Possible decreased digoxin effect (mechanism not established)

Manufacturer's package insert (miglitol)

Digoxin concentration decreased in study in healthy volunteers, but not in diabetic patients; clinical significance not established

Nefazodone

Possible digoxin toxicity (mechanism not established)

RC Dockens et al, Assessment of pharmacokinetic and pharmacodynamic drug interactions between nefazodone and digoxin in healthy male volunteers. J Clin Pharmacol, 36:160, 1996

Based on study in healthy men; monitor digoxin concentrations and clinical status

Neuromuscular blocking agents

Increased incidence of arrhythmias (mechanism not established)

EG Dowdy and LW Fabian, Ventricular arrhythmias induced by succinylcholine in digitalized patients: a preliminary report. Anesth Analg, 42:501, 1963; RS Bartolone and TLK Rao, Dysrhythmias following muscle relaxant administration in patients receiving digitalis. Anesthesiology, 58:567, 1983

Fewer arrhythmias with succinylcholine than with pancuronium; treat resulting arrhythmias with tubocurarine

Nifedipine

Possibility of both digoxin toxicity and decreased digoxin effect has been reported (mechanism not established)

JM De Vito and B Friedman, Evaluation of the pharmacodynamic and pharmacokinetic interaction between calcium antagonists and digoxin. Pharmacotherapy, 6:73, 1986

Clinical significance not established; monitor digoxin concentration

DIGOXIN, with: *(continued)*

Nitrates

Decreased digoxin effect with nitroprusside (increased renal excretion)

> JJ Cogan et al, Acute vasodilator therapy increases renal clearance of digoxin in patients with congestive heart failure. Circulation, 64:973, 1981

Monitor digoxin concentration

Nitrendipine

Digoxin toxicity (probably decreased metabolism)

> W Kirch et al, Nitrendipine/digoxin interaction. J Cardiovasc Pharmacol, 10 suppl 10:S74, 1987; W Kirch et al, Effect of two different doses of nitrendipine on steady-state plasma digoxin level and systolic time intervals. Eur J Clin Pharmacol, 31:391, 1986; R Ziegler et al, Study of pharmacokinetic and pharmacodynamic interaction between nitrendipine and digoxin. J Cardiovasc Pharmacol, 9 suppl 4:S101, 1987

Based on studies in healthy volunteers, one of whom developed toxicity

Nonsteroidal anti-inflammatory drugs

Possible digoxin toxicity with indomethacin in preterm infants and neonates (decreased renal excretion)

> G Koren et al, Effects of indomethacin on digoxin pharmacokinetics in preterm infants. Pediatr Pharmacol, 4:25, 1984; HS Jørgensen et al, Interaction between digoxin and indomethacin or ibuprofen. Br J Clin Pharmacol, 31:108, 1991; GM Haig and EG Brookfield, Increase in serum digoxin concentrations after indomethacin therapy in a full-term neonate. Pharmacotherapy, 12:334, 1992

Decrease digoxin dosage by 50% and monitor digoxin concentration; clinical significance in adults not established

Omeprazole

Possible digoxin toxicity (increased absorption)

> AF Cohen et al, Effects of gastric acidity on the bioavailability of digoxin. Evidence for a new mechanism for interactions with omeprazole. Br J Clin Pharmacol, 31:565P, 1991; M Hartmann et al, Lack of interaction between pantoprazole and digoxin at therapeutic doses in man. Int J Clin Pharmacol Ther, 33:481, 1995

Based on study in healthy young men; pantoprazole does not appear to affect digoxin

Penicillamine

Decreased digoxin effect (mechanism not established)

> B Moezzi et al, The effect of penicillamine on serum digoxin levels. Jpn Heart J, 19:366, 1978

Monitor digoxin concentration

Phenytoin

Decreased digoxin effect (increased metabolism)

> H Rameis, On the interaction between phenytoin and digoxin. Eur J Clin Pharmacol, 29:49, 1985

Monitor digoxin concentration

(continued)

DIGOXIN, with: *(continued)*

Prazosin
Possible digoxin toxicity (mechanism not established)
> S Copur et al, Effects of oral prazosin on total plasma digoxin levels. Fundam Clin Pharmacol, 2:13, 1988

Based on study in hypertensive patients

Procarbazine
Decreased digoxin effect (decreased intestinal absorption)
> TD Bjornsson et al, Effects of high-dose cancer chemotherapy on the absorption of digoxin in two different formulations. Clin Pharmacol Ther, 39:25, 1986

Clinical significance not established; monitor digoxin concentration

Propafenone
Possible digoxin toxicity (mechanism not established)
> E Zalzstein et al, Interaction between digoxin and propafenone in children. J Pediatr 116:310, 1990; M-C Bigot et al, Serum digoxin levels related to plasma propafenone levels during concomitant treatment. J Clin Pharmacol, 31:521, 1991

Monitor digoxin concentration

Quinidine
Possible digoxin toxicity (altered excretion; possibly P-glycoprotein; tissue binding)
> JT Bigger, Jr and EB Leahey, Jr, Quinidine and digoxin: an important interaction. Drugs, 24:229, 1982; MF Fromm et al, Inhibition of p-glycoprotein—mediated drug transport. A unifying mechanism to explain the interaction between digoxin and quinidine. Circulation, 99:552, 1999; I Rodriguez et al, P-glycoprotein in clinical cardiology. Circulation, 99:474, 1999

Monitor for signs of digoxin toxicity; digoxin concentration may not correlate with cardiac effects

> W Doering, The effect of coadministration of verapamil and quinidine on serum digoxin concentration. Eur J Clin Pharmacol, 25:517, 1983

Quinidine and verapamil may be synergistic in their effect on digoxin

> HI Bussey et al, The influence of rifampin on quinidine and digoxin. Arch Intern Med, 144:1021, 1984

Rifampin can increase the metabolism of both digoxin and quinidine, and either prevent or lessen the interaction or cause a decreased digoxin effect

> DJ Chapron et al, Apparent quinidine-induced digoxin toxicity after withdrawal of pentobarbital. A case of sequential drug interactions. Arch Intern Med, 139:363, 1979

Patients receiving barbiturates may not be affected unless the drugs are withdrawn, since barbiturates increase quinidine metabolism

> LB Polish et al, Digitoxin-quinidine interaction: potentiation during administration of cimetidine. South Med J, 74:633, 1981

The interaction may be potentiated by cimetidine, which inhibits quinidine metabolism

> PE Fenster et al, Digoxin-quinidine-spironolactone interaction. Clin

DIGOXIN, with: *(continued)*
>> Pharmacol Ther, 36:70, 1984
> *The effects of quinidine and spironolactone on digoxin may be additive*

Quinine
> Possible digoxin toxicity (mechanism not established)
>> KE Pedersen et al, Effect of quinine on plasma digoxin concentration and renal digoxin clearance. Acta Med Scand, 218:229, 1985
>
> *Monitor digoxin concentration*

Rabeprazole
> Possible digoxin toxicity (increased absorption)
>> Manufacturer's package insert (rabeprazole)
>
> *Based on study in normal subjects; monitor clinical status*

Rifampin
> Decreased digoxin effect (probably reduced bioavailability due to increased intestinal P-glycoprotein)
>> HI Bussey et al, The influence of rifampin on quinidine and digoxin. Arch Intern Med, 144:1021, 1984; H Gault et al, Digoxin-rifampin interaction. Clin Pharmacol Ther, 35:750, 1984; C Novi et al, Rifampin and digoxin: possible drug interaction in a dialysis patient. JAMA, 244:2521, 1980; B Greiner et al, The role of intestinal P-glycoprotein in the interaction of digoxin and rifampin. J Clin Invest, 104:147, 1999
>
> *Effect on digoxin may be increased in patients on dialysis; monitor digoxin concentration and clinical status*

Saint John's wort
> Possible decreased digoxin effect (probably induction of intestinal P-glycoprotein)
>> A Johne et al, Pharmacokinetic interaction of digoxin with an herbal extract from St. John's wort *(Hypericum perforatum)*. Clin Pharmacol Ther, 66:338, 1999
>
> *Based on study in healthy subjects; effect modest; monitor digoxin levels and clinical status*

Selective serotonin reuptake inhibitors (SSRIs)
> Possible digoxin toxicity with fluoxetine (mechanism not established)
>> A Leibovitz et al, Elevated serum digoxin level associated with coadministered fluoxetine. Arch Intern Med, 158:1152, 1998
>
> *Based on single case report (1998); monitor digoxin concentration and clinical status*

Spironolactone
> Possible digoxin toxicity (decreased renal clearance and possibly decreased metabolism)
>> PE Fenster et al, Digoxin-quinidine-spironolactone interaction. Clin Pharmacol Ther, 36:70, 1984; G Koren, Interaction between digoxin and commonly coadministered drugs in children. Pediatrics, 75:1032, 1985; A Hedman et al, Digoxin-interactions in man: Spironolactone reduces renal but not biliary digoxin clearance. Eur J Clin Pharmacol, 42:481, 1992

(continued)

DIGOXIN, with: *(continued)*

Monitor digoxin concentration; effects of spironolactone and quinidine on digoxin may be additive

Sucralfate

Decreased digoxin effect (possibly decreased absorption)

AM Rey and JG Gums, Altered absorption of digoxin, sustained-release quinidine, and warfarin with sucralfate administration. DICP Ann Pharmacother, 25:745, 1991

Single case report (1991); medications were taken 2 hours apart

Sulfonamides

Possible decreased digoxin effect with sulfasalazine (decreased absorption)

RP Juhl et al, Effect of sulfasalazine on digoxin bioavailability. Clin Pharmacol Ther, 20:387, 1976

Monitor digoxin concentration

Sympathomimetic amines

Increased tendency to cardiac arrhythmias (additive)

Manufacturer's package insert

Theoretical, but best to avoid concurrent use

Sympathomimetic bronchodilators

Possible digoxin toxicity with oral or IV albuterol (hypokalemia and possibly increase in intramyocardial digoxin concentration)

M Edner and T Jogestrand, Effect of salbutamol on digoxin concentration in serum and skeletal muscle. Eur J Clin Pharmacol, 36:235, 1989; M Edner and T Jogestrand, Oral salbutamol decreases serum digoxin concentration. Eur J Clin Pharmacol, 38:195, 1990; M Edner et al, Effect of salbutamol on digoxin pharmacokinetics. Eur J Clin Pharmacol, 42:197, 1992

Monitor cardiovascular status; digoxin concentration may be normal or low; based on studies in healthy men

Telmisartan

Possible digoxin toxicity

Manufacturer's package insert (telmisartan)

Monitor digoxin concentrations

Tetracyclines

Possible digoxin toxicity (decreased gut metabolism and increased absorption)

J Lindenbaum et al, Inactivation of digoxin by the gut flora: reversal by antibiotic therapy. N Engl J Med, 305:789, 1981

Monitor digoxin concentration

Thiazide diuretics

Digoxin toxicity (potassium and magnesium depletion)

FJ Ascione, Digitalis glycosides with potassium-depleting diuretics. Drug Ther (Hosp), 7:5, 1977; DC Brater and HF Morrelli, Digoxin toxicity in patients with normokalemic potassium depletion. Clin Pharmacol Ther, 22:21, 1977; E Steiness and KH Olesen, Cardiac arrhythmias induced by hypokalaemia and potassium loss during maintenance digoxin therapy. Br Heart J, 38:167, 1976

Monitor potassium and magnesium concentrations

DIGOXIN, with: *(continued)*

Torsemide
Possible increased toxicity with torsemide (mechanism not established)
   Manufacturer's package insert
Monitor clinical status

Trazodone
Digoxin toxicity (mechanism not established)
   PK Rauch and MA Jenike, Digoxin toxicity possibly precipitated by trazodone. Psychosomatics, 25:334, 1984
Single case report (1984)

Trimethoprim
Possible digoxin toxicity (decreased renal excretion and possibly decreased metabolism)
   P Petersen et al, Digoxin-trimethoprim interaction. Acta Med Scand, 217:423, 1985
Monitor for signs of digoxin toxicity; digoxin concentration may not correlate with cardiac effects

Vancomycin
Possible decreased digoxin effect (possibly decreased absorption)
   B Halawa, Interakcje digoksyny z cefradyna (Sefril), tetracyklina (Tetracyclinum), gentamycyna (Gentamycin) i wankomycyna (Vancocin). Pol Tyg Lek, 319:1717, 1984
Monitor digoxin concentration

Verapamil
Digoxin toxicity (probably decreased biliary excretion; inhibition P-glycoprotein)
   B Fichtl and W Doering, The quinidine-digoxin interaction in perspective. Clin Pharmacokinet, 8:137, 1983; I Maragno et al, Verapamil-induced changes in digoxin kinetics in cirrhosis. Eur J Clin Pharmacol, 32:309, 1987; A Hedman et al, Digoxin-verapamil interaction: reduction of biliary but not renal digoxin clearance in humans. Clin Pharmacol Ther, 49:256, 1991; M Verschraagen et al, P-glycoprotein system as a determinant of drug interactions: the case of digoxin-verapamil. Pharmacol Res, 40:301, 1999
Monitor digoxin concentration; quinidine and verapamil may be synergistic in their effect on digoxin; cirrhosis may increase likelihood of toxicity

Vincristine
Decreased digoxin effect (decreased intestinal absorption)
   TD Bjornsson et al, Effects of high-dose cancer chemotherapy on the absorption of digoxin in two different formulations. Clin Pharmacol Ther, 39:25, 1986
Clinical significance not established; monitor digoxin concentration

DIGOXIN IMMUNE FAB, with:

Anticoagulants, oral - See Anticoagulants, oral with Digoxin immune Fab, page 65

Dihydrocodeine, see Narcotics: morphine-like

Dihydroergotamine, see Ergot alkaloids

Dihydrotachysterol, see Vitamin D

Dihydroxyaluminum, see Antacids
DILTIAZEM, with:
  Amiodarone - See Amiodarone with Diltiazem, page 35
  Angiotensin-converting enzyme (ACE) inhibitors - See Angiotensin-converting enzyme (ACE) inhibitors with Diltiazem, page 44
  Antidepressants, tricyclic - See Antidepressants, tricyclic with Diltiazem, page 85
  Antihistamines, H$_2$-blockers - See Antihistamines, H$_2$-blockers with Diltiazem, page 117
  Benzodiazepines - See Benzodiazepines with Diltiazem, page 141
  Beta-adrenergic blockers - See Beta-adrenergic blockers with Diltiazem, page 154
  Buspirone - See Buspirone with Diltiazem, page 170
  Carbamazepine - See Carbamazepine with Diltiazem, page 178
  Cilostazol - See Cilostazol with Diltiazem, page 198
  Corticosteroids - See Corticosteroids with Diltiazem, page 220
  Cyclosporine - See Cyclosporine with Diltiazem, page 228
  Digitoxin - See Digitoxin with Diltiazem, page 250
  Digoxin - See Digoxin with Diltiazem, page 251
  Enflurane
    Cardiac arrhythmias (possibly additive)
      CB Hantler et al, Impaired myocardial conduction in patients receiving diltiazem therapy during enflurane anesthesia. Anesthesiology, 67:94, 1987
    Single case reports of sinus arrest and impaired A-V conduction (1987)
  HMG-COA Reductase Inhibitors
    Possible lovastatin or simvastatin toxicity (decreased metabolism; CYP3A4)
      NE Azie et al, The interaction of diltiazem with lovastatin and pravastatin. Clin Pharmacol Ther, 64:369, 1998; DR Jones et al, Oral but not intravenous (IV) diltiazem impairs lovastatin clearance. Clin Pharmacol Ther, 65:149, 1999; PJK Gruer et al, Concomitant use of cytochrome P450 3A4 inhibitors and simvastatin. Am J Cardiol, 84:811, 1999; KR Yeo et al, Enhanced cholesterol reduction by simvastatin in diltiazem-treated patients. Br J Clin Pharmacol, 48:610, 1999; O Mousa et al, The interaction of diltiazem with simvastatin. Clin Pharmacol Ther, 67:267, 2000
    Incidence probably low, but unpredictable; avoid concurrent use or if combination is used monitor creatine phosphokinase (CPK) for signs of rhabdomyolysis (muscle pain, weakness or dark urine); pravastatin not affected, and fluvastatin unlikely to interact (neither is metabolized by CYP3A4); IV diltiazem does not interact with lovastatin
  Insulin
    Decreased insulin effect (mechanism not established)
      HA Pershadsingh et al, Association of diltiazem therapy with increased insulin resistance in a patient with type I diabetes mellitus. JAMA, 257:930, 1987
    Single case report (1987)
  Lithium
    Parkinsonism (possibly additive)
      EF Binder et al, Diltiazem-induced psychosis and a possible diltiazem-lithium interaction. Arch Intern Med, 151:373, 1991

DILTIAZEM, with: *(continued)*

Two cases (1985,1991); poorly documented interaction

Moricizine

Possible moricizine toxicity and decreased diltiazem effect (probably decreased and increased metabolism, respectively)

> L Shum et al, Pharmacokinetic interactions of moricizine and diltiazem in healthy volunteers. J Clin Pharmacol, 36:1161, 1996

Based on study in healthy subjects; monitor clinical status

Narcotics: meperidine and congeners

Possible prolonged alfentanil effect (probably decreased metabolism)

> J Ahonen et al, Effect of diltiazem on midazolam and alfentanil disposition in patients undergoing coronary artery bypass grafting. Anesthesiology, 85:1246, 1996

Monitor clinical status

Nifedipine

Possible nifedipine or diltiazem toxicity (decreased metabolism)

> K Ohashi et al, Effects of diltiazem on the pharmacokinetics of nifedipine. J Cardiovasc Pharmacol, 15:96, 1990; T Tateishi et al, The effect of nifedipine on the pharmacokinetics and dynamics of diltiazem: the preliminary study in normal volunteers. J Clin Pharmacol, 33:738, 1993

Monitor nifedipine concentration; based on studies in healthy men (1993)

Nitrates

Hypotension with nitroglycerin (additive)

> RA Bruce et al, Excessive reduction in peripheral resistance during exercise and risk of orthostatic symptoms with sustained-release nitroglycerin and diltiazem treatment of angina. Am Heart J, 109:1020, 1985

One study with sustained-release nitroglycerin; avoid concurrent use

Quinidine

Possible quinidine toxicity (decreased metabolism)

> S Laganière et al, Pharmacokinetic and pharmacodynamic interactions between diltiazem and quinidine. Clin Pharmacol Ther, 60:255, 1996

Based on study in healthy subjects; monitor clinical status and quinidine concentration

Rifampin

Decreased diltiazem effect (increased metabolism)

> KD Drda et al, Effects of debrisoquine hydroxylation phenotype and enzyme induction with rifampin on diltiazem pharmacokinetics and pharmacodynamics. Pharmacotherapy, 11:278, 1991 abs 97; H Fujino et al, A case of refractory spastic angina with reduction of bioavailability of diltiazem by rifampin. Shinzo Heart, 26:732, 1994

Based on study in healthy subjects and a single case report (1994); monitor clinical response or diltiazem concentration

Sirolimus

Possible sirolimus toxicity (possible decreased metabolism)

> Manufacturer's package insert (sirolimus)

Monitor sirolimus concentrations

(continued)

DILTIAZEM, with: *(continued)*
  Tacrolimus
    Possible tacrolimus toxicity (decreased metabolism; CYP3A4; decreased P-glycoprotein transport)
      MF Hebert and AY Lam, Diltiazem increases tacrolimus concentrations. Ann Pharmacother, 33:680, 1999
    Single well documented case report (1999); avoid concurrent use or monitor tacrolimus concentration and clinical status
  Theophyllines
    Possible theophylline toxicity (decreased metabolism)
      K Ohashi et al, Effects of diltiazem and cimetidine on theophylline oxidative metabolism. J Clin Pharmacol, 33:1233, 1993
    Clinical significance not established

Dimenhydrinate, no documented interactions, see page 4, Criteria for Listing Interactions

DIMETHYL SULFOXIDE, with:
  Nonsteroidal anti-inflammatory drugs
    Peripheral neuropathy with sulindac (mechanism not established)
      BN Swanson et al, Peripheral neuropathy after concomitant administration of dimethyl sulfoxide and sulindac. Arthritis Rheum, 26:791, 1983; L Reinstein et al, Peripheral neuropathy after concomitant dimethyl sulfoxide use and sulindac therapy. Arch Phys Med Rehabil, 63:581, 1982
    Avoid concurrent use

    Decreased anti-inflammatory effect with sulindac (decreased formation of active metabolites)
      BN Swanson et al, Dimethyl sulfoxide inhibits bioactivation of sulindac. J Lab Clin Med, 102:95, 1983
    Avoid concurrent use

Diphenadione, see Anticoagulants, oral

Diphenhydramine, see Antihistamines, H_1-blockers: Diphenhydramine

Diphtheria-tetanus-acellular pertussis vaccine, no documented interactions, see page 4, Criteria for Listing Interactions

Diphtheria-tetanus-pertussis vaccine, no documented interactions, see page 4, Criteria for Listing Interactions

Dipivefrin, see Sympathomimetic amines

DIPYRIDAMOLE, with:
  Adenosine - See Adenosine with Dipyridamole, page 12
  Anticoagulants, oral - See Anticoagulants, oral with Dipyridamole, page 65
  Caffeine - See Caffeine with Dipyridamole, page 173
  Nonsteroidal anti-inflammatory drugs
    Water retention with indomethacin (mechanism not established)
      P Seideman et al, Additive renal effects of indomethacin and dipyridamole in man. Br J Clin Pharmacol, 23:323, 1987
    Monitor for edema

Dirithromycin, see Macrolide antibiotics

DISOPYRAMIDE, with:

Amrinone - See Amrinone with Disopyramide, page 40

Anticoagulants, oral - See Anticoagulants, oral with Disopyramide, page 65

Beta-adrenergic blockers - See Beta-adrenergic blockers with Disopyramide, page 154

Cyclosporine - See Cyclosporine with Disopyramide, page 229

Macrolide antibiotics

Disopyramide toxicity with erythromycin or clarithromycin (probably decreased metabolism)

> M Ragosta et al, Potentially fatal interaction between erythromycin and disopyramide. Am J Med, 86:465, 1989; T Kawamoto et al, A case of Torsade de pointes occurred by interaction between erythromycin and disopyramide. Shinzo Heart, 25:696, 1993; D Paar et al, Life-threatening interaction between clarithromycin and disopyramide. Lancet, 349:326, 1997; H Iida et al, Hypoglycemia induced by interaction between clarithromycin and disopyramide. Jpn Heart J. 40:91, 1999; N Morlet-Barla et al, Hypoglycémie grave et récidivante secondaire à l'interaction disopyramide-clarithromicine. Presse Med, 29:1351, 2000

Case reports of both cardiac arrhythmias and severe hypoglycemia; avoid concurrent use

Neuromuscular blocking agents

Prolonged neuromuscular blockade with vecuronium (possibly additive)

> M Baurain et al, Impairment of the antagonism of vecuronium-induced paralysis and intra-operative disopyramide administration. Anaesthesia, 44:34, 1989

Single case report (1989)

Nitrates

Decreased nitrate effect (failure to dissolve)

> LJ Robbins, Dry mouth and delayed dissolution of sublingual nitroglycerin. N Engl J Med, 309:985, 1983

Single case report with isosorbide dinitrate (1985) and nitroglycerin (1983); disopyramide caused dry mouth

Phenytoin

Decreased disopyramide effect and toxicity (increase in toxic metabolite)

> J Nightingale and JM Nappi, Effect of phenytoin on serum disopyramide concentrations. Clin Pharm, 6:46, 1987

Avoid concurrent use, if possible

Rifampin

Decreased disopyramide effect (probably increased metabolism)

> M-L Aitio et al, The effect of enzyme induction on the metabolism of disopyramide in man. Br J Clin Pharmacol, 11:279, 1981

Avoid concurrent use, if possible

DISULFIRAM, with:

Alcohol - See Alcohol with Disulfiram, page 17

Anticoagulants, oral - See Anticoagulants, oral with Disulfiram, page 65

Antidepressants, tricyclic - See Antidepressants, tricyclic with Disulfiram, page 85

(continued)

DISULFIRAM, with: *(continued)*
  Benzodiazepines - See Benzodiazepines with Disulfiram, page 142
  Caffeine - See Caffeine with Disulfiram, page 173
  Chlorzoxazone - See Chlorzoxazone with Disulfiram, page 195
  Cocaine - See Cocaine with Disulfiram, page 209
  Isoniazid
    Psychotic episodes, ataxia (altered dopamine metabolism)
      HG Whittington and L Grey, Possible interaction between disulfiram and isoniazid. Am J Psychiatry, 125:1725, 1969
    Avoid concurrent use
  Marijuana, smoking
    Psychotic episode (mechanism not established)
      RB Lacoursiere and R Swatek, Adverse interaction between disulfiram and marijuana: a case report. Am J Psychiatry, 140:243, 1983
    Single case report (1983)
  Metronidazole
    Organic brain syndrome (mechanism not established)
      WW Goodhue, Jr, Disulfiram-metronidazole (well identified) toxicity. N Engl J Med, 280:1482, 1969; E Rothstein and DD Clancy, Disulfiram-metronidazole (continued). N Engl J Med, 281:331, 1969
    Avoid concurrent use
  Omeprazole
    Confusion, catatonic reaction, and disorientation (mechanism not established)
      R Hajela et al, Catatonic reaction to omeprazole and disulfiram in a patient with alcohol dependence. Can Med Assoc J, 143:1207, 1990
    Single well-documented case report (1990)
  Phenothiazines
    Decreased perphenazine effect (increased hepatic metabolism)
      LB Hansen and N-E Larsen, Metabolic interaction between perphenazine and disulfiram. Lancet, 2:1472, 1982
    Avoid concurrent use or give perphenazine parenterally
  Phenytoin
    Possible phenytoin toxicity (decreased metabolism)
      DJ Birkett et al, Multiple drug interactions with phenytoin. Med J Aust, 2:467, 1977; JG Solomon, Drug interactions on an alcohol unit. Va Med, 109:220, 1981
    Avoid concurrent use, if possible
  Theophyllines
    Possible theophylline toxicity (possibly decreased metabolism)
      C-M Loi et al, Dose-dependent inhibition of theophylline metabolism by disulfiram in recovering alcoholics. Clin Pharmacol Ther, 45:476, 1989
    Monitor theophylline concentration
Divalproex sodium, see Valproate
DMSO, see Dimethyl sulfoxide
Dobutamine, see Sympathomimetic amines
Docetaxel, no documented interactions, see page 4, Criteria for Listing Interactions
Docosanol, no documented interactions, see page 4, Criteria for Listing Interactions

Docusate sodium, no documented interactions, see page 4, Criteria for Listing Interactions

DOFETILIDE, with:

Amiodarone - See Amiodarone with Dofetilide, page 35

Antidepressants, tricyclic - See Antidepressants, tricyclic with Dofetilide, page 85

Antifungals, imidazoles and triazoles - See Antifungals, imidazoles and triazoles with Dofetilide, page 101

Antihistamines, H$_2$-blockers - See Antihistamines, H$_2$-blockers with Dofetilide, page 117

Bepridil - See Bepridil with Dofetilide, page 151

Beta-adrenergic blockers - See Beta-adrenergic blockers with Dofetilide, page 154

Cisapride - See Cisapride with Dofetilide, page 199

Macrolide antibiotics

Increased risk of arrhythmias (additive effect on QTc interval)
Manufacturer's package insert (dofetilide)
Avoid concurrent use

Megestrol acetate

Increased risk of arrhythmias (decreased renal excretion of dofetilide)
Manufacturer's package insert (dofetilide)
Avoid concurrent use

Phenothiazines

Increased risk of arrhythmias with prochlorperazine (decreased renal excretion of dofetilide)
Manufacturer's package insert (dofetilide)
Avoid concurrent use

Trimethoprim

Increased risk of arrhythmias (decreased renal excretion of dofetilide)
Manufacturer's package insert (dofetilide)
Avoid concurrent use

Trimethoprim-sulfamethoxazole

Increased risk of arrhythmias (decreased renal excretion of dofetilide)
Manufacturer's package insert (dofetilide)
Avoid concurrent use

Verapamil

Increased risk of arrhythmias (decreased renal excretion of dofetilide)
Manufacturer's package insert (dofetilide)
Avoid concurrent use

DOLASETRON, with:

Antihistamines, H$_2$-blockers - See Antihistamines, H$_2$-blockers with Dolasetron, page 117

Beta-adrenergic blockers - See Beta-adrenergic blockers with Dolasetron, page 155

Rifampin

Possible decreased dolasetron effect (increased metabolism)
Manufacturer's package insert
Theoretical; monitor clinical status

(continued)

DOLASETRON, with: *(continued)*
  Verapamil
    Possible increased risk of cardiac conduction abnormalities (probably additive)
        Manufacturer's package insert
    Single case reported to manufacturer; monitor cardiac status

Domperidone, no documented interactions, see page 4, Criteria for Listing Interactions

DONEPEZIL, with:
  Antifungals, Imidazoles and Triazoles - See Antifungals, Imidazoles and Triazoles with Donepezil, page 101
  Neuromuscular blocking agents
    Potentially prolongs succinylcholine effects (decreased metabolism)
        G Lane, Potential donepezil - succinylcholine interaction. Can J Hosp Pharm, 51:272, 1998; manufacturers package insert
    Monitor clinical status or use non-depolarizing muscle relaxant if possible
  Risperidone
    Parkinsonism (possibly additive)
        TM Magnuson et al, Extrapyramidal side effects in a patient treated with risperidone plus donepezil. Am J Psychiatry, 155:1458, 1998
    Single case report (1998)
  Selective serotonin reuptake inhibitors (SSRIs)
    Possible donepezil toxicity with paroxetine (possible decreased metabolism
        L Carrier, Donepezil and paroxetine: possible drug interaction. J Am Geriatr Soc, 47:1037, 1999
    Two case reports (1999); monitor clinical status

DONG QUAI, with:
  Anticoagulants, oral - See Anticoagulants, oral with Dong Quai, page 65

Dopamine, see Sympathomimetic amines

Dorzolamide, no documented interactions, see page 4, Criteria for Listing Interactions

DOXAPRAM, with:
  Neuromuscular blocking agents
    Prolonged neuromuscular blockade with vecuronium (mechanism not established)
        R Cooper et al, Effect of doxapram on the rate of recovery from atracurium and vecuronium neuromuscular block. Br J Anaesth, 68:527, 1992
    Clinical significance not established

Doxazosin, no documented interactions, see page 4, Criteria for Listing Interactions

Doxepin, see Antidepressants, tricyclic

DOXORUBICIN, with:
  Cyclosporine - See Cyclosporine with Doxorubicin, page 229
  Streptozocin
    Doxorubicin toxicity (decreased hepatic inactivation and excretion)
        P Chang et al, Combination chemotherapy with adriamycin [doxorubicin] and streptozotocin. Clin Pharmacol Ther, 20:611, 1976
    Monitor doxorubicin concentration

Doxycycline, see Tetracyclines

Doxylamine, no documented interactions, see page 4, Criteria for Listing Interactions

Dromostanolone, see Anabolic and androgenic steroids

Dronabinol, no documented interactions, see page 4, Criteria for Listing Interactions

D-tubocurarine, see Neuromuscular blocking agents

DROPERIDOL, with:

  Cyclobenzaprine - See Cyclobenzaprine with Droperidol, page 226

  Lithium

    Neuroleptic malignant syndrome (mechanism not established)

      JS Bamrah, Neuroleptic-induced pyrexia. A benign variant. J Nerv Ment Dis, 176:741, 1988

    Single case report (1991)

Dyphylline, see Theophyllines

Econazole, no documented interactions, see page 4, Criteria for Listing Interactions

Edetate disodium, no documented interactions, see page 4, Criteria for Listing Interactions

Edrophonium, see Anticholinesterases

EFAVIRENZ, with:

  Amprenavir - See Amprenavir with Efavirenz, page 39

  Anticoagulants, oral - See Anticoagulants, oral with Efavirenz, page 66

  Antihistamines, H$_1$-blockers: astemizole, terfenadine - See Antihistamines, H$_1$-blockers: astemizole, terfenadine with Efavirenz, page 110

  Benzodiazepines - See Benzodiazepines with Efavirenz, page 142

  Cisapride - See Cisapride with Efavirenz, page 199

  Contraceptives, oral - See Contraceptives, oral with Efavirenz, page 213

  Ergot alkaloids

    Possible ergotism (decreased metabolism)

      Manufacturer's package insert (efavirenz)

    Manufacturer recommends avoiding concurrent use; theoretical

  Indinavir

    Decreased indinavir effect (increased metabolism)

      Manufacturer's package insert (efavirenz)

    The manufacturer recommends increasing indinavir dose from 800 mg to 1000 mg every 8 hours

  Lopinavir/Ritonavir

    Decreased lopinavir effect (increased metabolism)(*Kaletra*)

      Manufacturer's package insert (*Kaletra*)

    Manufacturer recommends increasing Kaletra dose to 533/133 mg bid with food

  Macrolide antibiotics

    Possible decreased clarithromycin effect; possible increased risk of skin rash (probably increased metabolism)

      Manufacturer's package insert (efavirenz)

    Clinical importance not established; monitor clinical status; azithromycin may not interact

(continued)

EFAVIRENZ, with: *(continued)*

Narcotics: methadone and congeners

Decreased methadone concentrations (increased metabolism)

K Tashima et al, The potential impact of efavirenz on methadone maintenance. 9th European Conference of Clinical Microbiology, Berlin, Germany, 1999, Poster P0552; S Clarke et al, The Pharmacokinetics and tolerability of methadone and efavirenz in injecting drug users with HIV infection. 7th European Conference on Clinical Aspects and Treatment of HIV-infection, Lisbon, Portugal, 1999, abstract 1210; V Pinzani et al, Methadone withdrawal symptoms with nevirapine and efavirenz. Ann Pharmacother, 34:405, 2000; C Marzolini, Efavirenz decreases methadone blood concentrations. AIDS, 14:1291, 2000

Possible withdrawal symptoms; monitor clinical status and increase methadone dose as needed

Rifampin

Possible decreased efavirenz effect (increased metabolism)

Manufacturer's package insert (efavirenz)

Based on study in healthy subjects; clinical significance not established

Saquinavir

Decreased saquinavir effect (increased metabolism)

Manufacturer's package insert (efavirenz)

Based on study in healthy subjects; add an additional protease inhibitor

Effervescent analgesics, see Citrates

Eflornithine, no documented interactions, see page 4, Criteria for Listing Interactions

Enalapril, see Angiotensin-converting enzyme (ACE) inhibitors

Enalaprilat, see Angiotensin-converting enzyme (ACE) inhibitors

ENCAINIDE, with:

Antihistamines, H_2-blockers - See Antihistamines, H_2-blockers with Encainide, page 117

Quinidine

Possible encainide toxicity (decreased metabolism in extensive metabolizers)

C Funck-Brentano et al, Effect of low dose quinidine on encainide pharmacokinetics and pharmacodynamics. Influence of genetic polymorphism. J Pharmacol Exp Ther, 249:134, 1989; J Turgeon et al, Genetically determined steady-state interaction between encainide and quinidine in patients with arrhythmias. J Pharmacol Exp Ther, 255:642, 1990

Based on study in healthy men; monitor encainide concentration or ECG; in patients no adverse effects, but enhanced therapeutic effect was observed

Ritonavir

Possible encainide toxicity (decreased metabolism)

Manufacturer's package insert (ritonavir)

Theoretical considerations; listed as contraindicated in product information

ENFLURANE, with:

Aminoglycoside antibiotics - See Aminoglycoside antibiotics with Enflurane, page 31

ENFLURANE, with: *(continued)*

Amiodarone - See Amiodarone with Enflurane, page 35

Angiotensin-converting enzyme (ACE) inhibitors - See Angiotensin-converting enzyme (ACE) inhibitors with Enflurane, page 44

Diltiazem - See Diltiazem with Enflurane, page 260

Guanethidine

Hypotension (additive)
> Manufacturer's package insert

Monitor blood pressure

Isoniazid

Possible nephrotoxicity (increased fluoride concentration derived from enflurane metabolism)
> RI Mazze et al, Isoniazid-induced enflurane defluorination in humans. Anesthesiology, 57:5, 1982

Avoid concurrent use; large variation in individual response

Narcotics: meperidine and congeners

Possible narcotic toxicity with fentanyl (decreased metabolism)
> KA Lehmann et al, Biotransformation of fentanyl II. Acute drug interactions in rats and men. Anaesthesist, 31:221, 1982

Monitor closely

Phenothiazines

Possible increase in risk of seizures with chlorpromazine
> SB Vohra, Convulsions after enflurane in a schizophrenic patient receiving neuroleptics. Can J Anaesth, 41:5, 1994

Single case report (1994)

Enoxacin, see Fluoroquinolones

Enoxaparin, no documented interactions, see page 4, Criteria for Listing Interactions

ENTACAPONE, with:

Bitolterol - See Bitolterol with Entacapone, page 166

Methyldopa

Possible tachycardia and hypertension (decreased metabolism; COMT)
> Manufacturer's package insert (entacapone)

Avoid concurrent use

Monoamine oxidase inhibitors

Possible cardiovascular toxicity (decreased metabolism; COMT and monoamine oxidase)
> Manufacturer's package insert (entacapone)

Avoid concurrent use; selegiline, an MAO-B inhibitor, does not appear to interact

Sympathomimetic amines

Tachycardia (mechanism not established)
> Manufacturer's package insert (entacapone)

Heart rate increased 50% with isoproterenol and 80% with epinephrine; ventricular tacycardia was reported in one healthy male volunteer

(continued)

ENTACAPONE, with: *(continued)*
   Sympathomimetic bronchodilators
      Tachycardia (mechanism not established)
         Manufacturer's package insert (entacapone)
      Heart rate increased 50% with isoproterenol and 80% with epinephrine; ventricular tacycardia was reported in one healthy male volunteer

Ephedrine, see Sympathomimetic amines; Sympathomimetic bronchodilators
Epinephrine, see Sympathomimetic amines; Sympathomimetic bronchodilators
EPIRUBICIN, with:
   Antihistamines, H$_2$-blockers - See Antihistamines, H$_2$-blockers with Epirubicin, page 117

EPOETIN, with:
   Anabolic and androgenic steroids - See Anabolic and androgenic steroids with Epoetin, page 41
   Angiotensin-converting enzyme (ACE) inhibitors - See Angiotensin-converting enzyme (ACE) inhibitors with Epoetin, page 44
   Interferon
      Decreased epoetin effect with interferon alpha (mechanism not established)
         RG Desai, Drug interaction between alpha interferon and erythropoietin. J Clin Oncol, 9:893, 1991; M Nordio et al, Interaction between α-interferon and erythropoietin in antiviral and antineoplastic therapy in uraemic patients on haemodialysis. Nephrol Dial Transplant, 8(11):1308, 1993
      Several case reports (1991,1992)
   Valproate
      Epoetin unresponsiveness (marrow suppression due to valproate toxicity)
         C Sungur et al, Unresponsiveness to human recombinant erythropoietin in an epileptic dialysis patient secondary to valproic acid toxicity. Ann Pharmacother, 26:1156, 1992
      Report of single patient on dialysis (1992); monitor valproate concentration - valproate is dialysed poorly

Epoprostenol, no documented interactions, see page 4, Criteria for Listing Interactions
Eprosartan, no documented interactions, see page 4, Criteria for Listing Interactions
EPTIFIBATIDE, with:
   Thrombolytics
      Increased bleeding (additive)
         Manufacturer's package insert (eptifibatide)
      Monitor prothrombin time

Ergocalciferol, see Vitamin D
Ergoloid Mesylates, see Ergot alkaloids
Ergonovine, see Ergot alkaloids
ERGOT ALKALOIDS, with:
   Amprenavir - See Amprenavir with Ergot alkaloids, page 39
   Antidepressants, tricyclic - See Antidepressants, tricyclic with Ergot alkaloids, page 85

ERGOT ALKALOIDS, with: *(continued)*

Beta-adrenergic blockers - See Beta-adrenergic blockers with Ergot alkaloids, page 155

Efavirenz - See Efavirenz with Ergot alkaloids, page 267

Indinavir

Ergotism (decreased metabolism; probably CYP3A4)

E Rosenthal et al, Ergotism related to concurrent administration of ergotamine tartrate and indinavir. JAMA, 281:987, 1999

Single case report with ergotamine (1999); avoid concurrent use

Lopinavir/Ritonavir

Acute ergot toxicity (decreased metabolism)

Manufacturer's package insert (*Kaletra*)

Avoid concurrent use

Macrolide antibiotics

Ergot toxicity with erythromycin (mechanism not established)

H Francis et al, Severe vascular spasm due to erythromycin – ergotamine interaction. Clin Rheumatol, 3:243, 1984; R Ghali et al, Erythromycin-associated ergotamine intoxication: arteriographic and electrophysiologic analysis of a rare cause of severe ischemia of the lower extremities and associated ischemic neuropathy. Ann Vasc Surg, 7:291, 1993

Avoid concurrent use

Ritonavir

Ergotism (decreased metabolism; probably CYP3A4)

FJ Caballero-Granado et al, Ergotism related to concurrent administration of ergotamine tartrate and ritonavir in an AIDS patient. Antimicrob Agents Chemother, 41:1207, 1997; L Liaudet et al, Severe ergotism associated with interaction between ritonavir and ergotamine. BMJ, 318:771, 1999; A Montero et al, Leg ischemia in a patient receiving ritonavir and ergotamine. Ann Intern Med, 130:329, 1999

Three case reports with ergotamine (1997, 1999); avoid concurrent use

Selective serotonin reuptake inhibitors (SSRIs)

Serotonin syndrome (additive)

NT Mathew et al, Serotonin syndrome complicating migraine pharmacotherapy. Cephalalgia, 16:323, 1996

Single case report (1996)

Sibutramine

Possible serotonin syndrome (additive serotonergic effect)

Manufacturer's package insert

Avoid concurrent use

Sympathomimetic amines

Gangrene with dopamine (additive)

N Buchanan et al, Symmetrical gangrene of the extremities associated with use of dopamine subsequent to ergometrine administration. Intensive Care Med, 3:55, 1977

Avoid concurrent use

(continued)

ERGOT ALKALOIDS, with: *(continued)*
   Triptans
   Possible excessive vasoconstriction (additive)
   Manufacturer's package insert; H Liston et al, The association of the combination of sumatriptan and methysergide in myocardial infarction in a premenopausal woman. Arch Intern Med, 159:511, 1999
   Single case report of myocardial infarction with sumatriptan and methysergide (1999); avoid concurrent use within 24 hours
   Troleandomycin
   Ergot toxicity (mechanism not established)
   AC Hayton, Precipitation of acute ergotism by triacetyloleandomycin. N Z Med J, 69:42, 1969; PhY Baudouy et al, Infarctus du myocarde provoqué par l'association tartrate d'ergotamine-troléandomycine. Rev Med Interne, 9:420, 1988
   Avoid concurrent use
Ergotamine, see Ergot alkaloids
Erythrityl tetranitrate, see Nitrates
Erythromycins, see Macrolide antibiotics
Erythropoietin, see Epoetin
Esmolol, see Beta-adrenergic blockers
Estazolam, see Benzodiazepines
Estradiol, see Estrogens
ESTROGENS, with:
   Antidepressants, tricyclic - See Antidepressants, tricyclic with Estrogens, page 85
   Corticosteroids - See Corticosteroids with Estrogens, page 220
   Grapefruit juice
   Increased ethinyl estradiol and 17β-estradiol effect (probably decreased first pass metabolism)
   W Schubert et al, Inhibition of 17β-estradiol metabolism by grapefruit juice in ovariectomized women. Maturitas, 20:155, 1995; A Weber et al, Can grapefruit juice influence ethinylestradiol bioavailability? Contraception, 53:41, 1996
   Based on studies in healthy subjects; clinical significance not established
   Phenytoin
   Decreased estrogen effect (increased metabolism)
   M Notelovitz et al, Interaction between estrogen and Dilantin in a menopausal woman. N Engl J Med, 304:788, 1981
   Monitor for symptoms of estrogen deficiency
   Raloxifene
   Possible alteration in estrogen effect (mechanism not established)
   Manufacturer's package insert
   Avoid concurrent use until clinical data are available
   Ropinirole
   Possible ropinirole toxicity with ethinyl estradiol (mechanism not established)
   Manufacturer's package insert
   Avoid concurrent use; effect of other estrogens unknown

ESTROGENS, with: *(continued)*

Tacrine

Increased tacrine effect (probably decreased metabolism; CYP1A2)

K Laine et al, Plasma tacrine concentrations are significantly increased by concomitant hormone replacement therapy. Clin Pharmacol Ther, 66:602, 1999

Based on study in healthy women taking hormone replacement therapy; monitor clinical status

Tobacco, smoking

Possible decreased estrogen effect (increased metabolism)

J Jensen et al, Cigarette smoking, serum estrogens, and bone loss during hormone-replacement therapy early after menopause. N Engl J Med, 313:973, 1985; DL Cassidenti et al, Short-term effects of smoking on the pharmacokinetic profiles of micronized estradiol in postmenopausal women. Am J Obstet Gynecol, 163:1953, 1990

Avoid concurrent use

Vitamin C

Increased serum concentration and possible toxicity of estrogens with 1 gram/day of vitamin C (decreased metabolism)

DJ Back et al, Interaction of ethinyloestradiol with ascorbic acid in man. Br Med J, 282:1516, 1981; MH Briggs, Megadose vitamin C and metabolic effects of the pill. Br Med J, 283:1547, 1981; JC Morris et al, Interaction of ethinyloestradiol with ascorbic acid in man. Br Med J, 283:503, 1981

Decrease vitamin C to 100 mg/day

Estrone, see Estrogens

Estropipate, see Estrogens

Etanercept, no documented interactions, see page 4, Criteria for Listing Interactions

ETHACRYNIC ACID, with:

Aminoglycoside antibiotics - See Aminoglycoside antibiotics with Ethacrynic acid, page 31

Anticoagulants, oral - See Anticoagulants, oral with Ethacrynic acid, page 66

Cephalosporins - See Cephalosporins with Ethacrynic acid, page 190

Corticosteroids - See Corticosteroids with Ethacrynic acid, page 220

Digitoxin - See Digitoxin with Ethacrynic acid, page 250

Digoxin - See Digoxin with Ethacrynic acid, page 252

Ethambutol, no documented interactions, see page 4, Criteria for Listing Interactions

Ethanol, see Alcohol

Ethaverine, see Papaverine

Ethchlorvynol, no documented interactions, see page 4, Criteria for Listing Interactions

ETHER, with:

Angiotensin-converting enzyme (ACE) inhibitors - See Angiotensin-converting enzyme (ACE) inhibitors with Ether, page 44

Beta-adrenergic blockers - See Beta-adrenergic blockers with Ether, page 155

(continued)

ETHER, with: *(continued)*
  Reserpine
    Hypotension (additive)
      CS Coakley et al, Circulatory responses during anesthesia of patients on rauwolfia therapy. JAMA, 161:1143, 1958; RL Katz et al, Anesthesia, surgery and rauwolfia. Anesthesiology, 25:142, 1964
    Monitor blood pressure

Ethinyl estradiol, see Estrogens

Ethionamide, no documented interactions, see page 4, Criteria for Listing Interactions

ETHOSUXIMIDE, with:
  Contraceptives, oral - See Contraceptives, oral with Ethosuximide, page 213
  Valproate
    Possible ethosuximide toxicity (decreased metabolism)
      F Pisani et al, Valproic acid-ethosuximide interaction: a pharmacokinetic study. Epilepsia, 25:229, 1984
    Highly variable; clinical significance not established; monitor ethosuximide concentration

    Possible decreased valproate effect (mechanism not established)
      RA Sälke-Kellermann et al, Influence of ethosuximide on valproic acid serum concentrations. Epilepsy Res, 26:345, 1997
    Based on study in 13 children; monitor valproate concentration

Ethoxzolamide, see Carbonic anhydrase inhibitors

Ethyl biscoumacetate, see Anticoagulants, oral

Ethylestrenol, see Anabolic and androgenic steroids

Ethynodiol diacetate, see Progestins

Etidronate, no documented interactions, see page 4, Criteria for Listing Interactions

Etodolac, see Nonsteroidal anti-inflammatory drugs

ETOMIDATE, with:
  Chloramphenicol - See Chloramphenicol with Etomidate, page 192
  Verapamil
    Prolonged anesthesia (mechanism not established)
      CA Moore et al, Potentiation of etomidate anesthesia by verapamil: a report of two cases. Hosp Pharm, 24:24, 1989
    Report of two cases (1989)

ETOPOSIDE, with:
  Anticoagulants, oral - See Anticoagulants, oral with Etoposide, page 66
  Cyclosporine - See Cyclosporine with Etoposide, page 229
  Irinotecan
    Hepatotoxicity (probably additive)
      T Ohtsu et al, Unexpected hepatotoxicities in patients with non-Hodgkin's lymphoma treated with irinotecan (CPT-11) and etoposide. Jpn J Clin Oncol, 28:502, 1998
    Based on study in 3 patients with refractory non-Hodgkins lymphoma; avoid concurrent use

ETOPOSIDE, with: *(continued)*
  Methotrexate
  Methotrexate toxicity (mechanism not established)
  > K Paál et al, Effect of etoposide on the pharmacokinetics of methotrexate *in vivo*. Anticancer Drugs, 9:765, 1998

  Based on study of patients with medulloblastoma; can be minimized by changing dosing protocol

  Tamoxifen
  Increased hematological toxicity (mechanism not established)
  > G Corona et al, Pharmacokinetic interaction between etoposide and tamoxifen in patients with hepatocellular carcinoma. Anti-Cancer Drugs, 10:815, 1999

  No pharmacokinetic interaction detected in patients with hepatocellular carcinoma; effect may be pharmacodynamic; monitor clinical status

ETRETINATE, with:
  Anticoagulants, oral - See Anticoagulants, oral with Etretinate, page 66
  Carbamazepine - See Carbamazepine with Etretinate, page 178
  Methotrexate
  Hepatotoxicity (mechanism not established)
  > H Zachariae, Dangers of methotrexate/etretinate combination therapy. Lancet, 1:422, 1988; FG Larsen et al, Interaction of etretinate with methotrexate pharmacokinetics in psoriatic patients. J Clin Pharmacol, 30:802, 1990

  Avoid concurrent use

Exemestane, no documented interactions, see page 4, Criteria for Listing Interactions

Factor VIII concentrates, no documented interactions, see page 4, Criteria for Listing Interactions

Famciclovir, no documented interactions, see page 4, Criteria for Listing Interactions

Famotidine, see Antihistamines, H_2-blockers

FELBAMATE, with:
  Anticoagulants, oral - See Anticoagulants, oral with Felbamate, page 66
  Barbiturates - See Barbiturates with Felbamate, page 133
  Carbamazepine - See Carbamazepine with Felbamate, page 178
  Contraceptives, oral - See Contraceptives, oral with Felbamate, page 213
  Phenytoin
  Possible phenytoin toxicity (decreased metabolism; probably CYP2C19)
  > RH Fuerst et al, Felbamate increases phenytoin but decreases carbamazepine concentrations. Epilepsia, 29:488, 1988; NM Graves et al, Effect of felbamate on phenytoin and carbamazepine serum concentrations. Epilepsia, 30:225, 1989; R Sachdeo et al, Stead-state pharmacokinetics of felbamate (Felbatol) when coadministered with phenytoin. Epilepsia, 33 suppl 3:84, 1992; R Sachdeo et al, Coadministration of phenytoin and felbamate: evidence of additional phenytoin dose-reduction requirements based on pharmacokinetics and tolerability with increasing doses of felbamate. Epilepsia, 40:1122, 1999

(continued)

FELBAMATE, with: *(continued)*

Monitor phenytoin concentration and clinical status; consider prophylactic 20% reduction in phenytoin dosage if felbamate is added

Valproate

Possible valproate toxicity (decreased metabolism)

> ML Wagner et al, The effect of felbamate on valproate disposition. Epilepsia, 32 suppl 3:15, 1993

Monitor valproate concentration

FELODIPINE, with:

Alcohol - See Alcohol with Felodipine, page 17

Antifungals, imidazoles and triazoles - See Antifungals, imidazoles and triazoles with Felodipine, page 101

Cyclosporine - See Cyclosporine with Felodipine, page 229

Digoxin - See Digoxin with Felodipine, page 252

Grapefruit juice

Possible felodipine toxicity (decreased metabolism; CYP3A4)

> KS Lown et al, Grapefruit juice increases felodipine oral availability in humans by decreasing intestinal CYP3A protein expression. J Clin Invest, 99:2545, 1997; J Lundahl et al, Effects of grapefruit juice ingestion-pharmacokinetics and haemodynamics of intravenously and orally administered felodipine in healthy men. Eur J Clin Pharmacol, 52:139, 1997; DG Bailey et al, Grapefruit juice—felodipine interaction: effect of naringin and 6',7'-dihydroxybergamottin in humans. Clin Pharmacol Ther, 64:248, 1998; DG Bailey et al, Grapefruit juice-felodipine interaction: effect of segments and an extract from unprocessed fruit. Clin Pharmacol Ther, 67:107, 2000, abs PI-71; H Takanaga et al, Pharmacokinetic analysis of felodipine-grapefruit juice interaction based on an irreversible enzyme inhibition model. Br J Clin Pharmacol, 49:49, 2000; GK Dresser et al, Grapefruit juice—felodipine interaction in the elderly. Clin Pharmacol Ther, 68:28, 2000

Based on several studies in healthy subjects; effect larger with multiple doses of grapefruit juice; monitor clinical status; effect of grapefruit juice may last 2 to 3 days

Macrolide antibiotics

Possible felodipine toxicity with erythromycin (decreased metabolism)

> DG Bailey et al, Erythromycin-felodipine interaction: magnitude, mechanism, and comparison with grapefruit juice. Clin Pharmacol Ther, 60:25, 1996

Based on study of healthy men; monitor clinical status and reduce felodipine dose as necessary

Oxcarbazepine

Possible decreased felodipine effect (increased metabolism)

> G Zaccara et al, Influence of single and repeated doses of oxcarbazepine on the pharmacokinetic profile of felodipine. Ther Drug Monit, 15:39, 1993

Felodipine concentration decreased 28%; monitor clinical status

Fenfluramine, see Sympathomimetic amines

FENOFIBRATE, with:
    Anticoagulants, oral - See Anticoagulants, oral with Fenofibrate, page 66
    Cholestyramine - See Cholestyramine with Fenofibrate, page 196
    Colestipol - See Colestipol with Fenofibrate, page 211
    HMG-CoA reductase inhibitors
        Possible myopathy (mechanism not established)
            Manufacturer's package insert (fenofibrate); W-J Pan et al, Lack of a clinically significant pharmacokinetic interaction between fenofibrate and pravastatin in healthy volunteers. J Clin Pharmacol, 40:316, 2000
        Theoretical; monitor clinical status; manufacturer believes benefit outweighs risk; pravastatin may be less likely to interact

FENOLDOPAM, with:
    Beta-adrenergic blockers - See Beta-adrenergic blockers with Fenoldopam, page 155

Fenoprofen, see Nonsteroidal anti-inflammatory drugs

Fenoterol, see Sympathomimetic bronchodilators

Fentanyl, see Narcotics: meperidine and congeners

Ferrous fumarate, see Iron

Ferrous gluconate, see Iron

Ferrous sulfate, see Iron

FEXOFENADINE, with:
    Rifampin
        Possible decreased fexofenadine effect (possibly induction of P-glycoprotein)
            MA Hamman et al, Effects of age, gender, and rifampin (RIF) on fexofenadine (FEX) disposition in humans. Clin Pharmacol Ther, 67:157, 2000, abs PIII-61
        Based on study of healthy subjects; interaction not affected by gender or age

FINASTERIDE, with:
    Terazosin
        Possible increase in finasteride concentration (mechanism not established)
            V Vashi et al, Pharmacokinetic interaction between finasteride and terazosin, but not finasteride and doxazosin. J Clin Pharmacol, 38:1072, 1998
        Based on study in healthy subjects; clinical significance not established

FK 506, see Tacrolimus

Flavoxate, no documented interactions, see page 4, Criteria for Listing Interactions

FLECAINIDE, with:
    Amiodarone - See Amiodarone with Flecainide, page 35
    Antihistamines, H$_2$-blockers - See Antihistamines, H$_2$-blockers with Flecainide, page 118
    Arbutamine - See Arbutamine with Flecainide, page 128
    Beta-adrenergic blockers - See Beta-adrenergic blockers with Flecainide, page 155
    Digoxin - See Digoxin with Flecainide, page 252
    Lopinavir/Ritonavir
        Increased flecainide toxicity including cardiac arrhythmias (decreased metabolism)
            Manufacturer's package insert (*Kaletra*)
        Avoid concurrent use

(continued)

FLECAINIDE, with: *(continued)*
  Quinidine
    Possible flecainide toxicity (decreased metabolism)
      A Munafo et al, Disposition of flecainide in subjects taking quinidine. Clin Pharmacol Ther, 47:156, 1990; UM Birgersdotter et al, Stereoselective genetically-determined interaction between chronic flecainide and quinidine in patients with arrhythmias. Br J Clin Pharmacol, 33:275, 1992; A Munafo et al, The effect of a low dose of quinidine on the disposition of flecainide in healthy volunteers. Eur J Clin Pharmacol, 43:441, 1992
    Based on studies in healthy subjects; monitor flecainide concentration or ECG
  Ritonavir
    Possible flecainide toxicity (decreased metabolism)
      Manufacturer's package insert (ritonavir)
    Theoretical; listed as contraindicated in product information
  Verapamil
    Asystole, cardiogenic shock (additive effects on conduction and contractility)
      JL Holtzman et al, The pharmacodynamic and pharmacokinetic interaction between single doses of flecainide acetate and verapamil: effects on cardiac function and drug clearance. Clin Pharmacol Ther, 46:26, 1989; J Buss et al, Asystole and cardiogenic shock due to combined treatment with verapamil and flecainide. Lancet, 340:546, 1992
    Case reports and studies in young healthy men; monitor ECG and cardiovascular status

Floxuridine, no documented interactions, see page 4, Criteria for Listing Interactions

Fluconazole, see Antifungals, Imidazoles and Triazoles

FLUCYTOSINE, with:
  Antifungals, Amphotericin B - See Antifungals, Amphotericin B with Flucytosine, page 94

Fludarabine, no documented interactions, see page 4, Criteria for Listing Interactions

Fludrocortisone, see Corticosteroids

Flumazenil, no documented interactions, see page 4, Criteria for Listing Interactions

Flunisolide, see Corticosteroids

Fluocinolone, no documented interactions, see page 4, Criteria for Listing Interactions

Fluocinonide, no documented interactions, see page 4, Criteria for Listing Interactions

FLUORIDE, with:
  Antacids - See Antacids with Fluoride, page 52
  Calcium - See Calcium with Fluoride, page 175
  Tamoxifen
    Fluorosis (mechanism not established)
      MF Odelin et al, Tamoxifen and fluoride: perhaps a dangerous association. J Exp Clin Cancer Res, 12:195, 1993
    Single case report (1993); requires further study

FLUOROQUINOLONES, with:
- **Amiodarone** - See Amiodarone with Fluoroquinolones, page 35
- **Antacids** - See Antacids with Fluoroquinolones, page 52
- **Anticoagulants, oral** - See Anticoagulants, oral with Fluoroquinolones, page 66
- **Antidepressants, tricyclic** - See Antidepressants, tricyclic with Fluoroquinolones, page 85
- **Antihistamines, H$_1$-blockers: astemizole, terfenadine** - See Antihistamines, H$_1$-blockers: astemizole, terfenadine with Fluoroquinolones, page 110
- **Antihistamines, H$_2$-blockers** - See Antihistamines, H$_2$-blockers with Fluoroquinolones, page 118
- **Benzodiazepines** - See Benzodiazepines with Fluoroquinolones, page 142
- **Bepridil** - See Bepridil with Fluoroquinolones, page 151
- **Beta-adrenergic blockers** - See Beta-adrenergic blockers with Fluoroquinolones, page 155
- **Caffeine** - See Caffeine with Fluoroquinolones, page 173
- **Cisapride** - See Cisapride with Fluoroquinolones, page 200
- **Clozapine** - See Clozapine with Fluoroquinolones, page 206
- **Cyclosporine** - See Cyclosporine with Fluoroquinolones, page 230
- **Didanosine** - See Didanosine with Fluoroquinolones, page 248
- **Digoxin** - See Digoxin with Fluoroquinolones, page 252
- **Foscarnet**

    Seizures with ciprofloxacin and norfloxacin (mechanism not established)
    P Fan-Havard et al, Concurrent use of foscarnet and ciprofloxacin may increase the propensity for seizures. Ann Pharmacother, 28:869, 1994
    Two patients with no predisposing factors (1994)

- **Iron**

    Decreased fluoroquinolone effect (decreased absorption)
    M Kara et al, Clinical and chemical interactions between iron preparations and ciprofloxacin. Br J Clin Pharmacol, 31:257, 1991; NRC Campbell et al, Clinical and chemical interactions between norfloxacin and clinically used metal ions. Clin Pharmacol Ther, 49:200, 1991 abs PIII-107; MM Cabarga et al, Effects of two cations on gastrointestinal absorption of ofloxacin. Antimicrob Agents Chemother, 35:2102, 1991; P Lehto et al, The effect of ferrous sulphate on the absorption of norfloxacin, ciprofloxacin and ofloxacin. Br J Clin Pharmacol, 37:82, 1994; P Lehto and KT Kivistö, Different effects of products containing metal ions on the absorption of lomefloxacin. Clin Pharmacol Ther, 56:477, 1994; manufacturer's package inserts
    Give fluoroquinolone 2 to 4 hours before or 6 hours after iron; based on studies in healthy volunteers

- **Macrolide antibiotics**

    Possible ventricular arrhythmia with grepafloxacin and erythromycin (possible additive effect on QTc interval; CYP3A4)
    Manufacturer's package insert
    Theoretical; manufacturer recommends avoiding concurrent use

(continued)

FLUOROQUINOLONES, with: *(continued)*
Magnesium citrate
Decreased ciprofloxacin effect (decreased absorption)
> SH Parpia et al, Sucralfate reduces the gastrointestinal absorption of norfloxacin. Antimicrob Agents Chemother, 33:99, 1989; JC Garrelts et al, Sucralfate significantly reduces ciprofloxacin concentrations in serum. Antimicrob Agents Chemother, 34:931, 1990; P Lehto and KT Kivistö, Effect of sucralfate on absorption of norfloxacin and ofloxacin. Antimicrob Agents Chemother, 38:248, 1994

Based on study in healthy nonsmoking subjects

Mexiletine
Possible mexiletine toxicity (decreased metabolism)
> L Labbé et al, Ciprofloxacin decreases mexiletine clearance in smokers and non-smokers. Clin Pharmacol Ther, 57:210, 1995

Based on study in healthy subjects, monitor mexiletine concentration

Narcotics: morphine-like
Decreased oral trovafloxacin effect with intravenous morphine (decreased absorption of trovafloxacin)
> Manufacturer's package insert

IV morphine can be given 2 hours after oral trovafloxacin when taken fasting or 4 hours after oral trovafloxacin when taken with food; potential interactions of other combinations of fluoroquinolones and narcotic analgesics not known

Olanzapine
Possible olanzapine toxicity (probably decreased metabolism; CYP1A2)
> JS Markowitz and CL DeVane, Suspected ciprofloxacin inhibition of olanzapine resulting in increased plasma concentration. J Clin Psychopharmacol, 19:289, 1999

Single case report (1999); monitor clinical status and olanzapine concentration

Penicillins
Possible ciprofloxacin toxicity with azlocillin (decreased metabolism)
> SL Barriere et al, Alteration in the pharmacokinetic disposition of ciprofloxacin by simultaneous administration of azlocillin. Antimicrob Agents Chemother, 34:823, 1990

Monitor ciprofloxacin concentration; based on study in 6 healthy men

Pentamidine
Possible ventricular arrhythmia with grepafloxacin (possible additive effect on QTc interval; CYP3A4)
> Manufacturer's package insert

Theoretical; manufacturer recommends avoiding concurrent use

Pentoxifylline
Headache probably due to pentoxifylline toxicity with ciprofloxacin (probably decreased metabolism)
> JD Cleary, Ciprofloxacin (CIPRO) and pentoxifylline (PTF): a clinically significant drug interaction. Pharmacotherapy, 12:259, 1992, abs 106

Avoid concurrent use

FLUOROQUINOLONES, with: *(continued)*
Phenothiazines
Possible ventricular arrhythmia with grepafloxacin (possible additive effect on QTc interval; CYP3A4)
    Manufacturer's package insert
Theoretical; manufacturer recommends avoiding concurrent use

Phenytoin
Altered phenytoin effect with ciprofloxacin (mechanism not established)
    D Schroeder et al, Effect of ciprofloxacin on serum phenytoin concentrations in epileptic patients. Pharmacotherapy, 11:275, 1991, abs 75; ML Dillard et al, Ciprofloxacin-phenytoin interaction. Ann Pharmacother, 26:263, 1992; ML Job et al, Effect of ciprofloxacin on the pharmacokinetics of multiple-dose phenytoin serum concentrations. Ther Drug Monit, 16:427, 1994; PT Pollak and KL Slayter, Hazards of doubling phenytoin dose in the face of an unrecognized interaction with ciprofloxacin. Ann Pharmacother, 31:61, 1997; PJ Brouwers et al, Ciprofloxacin-phenytoin interaction. Ann Pharmacother, 31:498, 1997; PT Pollak and KL Slayter, Comment: ciprofloxacin-phenytoin interaction. Ann Pharmacother, 31:1549, 1997; M-J Otero et al, Interaction between phenytoin and ciprofloxacin. Ann Pharmacother, 33:251, 1999
Possible decreased phenytoin effect; one study of 7 patients found increased phenytoin concentrations (1991); monitor phenytoin concentration and clinical status

Probenecid
Possible increased ciprofloxacin, ofloxacin, norfloxacin, lomefloxacin and gatifloxacin effect (decreased renal excretion)
    U Jaehde et al, Effect of probenecid on the distribution and elimination of ciprofloxacin in humans. Clin Pharmacol Ther, 58:532, 1995; B Nataraj et al, Probenecid affects the pharmacokinetics of ofloxacin in healthy volunteers. Clin Drug invest, 16:259, 1998; manufacturer's package insert
Based on studies in healthy subjects; clinical significance not established; effect of probenecid on ofloxacin elimination was modest

Procainamide
Possible procainamide toxicity with ofloxacin (mechanism not established)
    DE Martin et al, Effects of ofloxacin on the pharmacokinetics of procainamide. Clin Pharmacol Ther, 55:166, 1994
Monitor procainamide concentrations; based on studies of normal subjects

Possible ventricular arrhythmia with grepafloxacin (possible additive effect on QTc interval)
    Manufacturer's package insert
Theoretical; manufacturer recommends avoiding concurrent use

Quinidine
Possible ventricular arrhythmia with grepafloxacin (possible additive effect on QTc interval; CYP3A4)
    Manufacturer's package insert

(continued)

FLUOROQUINOLONES, with: *(continued)*
  Theoretical; manufacturer recommends avoiding concurrent use
Ropinirole
  Increased ropinirole effect with ciprofloxacin and probably enoxacin (decreased metabolism)
    Manufacturer's package insert
  Avoid concurrent use; little or no interaction would be expected with other fluoroquinolones
Sucralfate
  Decreased fluoroquinolone effect (decreased absorption)
    JC Garrelts et al, Sucralfate significantly reduces ciprofloxacin concentrations in serum. Antimicrob Agents Chemother, 34:931, 1990; P Lehto and KT Kivistö, Effect of sucralfate on absorption of norfloxacin and ofloxacin. Antimicrob Agents Chemother, 38:248, 1994; GR Granneman et al, Effect of antacid medication on the pharmacokinetics of temafloxacin. Clin Pharmacokinet, 22 suppl 1:83, 1992; P Lehto and KT Kivistö, Different effects of products containing metal ions on the absorption of lomefloxacin. Clin Pharmacol Ther, 56:477, 1994; J Kawakami et al, The effect of food on the interaction of ofloxacin with sucralfate in healthy volunteers. Eur J Clin Pharmacol, 47:67, 1994; manufacturer's inserts; L-J Lee et al, Effects of food and sucralfate on a single oral dose of 500 milligrams of levofloxacin in healthy subjects. Antimicrob Agents Chemother, 41:2196, 1997; JA Zix et al, Pharmacokinetics of sparfloxacin and interaction with cisapride and sucralfate. Antimicrob Agents Chemother, 41:1668, 1997; M Kamberi et al, The effect of staggered dosing of sucralfate on oral bioavailability of sparfloxacin. Br J Clin Pharmacol, 49:98, 2000
  Single report (1989) in an elderly patient and studies in healthy subjects; decrease in ofloxacin absorption caused by sucralfate is reduced by food; avoid concurrent use in patients with abnormal gastric emptying; give fluoroquinolones at least 2 hours before or 6 hours after sucralfate; because it is slowly absorbed, sparfloxacin may need to be given 4 hours before sulcralfate
Theophyllines
  Theophylline toxicity with ciprofloxacin, enoxacin, grepafloxacin, norfloxacin (decreased metabolism); levofloxacin, ofloxacin, sparfloxacin, temafloxacin, trovafloxacin and lomefloxacin may not interact; concurrent cimetidine may further increase theophylline toxicity
    J Beckmann et al, Enoxacin – a potent inhibitor of theophylline metabolism. Eur J Clin Pharmacol, 33:227, 1987; G Ho et al, Evaluation of the effect of norfloxacin on the pharmacokinetics of theophylline. Clin Pharmacol Ther, 44:35, 1988; WA Al-Turk et al, Effect of ofloxacin on the pharmacokinetics of a single intravenous theophylline dose. Ther Drug Monit, 10:160, 1988; RA Robson et al, Comparative effects of ciprofloxacin and lomefloxacin on the oxidative metabolism of theophylline. Br J Clin Pharmacol, 29:491, 1990; F Sörgel et al, Effects of 2 quinolone antibacterials, temafloxacin and enoxacin, on theophylline pharmacokinetics. Clin Pharmacokinet, 22 suppl 1:65, 1992; C-M Loi et al, Aging and drug interactions. III. Individual and combined effects of cimetidine and ciprofloxacin on

FLUOROQUINOLONES, with: *(continued)*
> theophylline metabolism in healthy male and female nonsmokers. J Pharmacol Exper Ther, 280:627, 1997; manufacturer's package inserts; Y Niki et al, Quinolone antimicrobial agents and theophylline. Chest, 101:881, 1992; PA Andrews, Interactions with ciprofloxacin and erythromycin leading to aminophylline toxicity. Nephrol Dial Transplant, 13:1005, 1998

Monitor theophylline concentration and avoid interacting fluoroquinolones

Ursodiol
Decreased ciprofloxacin effect (probably decreased absorption)
> PP Belliveau et al, Reduction in serum concentrations of ciprofloxacin after administration of ursodiol to a patient with hepatobiliary disease. Clin Infect Dis, 19:354, 1994

Single case report of a patient with hepatobiliary disease (1994)

Zinc
Decreased fluoroquinolone effect (decreased absorption)
> RE Polk et al, Effect of ferrous sulfate and multivitamins with zinc on absorption of ciprofloxacin in normal volunteers. Antimicrob Agents Chemother, 33:1841, 1989; NRC Campbell et al, Norfloxacin interaction with antacids and minerals. Br J Clin Pharmacol, 33:115, 1992; manufacturer's package insert

In healthy volunteers; also occurs with multivitamins containing zinc; avoid concurrent use or give fluoroquinolone 2 to 4 hours before

FLUOROURACIL, with:

Anticoagulants, oral - See Anticoagulants, oral with Fluorouracil, page 67
Antihistamines, H$_2$-blockers - See Antihistamines, H$_2$-blockers with Fluorouracil, page 118

Interferon
Possible fluorouracil toxicity (mechanism not established)
> MJ Czejka et al, Influence of different doses of interferon-α-2b on the blood plasma levels of 5-fluorouracil. Eur J Drug Metab Pharmacokinet, 18:247, 1993

Doubling of fluorouracil concentrations in patients with gastrointestinal carcinoma; monitor clinical status and adjust fluorouracil dosage if needed

Leucovorin
Deaths from enterocolitis, diarrhea, and dehydration reported in elderly subjects (mechanism not established)
> Manufacturer's package insert (capecitabine)

Avoid concurrent use in elderly

Methotrexate
Severe erythema and ulceration with topical fluorouracil (synergism)
> WD Blackburn, Jr and GS Alarcón, Toxic response to topical fluorouracil in two rheumatoid arthritis patients receiving low-dose, weekly methotrexate. Arthritis Rheum, 33:303, 1990

Avoid concurrent use with topical fluorouracil

Metronidazole
Metronidazole toxicity (decreased metabolism)
> Z Bardakji et al, 5-Fluorouracil-metronidazole combination therapy in

(continued)

FLUOROURACIL, with: *(continued)*
> metastatic colorectal cancer. Cancer Chemother Pharmacol, 18:140, 1986
>
> *Avoid concurrent use*

Sorivudine
Fatal fluorouracil toxicity (probably decreased fluorouracil metabolism)
> H Okuda et al, Lethal drug interactions of sorivudine, a new antiviral drug, with oral 5-fluorouracil prodrugs. Drug Metab Dispos, 25:270, 1997; T Watable, Strategic proposals for predicting drug-drug interactions during new drug development: based on sixteen deaths caused by interactions of the new antiviral sorivudine with 5-fluorouracil prodrugs. J Toxicol Sci, 21:299, 1996; H Okuda et al, Lethal drug interactions of sorivudine, a new antiviral drug, with oral 5-fluorouracil prodrugs, Drug Metab Dis, 25:270, 1997; RB Diasio, Sorivudine and 5-fluorouracil; a clinically significant drug-drug interaction due to inhibition of dihydropyrimidine dehydrogenase. Br J Clin Pharmacol, 46:1, 1998
>
> *Multiple fatalities in Japan; avoid concurrent use*

Fluoxetine, see Selective serotonin reuptake inhibitors (SSRIs)

Fluoxymesterone, see Anabolic and androgenic steroids

Fluphenazine, see Phenothiazines

Fluprednisolone, see Corticosteroids

Flurandrenolide, no documented interactions, see page 4, Criteria for Listing Interactions

Flurazepam, see Benzodiazepines

Flurbiprofen, see Nonsteroidal anti-inflammatory drugs

FLUTAMIDE, with:
> **Anticoagulants, oral** - See Anticoagulants, oral with Flutamide, page 67

Fluticasone, see Corticosteroids

Fluvastatin, see HMG-CoA Reductase Inhibitors

Fluvoxamine, see Selective serotonin reuptake inhibitors (SSRIs)

FOLIC ACID, with:

Phenytoin
Decreased phenytoin effect (increased metabolism); decreased folate effect (decreased absorption of possible increased metabolism)
> RG Strauss and R Bernstein, Folic acid and dilantin antagonism in pregnancy. Obstet Gynecol, 44:345, 1974; MP Rivey et al, Phenytoin-folic acid: a review. Drug Intell Clin Pharm, 18:292, 1984; PE MacCosbe and K Toomey, Interaction of phenytoin and folic acid. Clin Pharm, 2:362, 1983; MJ Berg et al, Phenytoin pharmacokinetics: before and after folic acid administration. Epilepsia, 33:712, 1992; DP Lewis et al, Phenytoin-folic acid interaction. Ann Pharmacother, 29:726, 1995; H Seligmann et al, Phenytoin-folic acid interaction: a lesson to be learned. Clin Neuropharmacol, 22:268, 1999
>
> *Monitor phenytoin concentration; phenytoin metabolism is folate dependent and addition of folate increases phenytoin metabolism; monitor folate concentration or provide folate supplements when phenytoin is given.*

Zinc
Decreased zinc availability (decreased absorption)
> DB Milne et al, Effect of oral folic acid supplements on zinc, copper, and

FOLIC ACID, with: *(continued)*
> iron absorption and excretion. Am J Clin Nutr, 39:535, 1984

Give as far apart as possible

Folinic acid, see Leucovorin

Foods, see Tyramine-rich foods and beverages

FOSCARNET, with:

Fluoroquinolones - See Fluoroquinolones with Foscarnet, page 279

Pentamidine

Hypocalcemia (additive)
> MS Youle et al, Severe hypocalcaemia in AIDS patients treated with foscarnet and pentamidine. Lancet, 1:1455, 1988

Monitor calcium concentration

FOSFOMYCIN, with:

Metoclopramide

Possible decreased fosfomycin effect (possibly increased gastrointestinal motility)
> Manufacturer's package insert

Monitor clinical status

Fosinopril, see Angiotensin-converting enzyme (ACE) inhibitors

Furazolidone, see Monoamine oxidase inhibitors

FUROSEMIDE, with:

Aminoglycoside antibiotics - See Aminoglycoside antibiotics with Furosemide, page 31

Angiotensin-converting enzyme (ACE) inhibitors - See Angiotensin-converting enzyme (ACE) inhibitors with Furosemide, page 45

Beta-adrenergic blockers - See Beta-adrenergic blockers with Furosemide, page 155

Carbamazepine - See Carbamazepine with Furosemide, page 178

Cephalosporins - See Cephalosporins with Furosemide, page 191

Chloral hydrate - See Chloral hydrate with Furosemide, page 192

Cholestyramine - See Cholestyramine with Furosemide, page 196

Colestipol - See Colestipol with Furosemide, page 211

Corticosteroids - See Corticosteroids with Furosemide, page 220

COX-2 inhibitors - See COX-2 inhibitors with Furosemide, page 225

Cyclosporine - See Cyclosporine with Furosemide, page 230

Digitoxin - See Digitoxin with Furosemide, page 250

Digoxin - See Digoxin with Furosemide, page 252

Ginseng

Possible decreased furosemide effect (mechanism not established)
> BN Becker et al, Ginseng-induced diuretic resistance. JAMA, 276:606, 1996

Single case report (1999); causal relationship not established; monitor clinical status

Lithium

Lithium toxicity (decreased renal excretion)
> RJ Kerry et al, Diuretics are dangerous with lithium. Br Med J, 281:371, 1980; S MacNeil et al, Diuretics during lithium therapy. Lancet, 1:1295, 1975

FUROSEMIDE, with: *(continued)*
  Monitor lithium concentration
  Neuromuscular blocking agents
    Increased d-tubocurarine blockade (mechanism not established)
      RD Miller et al, Enhancement of d-tubocurarine neuromuscular blockade by diuretics in man. Anesthesiology, 45:442, 1976; I Azar et al, Furosemide facilitates recovery of evoked twitch response after pancuronium. Anesth Analg, 59:55, 1980
    Monitor neuromuscular status; patients were undergoing renal transplants; in patients with normal renal function, furosemide can reverse pancuronium blockade
  Nonsteroidal anti-inflammatory drugs
    Decreased diuretic and antihypertensive effects (inhibition of renal prostaglandin synthesis)
      RV Patak et al, Antagonism of the effects of furosemide by indomethacin in normal and hypertensive man. Prostaglandins, 10:649, 1975; JC Frolich et al, Suppression of plasma renin activity by indomethacin in man. Circ Res, 39:447, 1976; DE Smith et al, Attenuation of furosemide's diuretic effect by indomethacin: pharmacokinetic evaluation. J Pharmacokinet Biopharm, 7:265, 1979; DE Baker, Piroxicam-furosemide drug interaction. Drug Intell Clin Pharm, 22:505, 1988; D Hartmann et al, Study on the possible interaction between tenoxicam and furosemide. Arzneimittelforschung, 37:1072, 1987; AP Passmore et al, A comparison of the effects of ibuprofen and indomethacin upon renal haemodynamics and electrolyte excretion in the presence and absence of frusemide. Br J Clin Pharmacol, 27:483, 1989; TC Li Kam Wa et al, Interaction of ketoprofen and frusemide in man. Postgrad Med J, 67:655, 1991; JG Motwani and AD Struthers, Interactive effects of indomethacin, angiotensin II and frusemide on renal haemodynamics and natriuresis in man. Br J Clin Pharmacol, 37:355, 1994
    Monitor blood pressure and diuretic effect
  Phenytoin
    Decreased furosemide effect (decreased absorption and renal insensitivity)
      A Fine et al, Malabsorption of furosemide caused by phenytoin. Br Med J, 2:1061, 1977
    Monitor diuretic effect
  Probenecid
    Decreased diuresis (decreased sodium excretion)
      Y-Y Hsieh et al, Probenecid interferes with the natriuretic action of furosemide. J Cardiovasc Pharmacol, 10:530, 1987; PE Walshaw et al, Diuretic and non-diuretic actions of furosemide: effects of probenecid. Clin Invest Med, 15:82, 1992; TB Vree et al, Probenecid inhibits the renal clearance of frusemide and its acyl glucuronide. Br J Clin Pharmacol, 39:692, 1995
    Avoid concurrent use, if possible; diuresis is decreased by one gram probenecid daily, but it may be enhanced with 2 grams daily
  Sympathomimetic amines
    Hypokalemia with epinephrine (intracellular uptake of potassium)
      JG Meechan and MD Rawlins, The effects of two different local anaesthetic

FUROSEMIDE, with: *(continued)*
>solutions administered for oral surgery on plasma potassium levels in patients taking kaliuretic diuretics. Eur J Clin Pharmacol, 42:155, 1992

Occurs with local anesthesia for oral surgery; use local anesthetic, such as prilocaine, without epinephrine

Sympathomimetic bronchodilators
>Hypokalemia with inhaled terbutaline (additive)
>>DM Newnham et al, The effects of frusemide and triamterene on the hypokalaemic and electrocardiographic responses to inhaled terbutaline. Br J Clin Pharmacol, 32:630, 1991
>
>*Monitor potassium concentration; based on study in healthy volunteers*

Theophyllines
>Decreased theophylline effect (mechanism not established)
>>PF Conlon et al, Effect of intravenous furosemide on serum theophylline concentration. Am J Hosp Pharm, 38:1345, 1981; JW Toback and ME Gilman, Theophylline-furosemide inactivation? Pediatrics, 71:140, 1983; G Carpentiere et al, Furosemide and theophylline. Ann Intern Med, 103:957, 1985; U-A Jänicke et al, Absence of a clinically significant interaction between theophylline and furosemide. Eur J Clin Pharmacol, 33:487, 1987
>
>*Monitor theophylline concentration; reports on IV furosemide with theophylline are conflicting; not confirmed in healthy volunteers, but dosing regimen differed*

Vancomycin
>Possible decreased vancomycin effect (possible increased renal elimination)
>>MY Yeung and JP Smyth, Concurrent frusemide-theophylline dosing reduces serum vancomycin concentrations in preterm infants. Aust J Hosp Pham, 29:269, 1999
>
>*Based on study in 10 preterm infants; patients also receiving theophylline; consider shorter dose intervals for vancomycin*

G-CSF, see Colony stimulating factors

GABAPENTIN, with:

Antacids - See Antacids with Gabapentin, page 53

Beta-adrenergic blockers - See Beta-adrenergic blockers with Gabapentin, page 156

Phenytoin
>Phenytoin toxicity (decreased metabolism)
>>F Tyndel, Interaction of gabapentin with other antiepileptics. Lancet, 343:1363, 1994
>
>*Single case documented by rechallenge (1994)*

GALLIUM, with:

Aminoglycoside antibiotics - See Aminoglycoside antibiotics with Gallium, page 31

Antifungals, Amphotericin B - See Antifungals, Amphotericin B with Gallium, page 94

GANCICLOVIR, with:

Didanosine - See Didanosine with Ganciclovir, page 248

GEMCITABINE, with:
   Anticoagulants, oral - See Anticoagulants, oral with Gemcitabine, page 68

GEMFIBROZIL, with:
   Anticoagulants, oral - See Anticoagulants, oral with Gemfibrozil, page 68
   Antitrypsin - See Antitrypsin with Gemfibrozil, page 127
   Bexarotene - See Bexarotene with Gemfibrozil, page 165
   Colestipol - See Colestipol with Gemfibrozil, page 211
   HMG-CoA reductase inhibitors

Rhabdomyolysis with lovastatin, simvastatin or cerivastatin (probably decreased lovastatin, simvastatin or cerivastatin metabolism)

    Manufacturer's package insert; GE Marais and KK Larson, Rhabdomyolysis and acute renal failure induced by combination lovastatin and gemfibrozil therapy. Ann Intern Med, 112:228, 1990; LR Pierce et al, Myopathy and rhabdomyolysis associated with lovastatin-gemfibrozil combination therapy. JAMA, 264:71, 1990; EP Van Puijenbroek et al, J Intern Med, 240:403, 1996; GW Pogson et al, Rhabdomyolysis and renal failure associated with cerivastatin-gemfibrozil combination therapy. Am J Cardiol, 83:1146, 1999; JR Guyton et al, Dual hepatic metabolism of cerivastatin—clarifications. Am J Cardiol, 84:497, 1999; RP Bermingham et al, Rhabdomyolysis in a patient receiving the combination of cerivastatin and gemfibrozil. Am J Health Syst Pharm, 57:461, 2000; G Alexandrisis et al, Rhabdomyolysis due to combination therapy with cerivastatin and gemfibrozil. Am J Med, 109:261, 2000

Monitor creatinine kinase and alanine aminotransferase concentrations while increasing lovastatin or simvastatin dosage gradually; concurrent use of cerivastatin and gemfibrozil is contraindicated by the manufacturer (cerivastatin)

Increased incidence of greater than four fold elevation of creatine kinase with pravastatin; no myopathy observed in this study (mechanism not established)

    O Wiklund et al, Pravastatin and gemfibrozil alone and in combination for the treatment of hypercholesterolemia. Am J Med, 94:13, 1993

Monitor creatine kinase

Hypoglycemics, sulfonylurea

Hypoglycemia with glyburide (mechanism not established)

    S Ahmad, Gemfibrozil: interaction with glyburide. South Med J, 84:102, 1991

Single case report (1991)

Insulin

Decreased hypoglycemic effect (gemfibrozil increases blood glucose)

    P Samuel, Effects of gemfibrozil on serum lipids. Am J Med, 74:23, 1983

Monitor blood glucose

Troglitazone

Increased triglyceridemia (mechanism not established)

    DSH Bell and F Ovalle, Troglitazone interferes with gemfibrozil's lipid-lowering action. Diabetes Care, 21:2028, 1998

GEMFIBROZIL, with: *(continued)*
> *Based on retrospective study in 18 patients; statins did not interact; troglitazone is no longer available*

Gemtuzumab, no documented interactions, see page 4, Criteria for Listing Interactions

Gentamicin, see Aminoglycoside antibiotics

Gestodene, see Contraceptives, oral

GINKGO BILOBA, with:
  Anticoagulants, oral - See Anticoagulants, oral with Ginkgo biloba, page 68
  Trazodone
    Possible increased sedative effect (possibly additive)
> S Galluzzi et al, Coma in a patient with Alzheimer's disease taking low dose trazodone and ginkgo biloba. J Neurol Neurosurg Psychiatry, 68:679, 2000

Single case report (2000); causal relationship not established; monitor clinical status

GINSENG, with:
  Anticoagulants, oral - See Anticoagulants, oral with Ginseng, page 68
  Digoxin - See Digoxin with Ginseng, page 252
  Furosemide - See Furosemide with Ginseng, page 285
  Monoamine oxidase inhibitors
    Euphoria (mechanism not established)
> BD Jones and AM Runikis, Interaction of ginseng with phenelzine. J Clin Psychopharmacol, 7:201, 1987; RI Shader and DJ Greenblatt, Bees, ginseng and MAOIs revisited. J Clin Psychopharmacol, 8:235, 1988

Two case reports (1987, 1988)

Glatiramer, no documented interactions, see page 4, Criteria for Listing Interactions

Glibenclamide, see Hypoglycemics, sulfonylurea

Glimepiride, no documented interactions, see page 4, Criteria for Listing Interactions

Glipizide, see Hypoglycemics, sulfonylurea

Glucocerebrosidase, no documented interactions, see page 4, Criteria for Listing Interactions

GLUTETHIMIDE, with:
  Anticoagulants, oral - See Anticoagulants, oral with Glutethimide, page 68

Glyburide, see Hypoglycemics, sulfonylurea

Glycopyrrolate, see Anticholinergics

GLYCYRRHIZA, with:
  Thiazide diuretics
    Hypokalemia (additive)
> L Pelner, Licorice and hypertension. JAMA, 208:1909, 1969

Avoid concurrent use; occurred with large amounts of natural licorice candy or natural licorice-containing chewing gum

GOLD SODIUM THIOMALATE, with:
  Angiotensin-converting enzyme (ACE) inhibitors - See Angiotensin-converting enzyme (ACE) inhibitors with Gold sodium thiomalate, page 45

(continued)

GOLD SODIUM THIOMALATE, with: *(continued)*
  Nonsteroidal anti-inflammatory drugs
    Pneumonitis with naproxen (possibly hypersensitivity)
      RG McFadden et al, Gold-naproxen pneumonitis; a toxic drug interaction? Chest, 96:216, 1989
    Single case report (1989)

Goserelin, no documented interactions, see page 4, Criteria for Listing Interactions
Granisetron, no documented interactions, see page 4, Criteria for Listing Interactions

GRAPEFRUIT JUICE, with:
  Amiodarone - See Amiodarone with Grapefruit juice, page 35
  Anticoagulants, oral - See Anticoagulants, oral with Grapefruit juice, page 68
  Antifungals, imidazoles and triazoles - See Antifungals, imidazoles and triazoles with Grapefruit juice, page 101
  Antihistamines, H$_1$-blockers: astemizole, terfenadine - See Antihistamines, H$_1$-blockers: astemizole, terfenadine with Grapefruit juice, page 110
  Artemether - See Artemether with Grapefruit juice, page 128
  Benzodiazepines - See Benzodiazepines with Grapefruit juice, page 142
  Buspirone - See Buspirone with Grapefruit juice, page 170
  Carbamazepine - See Carbamazepine with Grapefruit juice, page 178
  Cisapride - See Cisapride with Grapefruit juice, page 200
  Cyclosporine - See Cyclosporine with Grapefruit juice, page 231
  Estrogens - See Estrogens with Grapefruit juice, page 272
  Felodipine - See Felodipine with Grapefruit juice, page 276
  HMG-CoA reductase inhibitors
    Possible increased lovastatin or simvastatin toxicity (decreased metabolism in gut wall; CYP3A4)
      T Kantola et al, Grapefruit juice greatly increases serum concentrations of lovastatin and lovastatin acid. Clin Pharmacol Ther, 63:397, 1998; JJ Lilja et al, Grapefruit juice-simvastatin interaction: effect on serum concentrations of simvastatin, simvastatin acid, and HMG-CoA reductase inhibitors. Clin Pharmacol Ther, 64:477, 1998; JJ Lilja et al, Grapefruit juice increases serum concentrations of atorvastatin and has no effect on pravastatin. Clin Pharmacol Ther, 66:118, 1999; JD Rogers et al, Grapefruit juice has minimal effects on plasma concentrations of lovastatin-derived 3-hydroxy-3-methylglutaryl coenzyme A reductase inhibitors. Clin Pharmacol Ther, 66:358, 1999; DG Bailey and GK Dresser, Grapefruit juice—lovastatin interaction. Clin Pharmacol Ther, 67:690, 2000
    About 15-fold increase in lovastatin and simvastatin concentrations and about 3-fold increase in atorvastatin concentrations in healthy subjects with large amounts of grapefruit juice; cerivastatin probably interacts to a lesser degree; fluvastatin and pravastatin less likely to interact (not metabolized by CYP3A4)
  Nimodipine
    Possible nimodipine toxicity (decreased metabolism; CYP3A4)
      U Fuhr et al, Grapefruit juice increases oral nimodipine bioavailability. Int J Clin Pharmacol Ther, 36:126, 1998

GRAPEFRUIT JUICE, with: *(continued)*
Avoid concurrent use; based on study in healthy subjects
Nisoldipine
Possible increased nisoldipine toxicity (decreased metabolism; CYP3A4)
> DG Bailey et al, Effect of grapefruit juice and naringin on nisoldipine pharmacokinetics. Clin Pharmacol Ther, 54:589, 1993; H Takanaga et al, Relationship between time after intake of grapefruit juice and the effect on pharmacokinetics and pharmacodynamics of nisoldipine in healthy subjects. Clin Pharmacol Ther, 67:201, 2000

Based on studies in healthy subjects; effect may last for up to 3 days after intake of grapefruit juice; manufacturer recommends avoiding concurrent use

Pranidipine
Possible pranidipine toxicity (probably decreased metabolism; CYP3A4)
> K Hashimoto et al, Interaction of citrus juices with pranidipine, a new 1,4-dihydropyridine calcium antagonist, in healthy subjects. Eur J Clin Pharmacol, 54:753, 1998

Based on study in healthy subjects; monitor clinical status; orange juice had no effect

Saquinavir
Modest increase in saquinavir bioavailabilty (decreased first-pass metabolism; CYP3A4)
> HHT Kupferschmidt et al, Grapefruit juice enhances the bioavailability of the HIV protease inhibitor saquinavir in man. Br J Clin Pharmacol, 45:355, 1998; VA Eagling et al, Inhibition of the CYP3A4-mediated metabolism and P-glycoprotein-mediated transport of the HIV-1 protease inhibitor saquinavir by grapefruit juice components. Br J Clin Pharmacol, 48:543, 1999

Based on in vitro study and a study in healthy subjects with old formulation of saquinavir; modest effect, clinical significance unknown

Selective serotonin reuptake inhibitors (SSRIs)
Possible sertraline toxicity (probably increased bioavailability; CYP3A4)
> AJ Lee et al, The effects of grapefruit juice on sertraline metabolism: an in vitro and in vivo study. Clin Ther, 21:1890, 1999

Based on study in 5 patients with depression; clinical importance not established; monitor clinical status

Sirolimus
Possible sirolimus toxicity (decreased metabolism; CYP3A4)
> Manufacturer's package insert (sirolimus)

Avoid concurrent use

Theophyllines
Possible decreased theophylline effect (mechanism not established)
> MC Gupta et al, Effect of grapefruit juice on the pharmacokinetics of theophylline in healthy male volunteers. Methods Find Exp Clin Pharmacol, 21:679, 1999

Based on study in healthy subjects; effect small; clinical importance not established

GREEN TEA, with:
  Anticoagulants, oral - See Anticoagulants, oral with Green tea, page 68
Grepafloxacin, see Fluoroquinolones
Griseofulvin, see Antifungals, Griseofulvin
Growth hormone, recombinant, no documented interactions, see page 4, Criteria for Listing Interactions
Guanabenz acetate, no documented interactions, see page 4, Criteria for Listing Interactions
GUANADREL, with:
  Alcohol - See Alcohol with Guanadrel, page 17
  Antidepressants, tricyclic - See Antidepressants, tricyclic with Guanadrel, page 85
  Monoamine oxidase inhibitors
  Possible severe hypertension (additive effect on catecholamines)
    Manufacturer's package insert
  Give at least one week apart
  Phenothiazines
  Decreased antihypertensive effect of guanadrel (blockade of guanadrel uptake at target site)
    Manufacturer's package insert
  Avoid concurrent use
  Sympathomimetic amines
  Decreased antihypertensive effect (blockade of guanadrel uptake at target site)
    Manufacturer's package insert
  Avoid concurrent use
GUANETHIDINE, with:
  Antidepressants, tricyclic - See Antidepressants, tricyclic with Guanethidine, page 85
  Contraceptives, oral - See Contraceptives, oral with Guanethidine, page 214
  Enflurane - See Enflurane with Guanethidine, page 269
  Minoxidil
  Severe orthostatic hypotension (mechanism not established)
    Manufacturer's package insert
  Avoid concurrent use
  Phenothiazines
  Decreased antihypertensive effect (blockade of guanethidine uptake at target site)
    WE Fann et al, Chlorpromazine reversal of the antihypertensive action of guanethidine. Lancet, 2:436, 1971; DS Janowsky et al, Guanethidine antagonism by antipsychotic drugs. J Tenn Med Assoc, 65:620, 1972
  Avoid concurrent use, if possible
  Sympathomimetic amines
  Decreased antihypertensive effect (release of norepinephrine and blockade of reuptake of amines by neurons)
    MD Day, Effect of sympathomimetic amines on the blocking action of guanethidine, bretylium and xylocholine. Br J Pharmacol, 18:421, 1962; KF Ober and RIH Wang, Drug interactions with guanethidine. Clin Pharmacol

GUANETHIDINE, with: *(continued)*
> Ther, 14:190, 1973

Avoid concurrent use

GUANFACINE, with:

Antidepressants, tricyclic - See Antidepressants, tricyclic with Guanfacine, page 86

Barbiturates - See Barbiturates with Guanfacine, page 133

Bupropion - See Bupropion with Guanfacine, page 169

Narcotics: meperidine and congeners

Bradycardia with epidural fentanyl (probably additive)
> RG Burney, Bradycardia during epidural anesthesia in a patient receiving guanfacine. Anesthesiology, 77:1228, 1992

Single case report; also received epidural lidocaine

Valproate

Possible valproate toxicity (possible decreased metabolism)
> PJ Ambrosini and RM Sheikh, Increased plasma valproate concentrations when coadministered with guanfacine. J Child Adolesc Psychopharmacol, 8:143, 1998

Two case reports in children (1998); monitor clinical status and valproate concentrations

Venlafaxine

Possible dystonia (mechanism not established)
> Y Chong et al, Dystonia as a side effect of nonneuroleptics. J Am Acad Child Adolesc Psychiatry, 38:793, 1999

Single pediatric case report (1999); monitor clinical status

H_1-blockers, see Antihistamines, H_1-blockers

H_2-blockers, see Antihistamines, H_2-blockers

Halazepam, see Benzodiazepines

Halcinonide, no documented interactions, see page 4, Criteria for Listing Interactions

Halobetasol propionate, no documented interactions, see page 4, Criteria for Listing Interactions

HALOFANTRINE, with:

Antacids - See Antacids with Halofantrine, page 53

Mefloquine

QT prolongation (possibly additive)
> NJ White, Mefloquine in the prophylaxis and treatment of falciparum malaria. BMJ, 308:286, 1994; manufacturer's package insert

Manufacturer states that combination should not be used

Pyrimethamine

Possible halofantrine toxicity (mechanism not established)
> FW Hombhanje, Effect of a single oral dose of *Fansidar* on the pharmacokinetics of halofantrine in healthy volunteers: a preliminary report. Br J Clin Pharmacol, 49:283, 2000

Based on study in healthy subjects; monitor ECG (QTc) and clinical status; effect small

HALOPERIDOL, with:

Anticholinergics - See Anticholinergics with Haloperidol, page 58

Antidepressants, tricyclic - See Antidepressants, tricyclic with Haloperidol, page 86

Antifungals, imidazoles and triazoles - See Antifungals, imidazoles and triazoles with Haloperidol, page 101

Barbiturates - See Barbiturates with Haloperidol, page 134

Beta-adrenergic blockers - See Beta-adrenergic blockers with Haloperidol, page 156

Cabergoline - See Cabergoline with Haloperidol, page 172

Carbamazepine - See Carbamazepine with Haloperidol, page 179

Clozapine - See Clozapine with Haloperidol, page 206

Imipenem

Possible hypotensive episodes (mechanism not established)

K Franco-Bronson and P Gajwah, Hypotension associated with intravenous haloperidol and imipenem. J Clin Psychopharmacol, 19:480, 1999

Three case reports (1999); monitor blood pressure

Isoniazid

Possible haloperidol toxicity (possibly decreased metabolism)

M Takeda et al, Serum haloperidol levels of schizophrenics receiving treatment for tuberculosis. Clin Neuropharmacol, 9:386, 1986

Monitor haloperidol effect and, if necessary, concentration

Lithium

Encephalopathy, lethargy, fever, confusion, extrapyramidal symptoms (mechanism not established)

GI Keitner and S Rahman, Reversible neurotoxicity with combined lithium-haloperidol administration. J Clin Psychopharmacol, 4:104, 1984; CB Schaffer et al, The effect of haloperidol on serum levels of lithium in adult manic patients. Biol Psychiatry, 19:1495, 1984; JC-Y Chou et al, Acute mania: haloperiodol dose and augmentation with lithium or lorazepam. J Clin Psychopharmacol, 19:500, 1999

Monitor and discontinue both drugs if signs of toxicity occur; lithium may be useful when combined with low-dose haloperidol in manic patients

Marijuana, smoking

Possible decreased haloperidol effect (probably increased metabolism)

L Pan et al, Effects of smoking, CYP2D6 genotype, and concomitant drug intake on the steady state plasma concentrations of haloperidol and reduced haloperidol in schizophrenic inpatients. Ther Drug Monit, 21:489, 1999

Based on study in schizophrenic patients; monitor clinical status

Methyldopa

Dementia (mechanism not established)

WE Thornton, Dementia induced by methyldopa with haloperidol. N Engl J Med, 294:1222, 1976; I Nadel and M Wallach, Drug interaction between haloperidol and methyldopa. Br J Psychiatry, 135:484, 1979

Monitor for dementia and discontinue both drugs if it occurs

HALOPERIDOL, with: *(continued)*
  Metoclopramide
    Dystonia and parkinsonism on stopping or decreasing dosage of metoclopramide (mechanism not established)
      EC Lauterbach, Haloperidol-induced dystonia and parkinsonism on discontinuing metoclopramide: implications for differential thalamocortical activity. J Clin Psychopharmacol, 12:442, 1992
    Single case report (1992)
  Narcotics: morphine-like
    Increased psychomotor impairment with nalbuphine (mechanism not established)
      U Saarialho-Kere, Psychomotor, respiratory and neuroendocrinological effects of nalbuphine and haloperidol, alone and in combination, in healthy subjects. Br J Clin Pharmacol, 26:79, 1988
    Warn patients; based on study in healthy volunteers
  Nefazodone
    Possible haloperidol toxicity (mechanism not established)
      RH Barbhaiya et al, Investigation of pharmacokinetic and pharmacodynamic interactions after coadministration of nefazodone and haloperidol. J Clin Psychopharmacol, 16:26, 1996
    Based on study in healthy volunteers
  Nonsteroidal anti-inflammatory drugs
    Severe drowsiness with indomethacin (mechanism not established)
      HA Bird et al, Drowsiness due to haloperidol/indomethacin in combination. Lancet, 1:830, 1983
    Avoid concurrent use
  Olanzapine
    Possible increased risk of parkinsonian symptoms (mechanism not established)
      RF Gomberg, Interaction between olanzapine and haloperidol. J Clin Psychopharmacol, 19:272, 1999
    Single case report (1999); monitor clinical status
  Phenothiazines
    Agranulocytosis with chlorpromazine (mechanism not established)
      A Young and R Kehoe, Two cases of agranulocytosis on addition of a butyrophenone [haloperidol] to a long-standing course of phenothiazine treatment. Br J Psychiatry, 154:710, 1989; SA Allen, Effect of chlorpromazine and clozapine on plasma concentrations of haloperidol in a patient with schizophrenia. J Clin Pharmacol, 40:1296, 2000
    Two case reports (1989); phenothiazines alone tolerated for long periods

    Possible haloperidol toxicity (possibly decreased metabolism)
      SA Allen, Effect of chlorpromazine and clozapine on plasma concentrations of haloperidol in a patient with schizophrenia. J Clin Pharmacol, 40:1296, 2000

(continued)

HALOPERIDOL, with: *(continued)*
Single case report (2000); causal relationship not established; monitor clinical status

Phenytoin

Decreased haloperidol effect (increased metabolism)

M Linnoila et al, Effect of anticonvulsants on plasma haloperidol and thioridazine levels. Am J Psychiatry, 137:7, 1980; AW Marcoux, A phenytoin – thioridazine medication interaction. Hosp Pharm, 21:889, 1986

Monitor mental status

Pramipexole

Possible reduced pramipexole effect (dopamine antagonism)

Manufacturer's package insert

Avoid concurrent

Quinidine

Possible increased haloperidol effect (mechanism not established)

D Young et al, Effect of quinidine on the interconversion kinetics between haloperidol and reduced haloperidol in humans: implications for the involvement of cytochrome P450IID6. Eur J Clin Pharmacol, 44:433, 1993

Monitor clinical status or haloperidol concentration

Rifampin

Decreased haloperidol effect (increased metabolism)

M Takeda et al, Serum haloperidol levels of schizophrenics receiving treatment for tuberculosis. Clin Neuropharmacol, 9:386, 1986; Y-H Kim et al, Effect of rifampin on the plasma concentration and the clinical effect of haloperidol concomitantly administered to schizophrenic patients. J Clin Psychopharmacol, 16:247, 1996

Monitor clinical status and haloperidol concentration

Ropinirole

Possible reduced ropinirole effect (dopamine antagonism)

Manufacturer's package insert

Avoid concurrent use

Selective serotonin reuptake inhibitors (SSRIs)

Increased extrapyramidal symptoms with fluoxetine; one possible case of tardive dyskinesia with fluoxetine and low doses of haloperidol (1991) (mechanism not established)

MH Stein, Tardive dyskinesia in a patient taking haloperidol and fluoxetine. Am J Psychiatry, 148:683, 1991; DC Goff et al, Elevation of plasma concentrations of haloperidol after the addition of fluoxetine. Am J Psychiatry, 148:790, 1991; RH Bouchard et al, TM Brod, Fluoxetine and extrapyramidal side effects. Am J Psychiatry, 146:1352, 1989;

Monitor clinical status and haloperidol concentration if available

Possible toxicity with fluvoxamine (mechanism not established)

DG Daniel et al, Coadministration of fluvoxamine increases serum concentrations of haloperidol. J Clin Psychopharmacol, 14:340, 1994; S Vandel et al, Fluvoxamine and fluoxetine: interaction studies with amitriptyline, clomipramine and neuroleptics in phenotyped patients. Pharmacol Res,

HALOPERIDOL, with: *(continued)*

31:347, 1995; S-A Chong and A Cheong, Deliberate self-poisoning following fluvoxamine-neuroleptics combination. J Clin Psychiatry, 60:869, 1999

Monitor clinical status and haloperidol concentration if available

Tacrine

Possible parkinsonian symptoms (possibly additive)

MJ McSwain and LM Forman, Severe parkinsonian symptom development on combination treatment with tacrine and haloperidol. J Clin Psychopharmacol, 15:284, 1995; I Maany, Adverse interaction of tacrine and haloperidol. Am J Psychiatry, 153:1504, 1996

Two case reports (1995; 1996)

Tobacco, smoking

Possible decreased haloperidol effect (probably increased metabolism)

L Pan et al, Effects of smoking, CYP2D6 genotype, and concomitant drug intake on the steady state plasma concentrations of haloperidol and reduced haloperidol in schizophrenic inpatients. Ther Drug Monit, 21:489, 1999; K Shimoda et al, Lower plasma levels of haloperidol in smoking than in nonsmoking schizophrenic patients. Ther Drug Monit, 21:293, 1999

Based on studies in schizophrenic patients; monitor clinical status

Haloprogin, no documented interactions, see page 4, Criteria for Listing Interactions

HALOTHANE, with:

Amiodarone - See Amiodarone with Halothane, page 35

Angiotensin-converting enzyme (ACE) inhibitors - See Angiotensin-converting enzyme (ACE) inhibitors with Halothane, page 45

Beta-adrenergic blockers - See Beta-adrenergic blockers with Halothane, page 156

Narcotics: meperidine and congeners

Possible narcotic toxicity with fentanyl (decreased metabolism)

KA Lehmann et al, Biotransformation of fentanyl II. Acute drug interactions in rats and men. Anaesthesist, 31:221, 1982

Monitor closely

Reserpine

Hypotension (additive)

Manufacturer's package insert; CS Coakley et al, Circulatory responses during anesthesia of patients on rauwolfia therapy. JAMA, 161:1143, 1958; RL Katz et al, Anesthesia, surgery and rauwolfia. Anesthesiology, 25:142, 1964

Monitor blood pressure

Sympathomimetic amines

Possible fatal arrhythmias with epinephrine (probably additive)

SC Buzik, Fatal interaction? Halothane, epinephrine and tooth implant surgery. Can Pharm J, 123:68, 1990; CF Stannard, Ventricular fibrillation during examination of nose. Anaesthesia, 46:794, 1991

Avoid concurrent use

Sympathomimetic bronchodilators

Arrhythmias with terbutaline (mechanism not established)

S Thiagarajah et al, Ventricular arrhythmias after terbutaline administration

HALOTHANE, with: *(continued)*
> to patients anesthetized with halothane. Anesth Analg, 65:417, 1986
> *Avoid concurrent use*

Theophyllines
Increased ventricular arrhythmias (synergism)
> BL Zimmerman, Arrhythmogenicity of theophylline and halothane used in combination. Anesth Analg, 58:259, 1979; W Richards et al, Cardiac arrest associated with halothane anesthesia in a patient receiving theophylline. Ann Allergy, 61:83, 1988

Use with caution

Verapamil
Bradycardia and hypotension (additive)
> D Zuck and JJ Rao, Profound bradycardia with verapamil and halothane. Anaesthesia, 40:84, 1985; RG Merin, IW Møller, Cardiac arrest following i.v. verapamil may be related to concomitant digoxin therapy as well as halothane. Br J Anaesth, 61:366, 1988; IW Møller, Cardiac arrest following i.v. verapamil combined with halothane anaesthesia. Br J Anaesth, 59:522, 1987

Single case report (1985); cardiac arrest in one patient also taking digoxin (1988)

HEPARINS, with:

Aprotinin - See Aprotinin with Heparins, page 127
Cephalosporins - See Cephalosporins with Heparins, page 191
Hypoglycemics, sulfonylurea
Hypoglycemic episodes with glipizide (possibly displacement from binding)
> G McKillop et al, Possible interaction between heparin and a sulphonylurea a cause of prolonged hypoglycaemia? Br Med J, 293:1073, 1986

Single case report (1986)

Nitrates
Decreased heparin effect with IV nitroglycerin (mechanism not established)
> MA Habbab and JI Haft, Heparin resistance induced by intravenous nitroglycerin; a word of caution when both drugs are used concomitantly. Arch Intern Med, 147:857, 1987; L Pizzulli et al, Hemmung der heparinwirkung durch glyceroltrinitrat. Deutsch Med Wochenschr, 113:1837, 1988; NE Lepor et al, Does nitroglycerin induce heparin resistance? Clin Cardiol, 12:432, 1989; RC Becker et al, Intravenous nitroglycerin-induced heparin resistance: a qualitative antithrombin III abnormality. Am Heart J, 119:1254, 1990; V Bode et al, Absence of drug interaction between heparin and nitroglycerin; randomized placebo-controlled crossover study. Arch Intern Med, 150:2117, 1990; ER Gonzalez et al, Assessment of the drug interaction between intravenous nitroglycerin and heparin. Ann Pharmacother, 26:1512, 1992; M Pye et al, A clinical and in vitro study on the possible interaction of intravenous nitrates with heparin anticoagulation. Clin Cardiol, 17:658, 1994; SY Nottestad and AM Mascette, Nitroglycerin-induced heparin resistance: absence of interaction at clinically relevant doses. Mil Med, 159:569, 1994

HEPARINS, with: *(continued)*
> *Confirmed in 3 patient studies, but one study in healthy people and two studies in patients shows no interaction and one study in patients taking nitrates chronically given IV heparin during cardiac surgery showed no interaction. May affect only a minority of patients*

Nonsteroidal anti-inflammatory drugs
> Increased bleeding risk with aspirin (inhibition of platelet function)
>> HS Yett et al, The hazards of aspirin plus heparin. N Engl J Med, 298:1092, 1978; CJ Bang et al, Interaction between heparin and acetylsalicylic acid on gastric mucosal and skin bleeding in humans. Scand J Gastroenterol, 27:489, 1992
>
> *Avoid concurrent use*

Pentosan
> Increased bleeding risk (additive)
>> Manufacturer's package insert
>
> *Monitor prothrombin time*

Tirofiban
> Increased bleeding (additive)
>> Manufacturer's package insert (tirofiban)
>
> *Monitor prothrombin time*

Heroin, see Narcotics: morphine-like

Hexobarbital, see Barbiturates

HMG-COA REDUCTASE INHIBITORS, with:

Anabolic and androgenic steroids - See Anabolic and androgenic steroids with HMG-CoA reductase inhibitors, page 42

Anticoagulants, oral - See Anticoagulants, oral with HMG-CoA reductase inhibitors, page 69

Antifungals, imidazoles and triazoles - See Antifungals, imidazoles and triazoles with HMG-CoA reductase inhibitors, page 102

Antihistamines, H_2-blockers - See Antihistamines, H_2-blockers with HMG-CoA reductase inhibitors, page 118

Cholestyramine - See Cholestyramine with HMG-CoA reductase inhibitors, page 196

Cilostazol - See Cilostazol with HMG-COA reductase inhibitors, page 199

Colestipol - See Colestipol with HMG-CoA reductase inhibitors, page 211

Cyclosporine - See Cyclosporine with HMG-CoA reductase inhibitors, page 231

Digoxin - See Digoxin with HMG-CoA reductase inhibitors, page 252

Diltiazem - See Diltiazem with HMG-COA Reductase Inhibitors, page 260

Fenofibrate - See Fenofibrate with HMG-CoA reductase inhibitors, page 277

Gemfibrozil - See Gemfibrozil with HMG-CoA reductase inhibitors, page 288

Grapefruit juice - See Grapefruit juice with HMG-CoA reductase inhibitors, page 290

Isradipine
> Possible decreased lovastatin effect in men (mechanism not established)
>> JL Holtzman et al, Chronic isradipine increases lovastatin clearance in normal male, but not female volunteers. Clin Pharmacol Ther, 55:166, 1994

(continued)

HMG-COA REDUCTASE INHIBITORS, with: *(continued)*
Monitor blood lipids
Lopinavir/Ritonavir
Possible increased atorvastatin or cerivastatin toxicity (decreased metabolism)
> Manufacturer's package insert (*Kaletra*)

Use lowest effective dose; pravastatin and fluvastatin may not interact

Increased lovastatin and simvastatin toxicity including myopathy and rhabdomyolysis (decreased metabolism; CYP3A4)
> Manufacturer's package insert (*Kaletra*)

Avoid concurrent use with lovastatin or simvastatin

Macrolide antibiotics
Rhabdomyolysis with lovastatin or simvastatin and erythromycin or clarithromycin (decreased metabolism; CYP3A4)
> JZ Ayanian et al, Lovastatin and rhabdomyolysis. Ann Intern Med, 109:682, 1988; DH Spach et al, Rhabdomyolysis associated with lovastatin and erythromycin use. West J Med, 154:213, 1991; JW Grunden and KA Fisher, Lovastatin-induced rhabdomyolysis possibly associated with clarithromycin and azithromycin. Ann Pharmacother, 31:859, 1997; K Ochmann et al, Influence of erythromycin pre- and co-treatment on the single-dose pharmacokinetics of cerivastatin. Eur J Clin Pharmacol, 52:A139, 1997; W Mück et al, Influence of erythromycin pre- and co-treatment on single-dose pharmacokinetics of the HMG-CoA reductase inhibitor cerivastatin. Eur J Clin Pharmacol, 53:469, 1998; T Kantola et al, Erythromycin and verapamil considerably increase serum simvastatin and simvastatin acid concentrations. Clin Pharmacol Ther, 64:177, 1998; PWK Wong et al, Multiple organ toxicity from addition of erythromycin to long-term lovastatin therapy. South Med J, 91:202, 1998; PH Siedlik et al, Erythromycin coadministration increases plasma atorvastatin concentrations. J Clin Pharmacol, 39:501, 1999; JA Tobert et al, Calcium channel blocker-simvastatin interaction. Clin Pharmacol Ther, 65:583, 1999

Single lovastatin case report with IV (1988) and two with oral erythromycin (1991; 1998); single case report with clarithromycin and azithromycin (1997); small increases in cerivastatin and atorvastatin concentration with erythromycin in normal subjects were not clinically significant; simvastatin and lovastatin likely to interact similarly with macrolides; moderate inhibitors of CYP3A such as calcium-channel blockers are less likely to cause clinically significant interactions (1999)

Mianserin
Possible increased risk of myopathy with pravastatin (mechanism not established)
> A Takei and S Chiba, Rhabdomyolysis associated with pravastatin treatment for major depression. Psychiatry Clin Neurosci, 53:539, 1999

Single case report of rhabdomyolysis (1999); causal relationship not established; monitor for evidence of rhabdomyolysis (muscle pain and weakness, dark urine)

HMG-COA REDUCTASE INHIBITORS, with: *(continued)*

Nefazodone
Possible myopathy and rhabdomyolysis with simvastatin and probably lovastatin (decreased metabolism)

RH Jacobson et al, Myositis and Rhabdomyolysis associated with concurrent use of simvastatin and nefazodone. JAMA, 277:296, 1997; CP Alderman et al, Possible interaction between nefazodone and pravastatin. Ann Pharmacother, 33:871, 1999; MB Bottorf, Comment: possible interaction between nefazodone and pravastatin. Ann Pharmacother, 34:538, 2000

Single case report with simvastatin (1997); avoid concurrent use; if combination is used monitor for signs of rhabdomyolysis (muscle pain, weakness or dark urine); pravastatin or fluvastatin may be less likely to produce myopathy; single case report of creatine kinase elevations with pravastatin, but causal relationship not established

Nicotinic acid
Rhabdomyolysis with lovastatin (mechanism not established)

P Reaven and JL Witztum, Lovastatin, nicotinic acid, and rhabdomyolysis. Ann Intern Med, 109:597, 1988; manufacturer's package insert

Isolated case reports; monitor clinical status and CPK

Nonsteroidal anti-inflammatory drugs
Possible diclofenac toxicity (decreased metabolism)

C Transon et al, In vivo inhibition profile of cytochrome P450TB (CYP2C9) by (±)-fluvastatin. Clin Pharmacol Ther, 58:412, 1995

Based on study in healthy subjects; monitor clinical status

Oat bran
Decreased cholesterol-lowering effect (probably decreased absorption)

WO Richter et al, Interaction between fibre and lovastatin. Lancet, 338:706, 1991

Two case reports (1991); separation of intake by several hours might alleviate the problem

Pectin
Decreased cholesterol-lowering effect (probably decreased absorption)

WO Richter et al, Interaction between fibre and lovastatin. Lancet, 338:706, 1991

Three case reports (1991); separation of intake by several hours might alleviate the problem

Phenytoin
Possible decreased effect of HMG CoA reductase inhibitors (increased metabolism; CYP3A4; possible increased P-glycoprotein activity)

MJ Murphy and MH Dominiczak, Efficacy of statin therapy: possible effect of phenytoin. Postgrad Med J, 75:359, 1999

Single case report with simvastatin (1999); theoretically, pravastatin would be less likely to interact than other HMG-CoA reductase inhibitors

Rifampin
Decreased fluvastatin effect (increased metabolism)

Manufacturer's package insert

(continued)

HMG-COA REDUCTASE INHIBITORS, with: *(continued)*
  Monitor cholesterol and if available fluvastatin concentration
  Thyroid hormones
    Decreased thyroxine effect (mechanism not established)
      BP Lustgarten, Catabolic response to lovastatin therapy. Ann Intern Med, 109:171, 1988
    Single well-documented case report (1989)

    Hyperthyroidism with levothyroxine (mechanism not established)
      DM Demke, GJ Gormley and JA Tobert, Drug interaction between thyroxine and lovastatin. N Engl J Med, 321:1341, 1989
    Single case report in a patient on multiple drugs, including gemfibrozil and a beta-blocker (1988)
  Troglitazone
    Possible reduction in simvastatin hypolipidemic effect (possible enzyme induction)
      JC Lin and MK Ito, A drug interaction between troglitazone and simvastatin. Diabetes Care, 22:2104, 1999
    Based on retrospective study; monitor lipid concentrations; pravastatin may be less likely to interact; troglitazone is no longer available
  Verapamil
    Possible simvastatin toxicity: rhabdomyolysis (decreased metabolism; CYP3A4)
      T Kantola et al, Erythromycin and verapamil considerably increase serum simvastatin and simvastatin acid concentrations. Clin Pharmacol Ther, 64:177, 1998; S Donahue et al, Verapamil significantly increases serum concentrations of simvastatin but not pravastatin. Clin Pharmacol Ther, 65:179, 1999; JA Tobert et al, Calcium channel blocker-simvastatin interaction. Clin Pharmacol Ther, 65:583, 1999; PJK Gruer et al, Concomitant use of cytochrome P450 3A4 inhibitors and simvastatin. Am J Cardiol, 84:811, 1999
    Based on studies in healthy subjects; monitor clinical status, creatine phosphokinase (CPK) and for signs of rhabdomyolysis (muscle pain, weakness or dark urine); verapamil had no effect on pravastatin; fluvastatin theoretically would not interact

Homatropine, see Anticholinergics

Hyaluronan, no documented interactions, see page 4, Criteria for Listing Interactions

HYDRALAZINE, with:
  Beta-adrenergic blockers - See Beta-adrenergic blockers with Hydralazine, page 156
  Diazoxide - See Diazoxide with Hydralazine, page 246
  Digoxin - See Digoxin with Hydralazine, page 252
  Nonsteroidal anti-inflammatory drugs
    Decreased hypotensive effect of hydralazine with indomethacin (probably decreased prostaglandin synthesis)
      MP Cinquegrani and C-S Liang, Indomethacin attenuates the hypotensive action of hydralazine. Clin Pharmacol Ther, 39:564, 1986

HYDRALAZINE, with: *(continued)*
  Monitor blood pressure
Hydrochlorothiazide, see Thiazide diuretics
Hydrocodone, see Narcotics: morphine-like
Hydrocortisone, see Corticosteroids
Hydroflumethiazide, see Thiazide diuretics
Hydromorphone, see Narcotics: morphine-like
HYDROXYCHLOROQUINE, with:
  Beta-adrenergic blockers - See Beta-adrenergic blockers with Hydroxychloroquine, page 156
  Digoxin - See Digoxin with Hydroxychloroquine, page 253
  Rifampin
    Possible decreased hydroxychloroquine effect (probably increased metabolism)
      CJ Harvey et al, Influence of rifampicin on hydroxychloroquine. Clin Exper Rheumatol, 13:536, 1995
    Single case report (1995)
HYDROXYUREA, with:
  Didanosine - See Didanosine with Hydroxyurea, page 248
HYDROXYZINE, with:
  Antihistamines, H_2-blockers - See Antihistamines, H_2-blockers with Hydroxyzine, page 118
  Metoclopramide
    Neurotoxicity (possibly additive)
      JL Fouilladieu et al, Possible potentiation by hydroxyzine of metoclopramide's undesirable side effects. Anesth Analg, 64:1227, 1985
    Single case report (1985); needs confirmation
Hymenoptera, see Insect venom extracts
Hyoscyamine, see Anticholinergics
HYPOGLYCEMICS, SULFONYLUREA, with:
  Alcohol - See Alcohol with Hypoglycemics, sulfonylurea, page 18
  Amiloride - See Amiloride with Hypoglycemics, sulfonylurea, page 28
  Anabolic and androgenic steroids - See Anabolic and androgenic steroids with Hypoglycemics, sulfonylurea, page 42
  Angiotensin-converting enzyme (ACE) inhibitors - See Angiotensin-converting enzyme (ACE) inhibitors with Hypoglycemics, sulfonylurea, page 45
  Antacids - See Antacids with Hypoglycemics, sulfonylurea, page 53
  Anticoagulants, oral - See Anticoagulants, oral with Hypoglycemics, sulfonylurea, page 69
  Antidepressants, tricyclic - See Antidepressants, tricyclic with Hypoglycemics, sulfonylurea, page 86
  Antifungals, imidazoles and triazoles - See Antifungals, imidazoles and triazoles with Hypoglycemics, sulfonylurea, page 102
  Antihistamines, H_2-blockers - See Antihistamines, H_2-blockers with Hypoglycemics, sulfonylurea, page 118
  Beta-adrenergic blockers - See Beta-adrenergic blockers with Hypoglycemics, sulfonylurea, page 156

(continued)

HYPOGLYCEMICS, SULFONYLUREA, with: *(continued)*

Chloramphenicol - See Chloramphenicol with Hypoglycemics, sulfonylurea, page 193

Cholestyramine - See Cholestyramine with Hypoglycemics, sulfonylurea, page 196

Clofibrate - See Clofibrate with Hypoglycemics, sulfonylurea, page 203

Contraceptives, oral - See Contraceptives, oral with Hypoglycemics, sulfonylurea, page 214

Cyclosporine - See Cyclosporine with Hypoglycemics, sulfonylurea, page 232

Digoxin - See Digoxin with Hypoglycemics, sulfonylurea, page 253

Gemfibrozil - See Gemfibrozil with Hypoglycemics, sulfonylurea, page 288

Heparins - See Heparins with Hypoglycemics, sulfonylurea, page 298

Macrolide antibiotics

Cholestasis with chlorpropamide with erythromycin (mechanism not established)

AP Geubel et al, Prolonged cholestasis and disappearance of interlobular bile ducts following chlorpropamide and erythromycin ethylsuccinate. Case of drug interaction? Liver, 8:350, 1988

Single case report (1988)

Methyldopa

Increased hypoglycemia with tolbutamide (possibly decreased metabolism)

B Gachalyi et al, Effect of alphamethyldopa on the half-lives of antipyrine, tolbutamide and D-glucaric acid excretion in man. Int J Clin Pharmacol Ther Toxicol, 18:133, 1980

May not be clinically significant; monitor blood glucose

Monoamine oxidase inhibitors

Increased hypoglycemic effect (mechanism not established)

PI Adnitt, Hypoglycemic action of monoamineoxidase inhibitors (MAOI's). Diabetes, 17:628, 1968

Monitor blood glucose

Nonsteroidal anti-inflammatory drugs

Hypoglycemia with tolbutamide and azapropazone (displacement from binding)

DG Waller and D Waller, Hypoglycaemia due to azapropazone-tolbutamide interaction. Br J Rheumatol, 23:24, 1984; PB Andreasen et al, Hypoglycaemia induced by azapropazone-tolbutamide interaction. Br J Clin Pharmacol, 12:581, 1981

Avoid concurrent use; no reaction occurred with ketoprofen or ibuprofen

Possible hypoglycemia with glibenclamide and piroxicam (mechanism not established)

PV Diwan et al, Potentiation of hypoglycemic response of glibenclamide by piroxicam in rats and humans. Indian J Exp Biol, 30:317, 1992

Avoid concurrent use; no reaction occurred with ketoprofen or ibuprofen

Increased hypoglycemic effect, especially with salicylates and chlorpropamide (additive)

T Richardson et al, Enhancement by sodium salicylate of the blood glucose

HYPOGLYCEMICS, SULFONYLUREA, with: *(continued)*
> lowering effect of chlorpropamide – drug interaction or summation of similar effects? Br J Clin Pharmacol, 22:43, 1986

Usual therapeutic doses of aspirin have little effect; large doses may require decreased dosage of hypoglycemic drugs; monitor blood glucose

Phenylbutazone

Increased hypoglycemic effect (decreased metabolism or excretion)
> SM Pond et al, Mechanisms of inhibition of tolbutamide metabolism: phenylbutazone, oxyphenbutazone, sulfaphenazole. Clin Pharmacol Ther, 22:573, 1977; H Tannenbaum et al, Phenylbutazone-tolbutamide drug interaction. N Engl J Med, 290:344, 1974

Avoid concurrent use

Decreased phenylbutazone effect (increased metabolism)
> M Szita et al, Interaction of phenylbutazone and tolbutamide in man. Int J Clin Pharmacol Ther Toxicol, 18:378, 1980

Avoid concurrent use

Phenytoin

Phenytoin toxicity with tolbutamide (mechanism not established)
> E Beech et al, Phenytoin toxicity produced by tolbutamide. BMJ, 297:1613, 1988

Single case report (1988)

Rifampin

Decreased hypoglycemic effect of glyburide and tolbutamide (increased metabolism)
> W Zilly et al, Induction of drug metabolism in man after rifampicin treatment measured by increased hexobarbital and tolbutamide clearance. Eur J Clin Pharmacol, 9:219, 1975; TH Self et al, Interaction of rifampin and glyburide. Chest, 96:1443, 1989; V Surekha et al, Drug interaction: rifampicin and glibenclamide. Natl Med J India, 10:11, 1997

Monitor blood glucose

Selective serotonin reuptake inhibitors (SSRIs)

Possible hypoglycemia with sertraline and tolbutamide (possible inhibition of tolbutamide metabolism)
> LM Tremaine et al, A study of the potential effect of sertraline on the pharmacokinetics and protein binding of tolbutamide. Clin Pharmacokinet, 32 suppl 1:31, 1997

Based on study in healthy subjects with high dose sertraline and IV tolbutamide; monitor glucose concentration

Possible hypoglycemia with sertraline and glyburide (mechanism not established)
> J Takhar and P Williamson, Hypoglycemia associated with high doses of sertraline and sulphonylurea compound in a noninsulin-dependent diabetes mellitus patient. Can J Clin Pharmacol, 6:12, 1999

Single case report (1999); monitor glucose concentration

Sulfonamides

Increased hypoglycemic effect (mechanism not established)
> JB Field et al, Potentiation of acetohexamide hypoglycemia by

(continued)

HYPOGLYCEMICS, SULFONYLUREA, with: *(continued)*
    phenylbutazone. N Engl J Med, 277:889, 1967; SM Pond et al, Mechanisms of inhibition of tolbutamide metabolism: phenylbutazone, oxyphenbutazone, sulfaphenazole. Clin Pharmacol Ther, 22:573, 1977; E Schulz, Schwere hypoglykamische reaktionen nach den sulfonylharnstoffen tolbutamid, carbutamid und chlorpropamid. Arch Klin Med, 214:135, 1968; H StG Tucker, Jr and JI Hirsch, Sulfonamide-sulfonylurea interaction. N Engl J Med, 286:110, 1972; JF Johnson and ME Dobmeier, Symptomatic hypoglycemia secondary to a glipizide-trimethoprim/sulfamethoxazole drug interaction. DICP, 24:250, 1990

Monitor blood glucose; reaction infrequent but can be severe

Thiazide diuretics

Hyponatremia with chlorpropamide and an amiloride-thiazide combination (additive)
    AM Zalin et al, Hyponatraemia during treatment with chlorpropamide and Moduretic (amiloride plus hydrochlorothiazide). Br Med J, 289:659, 1984

Relative contribution of amiloride and thiazide to mild hyponatremia has not been established

Verapamil

Increased hypoglycemic effect (increased glucose metabolism)
    DEH Andersson and S Rojdmark, Improvement of glucose tolerance by verapamil in patients with non-insulin-dependent diabetes mellitus. Acta Med Scand, 210:27, 1981; CG Semple et al, Effect of oral verapamil on glibenclamide stimulated insulin secretion. Br J Clin Pharmacol, 22:187, 1986

Monitor blood glucose; glibenclamide may not interact

Ibuprofen, see Nonsteroidal anti-inflammatory drugs

Ibutilide, no documented interactions, see page 4, Criteria for Listing Interactions

IDARUBICIN, with:
  Cyclosporine - See Cyclosporine with Idarubicin, page 232

IFOSFAMIDE, with:
  Anticoagulants, oral - See Anticoagulants, oral with Ifosfamide, page 69
  Cisplatin - See Cisplatin with Ifosfamide, page 201

Imaging Agents, see Contrast Media

Imidazoles, see Antifungals, Imidazoles and Triazoles

IMIPENEM, with:
  Cyclosporine - See Cyclosporine with Imipenem, page 232
  Haloperidol - See Haloperidol with Imipenem, page 294
  Theophyllines

Seizures (mechanism not established)
    JD Semel and N Allen, Seizures in patients simultaneously receiving theophylline and imipenem or ciprofloxacin or metronidazole. South Med J, 84:465, 1991

Report of 3 patients (1991)

Imipramine, see Antidepressants, tricyclic

Imiquimod, no documented interactions, see page 4, Criteria for Listing Interactions

IMMUNE GLOBULIN, INTRAVENOUS, with:
Phenytoin
Fatal hypersensitivity myocarditis (mechanism not established)
> PJ Koehler and J Koudstaal, Lethal hypersensitivity myocarditis associated with the use of intravenous gammaglobulin for Guillain-Barré syndrome, in combination with phenytoin. J Neurol, 243:366, 1996

Single case report in patient with Guillain-Barré syndrome (1996); causal relationship not established

INDAPAMIDE, with:
Lithium
Lithium toxicity (decreased renal excretion)
> ME Hanna et al, Severe lithium toxicity associated with indapamide therapy. J Clin Psychopharmacol, 10:379, 1990

Monitor lithium concentration

INDINAVIR, with:
Amiodarone - See Amiodarone with Indinavir, page 36
Amprenavir - See Amprenavir with Indinavir, page 39
Anticoagulants, oral - See Anticoagulants, oral with Indinavir, page 70
Antifungals, imidazoles and triazoles - See Antifungals, imidazoles and triazoles with Indinavir, page 103
Antihistamines, H$_1$-blockers: astemizole, terfenadine - See Antihistamines, H$_1$-blockers: astemizole, terfenadine with Indinavir, page 111
Carbamazepine - See Carbamazepine with Indinavir, page 179
Cisapride - See Cisapride with Indinavir, page 200
Delavirdine - See Delavirdine with Indinavir, page 244
Didanosine - See Didanosine with Indinavir, page 248
Efavirenz - See Efavirenz with Indinavir, page 267
Ergot alkaloids - See Ergot alkaloids with Indinavir, page 271
Interleukin-2
Possible indinavir toxicity (possibly decreased metabolism)
> SC Piscitelli et al, Alteration in indinavir clearance during interleukin-2 infusions in patients infected with the human immunodeficiency virus. Pharmacotherapy, 18:1212, 1998

Based on study in patients with HIV; monitor clinical status

Isotretinoin
Possible isotretinoin toxicity (mechanism not established)
> J Padberg et al, Drug interaction of isotretinoin and protease inhibitors: support for the cellular retinoic acid-binding protein-1 theory of lipodystrophy? AIDS, 13:284, 1999; JO Sass and J Padberg, Human isotretinoin metabolism during indinavir therapy. AIDS Res Hum Retrovir, 16:1451, 2000

Single case report (1999); patient also receiving ritonavir, zidovudine and lamivudine; in this case, the plasma levels of isotretinoin were lower during antiviral therapy

Levodopa
Possible levodopa toxicity (mechanism not established)
> D Caparros-Lefebvre et al, Protease inhibitors enhance levodopa effects in parkinson's disease. Mov Disord, 14:535, 1999

(continued)

INDINAVIR, with: *(continued)*
Single case report (1999); monitor clinical status

Lopinavir/Ritonavir

Increased indinavir toxicity (decreased metabolim)
> Manufacturer's package insert (*Kaletra*)

Doses of the combination may need to be adjusted

Nelfinavir

Possible indinavir and nelfinavir toxicity (decreased metabolism; CYP3A)
> Manufacturer's package insert (nelfinavir); AL Tseng and MM Foisy, Significant interactions with new antiretrovirals and psychotropic drugs. Ann Pharmacother, 33:461, 1999; M Barry et al, Pharmacokinetics and potential interactions amongst antiretroviral agents used to treat patients with HIV infection. Clin Pharmacokinet, 36:289, 1999

Clinical significance remains to be established

Nevirapine

Possible decreased indinavir effect (increased metabolism; CYP3A)
> Manufacturer's package insert (nevirapine)

Indinavir manufacturer recommends dosage increase to 1000 mg q8h but combination has been used successfully with dosage adjustment

Rifabutin

Possible rifabutin toxicity (mechanism not established) and decreased indinavir concentration (increased metabolism)
> Manufacturer's package insert

Decrease rifabutin dosage to 150 mg q.d. and increase indinavir to 1000 mg q8h

Rifampin

Possible decreased indinavir effect (increased metabolism)
> Manufacturer's package insert (indinavir)

Theoretical; manufacturer recommends avoiding concurrent use

Rifapentine

Decreased indinavir effect (increased metabolism and increased clearance)
> Manufacturer's package insert (rifapentine)

Avoid concurrent use

Ritonavir

Possible indinavir toxicity (decreased metabolism; CYP3A4)
> A Hsu et al, Pharmacokinetic interaction between ritonavir and indinavir in healthy volunteers. Antimicrob Agents Chemother, 42:2784, 1998; AL Tseng and MM Foisy, Significant interactions with new antiretrovirals and psychotropic drugs. Ann Pharmacother, 33:461, 1999; M Barry et al, Pharmacokinetics and potential interactions amongst antiretroviral agents used to treat patients with HIV infection. Clin Pharmacokinet, 36:289, 1999

Based on study in healthy subjects; monitor clinical status

Saint John's wort

Decreased indinavir effect (possibly increased metabolism; possibly increased transport; P-glycoprotein)
> SC Piscitelli et al, Indinavir concentrations and St John's wort. Lancet, 355:547, 2000

INDINAVIR, with: *(continued)*

Based on study in healthy subjects; avoid combination if possible

Saquinavir

Possible saquinavir toxicity (decreased metabolism)

Manufacturer's package insert

Interaction may be therapeutically useful, but adverse effects may increase

Sildenafil

Possible sildenafil toxicity (decreased metabolism; CYP3A4)

C Merry et al, Interaction of sildenafil and indinavir when co-administered to HIV-positive patients. AIDS, 13:F101, 1999

Based on study in 6 HIV-positive patients; consider reduced dose of sildenafil

Indomethacin, see Nonsteroidal anti-inflammatory drugs

Infliximab, no documented interactions, see page 4, Criteria for Listing Interactions

INFLUENZA VACCINE, with:

Anticoagulants, oral - See Anticoagulants, oral with Influenza vaccine, page 70

Barbiturates - See Barbiturates with Influenza vaccine, page 134

Carbamazepine - See Carbamazepine with Influenza vaccine, page 179

Phenytoin

Possible decreased phenytoin effect or toxicity (mechanism not established)

RJ Sawchuk et al, Effect of influenza vaccination on plasma phenytoin concentrations. Ther Drug Monit, 1:285, 1979; M Levine et al, Increased serum phenytoin concentration following influenza vaccination. Clin Pharm, 3:505, 1984

Conflicting reports; clinical significance questionable

Theophyllines

Possible theophylline toxicity (decreased metabolism)

CG Meredith, Effects of influenza virus vaccine on hepatic drug metabolism. Clin Pharmacol Ther, 37:396, 1985; PA Winstanley et al, Lack of effect of highly purified subunit influenza vaccination on theophylline metabolism. Br J Clin Pharmacol, 20:47, 1985; JHG Jonkman et al, No effect of influenza vaccination on theophylline pharmacokinetics as studied by ultraviolet spectrophotometry, HPLC, and EMIT assay methods. Ther Drug Monit, 10:345, 1988

Recent vaccine formulations have not affected theophylline concentrations

INSECT VENOM EXTRACTS, with:

Angiotensin-converting enzyme (ACE) inhibitors - See Angiotensin-converting enzyme (ACE) inhibitors with Insect venom extracts, page 46

INSULIN, with:

Angiotensin-converting enzyme (ACE) inhibitors - See Angiotensin-converting enzyme (ACE) inhibitors with Insulin, page 46

Beta-adrenergic blockers - See Beta-adrenergic blockers with Insulin, page 157

Clonidine - See Clonidine with Insulin, page 204

Debrisoquine - See Debrisoquine with Insulin, page 243

Diltiazem - See Diltiazem with Insulin, page 260

Gemfibrozil - See Gemfibrozil with Insulin, page 288

(continued)

INSULIN, with: *(continued)*
Monoamine oxidase inhibitors
Possible increased hypoglycemic effect (mechanism not established)
> PI Adnitt, Hypoglycemic action of monoamineoxidase inhibitors (MAOI's). Diabetes, 17:628, 1968

Monitor blood glucose

Naltrexone
Possible increase in insulin requirements (mechanism not established)
> MA Marrazzi et al, A naltrexone-induced increase in insulin requirement. J Clin Psychopharmacol, 14:363, 1994

Single case report (1994)

Nefazodone
Possible hypoglycemia (mechanism not established)
> JK Warnock and F Biggs, Nefazodone-induced hypoglycemia in a diabetic patient with major depression. Am J Psychiatry, 154:288, 1997

Single case report (1997); monitor glucose concentration

Nonsteroidal anti-inflammatory drugs
Possible increased hypoglycemic effect with large doses of salicylates (mechanism not established)
> R Kaye et al, Antipyretics in patients with juvenile diabetes mellitus. Am J Dis Child, 112:52, 1966; JM Stowers et al, A clinical and pharmacological comparison of chlorpropamide and other sulfonylureas. Ann NY Acad Sci, 74:689, 1959; T Richardson et al, Enhancement by sodium salicylate of the blood glucose lowering effect of chlorpropamide – drug interaction or summation of similar effects? Br J Clin Pharmacol, 22:43, 1986

Monitor blood glucose

Sympathomimetic amines
Decreased insulin effect with dobutamine (increased glucose and fatty acid mobilization)
> SM Wood et al, Effect of dobutamine on insulin requirements in diabetic ketoacidosis. Br Med J, 282:946, 1981

Monitor blood glucose

Tobacco, smoking
Decreased insulin effect (decreased absorption from injection site)
> S Madsbad et al, Influence of smoking on insulin requirement and metabolic status in diabetes mellitus. Diabetes Care, 3:41, 1980; P Klemp et al, Smoking reduces insulin absorption from subcutaneous tissue. Br Med J, 284:237, 1982

Avoid concurrent use

INTERFERON, with:
Angiotensin-converting enzyme (ACE) inhibitors - See Angiotensin-converting enzyme (ACE) inhibitors with Interferon, page 46
Anticoagulants, oral - See Anticoagulants, oral with Interferon, page 70
Clozapine - See Clozapine with Interferon, page 206
Epoetin - See Epoetin with Interferon, page 270
Fluorouracil - See Fluorouracil with Interferon, page 283

INTERFERON, with: *(continued)*
  Selective serotonin reuptake inhibitors (SSRIs)
    Possible reduction in antidepressant effect with paroxetine (possible antagonism)
      RH McAllister-Williams et al, Antidepressant response reversed by interferon. Br J Psychiatry, 176:93, 2000
    Single case report (2000); patient also taking trazodone; monitor clinical status
  Theophyllines
    Possible theophylline toxicity with interferon alfa 2a (decreased metabolism)
      JHG Jonkman et al, Effects of α-interferon on theophylline pharmacokinetics and metabolism. Br J Clin Pharmacol, 27:795, 1989
    Monitor theophylline concentration
  Trazodone
    Possible reduction in antidepressant effect (possible antagonism)
      RH McAllister-Williams et al, Antidepressant response reversed by interferon. Br J Psychiatry, 176:93, 2000
    Single case report (2000); patient also taking paroxetine; monitor clinical status

INTERLEUKIN-2, with:
  Contrast media - See Contrast media with Interleukin-2, page 219
  Indinavir - See Indinavir with Interleukin-2, page 307

Iohexol, see Contrast media
Iothalamate meglumine, see Contrast media
Ioxaglate, see Contrast media

IRBESARTAN, with:
  Antifungals, imidazoles and triazoles - See Antifungals, imidazoles and triazoles with Irbesartan, page 103

IRINOTECAN, with:
  Etoposide - See Etoposide with Irinotecan, page 274
  Oxaliplatin
    Possible cholinergic symptoms such as hypersalivation and abdominal pain (probably additive inhibition of cholinesterase)
      HM Dodds et al, More about: irinotecan-related cholinergic syndrome induced by coadministration of oxaliplatin. J Natl Cancer Inst, 91:91, 1999
    May be prevented or reversed by atropine; monitor clinical status

IRON, with:
  Angiotensin-converting enzyme (ACE) inhibitors - See Angiotensin-converting enzyme (ACE) inhibitors with Iron, page 46
  Antacids - See Antacids with Iron, page 54
  Antihistamines, H$_2$-blockers - See Antihistamines, H$_2$-blockers with Iron, page 119
  Caffeine - See Caffeine with Iron, page 174
  Cephalosporins - See Cephalosporins with Iron, page 191
  Fluoroquinolones - See Fluoroquinolones with Iron, page 279
  Levodopa
    Possible decreased levodopa effect (decreased absorption)
      NRC Campbell and B Hasinoff, Ferrous sulfate reduces levodopa bioavailability: chelation as a possible mechanism. Clin Pharmacol Ther, 45:220,

(continued)

IRON, with: *(continued)*
>1989; NRC Campbell et al, Sinemet-ferrous sulphate interaction in patients with Parkinson's disease. Br J Clin Pharmacol, 30:599, 1990

With carbidopa, only a minority of patients are affected

Methyldopa
Decreased hypotensive effect (decreased absorption)
>N Campbell et al, Alteration of methyldopa absorption, metabolism, and blood pressure control caused by ferrous sulfate and ferrous gluconate. Clin Pharmacol Ther, 43:381, 1988

Monitor blood pressure

Penicillamine
Renal toxicity (penicillamine absorption decreases when iron is added and increases when iron is withdrawn)
>JAL Harkness and DR Blake, Penicillamine nephropathy and iron. Lancet, 2:1368, 1982

Increased dosage may be necessary to control symptoms when iron is added; decrease penicillamine dosage when iron is withdrawn

Tetracyclines
Decreased tetracycline effect (decreased absorption), but not with doxycycline
>G Gothoni et al, Iron-tetracycline interaction: effect of time interval between the drugs. Acta Med Scand, 191:409, 1972; PJ Neuvonen and H Turakka, Inhibitory effect of various iron salts on the absorption of tetracycline in man. Eur J Clin Pharmacol, 7:357, 1974; PJ Neuvonen and O Penttila, Effect of oral ferrous sulfate on the half-life of doxycycline in man. Eur J Clin Pharmacol, 7:361, 1974

If concurrent use cannot be avoided, give iron 3 hours before or 2 hours after tetracycline

Decreased iron effect (decreased absorption)
>HC Heinrich and KH Oppitz, Tetracycline inhibits iron absorption in man. Naturwissenschaften, 60:524, 1973

Absorption of iron-ascorbic acid combination may not be affected

Thyroid hormones
Decreased effect of thyroxine (possibly decreased absorption)
>NRC Campbell et al, Ferrous sulfate reduces thyroxine efficacy in patients with hypothyroidism. Ann Intern Med, 117:1010, 1992; JL Schlienger, Accroissement des besoins en throxine par le sulfate de fer. La Presse Med, 23:492, 1994

Give thyroid hormones at least two hours before or four hours after iron; monitor TSH

Zinc
Decreased zinc effect (decreased absorption)
>NJ Meadows et al, Oral iron and the bioavailability of zinc. Br Med J, 287:1013, 1983

Avoid concurrent use

Isocarboxazid, see Monoamine oxidase inhibitors

Isoetharine, see Sympathomimetic amines; Sympathomimetic bronchodilators

ISOFLURANE, with:
   Amiodarone - See Amiodarone with Isoflurane, page 36
   Angiotensin-converting enzyme (ACE) inhibitors - See Angiotensin-converting enzyme (ACE) inhibitors with Isoflurane, page 46
   Reserpine
      Hypotension (additive)
           CS Coakley et al, Circulatory responses during anesthesia of patients on rauwolfia therapy. JAMA, 161:1143, 1958; RL Katz et al, Anesthesia, surgery and rauwolfia. Anesthesiology, 25:142, 1964
      Monitor blood pressure

Isometheptene, see Sympathomimetic amines

ISONIAZID, with:
   Acetaminophen - See Acetaminophen with Isoniazid, page 9
   Alcohol - See Alcohol with Isoniazid, page 18
   Antacids - See Antacids with Isoniazid, page 54
   Anticoagulants, oral - See Anticoagulants, oral with Isoniazid, page 70
   Antifungals, imidazoles and triazoles - See Antifungals, imidazoles and triazoles with Isoniazid, page 103
   Benzodiazepines - See Benzodiazepines with Isoniazid, page 143
   Carbamazepine - See Carbamazepine with Isoniazid, page 179
   Cycloserine - See Cycloserine with Isoniazid, page 227
   Disulfiram - See Disulfiram with Isoniazid, page 264
   Enflurane - See Enflurane with Isoniazid, page 269
   Haloperidol - See Haloperidol with Isoniazid, page 294
   Phenytoin
      Phenytoin toxicity (decreased metabolism)
           J Johnson and HL Freeman, Death due to isoniazid (INH) and phenytoin. Br J Psychiatry, 129:511, 1976; RR Miller et al, Clinical importance of the interaction of phenytoin and isoniazid: a report from the Boston Collaborative Drug Surveillance Program. Chest, 75:356, 1979; WW Yew et al, Phenytoin toxicity in a patient with isoniazid-induced hepatitis. Tubercle, 72:309, 1991
      Monitor phenytoin concentration; effect of rifampin is opposite to that of isoniazid and tends to predominate when both drugs are given
   Rifampin
      Hepatotoxicity (possibly increased toxic metabolites)
           D Pessayre et al, Isoniazid-rifampin fulminant hepatitis. Gastroenterology, 72:284, 1977; H Tsagaropoulon-Stinga et al, Hepatotoxic reactions in children with severe tuberculosis treated with isoniazid-rifampin. Pediatr Infect Dis, 4:270, 1985; G Raghupati Sarma et al, Rifampin-induced release of hydrazine from isoniazid. Am Rev Respir Dis, 133:1072, 1986; DS Askgaard et al, Hepatotoxicity caused by the combined action of isoniazid and rifampicin. Thorax, 50:213, 1995
      Monitor for hepatotoxicity
   Stavudine
      Increased risk of peripheral neuropathy (possibly additive)
           RAM Breen et al, Increased incidence of peripheral neuropathy with co-

(continued)

ISONIAZID, with: *(continued)*
>> administration of stavudine and isoniazid in HIV-infected individuals. AIDS, 14:615, 2000
> *Twelve of 22 patients on combination developed peripheral neuropathy; avoid combination if possible*

> **Theophyllines**
>> Theophylline toxicity with isoniazid alone or isoniazid and rifampin (mechanism not established)
>>> R Dal Negro et al, Rifampicin-isoniazid and delayed elimination of theophylline: a case report. Int J Clin Pharm Res, 8:275, 1988; J Torrent et al, Theophylline-isoniazid interaction. DICP, 23:143, 1989; JR Thompson and TH Self, Theophylline and isoniazid. Br J Clin Pharmacol, 30:909, 1990; Samigun et al, Lowering of theophylline clearance by isoniazid in slow and rapid acetylators. Br J Clin Pharmacol, 29:570, 1990
>> *Two case reports (1988, 1989); liver function impaired in patient on rifampin and normal in other patient; probably requires dosage of more than 300 mg/day of isoniazid alone*

> **Tyramine-rich foods and beverages**
>> Palpitations, tachypnea, sweating, urticaria, headache, vomiting (mechanism not established)
>>> M Toutoungi et al, Cheese, wine, and isoniazid. Lancet, 2:671, 1985; LM Kahana and E Todd, Histamine poisoning in a patient on isoniazid. Can Dis Weekly Rep, 7-16:77, 1981; CG Uragoda and SR Kottegoda, Adverse reactions to isoniazid on ingestion of fish with a high histamine content. Tubercle, 58:83, 1977
>> *Reports in patients consuming cheese and wine and some species of fish including tuna; these foods also have high histamine concentrations and isoniazid inhibits histaminase*

> **Valproate**
>> Hepatic and CNS toxicity (possibly additive and decreased metabolism)
>>> U Dockweiler, Isoniazid-induced valproic-acid toxicity, or vice versa. Lancet, 2:152, 1987; AP Jonville et al, Interaction between isoniazid and valproate: a case of valproate overdosage. Eur J Clin Pharmacol, 40:197, 1991
>> *Two case reports (1987, 1991)*

> **Vincristine**
>> Neurotoxicity (probable decreased vincristine metabolism; possible additive toxicity)
>>> C Carrión et al, Possible vincristine-isoniazid interaction. Ann Pharmacother, 29:201, 1995; J Hildebrand and Y Kenis, Additive toxicity of vincristine and other drugs for the peripheral nervous system: three case reports. Acta Neurol Belg, 71:486, 1971
>> *Several case reports (1971, 1995); avoid concurrent use*

Isopropamide iodide, see Anticholinergics
Isoproterenol, see Sympathomimetic amines; Sympathomimetic bronchodilators
Isosorbide dinitrate, see Nitrates
Isosorbide mononitrate, see Nitrates

ISOTRETINOIN, with:
  Alcohol - See Alcohol with Isotretinoin, page 18
  Azathioprine - See Azathioprine with Isotretinoin, page 129
  Carbamazepine - See Carbamazepine with Isotretinoin, page 179
  Indinavir - See Indinavir with Isotretinoin, page 307
  Ritonavir
    Possible isotretinoin toxicity (mechanism not established)
      J Padberg et al, Drug interaction of isotretinoin and protease inhibitors: support for the cellular retinoic acid-binding protein-1 theory of lipodystrophy? AIDS, 13:284, 1999; JO Sass and J Padberg, Human isotretinoin metabolism during indinavir therapy. AIDS Res Hum Retrovir, 16:1451, 2000
    Single case report (1999); patient also receiving indinavir, zidovudine and lamivudine; in this case, the plasma levels of isotretinoin were lower during antiviral therapy
  Tetracyclines
    Possible increased risk of pseudotumor cerebri (possible additive effect)
      AG Lee, Pseudotumor cerebri after treatment with tetracycline and isotretinoin for acne. Cutis, 55:165, 1995
    Single case report in 14-year-old boy (1995); avoid combination or monitor for symptoms (headache, nausea, vomiting, visual disturbances)

ISRADIPINE, with:
  Beta-adrenergic blockers - See Beta-adrenergic blockers with Isradipine, page 157
  Digoxin - See Digoxin with Isradipine, page 253
  HMG-CoA reductase inhibitors - See HMG-CoA reductase inhibitors with Isradipine, page 299

Itraconazole, see Antifungals, Imidazoles and Triazoles

IVERMECTIN, with:
  Alcohol - See Alcohol with Ivermectin, page 18

IVIG, see Immune Globulin, Intravenous

Kanamycin, see Aminoglycoside antibiotics

KAOLIN OR KAOLIN-PECTIN, with:
  Chloroquine - See Chloroquine with Kaolin or Kaolin-pectin, page 194
  Digoxin - See Digoxin with Kaolin or Kaolin-pectin, page 253
  Lincomycin
    Decreased lincomycin effect (decreased absorption)
      JG Wagner, Design and data analysis of biopharmaceutical studies in man. Can J Pharm Sci, 1:62, 1966
    Give kaolin-pectin 2 hours after antibiotic
  Narcotics: morphine-like
    Decreased codeine effect (decreased absorption)
      SKS Yu et al, Codeine phosphate adsorbed by kaolin. Aust J Pharm, 57:468, 1976
    Single report of loss of effect of codeine on diarrhea (1976)
  Pyrimethamine
    Possible decreased pyrimethamine effect (decreased absorption)
      JC McElnay et al, *In vitro* experiments on chloroquine and pyrimethamine

(continued)

KAOLIN OR KAOLIN-PECTIN, with: *(continued)*
>absorption in the presence of antacid constituents or kaolin. J Trop Med Hyg, 85:153, 1982

Give at least 4 hours apart

Tetracyclines
>Decreased tetracycline effect (decreased absorption)
>>MW Gouda, Effect of an antidiarrhoeal mixture on the bioavailability of tetracycline. Int J Pharmaceutics, 89:75, 1993
>
>*Avoid concurrent use or give tetracycline at least 2 hours before or 6 hours after kaolin if alternative antibiotic is not available; based on study in healthy volunteers*

KAVA, with:
>**Benzodiazepines** - See Benzodiazepines with Kava, page 143

Ketamine, no documented interactions, see page 4, Criteria for Listing Interactions
Ketazolam, see Benzodiazepines
Ketoconazole, see Antifungals, Imidazoles and Triazoles
Ketoprofen, see Nonsteroidal anti-inflammatory drugs
Ketorolac, see Nonsteroidal anti-inflammatory drugs
Ketotifen, no documented interactions, see page 4, Criteria for Listing Interactions
Labetalol, see Beta-adrenergic blockers
Lactulose, no documented interactions, see page 4, Criteria for Listing Interactions

LAMIVUDINE, with:
>**Zidovudine**
>>Zidovudine toxicity (mechanism not established)
>>>Manufacturer's package insert; EK Hester and JE Peacock Jr, et al, Profound and unanticipated anemia with lamivudine—zidovudine combination therapy in zidovudine-experienced patients with HIV infection. AIDS, 12:439, 1998
>>
>>*Profound anemia in two patients (1998)*

LAMOTRIGINE, with:
>**Barbiturates** - See Barbiturates with Lamotrigine, page 134
>**Carbamazepine** - See Carbamazepine with Lamotrigine, page 180
>**Methsuximide**
>>Reduced lamotrigine effect (increased metabolism)
>>>TW May et al, Influence of oxcarbazepine and methsuximide on lamotrigine concentrations in epileptic patients with and without valproic acid comedication: results of a retrospective study. Ther Drug Monit, 21:175, 1999; FMC Besag et al, Methsuximide lowers lamotrigine blood levels: a pharmacokinetic antiepileptic drug interaction. Epilepsia, 41:624, 2000
>>
>>*Serum lamotrigine concentration substantially lower with methsuximide comedication; monitor lamotrigine levels and clinical status*
>
>**Oxcarbazepine**
>>Possible decreased lamotrigine effect (increased metabolism)
>>>TW May et al, Influence of oxcarbazepine and methsuximide on lamotrigine concentrations in epileptic patients with and without valproic acid comedication: results of a retrospective study. Ther Drug Monit, 21:175, 1999

LAMOTRIGINE, with: *(continued)*
Monitor lamotrigine concentration
Phenytoin
Decreased lamotrigine effect (probably increased metabolism)
> Y Böttiger et al, Lamotrigine drug interactions in a TDM material. Ther Drug Monit, 21:171, 1999; JA Armijo et al, Lamotrigine serum concentration-to-dose ratio: influence of age and concomitant antiepileptic drugs and dosage implications. Ther Drug Monit, 21:182, 1999

Monitor lamotrigine serum concentrations and clinical status; lamotrigine dosage may need to be adjusted
Primidone
Decreased lamotrigine effect (probably increased metabolism)
> Manufacturer's package insert (lamotrigine)

Monitor lamotrigine serum concentrations and clinical status; lamotrigine dosage may need to be adjusted
Rifampin
Decreased lamotrigine effect (increased metabolism)
> A Armijo et al, Lamotrigine interaction with rifampicin and isoniazid. Methods Find Exp Clin Pharmacol, 8 suppl 3:59, 1996; U Ebert et al, Effects of rifampicin and cimetidine on pharmacokinetics and pharmacodynamics of lamotrigine in healthly subjects. Eur J Clin Pharmacol, 56:299, 2000

Single case report (1996) and pharmacokinetic study in healthy subjects; monitor lamotrigine concentration and clinical status
Selective serotonin reuptake inhibitors (SSRIs)
Possible lamotrigine toxicity (mechanism not established)
> KR Kaufman and R Gerner, Lamotrigine toxicity secondary to sertraline. Seizure, 7:163, 1998

Two case reports (1998); monitor clinical status and lamotrigine concentration
Valproate
Severe tremor due to lamotrigine toxicity (probably decreased metabolism)
> DC Reutens et al, Disabling tremor after lamotrigine with sodium valproate. Lancet, 342:185, 1993; GD Anderson et al, Bidirectional interaction of valproate and lamotrigine in healthy subjects. Clin Pharmacol Ther, 60:145, 1996; F Pisani et al, The efficacy of valproate-lamotrigine comedication in refractory complex partial seizures: evidence for a pharmacodyamic interaction. Epilepsia, 40:1141, 1999; TW May et al, Influence of oxcarbazepine and methsuximide on lamotrigine concentrations in epileptic patients with and without valproic acid comedication: results of a retrospective study. Ther Drug Monit, 21:175, 1999; Y Böttiger et al, Lamotrigine drug interactions in a TDM material. Ther Drug Monit, 21:171, 1999; JA Armijo et al, Lamotrigine serum concentration-to-dose ratio: influence of age and concomitant antiepileptic drugs and dosage implications. Ther Drug Monit, 21:182, 1999; MA Meyer, Valproic acid dosing recommendations questioned. Geriatrics, 55:16, 2000; LF Ferriols et al, Farmacocinética del ácido valproico tras la administración de lamotrigina. Farm Hosp, 23:64, 1999; AM Kanner et al, Addidng valproate to lamotrigine: a study of their pharmacokinetic interaction. Neurology, 55:588, 2000; BE Gidal et al, Lack

(continued)

LAMOTRIGINE, with: *(continued)*
of an effect of valproate concentration on lamotrigine pharmacokinetics in developmentally disabled patients with epilepsy. Epilepsy Res, 42:23, 2000
Monitor lamotrigine concentration and clinical status; consider decreased lamotrigine starting dose if patient on valproate; combination has been used successfully in refractory complex partial seizures when dosage of both drugs was lowered; valproate levels may not be affected by lamotrigine

Possible multiorgan failure and disseminated intravascular coagulation due to lamotrigine toxicity (probably decreased metabolism)
DS Chattergoon et al, Multiorgan dysfunction and disseminated intravascular coagulation in children receiving lamotrigine and valproic acid. Neurology, 19:14442, 1997
Two case reports in children (1997)

Stevens-Johnson syndrome and toxic epidermal necrolysis (probably decreased metabolism; glucuronidation)
RL Page II et al, Fatal toxic epidermal necrolysis related to lamotrigine administration. Pharmacotherapy, 18:392, 1998; M Bhushan et al, Prolonged toxic epidermal necrolysis due to lamotrigine. Clin Exp Dermatol, 25:349, 2000
Monitor clinical status

LANSOPRAZOLE, with:
Macrolide antibiotics
Possible glossitis, black tongue, or stomatitis with clarithromycin (mechanism not established)
S Greco et al, Glossitis, stomatitis, and black tongue with lansoprazole plus clarithromycin and other antibiotics. Ann Pharmacother, 31:1548, 1997
Reports of six cases (1997)

Sucralfate
Decreased lansoprazole effect (decreased absorption)
Manufacturer's package insert
Lansoprazole should be taken at least 30 minutes before sucralfate

Theophyllines
Possible decreased theophylline effect in some patients (increased metabolism)
T Kokufu et al, Effects of lansoprazole on pharmacokinetics and metabolism of theophylline. Eur J Clin Pharmacol, 48:391, 1995; J-W Ko et al, Theophylline pharmacokinetics are not altered by lansoprazole in CYP2C19 poor metabolizers. Clin Pharmacol Ther, 65:606, 1999; K Dilger et al, Lack of drug interaction between omeprazole, lansoprazole, and theophylline. Br J Clin Pharmacol, 48:438, 1999
Effect small; clinical significance probably minimal; no interaction found in healthy subjects given intravenous theophylline; no interaction found in healthy subjects given oral theophylline

Latanoprost, no documented interactions, see page 4, Criteria for Listing Interactions

L-carnitine, see Levocarnitine

LEFLUNOMIDE, with:
  Cholestyramine - See Cholestyramine with Leflunomide, page 196
  Methotrexate
    Possible hepatotoxicity (possibly additive)
      ME Weinblatt et al, Pharmacokinetics, safety, and efficacy of combination treatment with methotrexate and leflunomide in patients with active rheumatoid arthritis. Arthritis Rheum, 42:1322, 1999
    Based on study in 30 patients; monitor aminotransferase activities
  Rifampin
    Possible leflunomide toxicity (enzyme induction; increased concentration of active metabolite)
      Manufacturer's package insert
    Based on single-dose study; clinical significance not established

Letrozole, no documented interactions, see page 4, Criteria for Listing Interactions

LEUCOVORIN, with:
  Fluorouracil - See Fluorouracil with Leucovorin, page 283
  Methotrexate
    Deterioration of rheumatoid arthritis (mechanism not established)
      M Tishler et al, The effects of leucovorin (folinic acid) on methotrexate therapy in rheumatoid arthritis patients. Arthritis Rheum, 31:906, 1988
    Avoid concurrent use in rheumatoid arthritis, unless leucovorin is being used to treat severe methotrexate toxicity

Leuprolide, no documented interactions, see page 4, Criteria for Listing Interactions

Levalbuterol, see Sympathomimetic amines

Levamphetamine, see Sympathomimetic amines

Levetiracetam, no documented interactions, see page 4, Criteria for Listing Interactions

Levobunolol, see Beta-adrenergic blockers

Levocabastine, no documented interactions, see page 4, Criteria for Listing Interactions

LEVOCARNITINE, with:
  Anticoagulants, oral - See Anticoagulants, oral with Levocarnitine, page 70

LEVODOPA, with:
  Anticholinergics - See Anticholinergics with Levodopa, page 58
  Antidepressants, tricyclic - See Antidepressants, tricyclic with Levodopa, page 86
  Benzodiazepines - See Benzodiazepines with Levodopa, page 143
  Bupropion - See Bupropion with Levodopa, page 169
  Clonidine - See Clonidine with Levodopa, page 204
  Dacarbazine - See Dacarbazine with Levodopa, page 241
  Indinavir - See Indinavir with Levodopa, page 307
  Iron - See Iron with Levodopa, page 311
  Methionine
    Decreased levodopa effect (mechanism not established)
      LA Pearce and LD Waterbury, L-methionine: a possible levodopa antagonist. Neurology, 21:410, 1971; 24:640, 1974
    Avoid large doses of methionine

(continued)

LEVODOPA, with: *(continued)*

Mirtazapine
Possible psychosis (mechanism not established)
> C Normann et al, Psychosis during chronic levodopa therapy triggered by the new antidepressive drug mirtazapine. Pharmacopsychiatria, 30:263, 1997

Single case report (1997)

Monoamine oxidase inhibitors
Hypertensive crisis, but not if taking carbidopa (increase in storage and release of dopamine, norepinephrine, or both)
> PF Teychenne et al, Interactions of levodopa with inhibitors of monoamine oxidase and L-aromatic amino acid decarboxylase. Clin Pharmacol Ther, 18:273, 1975

Always use carbidopa if monoamine oxidase inhibitors must be used

Prolonged dyskinesias with selegiline, an MAO B inhibitor (probably decreased levodopa metabolism)
> F Baronti et al, Deprenyl (selegiline) effects on levodopa pharmacodynamics, mood, and free radical scavenging. Neurology, 42:541, 1992

Monitor clinical status

Orphenadrine
Decreased levodopa effect (decreased absorption)
> M Contin et al, Combined levodopa-anticholinergic therapy in the treatment of Parkinson's disease. Clin Neuropharmacol, 14:148, 1991

Monitor clinical status; due to anticholinergic effects of orphenadrine, which is also a muscle relaxant

Papaverine
Decreased levodopa effect (mechanism not established)
> DM Posner, Antagonism of levodopa by papaverine. JAMA, 233:768, 1975; RC Duvoisin, Antagonism of levodopa by papaverine. JAMA, 231:845, 1975; JL Montastruc et al, Does papaverine interact with levodopa in Parkinson's disease? Ann Neurol, 22:558, 1987

Avoid concurrent use; controlled trial failed to confirm

Phenothiazines
Decreased levodopa effect (inhibition of dopamine uptake); decreased antipsychotic effect (mechanism not established)
> MD Yahr and RC Duvoisin, Drug therapy of parkinsonism. N Engl J Med, 287:20, 1972; GC Cotzias et al, L-Dopa in parkinson's syndrome. N Engl J Med, 281:272, 1969

Avoid concurrent use, if possible

Phenytoin
Decreased levodopa effect (mechanism not established)
> JS Mendez et al, Diphenylhydantoin: blocking of levodopa effects. Arch Neurol, 32:44, 1975

LEVODOPA, with: *(continued)*
Use alternative anticonvulsant; do not treat dyskinesias with phenytoin in patients with Parkinsonism receiving levodopa

Pyridoxine
Decreased levodopa effect, but not if taking carbidopa (enhanced decarboxylation of levodopa at periphery)
> H Mars, Levodopa, carbidopa, and pyridoxine in parkinson disease. Arch Neurol, 30:444, 1974; RC Duvoisin et al, Pyridoxine reversal of L-dopa effects in parkinsonism. Trans Am Neurol Assoc, 94:81, 1969

Avoid pyridoxine supplements or vitamin preparations containing pyridoxine if carbidopa is not used

Quetiapine
Possible decreased levodopa effect (antagonism)
> Manufacturer's package insert

Avoid concurrent use, if possible

Spiramycin
Possible decreased antiparkinson effect with carbidopa-levodopa (possibly decreased absorption)
> N Brion et al, Effect of a macrolide (spiramycin) on the pharmacokinetics of L-dopa and carbidopa in healthy volunteers. Clin Neuropharmacol, 15:229, 1992

Monitor clinical status

Levofloxacin, see Fluoroquinolones

Levomethadyl, no documented interactions, see page 4, Criteria for Listing Interactions

Levonorgestrel, see Contraceptives, implant; Contraceptives, oral

Levorphanol, see Narcotics: morphine-like

Levothyroxine, see Thyroid hormones

Licorice, see Glycyrrhiza

LIDOCAINE, with:

Amiodarone - See Amiodarone with Lidocaine, page 36

Amprenavir - See Amprenavir with Lidocaine, page 39

Antifungals, imidazoles and triazoles - See Antifungals, imidazoles and triazoles with Lidocaine, page 103

Antihistamines, H$_2$-blockers - See Antihistamines, H$_2$-blockers with Lidocaine, page 119

Arbutamine - See Arbutamine with Lidocaine, page 128

Beta-adrenergic blockers - See Beta-adrenergic blockers with Lidocaine, page 157

Bupivacaine - See Bupivacaine with Lidocaine, page 168

Macrolide antibiotics
Possible oral lidocaine toxicity with erythromycin (probably decreased first-pass metabolism; CYP3A4)
> MH Isohanni et al, Effect of erythromycin and itraconazole on the pharmacokinetics of oral lignocaine. Pharmacol Toxicol, 84:143, 1999

(continued)

LIDOCAINE, with: *(continued)*
> *Based on study in healthy subjects; monitor clinical status; theoretically clarithromycin would interact similarly, while azithromycin and dirithromycin would not*

Mexiletine
> Oral lidocaine toxicity (mechanism not established)
>> DR Geraets et al, Toxicity potential of oral lidocaine in a patient receiving mexiletine. Ann Pharmacother, 26:1380, 1992
>
> *Single case report (1992); cachectic patient also receiving ranitidine*
>
> Myoclonus with IV lidocaine (mechanism not established)
>> JM Christie et al, Neurotoxicity of lidocaine combined with mexiletine. Anesth Analg, 77:1291, 1993
>
> *Single case report (1993)*

Narcotics: meperidine and congeners
> Possible CNS and respiratory depression with fentanyl (additive)
>> E Jensen and ND Nader, Potentiation of narcosis after intravenous lidocaine in a patient given spinal opioids. Anesth Analg, 89:758, 1999
>
> *Single case report (1999); in a patient given intravenous bolus and constant infusion of lidocaine; monitor clinical status*

Narcotics: morphine-like
> Possible CNS and respiratory depression with morphine (additive)
>> E Jensen and ND Nader, Potentiation of narcosis after intravenous lidocaine in a patient given spinal opioids. Anesth Analg, 89:758, 1999
>
> *Single case report (1999); in a patient given intravenous bolus and constant influsion of lidocaine; monitor clinical status*

Propafenone
> CNS toxicity (possibly additive)
>> MR Ujhelyi et al, The pharmacokinetic and pharmacodynamic interaction between propafenone and lidocaine. Clin Pharmacol Ther, 53:38, 1993
>
> *Monitor clinical status; based on study in 12 healthy men*

Tocainide
> Seizures (possibly additive neurotoxicity)
>> E Forrence et al, A seizure induced by concurrent lidocaine-tocainide therapy – is it just a case of additive toxicity? Drug Intell Clin Pharm, 20:56, 1986
>
> *Single case report (1986); patient received IV lidocaine for 10 days before oral tocainide was started; alternative antiarrhythmic agent may be preferable after prolonged IV lidocaine*

Trimethoprim-sulfamethoxazole
> Methemoglobinemia (probably additive)
>> B Jakobson and A Nilsson, Methemoglobinemia associated with a prilocaine – lidocaine cream and trimethoprim-sulphamethoxazole. A case report. Acta Anaesthesiol Scand, 29:453, 1985
>
> *Single case report in an infant with prilocaine-lidocaine cream (1985)*

LINCOMYCIN, with:
  Kaolin or Kaolin-pectin - See Kaolin or Kaolin-pectin with Lincomycin, page 315
  Neuromuscular blocking agents
    Increased neuromuscular blockade (additive)
      JT Rubbo et al, Comparative neuromuscular effects of lincomycin and clindamycin. Anesth Analg, 56:329, 1977
    Monitor neuromuscular status

Lindane, no documented interactions, see page 4, Criteria for Listing Interactions

LINEZOLID, with:
  Sympathomimetic amines
    Hypertension (mechanism not established)
      Manufacturer's package insert (linezolid)
    In one study in normotensive volunteers, blood pressure increased with co-administration of phenylpropanolamine or pseudoephedrine; monitor clinical status
  Tyramine-rich foods and beverages
    Hypertension (mechanism not established)
      Manufacturer's package insert (linezolid)
    Increased hypertensive response in normal adults eating large amounts of tyramine (100 mg or more)

Liothyronine, see Thyroid hormones

Liotrix, see Thyroid hormones

LIPIDS, INTRAVENOUS PREPARATIONS, with:
  Cyclosporine - See Cyclosporine with Lipids, intravenous preparations, page 233

Lisinopril, see Angiotensin-converting enzyme (ACE) inhibitors

LITHIUM, with:
  Alcohol - See Alcohol with Lithium, page 18
  Angiotensin-converting enzyme (ACE) inhibitors - See Angiotensin-converting enzyme (ACE) inhibitors with Lithium, page 46
  Anticholinergics - See Anticholinergics with Lithium, page 59
  Antidepressants, tricyclic - See Antidepressants, tricyclic with Lithium, page 86
  Benzodiazepines - See Benzodiazepines with Lithium, page 143
  Beta-adrenergic blockers - See Beta-adrenergic blockers with Lithium, page 157
  Caffeine - See Caffeine with Lithium, page 174
  Calcitonin - See Calcitonin with Lithium, page 175
  Carbamazepine - See Carbamazepine with Lithium, page 180
  Carbonic anhydrase inhibitors - See Carbonic anhydrase inhibitors with Lithium, page 188
  Cisplatin - See Cisplatin with Lithium, page 201
  Clozapine - See Clozapine with Lithium, page 206
  COX-2 inhibitors - See COX-2 inhibitors with Lithium, page 225
  Diltiazem - See Diltiazem with Lithium, page 260
  Droperidol - See Droperidol with Lithium, page 267
  Furosemide - See Furosemide with Lithium, page 285
  Haloperidol - See Haloperidol with Lithium, page 294
  Indapamide - See Indapamide with Lithium, page 307

(continued)

LITHIUM, with: *(continued)*
  Losartan
    Lithium toxicity with losartan (possible increased renal reabsorption of lithium)
      P Blanche et al, Lithium intoxication in an elderly patient after combined treatment with losartan. Eur J Clin Pharmacol, 52:501, 1997
    Single case report (1997); avoid concurrent use
  Mazindol
    Lithium toxicity (mechanism not established)
      MS Hendy et al, Mazindol-induced lithium toxicity. Br Med J, 280:684, 1980
    Avoid concurrent use
  Methyldopa
    Lithium toxicity (mechanism not established)
      JB O'Regan, Adverse interaction of lithium carbonate and methyldopa. Can Med Assoc J, 115:385, 1976; GJ Byrd, Lithium carbonate and methyldopa: apparent interaction in man. Clin Toxicol, 11:1, 1977; R Yassa, Lithium-methyldopa interaction. Can Med Assoc J, 134:141, 1986
    Monitor lithium concentration and clinical status; lithium concentration may remain near upper normal limit
  Metronidazole
    Lithium toxicity (mechanism not established)
      MH Teicher et al, Possible nephrotoxic interaction of lithium and metronidazole. JAMA, 257:3365, 1987
    Monitor lithium concentration and clinical status
  Monoamine oxidase inhibitors
    Neuroleptic malignant syndrome with phenelzine (mechanism not established)
      D Brennan et al, 'Neuroleptic malignant syndrome' without neuroleptics. Br J Psychiatry, 152:578, 1988
    Single case report (1988)
  Neuromuscular blocking agents
    Prolonged neuromuscular blockade (mechanism not established)
      FW Reimherr et al, Prolongation of muscle relaxant effects by lithium carbonate. Am J Psychiatry, 134:205, 1977; GE Hill et al, Potentiation of succinylcholine neuromuscular blockade by lithium carbonate. Anesthesiology, 44:439, 1976; H Borden et al, The use of pancuronium bromide in patients receiving lithium carbonate. Can Anaesthesiol Soc J, 21:79, 1974; G Jephcott and RJ Kerry, Lithium: an anaesthetic risk. Br J Anaesth, 46:389, 1974
    Monitor neuromuscular status
  Nonsteroidal anti-inflammatory drugs
    Lithium toxicity with NSAIDs (decreased renal excretion)
      JC Frolich et al, Indomethacin increases plasma lithium. Br Med J, 1:1115, 1979; CA Kristoff et al, Effect of ibuprofen on lithium plasma and red blood cell concentrations. Clin Pharm, 5:51, 1986; MM Furnell and J Davies, The effect of sulindac on lithium therapy. Drug Intell Clin Pharm, 19:374, 1985; J Nadarajah and GS Stein, Piroxicam induced lithium toxicity. Ann Rheum Dis, 44:502, 1985; MA Ragheb and AL Powell, Failure of sulindac to increase serum lithium levels. J Clin Psychiatry, 47:33, 1986; M Ragheb and AL Powell, Lithium interaction with sulindac and naproxen. J Clin Psycho-

LITHIUM, with: *(continued)*

pharmacol, 6:150, 1986; IW Reimann and JC Frölich, Effects of diclofenac on lithium kinetics. Clin Pharmacol Ther, 30:348, 1981; IH Khan, Lithium and non-steroidal anti-inflammatory drugs. BMJ, 302:1537, 1991; TM Harrison et al, Lithium carbonate and piroxicam. Br J Psychiatry, 149:124, 1986; H Bendz and M Feinberg, Aspirin increases serum lithium ion levels. Arch Gen Psychiatry, 41:310, 1984; I Reimann, In reply. Arch Gen Psychiatry 41:311, 1984; V Iyer, Ketorolac *(Toradol)* induced lithium toxicity. Headache, 34:442, 1994; BM Hughes et al, The effect of flurbiprofen on steady-state plasma lithium levels. Pharmacotherapy, 17:113, 1997; GM Levin et al, Effect of over-the-counter dosages of naproxen sodium and acetaminophen on plasma lithium concentrations in normal volunteers. J Clin Psychopharmacol, 18:237, 1998; SS Chandragiri et al, Lithium, ACE inhibitors, NSAIDs, and verapamil: a possible fatal combination. Psychosomatic, 39:281, 1998; MT Jones and SC Stoner, Increased lithium concentrations reported in patients treated with sulindac. J Clin Psychiatry, 61:527, 2000

Monitor lithium concentration; OTC doses of naproxen did not interact in 12 healthy subjects; although sulindac has been reported not to affect lithium, two cases of possible sulindac-induced lithium toxicity have been reported (2000)

Possible renal toxicity (mechanism not established)

J MacDonald and TJ Neale, Toxic interaction of lithium carbonate and mefenamic acid. Br Med J, 297:1339, 1988

Single case report with mefenamic acid (1988)

Penicillins

Hypernatremia with ticarcillin (large sodium load from ticarcillin and decreased renal excretion)

RA Finch, Hypernatremia during lithium and ticarcillin therapy. South Med J, 74:376, 1981

Avoid penicillins with high sodium content

Phenothiazines

Neurotoxicity (mechanism not established)

GK Spring, Neurotoxicity with combined use of lithium and thioridazine. J Clin Psychiatry, 40:135, 1979; SV Singh, Lithium carbonate/fluphenazine decanoate producing irreversible brain damage. Lancet, 2:278, 1982; F Miller et al, Lithium-neuroleptic neurotoxicity in the elderly bipolar patient. J Clin Psychopharmacol, 6:176, 1986; J de la Gandara and RA Dominguez, Lithium and loxapine: a potential interaction. J Clin Psychiatry, 49:126, 1988; G Addonizio et al, Increased extrapyramidal symptoms with addition of lithium to neuroleptics. J Nerv Ment Dis, 176:682, 1988

Monitor EEG and neurological status

Decreased chlorpromazine effect (mechanism not established)

L Rivera-Calimlim et al, Effect of lithium on plasma chlorpromazine levels. Clin Pharmacol Ther, 23:451, 1978; R Yassa, A case of lithium-chlorpromazine interaction. J Clin Psychiatry, 47:90, 1986; RN Stevenson et al, Ventricular fibrillation due to lithium withdrawal – an interaction with

LITHIUM, with: *(continued)*

chlorpromazine? Postgrad Med J, 65:936, 1989

Monitor for decreased chlorpromazine response; single case report of ventricular fibrillation with chlorpromazine on withdrawal of lithium (1989)

Acute hypotension (mechanism not established)

A Byrne et al, Severe hypotension associated with combined lithium and chlorpromazine therapy: a case report and a review. Can J Psychiatry, 39:294, 1994

Single case report (1994)

Phenytoin

Lithium toxicity (possibly synergism)

J Speirs and SR Hirsch, Severe lithium toxicity with "normal" serum concentrations. Br Med J, 1:815, 1978; WAG MacCallum, Interaction of lithium and phenytoin. Br Med J, 280:610, 1980; DE Raskin, Lithium and phenytoin interaction. J Clin Psychopharmacol, 4:120, 1984

Monitor for renal and CNS effects; lithium concentration normal

Psyllium

Decreased lithium effect (probably decreased absorption)

BB Perlman, Interaction between lithium salts and ispaghula husk. Lancet, 335:416, 1990; M Toutoungi et al, Probable interaction entre le psyllium et le lithium. Therapie, 45:357, 1990

Single case report (1990); confirmed in healthy subjects (1990)

Selective serotonin reuptake inhibitors (SSRIs)

Lithium toxicity with fluoxetine (mechanism not established)

AA Salama and M Shafey, A case of severe lithium toxicity induced by combined fluoxetine and lithium carbonate. Am J Psychiatry, 146:278, 1989; A Hadley and MP Cason, Mania resulting from lithium-fluoxetine combination. Am J Psychiatry, 146:1637, 1989; JA Sacristan et al, Absence seizures induced by lithium: possible interaction with fluoxetine. Am J Psychiatry, 148:146, 1991

Monitor lithium concentration; several case reports of lithium toxicity;

Mania with fluvoxamine (mechanism not established)

C Burrai et al, Mania and fluvoxamine. Am J Psychiatry, 148:1263, 1991

Patients with mania and elevated lithium concentrations

Tremor, incoordination, hyperreflexia - serotonin syndrome - with fluvoxamine, fluoxetine, paroxetine or citalopram (probably additive)

R Öhman and O Spigset, Serotonin syndrome induced by fluvoxamine-lithium interaction. Pharmacopsychiatry, 26:263, 1993; EC Muly et al, Serotonin syndrome produced by a combination of fluoxetine and lithium. Am J Psychiatry, 150:1565, 1993; J Karle and F Bjørndal, Serotonergt syndrom — ved kombineret behandling med litium og fluoxetin. Ugeskr Laeger, 27:1204, 1995; T Sobanski et al, Serotonin syndrome after lithium add-on medication to paroxetine. Pharmacopsychiatry, 30:106, 1997; manufacturer's package insert; R Grohmann et al, Assessment of adverse drug reactions in psychiatric inpatients with the AMSP drug safety program: methods and first results for tricyclic antidepressants and SSRI.

LITHIUM, with: *(continued)*
> Pharmacopsychiatry, 32:21, 1999; M Bauer et al, Paroxetine and amitriptyline augmentation of lithium in the treatment of major depression: a double-blind study. J Clin Psychopharmacol, 19:164, 1999

Single case reports with fluvoxamine (1993) and paroxetine (1997) and 2 case reports with fluoxetine (1993, 1995); two case reports with unspecified SSRI (1999); theoretically could occur with any SSRI; addition of paroxetine to lithium may produce more rapid improvement of major depression in some patients

Sibutramine

Possible serotonin syndrome (additive serotonergic effect)
> Manufacturer's package insert

Avoid concurrent use

Spectinomycin

Lithium toxicity (decreased renal excretion)
> RW Conroy, Personal communication, cited in Anonymous, Possible adverse drug-drug interaction report: lithium intoxication in a spectinomycin-treated patient. Int Drug Ther Newslett, 13:15, 1978

Monitor lithium concentration

Tetracyclines

Lithium toxicity (decreased renal excretion)
> U Malt, Lithium carbonate and tetracycline interaction. Br Med J, 2:502, 1978; AJ McGennis, Lithium carbonate and tetracycline interaction. Br Med J, 1:1183, 1978; SC Miller, Doxycycline-induced lithium toxicity. J Clin Psychopharmacol, 17:54, 1997

Monitor clinical status and lithium concentration

Theophyllines

Decreased lithium effect (probably increased renal clearance)
> PJ Perry et al, Theophylline precipitated alterations of lithium clearance. Acta Psychiatr Scand, 69:528, 1984; BL Cook et al, Theophylline – lithium interaction. J Clin Psychiatry, 46:278, 1985

Monitor lithium concentration

Thiazide diuretics

Lithium toxicity (decreased renal excretion)
> RJ Kerry et al, Diuretics are dangerous with lithium. Br Med J, 281:371, 1980; S MacNeil et al, Diuretics during lithium therapy. Lancet, 1:1295, 1975

Monitor lithium concentration

Venlafaxine

Serotonin syndrome (additive)
> G Mekler and B Woggon, A case of serotonin syndrome caused by venlafaxine and lithium. Pharmacopsychiatria, 30:272, 1997; E Hoencamp et al, Lithium augmentation of venlafaxine: an open-label trial. J Clin Psychopharmacol, 20:538, 2000

Single case report (1997); some have used combination with good results

(continued)

LITHIUM, with: *(continued)*
  Verapamil
    Decreased lithium effect (mechanism not established)
      LA Weinrauch et al, Decreased serum lithium during verapamil therapy. Am Heart J, 108:1378, 1984
    Avoid concurrent use

    Neurotoxicity (mechanism not established)
      WA Price and AJ Giannini, Neurotoxicity caused by lithium-verapamil synergism. J Clin Pharmacol, 26:717, 1986; BA Wright and DB Jarrett, Lithium and calcium channel blockers: possible neurotoxicity. Biol Psychiatry, 30:635, 1991; SS Chandragiri et al, Lithium, ACE inhibitors, NSAIDs, and verapamil: a possible fatal combination. Psychosomatic, 39:281, 1998
    Avoid concurrent use

    Bradycardia (mechanism not established)
      SL Dubovsky et al, Verapamil: a new antimanic drug with potential interactions with lithium. J Clin Psychiatry, 48:371, 1987
    Avoid concurrent use

Lodoxamide, no documented interactions, see page 4, Criteria for Listing Interactions

Lomustine, see Alkylating agents

Loperamide, see Narcotics: meperidine and congeners

LOPINAVIR/RITONAVIR, with:
  Amiodarone - See Amiodarone with Lopinavir/Ritonavir, page 36
  Amprenavir - See Amprenavir with Lopinavir/Ritonavir, page 39
  Anticoagulants, oral - See Anticoagulants, oral with Lopinavir/Ritonavir, page 70
  Antifungals, imidazoles and triazoles - See Antifungals, imidazoles and triazoles with Lopinavir/Ritonavir, page 103
  Atovaquone - See Atovaquone with Lopinavir/Ritonavir, page 129
  Benzodiazepines - See Benzodiazepines with Lopinavir/Ritonavir, page 143
  Bepridil - See Bepridil with Lopinavir/Ritonavir, page 152
  Cisapride - See Cisapride with Lopinavir/Ritonavir, page 200
  Contraceptives, oral - See Contraceptives, oral with Lopinavir/Ritonavir, page 214
  Delavirdine - See Delavirdine with Lopinavir/Ritonavir, page 244
  Efavirenz - See Efavirenz with Lopinavir/Ritonavir, page 267
  Ergot alkaloids - See Ergot alkaloids with Lopinavir/Ritonavir, page 271
  Flecainide - See Flecainide with Lopinavir/Ritonavir, page 277
  HMG-CoA reductase inhibitors - See HMG-CoA reductase inhibitors with Lopinavir/Ritonavir, page 300
  Indinavir - See Indinavir with Lopinavir/Ritonavir, page 308
  Macrolide antibiotics
    Possible clarithromycin toxicity (decreased metabolism)
      Manufacturer's package insert (*Kaletra*)
    Manufacturer recommends decreasing clarithromycin dosage in patients with renal impairment; monitor clinical status

LOPINAVIR/RITONAVIR, with: *(continued)*
  Narcotics: methadone and congeners
    Decreased methadone effect (increased metabolism)
      Manufacturer's package insert (*Kaletra*)
    Dosage of methadone may need to be increased
  Nevirapine
    Decreased lopinavir effect (increased metabolism)
      Manufacturer's package insert (*Kaletra*)
    Manufacturer recommends increasing Kaletra dose to 533/133 mg bid with food
  Pimozide
    Increased pimozide toxicity including cardiac arrhythmias (decreased metabolism; CYP3A4)
      Manufacturer's package insert (*Kaletra*)
    Avoid concurrent use
  Propafenone
    Increased propafenone toxicity including cardiac arrhythmias (decreased metabolism)
      Manufacturer's package insert (*Kaletra*)
    Avoid concurrent use
  Rifabutin
    Possible rifabutin toxicity (decreased metabolism)
      Manufacturer's package insert (*Kaletra*)
    Manufacturer recommends decreasing rifabutin dosage by at least 75% to 150 mg every other day or 3 times/week
  Rifampin
    Decreased virologic effectiveness of lopinavir/ritonavir (increased metabolism)
      Manufacturer's package insert (*Kaletra*)
    Avoid concurrent use
  Ritonavir
    Increased lopinavir toxicity (decreased metabolism)
      Manufacturer's package insert (*Kaletra*)
    Doses of the combination may need to be adjusted
  Saint John's wort
    Decreased virologic effectiveness of lopinavir/ritonavir (increased metabolism)
      Manufacturer's package insert (*Kaletra*)
    Avoid concurrent use
  Saquinavir
    Increased saquinavir toxicity (decreased metabolism
      Manufacturer's package insert (*Kaletra*)
    Doses of the combination may need to be adjusted
  Sildenafil
    Possible sildenafil toxicity (decreased metabolism)
      Manufacturer's package insert (*Kaletra*)
    Manufacturer recommends decreasing sildenafil dose to 25 mg every 48 hours; monitor clinical status

(continued)

LOPINAVIR/RITONAVIR, with: *(continued)*
  Tacrolimus
    Possible tacrolimus toxicity (decreased metabolism)
      Manufacturer's package insert (*Kaletra*)
    Single case report with ritonavir alone; monitor tacrolimus concentrations and clinical status
Loracarbef, no documented interactions, see page 4, Criteria for Listing Interactions
Loratadine, see Antihistamines, H$_1$-blockers: Loratadine
Lorazepam, see Benzodiazepines
LOSARTAN, with:
  Antifungals, imidazoles and triazoles - See Antifungals, imidazoles and triazoles with Losartan, page 103
  Cyclosporine - See Cyclosporine with Losartan, page 233
  Lithium - See Lithium with Losartan, page 324
  Nonsteroidal anti-inflammatory drugs
    Reduced antihypertensive effect of losartan (mechanism not established)
      PR Conlin et al, Effect of indomethacin on blood pressure lowering by captopril and losartan in hypertensive patients. Hypertension, 36:461, 2000
    Monitor blood pressure
  Phenytoin
    Possible decreased losartan effect (possible decreased metabolism; CYP2C9)
      TL Allen et al, In vivo inhibitory effect of phenytoin on losartan disposition. Clin Pharmacol Ther, 65:149, 1999
    Based on study in healthy subjects; monitor clinical status
  Rifampin
    Possible decreased losartan antihypertensive effect (increased metabolism)
      KM Williamson et al, Effects of erythromycin or rifampin on losartan pharmacokinetics in healthy volunteers. Clin Pharmacol Ther, 63:316, 1998
    Based on study in healthy subjects; monitor blood pressure
Lovastatin, see HMG-CoA Reductase Inhibitors
LOXAPINE, with:
  Benzodiazepines - See Benzodiazepines with Loxapine, page 144
  Carbamazepine - See Carbamazepine with Loxapine, page 180
Lyme disease vaccine, no documented interactions, see page 4, Criteria for Listing Interactions
MACROLIDE ANTIBIOTICS, with:
  Alcohol - See Alcohol with Macrolide antibiotics, page 19
  Anticoagulants, oral - See Anticoagulants, oral with Macrolide antibiotics, page 70
  Antifungals, imidazoles and triazoles - See Antifungals, imidazoles and triazoles with Macrolide antibiotics, page 104
  Antihistamines, H$_1$-blockers: astemizole, terfenadine - See Antihistamines, H$_1$-blockers: astemizole, terfenadine with Macrolide antibiotics, page 111
  Antihistamines, H$_1$-blockers: loratadine - See Antihistamines, H$_1$-blockers: loratadine with Macrolide antibiotics, page 113

MACROLIDE ANTIBIOTICS, with: *(continued)*
   Antihistamines, H$_2$-blockers - See Antihistamines, H$_2$-blockers with Macrolide antibiotics, page 119
   Benzodiazepines - See Benzodiazepines with Macrolide antibiotics, page 144
   Bromocriptine - See Bromocriptine with Macrolide antibiotics, page 167
   Buspirone - See Buspirone with Macrolide antibiotics, page 170
   Carbamazepine - See Carbamazepine with Macrolide antibiotics, page 180
   Cilostazol - See Cilostazol with Macrolide antibiotics, page 199
   Cisapride - See Cisapride with Macrolide antibiotics, page 200
   Clozapine - See Clozapine with Macrolide antibiotics, page 207
   Colchicine - See Colchicine with Macrolide antibiotics, page 211
   Contraceptives, oral - See Contraceptives, oral with Macrolide antibiotics, page 214
   Corticosteroids - See Corticosteroids with Macrolide antibiotics, page 220
   Cyclosporine - See Cyclosporine with Macrolide antibiotics, page 233
   Delavirdine - See Delavirdine with Macrolide antibiotics, page 244
   Digitoxin - See Digitoxin with Macrolide antibiotics, page 250
   Digoxin - See Digoxin with Macrolide antibiotics, page 253
   Disopyramide - See Disopyramide with Macrolide antibiotics, page 263
   Dofetilide - See Dofetilide with Macrolide antibiotics, page 265
   Efavirenz - See Efavirenz with Macrolide antibiotics, page 267
   Ergot alkaloids - See Ergot alkaloids with Macrolide antibiotics, page 271
   Felodipine - See Felodipine with Macrolide antibiotics, page 276
   Fluoroquinolones - See Fluoroquinolones with Macrolide antibiotics, page 279
   HMG-CoA reductase inhibitors - See HMG-CoA reductase inhibitors with Macrolide antibiotics, page 300
   Hypoglycemics, sulfonylurea - See Hypoglycemics, sulfonylurea with Macrolide antibiotics, page 304
   Lansoprazole - See Lansoprazole with Macrolide antibiotics, page 318
   Lidocaine - See Lidocaine with Macrolide antibiotics, page 321
   Lopinavir/Ritonavir - See Lopinavir/Ritonavir with Macrolide antibiotics, page 328
   Monoamine oxidase inhibitors
     Severe hypotension, syncope with phenelzine and erythromycin (possibly increased absorption)
        AE Bernstein, Drug interaction. Hosp Community Psychiatr, 41:806, 1990
     Single case report (1990)
   Narcotics: meperidine and congeners
     Possible alfentanil toxicity with erythromycin (decreased metabolism)
        RR Bartkowski et al, Inhibition of alfentanil metabolism by erythromycin. Clin Pharmacol Ther, 46:99, 1989; RR Bartkowski and TE McDonnell, Prolonged alfentanil effect following erythromycin administration. Anesthesiology, 73:566, 1990
     Based on study in healthy men and case reports
   Phenytoin
     Possible decreased phenytoin effect or toxicity with erythromycin (altered metabolism)
        K Bachmann et al, Single dose phenytoin clearance during erythromycin

MACROLIDE ANTIBIOTICS, with: *(continued)*
> treatment. Res Commun Chem Pathol Pharmacol, 46:207, 1984; RW Milne et al, Lack of effect of erythromycin on the pharmacokinetics of single oral doses of phenytoin. Br J Clin Pharmacol, 26:330, 1988

One study in healthy volunteers showed large individual variation and a second was negative; monitor phenytoin concentration

Pimozide

Pimozide toxicity (ventricular arrhythmias) with clarithromycin (probably decreased metabolism; CYP3A4)
> DA Flockhart et al, A metabolic interaction between clarithromycin and pimozide may result in cardiac toxicity. Clin Pharmacol Ther, 59:189, 1996; Z Desta et al, Effect of clarithromycin on the pharmacokinetics and pharmacodynamics of pimozide in healthy poor and extensive metabolizers of cytochrome P450 2D6 (CYP2D6). Clin Pharmacol Ther, 65:10, 1999; DA Flockhart et al, Studies on the mechanism of a fatal clarithromycin-pimozide interaction in a patient with Tourette syndrome. J Clin Psychopharmacol, 20:317, 2000

Two fatal case reports (1996; 2000); avoid concurrent use; similar effect likely with erythromycin and other CYP3A4 inhibitors

Quinidine

Quinidine toxicity with erythromycin (decreased metabolism; CYP3A4 and decreased biliary and renal excretion; P-glycoprotein)
> SA Spinler et al, Possible inhibition of hepatic metabolism of quinidine by erythromycin. Clin Pharmacol Ther, 57:89, 1995; JC Lin and HA Quasny, QT prolongation and development of torsades de pointes with the concomitant administration of oral erythromycin base and quinidine. Pharmacotherapy, 17:626, 1997; P Damkier et al, Effect of diclofenac, disulfiram, itraconazole, grapefruit juice and erythromycin on the pharmacokinetics of quinidine. Br J Clin Pharmacol, 48:829, 1999

Based on two case reports (1995, 1997) and pharmacokinetic study in healthy subjects

Rifabutin

Rifabutin toxicity (uveitis; leukopenia) with clarithromycin (probably decreased metabolism) and decreased clarithromycin effect (increased metabolism; CYP3A4)
> P Kelleher et al, Uveitis associated with rifabutin and macrolide therapy for *Mycobacterium avium intracellulare* infection in AIDS patients. Genitourin Med, 72:419, 1996; R Hafner et al, Tolerance and pharmacokinetic interactions of rifabutin and clarithromycin in human immunodeficiency virus-infected volunteers. Antimicrob Agents Chemother, 42:631, 1998; G Apseloff et al, Comparison of azithromycin and clarithromycin in their interactions with rifabutin in healthy volunteers. J Clin Pharmacol, 38:830, 1998; C Figueras et al, Hyperpigmentaton in a patient with aids, receiving rifabutin for disseminated *mycobacterium genavense* infection. Eur J Pediatr, 157:612, 1998; DL Cohn et al, A prospective randomized trial of four three-drug regimens in the treatment of disseminated *Mycobacterium avium* complex disease in AIDS patients: Excess mortality associated with

MACROLIDE ANTIBIOTICS, with: *(continued)*
>high-dose clarithromycin. Clin Infect Dis, 29:125, 1999

Based on studies in HIV(+) patients; possibly similar effect with other macrolides that inhibit CYP3A4 (e.g., erythromycin, troleandomycin); neutropenia reported in healthy subjects receiving clarithromycin; single case report of hyperpigmentation with clarithromycin (1998), but a causal relationship was not established; avoid concurrent use

Ritonavir
Increased plasma clarithromycin concentrations (probable decreased metabolism)
>D Ouellet et al, Pharmacokinetic interaction between ritonavir and clarithromycin. Clin Pharmacol Ther, 64:355, 1998

Based on study in healthy subjects; may need to reduce clarithromycin dose in patients with renal impairment

Selective serotonin reuptake inhibitors (SSRIs)
Possible serotonin syndrome (possibly decreased metabolism; CYP3A4)
>DO Lee and CD Lee, Serotonin syndrome in a child associated with erythromycin and sertraline. Pharmacotherapy, 19:894, 1999

Single case report (1999); monitor clinical status

Sildenafil
Possible sildenafil toxicity with erythromycin (probably decreased metabolism; CYP3A4)
>Manufacturer's package insert; MD Cheitlin et al, Use of sildenafil (Viagra) in patients with cardiovascular disease. Circulation, 99:168, 1999

Theoretical; monitor clinical status

Tacrolimus
Tacrolimus toxicity with erythromycin or clarithromycin (decreased metabolism; CYP3A4; possibly decreased transport; P-glycoprotein)
>MS Shaeffer et al, Interaction between FK506 and erythromycin. Ann Pharmacother, 28:280, 1994; C Jensen et al, Interaction between tacrolimus and erythromycin. Lancet, 344:825, 1994; V Furlan et al, Interactions between FK506 and rifampicin or erythromycin in pediatric liver recipients. Transplantation, 59:1217, 1995; ID Padhi et al, Interaction between tacrolimus and erythromycin. Ther Drug Monit, 19:120, 1997; M Moreno et al, Clinical management of tacrolimus drug interactions in renal transplant patients. Transplant Proc, 31:2252, 1999; G Gómez et al, Acute tacrolimus nephrotoxicity in renal transplant patients treated with clarithromycin. Transplant Proc, 31:2250, 1999

Several reports; avoid concurrent use or monitor tacrolimus concentrations and clinical status; theoretically, azithromycin would not interact

Theophyllines
Possible theophylline toxicity with erythromycin, clarithromycin and azithromycin (decreased metabolism); dirithromycin may not interact
>CF LaForce et al, Effect of erythromycin on theophylline clearance in asthmatic children. J Pediatr, 99:153, 1981; DC May et al, The effects of erythromycin on theophylline elimination in normal males. J Clin Pharmacol, 22:125, 1982; G Reisz et al, The effect of erythromycin on theophylline phar-

MACROLIDE ANTIBIOTICS, with: *(continued)*
>macokinetics in chronic bronchitis. Am Rev Respir Dis, 127:581, 1983; J Pasic et al, The interaction between chronic oral slow-release theophylline and single-dose intravenous erythromycin. Xenobiotica, 17:493, 1987; R Hildebrandt et al, Lack of clinically important interaction between erythromycin and theophylline. Eur J Clin Pharmacol, 26:485, 1984; VS Watkins et al, Drug interactions of macrolides: emphasis on dirithromycin. Ann Pharmacother, 31:349, 1997; PT Pollak and KL Slayter, Reduced serum theophylline concentrations after discontinuation of azithromycin: evidence for an unusual interaction. Pharmacotherapy, 17:827, 1997; PT Pollak and DM MacNeil, Azithromycin-theophylline inhibition-induction interaction. Clin Pharmacol Ther, 65:144, 1999; SA McConnell et al, Lack of effect of dirithromycin on theophylline pharmacokinetics in healthy volunteers. J Antimicrob Chemother, 43:733, 1999; N Shimada et al, Theophylline and clarithromycin. Jpn J Nephrol, 41:460, 1999

Monitor theophylline concentration; large individual variation; conflicting reports; IV theophylline may not interact; effect of azithromycin usually small, but azithromycin is long-acting and close monitoring of theophylline concentration is necessary on withdrawal

Valproate

Valproate toxicity with erythromycin (probably decreased metabolism)
>K Redington et al, Erythromycin and valproate interaction. Ann Intern Med, 116:877, 1992

Monitor valproate concentration

Verapamil

Cardiovascular toxicity with clarithromycin (decreased metabolism)
>YA Kaeser et al, Severe hypotension and bradycardia associated with verapamil and clarithromycin. Am J Health Syst Pharm, 55:2417, 1998

Single case report (1998); other calcium-channel blockers probably affected similarly by clarithromycin and erythromycin; azithromycin theoretically would not interact

Zidovudine

Possible decreased zidovudine effect with clarithromycin (mechanism not established)
>MA Polis et al, Clarithromycin lowers plasma zidovudine levels in persons with human immunodeficiency virus infection. Antimicrob Agents Chemother, 41:1709, 1997

Modest reduction in zidovudine concentrations in 15 patients; clinical significance not established

Magaldrate, see Antacids

Magnesium carbonate, see Antacids

MAGNESIUM CITRATE, with:

Fluoroquinolones - See Fluoroquinolones with Magnesium citrate, page 280

Magnesium hydroxide, see Antacids

Magnesium salicylate, see Nonsteroidal anti-inflammatory drugs

MAGNESIUM SULFATE, with:

Amiloride - See Amiloride with Magnesium sulfate, page 28

Aminoglycoside antibiotics - See Aminoglycoside antibiotics with Magnesium sulfate, page 31

Neuromuscular blocking agents

Prolonged neuromuscular blockade (mechanism not established)

> MM Ghoneim and JP Long, The interaction between magnesium and other neuromuscular blocking agents. Anesthesiology, 32:23, 1970; AH Giesecke, Jr et al, Of magnesium, muscle relaxants, toxemic parturients, and cats. Anesth Analg, 47:689, 1968; T Fuchs-Buder et al, Antagonism of vecuronium-induced neuromuscular block in patients pretreated with magnesium sulphate: dose-effect relationship of neostigmine. Br J Anaesth, 82:61, 1999

Two case reports (1968, 1970) and study in 48 patients undergoing elective surgery (1999)

Nifedipine

Hypotension (possibly synergism)

> GD Waisman et al, Magnesium plus nifedipine: potentiation of hypotensive effect in preeclampsia? Am J Obstet Gynecol, 159:308, 1988

Two case reports (1988); monitor blood pressure

Neuromuscular blockade (possibly synergism)

> SW Snyder and MS Cardwell, Neuromuscular blockade with magnesium sulfate and nifedipine. Am J Obstet Gynecol, 161:35, 1989; M Ben-Ami et al, The combination of magnesium sulphate and nifedipine: a cause of neuromuscular blockade. Br J Obstet Gynaecol, 101:262, 1994

Two case reports (1989; 1994); monitor blood pressure and neuromuscular status

Magnesium trisilicate, see Antacids

MALATHION, with:

Aminoglycoside antibiotics - See Aminoglycoside antibiotics with Malathion, page 31

Neuromuscular blocking agents

Possible prolonged neuromuscular blockade with succinylcholine (inhibition of plasma cholinesterase)

> United States Pharmacopeial Convention, *Drug Information for the Health Care Professional* (USP DI), Vol I, 18th ed., Rockville, MD: Authors, 1998, page 1914

Topical malathion not significantly absorbed unless skin damaged

MAO inhibitors, see Monoamine oxidase inhibitors

MAPROTILINE, with:

Alcohol - See Alcohol with Maprotiline, page 19

Beta-adrenergic blockers - See Beta-adrenergic blockers with Maprotiline, page 157

Propofol

Possible increase in risk of seizures (possibly additive epileptogenic effect)

> B Orser et al, Propofol, seizure and antidepressants. Can J Anaesth, 41:3,

(continued)

MAPROTILINE, with: *(continued)*
    1994
    Single case report with maprotiline (1994); use propofol with caution in patients on tetracyclic-type antidepressants

MARIJUANA, SMOKING, with:
  Antidepressants, tricyclic - See Antidepressants, tricyclic with Marijuana, smoking, page 86
  Disulfiram - See Disulfiram with Marijuana, smoking, page 264
  Haloperidol - See Haloperidol with Marijuana, smoking, page 294
  Selective serotonin reuptake inhibitors (SSRIs)
    Mania with fluoxetine (possibly additive)
      AL Stoll et al, A case of mania as a result of fluoxetine-marijuana interaction. J Clin Psychiatry, 52:280, 1991
    Single case report (1991); poorly documented
  Theophyllines
    Decreased theophylline effect (increased metabolism)
      WJ Jusko et al, Enhanced biotransformation of theophylline in marijuana and tobacco smokers. Clin Pharmacol Ther, 24:406, 1978
    Monitor theophylline concentration

Masoprocol, no documented interactions, see page 4, Criteria for Listing Interactions

MAZINDOL, with:
  Lithium - See Lithium with Mazindol, page 324
  Sympathomimetic amines
    Cardiomyopathy with fenfluramine (mechanism not established)
      D Gillis et al, Fenfluramine and mazindol: acute reversible cardiomyopathy associated with their use. Int J Psychiatry Med, 15:197, 1985-6
    Single case report (1985-1986)

MDMA, see Methylenedioxymethamphetamine

Mebendazole, no documented interactions, see page 4, Criteria for Listing Interactions

Mechlorethamine, see Alkylating agents

Meclizine hydrochloride, no documented interactions, see page 4, Criteria for Listing Interactions

Meclofenamate, see Nonsteroidal anti-inflammatory drugs

Medroxyprogesterone, see Progestins

Mefenamic acid, see Nonsteroidal anti-inflammatory drugs

MEFLOQUINE, with:
  Beta-adrenergic blockers - See Beta-adrenergic blockers with Mefloquine, page 158
  Chloroquine - See Chloroquine with Mefloquine, page 194
  Halofantrine - See Halofantrine with Mefloquine, page 293
  Quinidine
    Possible increased risk of ECG abnormalities or cardiac arrest (mechanism not established)
      Manufacturer's package insert; W Supanaranond et al, lack of a significant adverse cardiovascular effect of combined quinine and mefloquine therapy

MEFLOQUINE, with: *(continued)*
> for uncomplicated malaria. Trans R Soc Trop Med Hyg, 91:694, 1997; K Nabangchang et al, Pharmacokinetic and pharmacodynamic interactions of mefloquine and quinine. Int J Clin Pharm Res, 19:73, 1999

Manufacturer recommends avoiding concurrent use; delay starting mefloquine until 12 hours after quinidine is stopped; monitor ECG for prolonged QTc interval; study in 13 patients found no evidence of adverse drug interaction

Quinine
Possible increased risk of convulsions, ECG abnormalities or cardiac arrest (mechanism not established)
> Manufacturer's package insert; W Supanaranond et al, Lack of a significant adverse cardiovascular effect of combined quinine and mefloquine therapy for uncomplicated malaria. Trans R Soc Trop Med Hyg, 91:694, 1997; K Na-Bangchang et al, Pharmacokinetic and pharmacodynamic interactions of mefloquine and quinine. Int J Clin Pharm Res, 19:73, 1999

Manufacturer recommends avoiding concurrent use; delay starting mefloquine until 12 hours after quinine is stopped; monitor ECG for prolonged QTc interval; study in 13 patients found no evidence of adverse drug interaction

MEGESTROL ACETATE, with:
Dofetilide - See Dofetilide with Megestrol acetate, page 265

MELATONIN, with:
Selective serotonin reuptake inhibitors (SSRIs)
Possible melatonin toxicity with fluvoxamine (probably decreased metabolism)
> S Härtter et al, Increased bioavailability of oral melatonin after fluvoxamine coadministration. Clin Pharmacol Ther, 67:1, 2000

Based on study in healthy subjects; marked increase in melatonin serum concentrations; monitor clinical status

Melphalan, see Alkylating agents

Menadione, no documented interactions, see page 4, Criteria for Listing Interactions

Mepenzolate bromide, see Anticholinergics

Meperidine, see Narcotics: meperidine and congeners

MEPHENYTOIN, with:
Rifampin
Decreased mephenytoin effect (increased metabolism)
> HH Zhou et al, Induction of polymorphic 4'-hydroxylation of S-mephenytoin by rifampicin. Br J Clin Pharmacol, 30:471, 1990

Monitor mephenytoin concentration

Mephobarbital, see Barbiturates

MEPIVACAINE, with:
Bupivacaine - See Bupivacaine with Mepivacaine, page 168

Meprednisone, see Corticosteroids

MEPROBAMATE, with:
Alcohol - See Alcohol with Meprobamate, page 19

Merbromin, see Antiseptics, mercurial

MERCAPTOPURINE, with:
  Allopurinol - See Allopurinol with Mercaptopurine, page 25
  Anticoagulants, oral - See Anticoagulants, oral with Mercaptopurine, page 71
  Phenytoin
    Decreased phenytoin effect with prednisone, methotrexate, mercaptopurine, and vincristine combination therapy (increased metabolism)
        PF Jarosinski et al, Altered phenytoin clearance during intensive chemotherapy for acute lymphoblastic leukemia. J Pediatr, 112:996, 1988
    Single well-studied case (1988); monitor
  Sulfonamides
    Possible mercaptopurine toxicity with sulfasalazine (decreased metabolism)
        CL Szumlanski and RM Weinshilboum, Sulphasalazine inhibition of thiopurine methyltransferase: possible mechanism for interaction with 6-mercaptopurine and azathioprine. Br J Clin Pharmacol, 39:456, 1995
    Based on an in vitro study showing inhibition of thiopurine methyltransferase (TPMT) by sulfasalazine; patients with genetically reduced TPMT are reported to have more severe thiopurine toxicity
  Trimethoprim-sulfamethoxazole
    Decreased antileukemic effect (mechanism not established)
        CA Rees et al, Disturbance of 6-mercaptopurine metabolism by cotrimoxazole in childhood lymphoblastic leukaemia. Cancer Chemother Pharmacol, 12:87, 1984
    Avoid concurrent use, pending further study

Mercurials, see Antiseptics, mercurial

Meropenem, no documented interactions, see page 4, Criteria for Listing Interactions

Merthiolate, see Antiseptics, mercurial

MESALAMINE, with:
  Anticoagulants, oral - See Anticoagulants, oral with Mesalamine, page 71

MESNA, with:
  Anticoagulants, oral - See Anticoagulants, oral with Mesna, page 71

Mesoridazine, see Phenothiazines

Mestranol, see Contraceptives, oral

Metaproterenol, see Sympathomimetic bronchodilators

Metaraminol, see Sympathomimetic amines

Metaxalone, no documented interactions, see page 4, Criteria for Listing Interactions

METFORMIN, with:
  Acarbose - See Acarbose with Metformin, page 6
  Alcohol - See Alcohol with Metformin, page 19
  Contrast media - See Contrast media with Metformin, page 219
  Nonsteroidal anti-inflammatory drugs
    Lactic acidosis with indomethacin (possibly NSAID-induced renal impairment)
        NN Chan et al, Non-steroidal anti-inflammatory drugs and metformin: a cause for concern? Lancet, 352:201, 1998
    Single case report (1998); monitor lactic acid concentration

Methacycline, see Tetracyclines

Methadone, see Narcotics: methadone and congeners
Methamphetamine, see Sympathomimetic amines
Methandriol, see Anabolic and androgenic steroids
Methandrostenolone, see Anabolic and androgenic steroids
Methantheline, see Anticholinergics
Methaqualone, no documented interactions, see page 4, Criteria for Listing Interactions
Metharbital, see Barbiturates
Methazolamide, see Carbonic anhydrase inhibitors
Methicillin, see Penicillins
METHIONINE, with:
   Levodopa - See Levodopa with Methionine, page 319
Methocarbamol, no documented interactions, see page 4, Criteria for Listing Interactions
Methohexital, see Barbiturates
METHOTREXATE, with:
   Acitretin - See Acitretin with Methotrexate, page 10
   Alcohol - See Alcohol with Methotrexate, page 19
   Aminoglycoside antibiotics - See Aminoglycoside antibiotics with Methotrexate, page 31
   Amiodarone - See Amiodarone with Methotrexate, page 36
   Azathioprine - See Azathioprine with Methotrexate, page 130
   Bentiromide - See Bentiromide with Methotrexate, page 138
   Blood transfusion - See Blood transfusion with Methotrexate, page 166
   Chloroquine - See Chloroquine with Methotrexate, page 194
   Cisplatin - See Cisplatin with Methotrexate, page 201
   Corticosteroids - See Corticosteroids with Methotrexate, page 221
   COX-2 inhibitors - See COX-2 inhibitors with Methotrexate, page 225
   Cyclosporine - See Cyclosporine with Methotrexate, page 233
   Etoposide - See Etoposide with Methotrexate, page 275
   Etretinate - See Etretinate with Methotrexate, page 275
   Fluorouracil - See Fluorouracil with Methotrexate, page 283
   Leflunomide - See Leflunomide with Methotrexate, page 319
   Leucovorin - See Leucovorin with Methotrexate, page 319
   Nonsteroidal anti-inflammatory drugs
     Possible methotrexate toxicity (decreased renal excretion)
       TS Tracy et al, Methotrexate disposition following concomitant administration of ketoprofen, piroxicam and flurbiprofen in patients with rheumatoid arthritis. Br J Clin Pharmacol, 37:453, 1994; ML Frenia and KS Long, Methotrexate and nonsteroidal antiinflammatory drug interactions. Ann Pharmacother, 26:234, 1992; J-M Anaya et al, Effect of etodolac on methotrexate pharmacokinetics in patients with rheumatoid arthritis. J Rheumatol, 21:203, 1994; B Combe et al, Total and free methotrexate pharmacokinetics, with and without piroxicam, in rheumatoid arthritis patients. Br J Rheumatol, 34:421, 1995; JM Kremer and RA Hamilton, The effects of nonsteroidal antiinflammatory drugs on methotrexate (MTX) pharmacokinetics: impairment of renal clearance of MTX at weekly maintenance doses but not at 7.5

(continued)

METHOTREXATE, with: *(continued)*

mg. J Rheumatol, 22:11, 1995; MP Iqbal et al, The effects of non-steroidal anti-inflammatory drugs on the disposition of methotrexate in patients with rheumatoid arthritis. Biopharm Drug Dispos, 19:163, 1998

Stop NSAIDs 2 to 3 days before methotrexate in elderly and others with decreased renal function; this interaction has been avoided when the drugs were given 12 hours apart; flurbiprofen, ketoprofen and piroxicam did not interact in one study of 10 patients; danger probably greater with high-dose methotrexate than with the lower doses used for rheumatoid arthritis; monitor for methotrexate toxicity

Omeprazole

Possible methotrexate toxicity (probably decreased renal tubular secretion)

B Beorlegui et al, Potential interaction between methotrexate and omeprazole. Ann Pharmacother, 34:1024, 2000

Single case report with high-dose methotrexate (2000); monitor methotrexate concentrations and clinical status

Penicillins

Possible methotrexate toxicity (decreased excretion)

DL Gibson et al, Carbenicillin potentiation of methotrexate plasma concentration during high dose methotrexate therapy. Am Soc Hosp Pharmacists, Midyear Clin Meet, New Orleans, Dec 6-10, 1981, Abstr P-305, page 111; KL Melmon, Drugs will interact. Emergency Med, 17:18, 1985; B Mayall et al, Neutropenia due to low-dose methotrexate therapy for psoriasis and rheumatoid arthritis may be fatal. Med J Aust, 155:480, 1991; R Dean et al, Possible methotrexate-mezlocillin interaction. Am J Pediatr Hematol Oncol, 14:88, 1992; K Yamamoto et al, Delayed elimination of methotrexate associated with piperacillin administration. Ann Pharmacother, 31:1261, 1997; AL Herrick et al, Lack of interaction between methotrexate and penicillins. Rheumatology, 38:284, 1999

Several case reports, including fatalities with neutropenia; flucloxacillin may not interact

Phenylbutazone

Methotrexate toxicity (mechanism not established)

JD Adams and GA Hunter, Drug interaction in psoriasis. Aust J Dermatol, 17:39, 1976

Avoid concurrent use

Phenytoin

Decreased phenytoin effect with prednisone, methotrexate, mercaptopurine, and vincristine combination therapy (increased metabolism)

PF Jarosinski et al, Altered phenytoin clearance during intensive chemotherapy for acute lymphoblastic leukemia. J Pediatr, 112:996, 1988

Single well-studied case (1988); monitor

Possible decreased methotrexate effect (mechanism not established)

MV Relling et al, Adverse effect of anticonvulsants on efficacy of chemotherapy for acute lymphoblastic leukaemia. Lancet, 356:285, 2000

METHOTREXATE, with: *(continued)*
> *Evidence of reduced methotrexate efficacy in children with acute lymphoblastic leukemia; monitor clinical status and methotrexate concentration if available*

Probenecid
> Methotrexate toxicity (decreased renal excretion)
>> JW Paxton, Interaction of probenecid with the protein binding of methotrexate. Pharmacology, 28:86, 1984; KS Basin et al, Severe pancytopenia in a patient taking low dose methotrexate and probenecid. J Rheumatol, 18:609, 1991
>
> *Avoid concurrent use*

Procarbazine
> Renal toxicity, methotrexate given immediately after a course of procarbazine (mechanism not established)
>> P Price et al, Renal impairment following the combined use of high-dose methotrexate and procarbazine. Cancer Chemother Pharmacol, 21:265, 1988
>
> *Wait at least 72 hours after a 14-day course of procarbazine before giving high-dose methotrexate (2 grams/m^2)*

Sulfonamides
> Possible methotrexate toxicity (displacement from binding and decreased renal excretion)
>> DS Zaharko et al, Antibiotics alter methotrexate metabolism and excretion. Science, 166:887, 1969; SL Morgan et al, Methotrexate and sulfasalazine combination therapy: Is it worth the risk? Arthritis Rheum, 36:281, 1993
>
> *Several case reports. Both drugs cause folate deficiency and an additive effect has been suggested, but not proven.*

Tetracyclines
> Possible methotrexate toxicity (mechanism not established)
>> JJ Tortajada-Ituren et al, High-dose methotrexate-doxycycline interaction. Ann Pharmacother, 33:804, 1999
>
> *Single case report of severe methotrexate toxicity in patient on high-dose methotrexate (1999); avoid concurrent use or carefully monitor clinical status*

Theophyllines
> Theophylline toxicity (decreased metabolism)
>> AM Glynn-Barnhart et al, Effect of low-dose methotrexate on the disposition of glucocorticoids and theophylline. J Allergy Clin Immunol, 88:180, 1991
>
> *Monitor theophylline concentration; large patient variability*

Triamterene
> Possible increased methotrexate toxicity (additive)
>> R Richmond et al, Methotrexate and triamterene-a potentially fatal combination? Ann Rheum Dis, 56:209, 1997
>
> *Single case report (1997); avoid concurrent use*

Trimethoprim-sulfamethoxazole
> Megaloblastic anemia and pancytopenia (probably additive inhibition of folate metabolism)
>> M Dan and I Shapira, Possible role of methotrexate in trimethoprim-sulfa-

(continued)

METHOTREXATE, with: *(continued)*
>methoxazole-induced acute megaloblastic anemia. Isr J Med Sci, 20:262, 1984; NL Kobrinsky and NKC Ramsay, Acute megaloblastic anemia induced by high-dose trimethoprim-sulfamethoxazole. Ann Intern Med, 94:780, 1981; G Ferrazzini et al, Interaction between trimethoprim-sulfamethoxazole and methotrexate in children with leukemia. J Pediatr, 117:823, 1990; JA Govert et al, Pancytopenia from using trimethoprim and methotrexate. Ann Intern Med, 117:877, 1992

>*Avoid concurrent use; leucovorin rescue was effective in one patient (1992); clinical significance not established*

METHOXSALEN, with:
Phenytoin
Failure of psoralen-ultraviolet A (PUVA) therapy (possibly increased methoxsalen metabolism)
>B Staberg and B Hueg, Interaction between 8-methoxypsoralen and phenytoin. Acta Dermatol Venereol, 65:553, 1985

>*Single case report (1985); monitor methoxsalen concentration*

Methscopolamine, see Anticholinergics

METHSUXIMIDE, with:
Barbiturates - See Barbiturates with Methsuximide, page 134
Lamotrigine - See Lamotrigine with Methsuximide, page 316
Phenytoin
Possible toxicity of both drugs (decreased metabolism)
>B Rambeck, Pharmacological interactions of mesuximide with phenobarbital and phenytoin in hospitalized epileptic patients. Epilepsia, 20:147, 1979

>*Monitor methsuximide and phenytoin concentrations*

Methyclothiazide, see Thiazide diuretics

Methylatropine, see Anticholinergics

METHYLDOPA, with:
Alpha-adrenergic blockers - See Alpha-adrenergic blockers with Methyldopa, page 26
Beta-adrenergic blockers - See Beta-adrenergic blockers with Methyldopa, page 158
Cephalosporins - See Cephalosporins with Methyldopa, page 191
Contraceptives, oral - See Contraceptives, oral with Methyldopa, page 214
Diazoxide - See Diazoxide with Methyldopa, page 246
Digoxin - See Digoxin with Methyldopa, page 254
Entacapone - See Entacapone with Methyldopa, page 269
Haloperidol - See Haloperidol with Methyldopa, page 294
Hypoglycemics, sulfonylurea - See Hypoglycemics, sulfonylurea with Methyldopa, page 304
Iron - See Iron with Methyldopa, page 312
Lithium - See Lithium with Methyldopa, page 324
Monoamine oxidase inhibitors
Hallucinations with pargyline (mechanism not established)
>ES Paykel, Hallucinosis on combined methyldopa and pargyline. Br Med J, 1:803, 1966

METHYLDOPA, with: *(continued)*
Avoid concurrent use
Thiazide diuretics
Hemolytic anemia with hydrochlorothiazide (mechanism not established)
Manufacturer's package insert
Apparently rare; monitor RBC parameters

METHYLENEDIOXYMETHAMPHETAMINE, with:
Ritonavir
Possible increased MDMA toxicity (probably decreased metabolism)
R de la Torre et al, Fatal MDMA intoxication. Lancet, 353:593, 1999; RD Harrington et al, Life-threatening interactions between HIV-1 protease inhibitors and the illicit drugs MDMA and γ-hydroxybutyrate. Arch Intern Med, 159:2221, 1999
Based on limited clinical evidence; avoid concurrent use

Methylergonovine, see Ergot alkaloids
Methylphenidate, see Sympathomimetic amines
Methylprednisolone, see Corticosteroids
Methylsalicylate, see Salicylates, topical
Methyltestosterone, see Anabolic and androgenic steroids
Methysergide, see Ergot alkaloids

METOCLOPRAMIDE, with:
Antihistamines, H_2-blockers - See Antihistamines, H_2-blockers with Metoclopramide, page 119
Atovaquone - See Atovaquone with Metoclopramide, page 129
Beta-adrenergic blockers - See Beta-adrenergic blockers with Metoclopramide, page 158
Cabergoline - See Cabergoline with Metoclopramide, page 172
Carbamazepine - See Carbamazepine with Metoclopramide, page 181
Cyclosporine - See Cyclosporine with Metoclopramide, page 234
Dantrolene - See Dantrolene with Metoclopramide, page 242
Digoxin - See Digoxin with Metoclopramide, page 254
Fosfomycin - See Fosfomycin with Metoclopramide, page 285
Haloperidol - See Haloperidol with Metoclopramide, page 295
Hydroxyzine - See Hydroxyzine with Metoclopramide, page 303
Narcotics: morphine-like
Oversedation or possibly other toxicity with oral controlled-release morphine (probably increased absorption)
AR Manara et al, The effect of metoclopramide on the absorption of oral controlled release morphine. Br J Clin Pharmacol, 25:518, 1988
Monitor clinical status
Neuromuscular blocking agents
Prolonged neuromuscular blockade with succinylcholine or mivacurium (possible metoclopramide inhibition of plasma cholinesterase)
JR Kambam et al, The inhibitory effect of metoclopramide on plasma cholinesterase activity. Anesth Analg, 67:S107, 1988; DR Turner et al, Neuromuscular block by suxamethonium following treatment with histamine type 2 antagonists or metoclopramide. Br J Anaesth, 63:348, 1989; YJ Kao

METOCLOPRAMIDE, with: *(continued)*

and DR Turner, Prolongation of succinylcholine block by metoclopramide. Anesthesiology, 70:905, 1989; HJ Skinner et al, Influence of metoclopramide on plasma cholinesterase and duration of action of mivacurium. Br J Anaesth, 82:542, 1999

Administer with caution

Phenothiazines

Priapism with metoclopramide and thioridazine (mechanism not established)

M Velek et al, Priapism associated with concurrent use of thioridazine and metoclopramide. Am J Psychiatry, 144:827, 1987

Single case report (1987); patient had sickle-cell trait

Enlarged blue tongue and partial upper airways obstruction with prochlorperazine (probably additive)

C Alroe and P Bowen, Metoclopramide and prochlorperazine: "the blue-tongue sign." Med J Aust, 150:724, 1989

Single case report (1989)

Tardive dyskinesia, parkinsonism with prochlorperazine (mechanism not established)

SA Factor and MK Matthews, Persistent extrapyramidal syndrome with dystonia and rigidity caused by combined metoclopramide and prochlorperazine therapy. South Med J, 84:626, 1991

Single case report (1991)

Pramipexole

Possible reduced pramipexole effect (dopamine antagonism)

Manufacturer's package insert

Avoid concurrent use

Quinidine

Possible decreased quinidine effect with sustained-release preparations (decreased absorption)

GJ Yuen et al, Effect of metoclopramide on the absorption of an oral sustained-release quinidine product. Clin Pharm, 6:722, 1987

Monitor quinidine concentration

Ropinirole

Possible decrease in ropinirole effect (dopamine antagonism)

Manufacturer's package insert

Avoid concurrent use

Selective serotonin reuptake inhibitors (SSRIs)

Possible extrapyramidal symptoms (possible additive effect)

RC Christensen and MJ Byerly, Mandibular dystonia associated with the combination of sertraline and metoclopramide. J Clin Psychiatry, 57:596, 1996; V Palop et al, Acute dystonia associated with fluvoxamine-metoclopramide. Ann Pharmacother, 33:382, 1999

Single case reports with sertraline (1996) and fluvoxamine (1999); monitor clinical status

Metocurine, see Neuromuscular blocking agents

Metolazone, see Thiazide diuretics

Metoprolol, see Beta-adrenergic blockers
METRONIDAZOLE, with:
  Alcohol - See Alcohol with Metronidazole, page 19
  Antacids - See Antacids with Metronidazole, page 54
  Anticoagulants, oral - See Anticoagulants, oral with Metronidazole, page 71
  Antihistamines, H$_2$-blockers - See Antihistamines, H$_2$-blockers with Metronidazole, page 119
  Barbiturates - See Barbiturates with Metronidazole, page 134
  Carbamazepine - See Carbamazepine with Metronidazole, page 181
  Chloroquine - See Chloroquine with Metronidazole, page 194
  Cholestyramine - See Cholestyramine with Metronidazole, page 197
  Contraceptives, oral - See Contraceptives, oral with Metronidazole, page 214
  Corticosteroids - See Corticosteroids with Metronidazole, page 221
  Cyclosporine - See Cyclosporine with Metronidazole, page 234
  Disulfiram - See Disulfiram with Metronidazole, page 264
  Fluorouracil - See Fluorouracil with Metronidazole, page 283
  Lithium - See Lithium with Metronidazole, page 324
  Phenytoin
    Possible phenytoin toxicity (decreased metabolism)
      GT Blyden et al, Metronidazole impairs clearance of phenytoin but not of alprazolam or lorazepam. J Clin Pharmacol, 28:240, 1988
    Monitor phenytoin concentration
  Tacrolimus
    Possible tacrolimus toxicity (probably decreased metabolism; CYP3A4)
      K Herzig and DW Johnson, Marked elevation of blood cyclosporin and tacrolimus levels due to concurrent metronidazole therapy. Nephrol Dial Transplant, 14:521, 1999
    Single case report (1999); monitor tacrolimus serum concentration while on metronidazole therapy
METYRAPONE, with:
  Narcotics: methadone and congeners
    Methadone withdrawal symptoms (mechanism not established)
      JA Kennedy et al, Metyrapone-induced withdrawal symptoms. Br J Addict, 85:1133, 1990
    Monitor clinical status
MEXILETINE, with:
  Fluoroquinolones - See Fluoroquinolones with Mexiletine, page 280
  Lidocaine - See Lidocaine with Mexiletine, page 322
  Phenytoin
    Decreased mexiletine effect (increased metabolism)
      EJ Begg et al, Enhanced metabolism of mexiletine after phenytoin administration. Br J Clin Pharmacol, 14:219, 1982
    Monitor mexiletine concentration
  Propafenone
    Possible increased mexilitine toxicity (probably decreased metabolism)
      L Labbé et al, Propafenone decreases mexiletine clearance in subjects with extensive CYP2D6 activity. Clin Pharmacol Ther, 67:117, 2000, abs PII-11; L

(continued)

MEXILETINE, with: *(continued)*
> Labbé et al, Pharmacokinetic and pharmacodynamic interactions between propafenone and mexiletine. Clin Pharmacol Ther, 67:117, 2000, abs PII-12; L Labbé et al, Pharmacokinetic and pharmacodynamic interaction between mexiletine and propafenone in human beings. Clin Pharmacol Ther, 68:44, 2000

Based on study in healthy subjects; CYP2D6-deficient subjects have higher mexiletine levels even in the absence of propafenone; no effect on propafenone pharmacokinetics; monitor clinical status

Rifampin
Decreased antiarrhythmic effect (increased metabolism)
> PJ Pentikainen et al, Effect of rifampicin treatment on the kinetics of mexiletine. Eur J Clin Pharmacol, 23:261, 1982

Monitor mexiletine concentration

Theophyllines
Theophylline toxicity (decreased metabolism)
> KM Kessler et al, Proarrhythmia related to a kinetic and dynamic interaction of mexiletine and theophylline. Am Heart J, 117:964, 1989; A Hurwitz et al, Mexiletine effects on theophylline disposition. Clin Pharmacol Ther, 50:299, 1991

Case reports confirmed by studies in healthy subjects; monitor theophylline concentrations; one case report suggests a proarrhythmic effect of the combination (1989)

Tobacco, smoking
Possible decreased mexiletine effect (increased metabolism)
> O Grech-Belanger et al, Effect of cigarette smoking on mexiletine kinetics. Clin Pharmacol Ther, 37:638, 1985

Monitor mexiletine concentration

Mezlocillin, see Penicillins

MIANSERIN, with:
- **Alcohol** - See Alcohol with Mianserin, page 20
- **Anticoagulants, oral** - See Anticoagulants, oral with Mianserin, page 71
- **Carbamazepine** - See Carbamazepine with Mianserin, page 181
- **HMG-CoA reductase inhibitors** - See HMG-CoA reductase inhibitors with Mianserin, page 300

Miconazole, see Antifungals, imidazoles and triazoles

Midazolam, see Benzodiazepines

MIDODRINE, with:
- **Digoxin** - See Digoxin with Midodrine, page 254
- **Sympathomimetic amines**
  Risk of severe hypertension (additive)
  > Manufacturer's package insert

  Monitor cardiovascular status

MIFEPRISTONE, with:
- **Acetaminophen** - See Acetaminophen with Mifepristone, page 9
- **Cyclosporine** - See Cyclosporine with Mifepristone, page 234

MIGLITOL, with:
    Antihistamines, H$_2$-blockers - See Antihistamines, H$_2$-blockers with Miglitol, page 119
    Beta-adrenergic blockers - See Beta-adrenergic blockers with Miglitol, page 158
    Digoxin - See Digoxin with Miglitol, page 254

Milk of magnesia, see Antacids

Minocycline, see Tetracyclines

MINOXIDIL, with:
    Cyclosporine - See Cyclosporine with Minoxidil, page 234
    Diazoxide - See Diazoxide with Minoxidil, page 246
    Guanethidine - See Guanethidine with Minoxidil, page 292

MIRTAZAPINE, with:
    Alcohol - See Alcohol with Mirtazapine, page 20
    Antihistamines, H$_2$-blockers - See Antihistamines, H$_2$-blockers with Mirtazapine, page 120
    Benzodiazepines - See Benzodiazepines with Mirtazapine, page 144
    Clonidine - See Clonidine with Mirtazapine, page 204
    Levodopa - See Levodopa with Mirtazapine, page 320
    Monoamine oxidase inhibitors

        Possible cardiovascular and neurological toxicity (mechanism not established)
            Manufacturer's package insert

        Mirtazapine should not be started for at least 14 days after stopping an MAOI and an MAOI should not be started for at least 14 days after stopping mirtazapine

    Selective serotonin reuptake inhibitors (SSRIs)

        Possible increased risk of mania with mirtazapine and sertraline (mechanism not established)
            CA Soutullo et al, Hypomania associated with mirtazapine augmentation of sertraline. J Clin Psychiatry, 59:320, 1998

        Single case report (1998); causal relationship not established

MISOPROSTOL, with:
    Nonsteroidal anti-inflammatory drugs

        Ataxia with naproxen (mechanism not established)
            M Huq, Neurological adverse effects of naproxen and misoprostol combination. Br J Gen Pract, 40:432, 1990

        Single case report (1990); monitor clinical status

        Decreased diclofenac effect and indomethacin concentration (decreased absorption)
            HG Dammann et al, The effects of misoprostol and of ranitidine on the pharmacokinetics of diclofenac. Gastroenterology, 102:A55, 1992, abs; MJ Kendall et al, Co-administration of misoprostol or ranitidine with indomethacin: effects on pharmacokinetics, abdominal symptoms and bowel habit. Aliment Pharmacol Ther, 6:437, 1992; A Karim, Pharmacokinetics of diclofenac and misoprostol when administered alone or as a combination product. Drugs, 45 suppl 1:7, 1993

(continued)

MISOPROSTOL, with: *(continued)*
> *A single dose study using a combination of diclofenac and misoprostol showed no significant interaction, but large interindividual variation; abdominal pain with diclofenac or indomethacin.*

Phenylbutazone

Neurological symptoms (mechanism not established)
> JM Jacquemier et al, Neurosensory adverse effects after phenylbutazone and misoprostol combined treatment. Lancet, 2:1283, 1989; Ph Chassagne et al, Neurosensory adverse effects after combined phenylbutazone and misoprostol. Br J Rheumatol, 30:392, 1991

Two well-documented cases

MITOMYCIN C, with:

Tamoxifen

Hemolytic uremic syndrome (mechanism not established)
> A Montes et al, A toxic interaction between mitomycin C and tamoxifen causing the haemolytic uraemic syndrome. Eur J Cancer, 29:1854, 1993

Avoid concurrent use if possible; monitor clinical status; reported in patients receiving mitomycin C, mitozantrone and methotrexate; has been reported in patients receiving high doses of mitomycin C alone

MITOTANE, with:

Anticoagulants, oral - See Anticoagulants, oral with Mitotane, page 71

Mitozoxane, no documented interactions, see page 4, Criteria for Listing Interactions

Mivacurium, see Neuromuscular blocking agents

Moclobemide, see Monoamine oxidase inhibitors

MODAFINIL, with:

Antidepressants, tricyclic - See Antidepressants, tricyclic with Modafinil, page 87

Cyclosporine - See Cyclosporine with Modafinil, page 234

MOLINDONE, with:

Phenytoin

Decreased phenytoin effect (calcium as an excipient inhibits absorption)
> Manufacturer's package insert

Give at least 2 hours apart

Tetracyclines

Decreased tetracycline effect (calcium as an excipient inhibits absorption)
> Manufacturer's package insert

Give at least 2 hours apart

Mometasone, see Corticosteroids

MONOAMINE OXIDASE INHIBITORS, with:

Altretamine - See Altretamine with Monoamine oxidase inhibitors, page 26

Amantadine - See Amantadine with Monoamine oxidase inhibitors, page 27

Antidepressants, tricyclic - See Antidepressants, tricyclic with Monoamine oxidase inhibitors, page 87

Benzodiazepines - See Benzodiazepines with Monoamine oxidase inhibitors, page 145

MONOAMINE OXIDASE INHIBITORS, with: *(continued)*

Beta-adrenergic blockers - See Beta-adrenergic blockers with Monoamine oxidase inhibitors, page 158

Brimonidine - See Brimonidine with Monoamine oxidase inhibitors, page 167

Bupropion - See Bupropion with Monoamine oxidase inhibitors, page 169

Buspirone - See Buspirone with Monoamine oxidase inhibitors, page 170

Carbamazepine - See Carbamazepine with Monoamine oxidase inhibitors, page 182

Contraceptives, oral - See Contraceptives, oral with Monoamine oxidase inhibitors, page 214

Cyproheptadine - See Cyproheptadine with Monoamine oxidase inhibitors, page 241

Entacapone - See Entacapone with Monoamine oxidase inhibitors, page 269

Ginseng - See Ginseng with Monoamine oxidase inhibitors, page 289

Guanadrel - See Guanadrel with Monoamine oxidase inhibitors, page 292

Hypoglycemics, sulfonylurea - See Hypoglycemics, sulfonylurea with Monoamine oxidase inhibitors, page 304

Insulin - See Insulin with Monoamine oxidase inhibitors, page 310

Levodopa - See Levodopa with Monoamine oxidase inhibitors, page 320

Lithium - See Lithium with Monoamine oxidase inhibitors, page 324

Macrolide antibiotics - See Macrolide antibiotics with Monoamine oxidase inhibitors, page 331

Methyldopa - See Methyldopa with Monoamine oxidase inhibitors, page 342

Mirtazapine - See Mirtazapine with Monoamine oxidase inhibitors, page 347

Narcotics: dextromethorphan

Neurological symptoms with dextromethorphan and isocarboxazid or phenelzine (mechanism not established)

R Sovner and J Wolfe, Interaction between dextromethorphan and monoamine oxidase inhibitor therapy with isocarboxazid. N Engl J Med, 319:1671, 1988; D Sauter et al, Phenelzine sulfate-dextromethorphan interaction: a case report. Vet Hum Toxicol, 33:365, 1991

Single case reports (1988, 1991); may occur with over-the-counter products

Possible dextromethorphan and moclobemide toxicity (decreased metabolism; CYP2D6)

S Härtter et al, Inhibition of dextromethorphan metabolism by moclobemide. Psychopharmacology, 135:22, 1998

Based on study in four healthy subjects; monitor clinical status

Narcotics: meperidine and congeners

Toxicity with both MAO and MAO-B (selegiline) inhibitor (mechanism not established)

D Meyer and V Halfin, Toxicity secondary to meperidine in patients on monoamine oxidase inhibitors: a case report and critical review. J Clin Psychopharmacol, 1:319, 1981; IM Vigran, Dangerous potentiation of meperidine hydrochloride by pargyline hydrochloride. JAMA, 187:953, 1964; JC Garbutt, Potentiation of propoxyphene by phenelzine. Am J Psychiatry, 144:251, 1987; GL Zornberg et al, Severe adverse interaction

(continued)

MONOAMINE OXIDASE INHIBITORS, with: *(continued)*
   between pethidine and selegiline. Lancet, 337:246, 1991
   Avoid concurrent use

Narcotics: methadone and congeners
   Increased sedation and somnolence with propoxyphene and phenelzine (mechanism not established)
      JC Garbutt, Potentiation of propoxyphene by phenelzine. Am J Psychiatry, 144:251, 1987
   Single case report (1987)

Narcotics: tramadol
   Increased risk of serotonin syndrome (reduced reuptake of monoamines)
      V Calvisi and M Ansseau, Confusion mentale liée à l'administration de tramadol chez une patiente sous IMAO. Rev Med Liege, 54:912, 1999; manufacturer's package insert
   Avoid concurrent use

Neuromuscular blocking agents
   Prolonged neuromuscular blockade with phenelzine and succinylcholine (inhibition of plasma cholinesterase)
      PO Bodley et al, Low serum pseudocholinesterase levels complicating treatment with phenelzine. Br Med J, 3:510, 1969
   Measure plasma cholinesterase and reduce succinylcholine dosage accordingly

Phenformin
   Increased hypoglycemic effect (mechanism not established)
      PI Adnitt, Hypoglycemic action of monoamineoxidase inhibitors (MAOI's). Diabetes, 17:628, 1968
   Monitor blood glucose

Reserpine
   Precipitation of mania (release of accumulated 5-hydroxytryptamine)
      AH Esser, Clinical observations on reserpine reversal after prolonged MAO inhibition. Psychiatr Neurol Neurochir, 70:59, 1967
   Avoid concurrent use

Selective serotonin reuptake inhibitors (SSRIs)
   Varied cardiovascular, GI, neurological, and psychiatric symptoms — serotonin syndrome (mechanism not established)
      H Sternbach, Danger of MAOI therapy after fluoxetine withdrawal. Lancet, 2:850, 1988; JP Feighner et al, Adverse consequences of fluoxetine-MAOI combination therapy. J Clin Psychiatry, 51:222, 1990; O Suchowersky and J deVries, Possible interactions between Deprenyl and Prozac. Can J Neurol Sci, 17:352, 1990; VS Bhatara and FC Bandettini, Possible interaction between sertraline and tranylcypromine. Clin Pharm, 12:222, 1993; JL Montastruc et al, Pseudophaeochromocytoma in parkinsonian patient treated with fluoxetine plus selegiline. Lancet, 341:555, 1993; SK Brannan et al, Sertraline and isocarboxazid cause a serotonin syndrome. J Clin Psychopharmacol, 14(2):144, 1994; SC Toyama and RP Iacono, Is it safe to combine a selective serotonin reuptake inhibitor with selegiline? Ann Pharmacother, 28:405, 1994; D Taylor and D Duncan, Moclobemide and SSRIs. Pharm J, 253:330, 1994; CJ Hawley et al, Safety and tolerability of

MONOAMINE OXIDASE INHIBITORS, with: *(continued)*
>   combined treatment with moclobemide and SSRIs: a systematic study of
>   50 patients. Int Clin Psychopharmacol, 11:187, 1996; SV Patel et al, L-
>   deprenyl augmentation of fluoxetine in a patient with Huntington's
>   disease. Ann Clin Psychiatry, 8:23, 1996; manufacturer's package insert; K
>   Laine et al, Lack of adverse interactions between concomitantly admin-
>   istered selegiline and citalopram. Clin Neuropharmacol, 20:419, 1997; BSH
>   Chan et al, Serotonin syndrome resulting from drug interactions. MJA,
>   169:523, 1998
>
>   *A drug-free interval of 5 weeks may be safest when switching to an MAOI and
>   2 weeks when switching from an MAOI to an SSRI; occurs with both MAO-A
>   and MAO-B inhibitors; unlikely with MAO-B inhibitors (e.g. selegiline) at usual
>   dosages; at carefully selected dosage, MAO-A inhibitors together with SSRIs
>   can be tolerated in intractable situations, but adverse effects increase;
>   citalopram may not interact significantly with selegiline*

Sibutramine
>   Possible serotonin syndrome (additive serotonergic effect)
>   Manufacturer's package insert
>   *Avoid concurrent use*

Sulfonamides
>   Possible phenelzine toxicity with sulfisoxazole (decreased metabolism)
>   WF Boyer and CR Lake, Interaction of phenelzine and sulfisoxazole. Am J
>   Psychiatry, 140:264, 1983
>   *Single case report (1983)*

Sympathomimetic amines
>   Severe hypertension and possible crisis except with isoproterenol or probably
>   epinephrine (increase in storage and release of norepinephrine)
>   SP Wright, Hazards with monoamine-oxidase inhibitors: a persistent prob-
>   lem. Lancet, 1:284, 1978; MF Cuthbert and DW Vere, Potentiation of the car-
>   diovascular effects of some catecholamines by a monoamine oxidase inhi-
>   bitor. Br J Pharmacol, 43:471P, 1971; AJ Boakes et al, Interactions between
>   sympathomimetic amines and antidepressant agents in man. Br Med J,
>   1:311, 1973; D Horwitz et al, Increased blood pressure responses to dopa-
>   mine and norepinephrine produced by monoamine oxidase inhibitors in
>   man. J Lab Clin Med, 56:747, 1960; I Krisko et al, Severe hyperpyrexia due
>   to tranylcypromine-amphetamine toxicity. Ann Intern Med, 70:559, 1969;
>   DS Thompson et al, Lack of interaction of monoamine oxidase inhibitors
>   and epinephrine in an older patient. J Clin Psychopharmacol, 17:322, 1997;
>   MJ Wahl, Drug interactions, J Am Dent Assoc, 130:1270, 1999; LM Rose et
>   al, A hypertensive reaction induced by concurrent use of selegiline and do-
>   pamine. Ann Pharmacother, 34:1020, 2000
>   *Avoid concurrent use; may occur with over-the-counter products*

Sympathomimetic bronchodilators
>   Hypomania with phenelzine and isoetharine (mechanism not established)
>   LS Goldman and JA Tiller, Hypomania related to phenelzine and isoetha-
>   rine interaction in one patient. J Clin Psychiatry, 48:170, 1987

(continued)

MONOAMINE OXIDASE INHIBITORS, with: *(continued)*
Single case report (1987)

Tolcapone

Possible tolcapone toxicity (decreased metabolism)

Manufacturer's package insert (tolcapone)

Avoid concurrent use of tolcapone and a non-selective MAO inhibitor; selegeline at recommended dosage does not interact.

Triptans

Possible rizatriptan, sumatriptan or zolmitriptan toxicity (possible decreased metabolism)

Manufacturer's package insert; P Rolan, Potential drug interactions with the novel antimigraine compound zolmitriptan (*Zomig*(tm), 311C90). Cephalalgia, 17 suppl 18:21, 1997; AD van Haarst et al, The effects of moclobemide on the pharmacokinetics of the 5-HT$_{IB/ID}$ agonist rizatriptan in healthy volunteers. Br J Clin Pharmacol, 48:190, 1999

Avoid concurrent use or use of triptan within 2 weeks of discontinuing an MAO inhibitor; selegeline, an MAO-B inhibitor does not appear to interact at usual doses; naratriptan is not expected to interact with an MAO inhibitor

Tryptophan

Adverse behavioral and neurological effects with phenelzine or tranylcypromine (mechanism not established)

HG Pope, Jr et al, Toxic reactions to the combination of monoamine oxidase inhibitors and tryptophan. Am J Psychiatry, 142:491, 1985; AB Levy et al, Myoclonus, hyperreflexia and diaphoresis in patients on phenelzine-tryptophan combination treatment. Can J Psychiatry, 30:434, 1985; G Alvine et al, Case of delirium secondary to phenelzine/L-tryptophan combination. J Clin Psychiatry, 51:311, 1990

Monitor clinical status

Tyramine-rich foods and beverages

Hypertensive crisis (increased storage and release of norepinephrine)

J Dingemanse et al, Pharmacokinetic—pharmacodynamic interactions between two selective monoamine oxidase inhibitors: moclobemide and selegiline. Clin Neuropharmacol, 19:399, 1996; JS Barrett et al, Pressor response to tyramine after single 24-hour application of a selegiline transdermal system in healthy males. J Clin Pharmacol, 37:238, 1997; AJ Gelenberg, Pizza and soy and MAOIs. Biol Ther Psychiatry, 22:49, 1999

Tyramine-containing foods are listed in the table on page 355; avoid concurrent use; several cases of interaction with MAO-B inhibitors (selegiline) have been reported to the manufacturer and concurrent use of tyramine-containing foods should be avoided; transdermal selegiline may be less likely to enhance pressor response to tyramine; reversible MAO-A inhibitors (moclobemide) may not interact with usual food intake; however, patients receiving both an MAO-A inhibitor and an MAO-B inhibitor can develop a hypertensive crisis with tyramine intake

MONOAMINE OXIDASE INHIBITORS, with: *(continued)*
  Venlafaxine
  Cardiovascular and neurological toxicity [serotonin syndrome] with phenelzine or tranylcypromine and possibly selegiline or moclobemide (additive inhibition of neurotransmitter reuptake)

  > SD Phillips and P Ringo, Phenelzine and venlafaxine interaction. Am J Psychiatry, 152:9, 1995; MA Heisler et al, Serotonin syndrome induced by administration of venlafaxine and phenelzine. Ann Pharmacother, 30:84, 1996; JF Brubacher et al, Serotonin syndrome from venlafaxine-tranylcypromine interaction. J Toxicol Clin Toxicol, 35:523, 1995; M Hodgman et al, Severe serotonin syndrome secondary to venlafaxine and maintenance tranylcypromine therapy. J Toxicol Clin Toxicol, 33:554, 1995; MJ Gitlin, Venlafaxine, monoamine oxidase inhibitors, and the serotonin syndrome. J Clin Psychopharmacol, 17:66, 1997; MJ Hodgman et al, Serotonin syndrome due to venlafaxine and maintenance tranylcypromine therapy. Human Exp Toxicol, 16:14, 1997; P Kolecki, Venlafaxine induced serotonin syndrome occurring after abstinence from phenelzine for more than two weeks. Clin Toxicol, 35:211, 1997; MG Roxanas et al, Serotonin syndrome in combined moclobemide and venlafaxine ingestion. Med J Aust, 168:523, 1998; S Diamond et al, Serotonin syndrome induced by transitioning from phenelzine to venlafaxine: four patient reports. Neurology, 51:274, 1998; BSH Chan et al, Serotonin syndrom resulting from drug interactions. MJA, 169:523, 1998

  Venlafaxine should not be started for 14 days after an MAOI is stopped (however, three patients developed serotonin syndrome when venlafaxine was given 14 to 16 days after an MAOI) and should be stopped 7 days before an MAOI is started; single case report with selegiline (1997); Two case reports with moclobemide, one involving a maclobemide overdose (1998)

Monoclonal antibody, see Muromonab-CD3
MONTELUKAST, with:
  Barbiturates - See Barbiturates with Montelukast, page 134
  Corticosteroids - See Corticosteroids with Montelukast, page 221
MORICIZINE, with:
  Anticoagulants, oral - See Anticoagulants, oral with Moricizine, page 71
  Antihistamines, H$_2$-blockers - See Antihistamines, H$_2$-blockers with Moricizine, page 120
  Diltiazem - See Diltiazem with Moricizine, page 261
  Theophyllines
  Possible decreased theophylline effect (increased metabolism)

  > LA Siddoway et al, Clinical pharmacokinetics of moricizine. Am J Cardiol, 65:21D, 1990; HJ Pieniaszek et al, Effect of moricizine on the pharmacokinetics of single-dose theophylline in healthy subjects. Ther Drug Monit, 15:199, 1993

  Monitor theophylline concentration
Morphine, see Narcotics: morphine-like
Moxalactam, see Cephalosporins
Murine monoclonal antibody, see Muromonab-CD3

MUROMONAB-CD3, with:
   Cyclosporine - See Cyclosporine with Muromonab-CD3, page 234

MYCOPHENOLATE MOFETIL, with:
   Antacids - See Antacids with Mycophenolate mofetil, page 54
   Cholestyramine - See Cholestyramine with Mycophenolate mofetil, page 197
   Colestipol - See Colestipol with Mycophenolate mofetil, page 211
   Cyclosporine - See Cyclosporine with Mycophenolate mofetil, page 234
   Sulfinpyrazone
      Possible mycophenolate mofetil toxicity (possibly reduced renal excretion)
         C Catalano et al, Mycophenolate mofetil toxicity in an anorexic kidney transplant patient treated with sulphinpirazone. Nephrol Dial Transplant, 12:2467, 1997
      Single case report (1997)
   Tacrolimus
      Possible mycophenolate mofetil toxicity (mechanism not established)
         GI Hübner et al, Drug interaction between mycophenolate mofetil and tacrolimus detectable within therapeutic mycophenolic acid monitoring in renal transplant patients. Ther Drug Monit, 21:536, 1999
      Based on study in renal transplant patients; tacrolimus appears to increase levels of the active metabolite, mycophenolic acid (MPA); monitor mycophenolate mofetil plasma levels and clinical status

Nabilone, no documented interactions, see page 4, Criteria for Listing Interactions
Nabumetone, see Nonsteroidal anti-inflammatory drugs
Nadolol, see Beta-adrenergic blockers
Nafcillin, see Penicillins
Naftifine, no documented interactions, see page 4, Criteria for Listing Interactions
Nalbuphine, see Narcotics: morphine-like

NALIDIXIC ACID, with:
   Anticoagulants, oral - See Anticoagulants, oral with Nalidixic acid, page 72
   Probenecid
      Possible nalidixic acid toxicity (decreased renal excretion)
         TB Vree et al, Probenecid inhibits the renal clearance and renal glucuronidation of nalidixic acid. Pharm World Sci, 15:165, 1993
      Avoid concurrent use

Nalmefene, no documented interactions, see page 4, Criteria for Listing Interactions

NALOXONE, with:
   Clonidine - See Clonidine with Naloxone, page 205

NALTREXONE, with:
   Insulin - See Insulin with Naltrexone, page 310
   Phenothiazines
      Increased sedation with thioridazine (mechanism not established)
         I Maany et al, Interaction between thioridazine and naltrexone. Am J Psychiatry, 144:966, 1987; R Malcolm et al, I Maany and CP O'Brien, Idiosyncratic reaction to naltrexone augmented by thioridazine. Am J Psychiatry, 145:773, 1988

NALTREXONE, with: *(continued)*
>*Avoid concurrent use; symptoms may result from thioridazine alone, but usually tolerance develops to the single drug*

Nandrolone, see Anabolic and androgenic steroids

Naproxen, see Nonsteroidal anti-inflammatory drugs

Naratriptan, see Triptans

NARCOTICS: DEXTROMETHORPHAN, with:

Amiodarone - See Amiodarone with Narcotics: dextromethorphan, page 36

Monoamine oxidase inhibitors - See Monoamine oxidase inhibitors with Narcotics: dextromethorphan, page 349

Narcotics: methadone and congeners

Possible dextromethorphan toxicity with methadone (decreased metabolism)
> D Wu et al, Inhibition of human cytochrome P450 2D6 (CYP2D6) by methadone. Br J Clin Pharmacol, 35:30, 1993

Avoid concurrent use

Quinidine

Dextromethorphan toxicity (decreased metabolism)
> Y Zhang et al, Dextromethorphan: enhancing its systemic availability by way of low-dose quinidine-mediated inhibition of cytochrome P4502D6. Clin Pharmacol Ther, 51:647, 1992; DA Capon et al, The influence of CYP2D6 polymorphism and quinidine on the disposition and antitussive effect of dextromethorphan in humans. Clin Pharmacol Ther, 60:295, 1996

Avoid concurrent use

Selective serotonin reuptake inhibitors (SSRIs)

Visual hallucinations with fluoxetine (probably decreased metabolism)
> NS Achamallah, Visual hallucinations after combining fluoxetine and dextromethorphan. Am J Psychiatry, 149:1406, 1992

Single case report (1992)

Sibutramine

Possible serotonin syndrome (additive serotonergic effect)
> Manufacturer's package insert

Avoid concurrent use

NARCOTICS: MEPERIDINE AND CONGENERS, with:

Acyclovir - See Acyclovir with Narcotics: meperidine and congeners, page 11

Amiodarone - See Amiodarone with Narcotics: meperidine and congeners, page 36

Antifungals, imidazoles and triazoles - See Antifungals, imidazoles and triazoles with Narcotics: meperidine and congeners, page 104

Antihistamines, H_2-blockers - See Antihistamines, H_2-blockers with Narcotics: meperidine and congeners, page 120

Barbiturates - See Barbiturates with Narcotics: meperidine and congeners, page 134

Benzodiazepines - See Benzodiazepines with Narcotics: meperidine and congeners, page 145

Beta-adrenergic blockers - See Beta-adrenergic blockers with Narcotics: meperidine and congeners, page 158

(continued)

NARCOTICS: MEPERIDINE AND CONGENERS, with: *(continued)*

Cholestyramine - See Cholestyramine with Narcotics: meperidine and congeners, page 197

Diltiazem - See Diltiazem with Narcotics: meperidine and congeners, page 261

Enflurane - See Enflurane with Narcotics: meperidine and congeners, page 269

Guanfacine - See Guanfacine with Narcotics: meperidine and congeners, page 293

Halothane - See Halothane with Narcotics: meperidine and congeners, page 297

Lidocaine - See Lidocaine with Narcotics: meperidine and congeners, page 322

Macrolide antibiotics - See Macrolide antibiotics with Narcotics: meperidine and congeners, page 331

Monoamine oxidase inhibitors - See Monoamine oxidase inhibitors with Narcotics: meperidine and congeners, page 349

Nifedipine

Toxic megacolon with loperamide (possibly synergism)
S Lelouch et al, Syndrome d'Ogilvie associé à un traitement par lopéramide et nifédipine. Gastroenterol Clin Biol, 15:455, 1991

Single case report (1991)

Phenothiazines

Narcotic toxicity with chlorpromazine or thioridazine (toxic metabolite)
JE Stambaugh, Jr and IW Wainer, Drug interaction: meperidine and chlorpromazine, a toxic combination. J Clin Pharmacol, 21:140, 1981; DR Grothe et al, Clinical implications of the neuroleptic-opioid interaction. Drug Intell Clin Pharm, 20:75, 1986

Monitor closely

Phenytoin

Decreased meperidine effect (increased metabolism)
SM Pond and KM Kretschzmar, Effect of phenytoin on meperidine clearance and normeperidine formation. Clin Pharmacol Ther, 30:680, 1981

Monitor analgesia

Ritonavir

Possible decreased meperidine effect (increased metabolism)
SC Piscitelli et al, The effect of ritonavir on the pharmacokinetics of meperidine and normeperidine. Pharmacotheray, 20:549, 2000; manufacturer's package insert (ritonavir)

Based on study in 8 healthy subjects; monitor for reduced meperidine effect; listed as contraindicated in product information based on theoretical increase in meperidine effect; subjects on chronic ritonavir therapy appear to eliminate meperidine more efficiently, probably due to enzyme induction

Possible increased fentanyl effect (probably decreased metabolism: CYP3A4)
KT Olkkola et al, Ritonavir's role in reducing fentanyl clearance and prolonging its half-life. Anesthesiology, 91:681, 1999

Based on study in 11 healthy subjects; monitor for increased fentanyl effect; reduce fentanyl dose as needed

NARCOTICS: MEPERIDINE AND CONGENERS, with: *(continued)*

Saint John's wort
Possible increased risk of delirium (mechanism not established)
> I Khawaja et al, Herbal medicines as a factor in delirium. Psychiatr Serv, 50:969, 1999

Single case report (1999); patient also taking valerian root; causal relationship not established

Sibutramine
Possible serotonin syndrome with meperidine (additive serotonergic effect)
> Manufacturer's package insert

Avoid concurrent use

Trimethoprim-sulfamethoxazole
Possible loperamide toxicity (possibly decreased metabolism)
> F Kamali and ML Huang, Increased systemic availability of loperamide after oral administration of loperamide and loperamide oxide with cotrimoxazole. Br J Clin Pharmacol, 41:125, 1996

Monitor clinical status; adjust dose as needed

Valerian root
Possible increased risk of delirium (mechanism not established)
> I Khawaja et al, Herbal medicines as a factor in delirium. Psychiatr Serv, 50:969, 1999

Single case report (1999); patient also taking Saint John's wort; causal relationship not established

NARCOTICS: METHADONE AND CONGENERS, with:

Anticoagulants, oral - See Anticoagulants, oral with Narcotics: methadone and congeners, page 72

Antidepressants, tricyclic - See Antidepressants, tricyclic with Narcotics: methadone and congeners, page 87

Antifungals, imidazoles and triazoles - See Antifungals, imidazoles and triazoles with Narcotics: methadone and congeners, page 104

Antihistamines, H_2-blockers - See Antihistamines, H_2-blockers with Narcotics: methadone and congeners, page 120

Barbiturates - See Barbiturates with Narcotics: methadone and congeners, page 135

Benzodiazepines - See Benzodiazepines with Narcotics: methadone and congeners, page 145

Carbamazepine - See Carbamazepine with Narcotics: methadone and congeners, page 182

Didanosine - See Didanosine with Narcotics: methadone and congeners, page 249

Efavirenz - See Efavirenz with Narcotics: methadone and congeners, page 268

Lopinavir/Ritonavir - See Lopinavir/Ritonavir with Narcotics: methadone and congeners, page 329

Metyrapone - See Metyrapone with Narcotics: methadone and congeners, page 345

(continued)

NARCOTICS: METHADONE AND CONGENERS, with: *(continued)*
  Monoamine oxidase inhibitors - See Monoamine oxidase inhibitors with Narcotics: methadone and congeners, page 350
  Narcotics: dextromethorphan - See Narcotics: dextromethorphan with Narcotics: methadone and congeners, page 355
  Nelfinavir
    Possible decreased methadone effect (probably increased metabolism)
      P Beauverie et al, Therapeutic drug monitoring of methadone in HIV-infected patients receiving protease inhibitors. AIDS, 12:2510, 1998; EF McCance-Katz et al, Decrease in methodone levels with nelfinavir mesylate. Am J Psychiatry, 157:481, 2000
      Three case reports (1998; 2000); monitor clinical status; similar effect with ritonavir but indinavir and saquinavir did not appear to interact
  Nevirapine
    Decreased methadone effect (probably increased metabolism; CYP3A4)
      MW Heelon and LB Meade, Methadone withdrawal when starting an antiretroviral regimen including nevirapine. Pharmacotherapy, 19:471, 1999; M-J Otero et al, Nevirapine-induced withdrawal symptoms in HIV patients on methadone maintenance programme: an alert. AIDS, 13:1004, 1999; FL Altice et al, Nevirapine induced opiate withdrawal among injection drug users with HIV infection receiving methadone. AIDS, 13:957, 1999; V Pinzani et al, Methadone withdrawal symptoms with nevirapine and efavirenz. Ann Pharmacother, 34:405, 2000; MDB Rodrigo et al, La nevirapina induce síntomas de abstenencia en pacientes en programa de mantenimiento con metadona con infección por VIH. Rev Clin Esp, 200:18, 2000
      Numerous case reports of methadone withdrawal, usually 5 to 10 days after starting nevirapine; monitor clinical status and increase methadone dose as needed
  Phenytoin
    Decreased methadone effect (increased metabolism)
      PF Finelli, Phenytoin and methadone tolerance. N Engl J Med, 294:227, 1976; TG Tong et al, Phenytoin-induced methadone withdrawal. Ann Intern Med, 94:349, 1981
      Monitor patients on methadone maintenance for withdrawal symptoms
  Rifampin
    Methadone withdrawal symptoms (increased metabolism)
      MJ Kreek et al, Rifampin-induced methadone withdrawal. N Engl J Med, 294:1104, 1976; MR Bending and PO Skacel, Rifampicin and methadone withdrawal. Lancet, 1:1211, 1977; VF Holmes, Rifampin-induced methadone withdrawal in AIDS. J Clin Psychopharmacol, 10:443, 1990
      Monitor patients on methadone maintenance for withdrawal symptoms
  Ritonavir
    Possible propoxyphene toxicity (decreased metabolism)
      Manufacturer's package insert (ritonavir)
      Theoretical; listed as contraindicated in product information

NARCOTICS: METHADONE AND CONGENERS, with: *(continued)*
    Possible decreased methadone effect (probably increased metabolism)
        P Beauverie et al, Therapeutic drug monitoring of methadone in HIV-infected patients receiving protease inhibitors. AIDS, 12:2510, 1998; SM Geletko and AD Erickson, Decreased methadone effect after ritonavir initiation. Pharmacotherapy, 20:93, 2000
    Two case reports (1998, 2000); monitor clinical status; similar effect with nelfinavir but indinavir and saquinavir did not appear to interact
  Selective serotonin reuptake inhibitors (SSRIs)
    Methadone toxicity with fluvoxamine and possibly fluoxetine (decreased methadone metabolism)
        G Bertschy et al, Probable metabolic interaction between methadone and fluvoxamine in addict patients. Ther Drug Monit,16:42, 1994; CB Eap et al, Fluvoxamine and fluoxetine do not interact in the same way with the metabolism of the enantiomers of methadone. J Clin Psychopharmacol, 17:113, 1997; G Bertschy et al, Fluoxetine addition to methadone in addicts: pharmacokinetic aspects. Ther Drug Monit, 18:570, 1996; CP Alderman and PA Frith, Fluvoxamine-methadone interaction. Aust N Z J Psychiatry, 33:99, 1999; PA DeMaria, Jr and RD Serota, A therapeutic use of the methadone fluvoxamine drug interaction. J Addict Dis, 18:5, 1999
    Based on studies in male and female addicts maintained on methadone; monitor methadone concentration; signs of opiate withdrawal when fluvoxamine or fluoxetine stopped; interaction has been used intentionally to maintain methadone serum concentrations
  Stavudine
    Possible decreased stavudine effect (probably decreased bioavailability)
        PM Rainey et al, Interaction of methadone with didanosine and stavudine. J Acquir Immune Defic Syndr, 24:241, 2000
    Based on study in HIV(+) patients; clinical importance not established; monitor clinical status and adjust stavudine dosage as needed
  Zidovudine
    Possible zidovudine toxicity with methadone (probable decreased metabolism-glucuronidation; possible decreased renal clearance)
        EL Schwartz et al, Pharmacokinetic interactions of zidovudine and methadone in intravenous drug-using patients with HIV infection. J Acquir Immune Defic Syndr, 5:619, 1992; DM Burger et al, Pharmacokinetic variability of zidovudine in HIV-infected individuals: subgroup analysis and drug interactions. AIDS, 8:1683, 1994; E Cretton-Scott et al, Methadone and its metabolite N-demethyl methadone, inhibit AZT glucuronidation in vitro. Clin Pharmacol Ther, 59:168, 1996; EF McCance-Katz et al, Methadone effects on zidovudine disposition (AIDS Clinical Trials Group 262). J Acq Immune Defic Syndr, 18:435, 1998
    Monitor clinical status and zidovudine concentrations if available
NARCOTICS: MORPHINE-LIKE, with:
  Alcohol - See Alcohol with Narcotics: morphine-like, page 20

(continued)

NARCOTICS: MORPHINE-LIKE, with: *(continued)*

Antihistamines, H$_2$-blockers - See Antihistamines, H$_2$-blockers with Narcotics: morphine-like, page 120

Bupivacaine - See Bupivacaine with Narcotics: morphine-like, page 168

Contraceptives, oral - See Contraceptives, oral with Narcotics: morphine-like, page 215

Fluoroquinolones - See Fluoroquinolones with Narcotics: morphine-like, page 280

Haloperidol - See Haloperidol with Narcotics: morphine-like, page 295

Kaolin or Kaolin-pectin - See Kaolin or Kaolin-pectin with Narcotics: morphine-like, page 315

Lidocaine - See Lidocaine with Narcotics: morphine-like, page 322

Metoclopramide - See Metoclopramide with Narcotics: morphine-like, page 343

Neuromuscular blocking agents

Central respiratory depression and respiratory muscle paralysis with tubocurarine (additive)

JW Bellville et al, The interaction of morphine and d-tubocurarine on respiration and grip strength in man. Clin Pharmacol Ther, 5:35, 1964

May require respiratory support postoperatively; use with caution

Octreotide

Possible decreased codeine effect (decreased conversion of codeine to morphine; CYP2D6)

E Rasmussen et al, Selective effects of somatostatin analogs on human drug-metabolizing enzymes. Clin Pharmacol Ther, 64:150, 1998

Based on study in patients with carcinoid syndrome; lanreotide has similar effect; monitor clinical status

Quinidine

Absence of codeine analgesia (blocked conversion to morphine in rapid metabolizers; CYP2D6)

J Desmeules et al, Impact of environmental and genetic factors on codeine analgesia. Eur J Clin Pharmacol, 41:23, 1991; SH Sindrup et al, The effect of quinidine on the analgesic effect of codeine. Eur J Clin Pharmacol, 42:587, 1992; Y Caraco et al, Pharmacogenetic determination of the effects of codeine and prediction of drug interactions. J Pharmacol Exper Ther, 278:1165, 1996; T Heiskanen et al, Effects of blocking CYP2D6 on the pharmacokinetics and pharmacodynamics of oxycodone. Clin Pharmacol Ther, 64:603, 1998

Based on studies in healthy subjects; hydrocodone and dihydrocodeine may also interact; codeine provides little or no analgesia for poor metabolizers; monitor analgesic effect; preliminary evidence suggests that oxycodone may not be dependent upon CYP2D6 for activity

Rifampin

Possible decreased codeine or morphine response (mechanism not established)

Y Caraco et al, Pharmacogenetic determinants of codeine induction by rifampin: the impact on codeine's respiratory, psychomotor and miotic effects. J Pharmacol Exp Ther, 281:330, 1997; MF Fromm et al, Loss of

NARCOTICS: MORPHINE-LIKE, with: *(continued)*
> analgesic effect of morphine due to coadministration of rifampin. Pain, 72:261, 1997
>
> *Avoid concurrent use; based on studies in healthy subjects*
> **Somatostatin**
> Possible decreased analgesic effect of morpine (mechanism not established)
>> C Ripamonti et al, Can somatostatin be administered in association with morphine in advanced cancer patients with pain? Ann Oncol, 8:921, 1998
>
> *Based on study of 3 cancer patients (1998); monitor clinical status*

NARCOTICS: PENTAZOCINE, with:
> **Antidepressants, tricyclic** - See Antidepressants, tricyclic with Narcotics: pentazocine, page 88
> **Selective serotonin reuptake inhibitors (SSRIs)**
> Hypertension, nausea, lightheadedness, anxiety, paresthesias, ataxia with fluoxetine (mechanism not established)
>> TE Hansen et al, Interaction of fluoxetine and pentazocine. Am J Psychiatry, 147:949, 1990
>
> *Single case report (1990); patient given pentazocine-naloxone combination orally; could have been due to pentazocine alone*

NARCOTICS: TRAMADOL, with:
> **Anticoagulants, oral** - See Anticoagulants, oral with Narcotics: tramadol, page 72
> **Carbamazepine** - See Carbamazepine with Narcotics: tramadol, page 182
> **Monoamine oxidase inhibitors** - See Monoamine oxidase inhibitors with Narcotics: tramadol, page 350
> **Selective serotonin reuptake inhibitors (SSRIs)**
> Nightmares and hallucinations with paroxetine (mechanism not established)
>> J Devulder et al, Nightmares and hallucinations after long term intake of tramadol combined with antidepressants. Acta Clin Belg, 51:184, 1996
>
> *Single case report (1996); patient also taking dothiepin (dosulepine); causal relationship not established*
>
> Serotonin syndrome (possible additive serotonergic effect)
>> BJ Mason and KH Blackburn, Possible serotonin syndrome associated with tramadol and sertraline coadministration. Ann Pharmacother, 31:175, 1997; ACG Egberts et al, Serotonin syndrome attributed to tramadol addition to paroxetine therapy. Int Clin Psychopharmacol, 12:181, 1997; MS Lantz et al, Int J Geriatr Psychiatry, 13:343, 1998
>
> *Four case reports (1997, 1998)*

Nedocromil, no documented interactions, see page 4, Criteria for Listing Interactions

NEFAZODONE, with:
> **Antihistamines, H$_1$-blockers: astemizole, terfenadine** - See Antihistamines, H$_1$-blockers: astemizole, terfenadine with Nefazodone, page 111
> **Benzodiazepines** - See Benzodiazepines with Nefazodone, page 145
> **Carbamazepine** - See Carbamazepine with Nefazodone, page 182
> **Cisapride** - See Cisapride with Nefazodone, page 200

(continued)

NEFAZODONE, with: *(continued)*
    Cyclosporine - See Cyclosporine with Nefazodone, page 235
    Digoxin - See Digoxin with Nefazodone, page 254
    Haloperidol - See Haloperidol with Nefazodone, page 295
    HMG-CoA reductase inhibitors - See HMG-CoA reductase inhibitors with Nefazodone, page 301
    Insulin - See Insulin with Nefazodone, page 310
    Saint John's wort
        Possible nausea, vomiting, confusion and anxiety (mechanism not established)
            MS Lantz et al, St. John's wort and antidepressant drug interactions in the elderly. J Geriatr Psychiatry Neurol, 12:7, 1999
        One case report (1999); monitor clinical status; avoid St. John's wort
    Tacrolimus
        Tacrolimus toxicity (decreased metabolism; CYP3A4)
            AJ Olyaei et al, Interaction between tacrolimus and nefazodone in a stable renal transplant recipient. Pharmacotherapy, 18:1356, 1998
        Single case report (1998)
    Trazodone
        Possible increased risk of serotonin syndrome (probably additive)
            HC Margolese and G Chouinard, Serotonin syndrome from addition of low-dose trazodone to nefazodone. Am J Psychiatry, 157:1022, 2000
        Single case report (2000); causal relationship not established; monitor clinical status

NELFINAVIR, with:
    Antihistamines, H$_1$-blockers: astemizole, terfenadine - See Antihistamines, H$_1$-blockers: astemizole, terfenadine with Nelfinavir, page 111
    Barbiturates - See Barbiturates with Nelfinavir, page 135
    Benzodiazepines - See Benzodiazepines with Nelfinavir, page 146
    Carbamazepine - See Carbamazepine with Nelfinavir, page 182
    Cisapride - See Cisapride with Nelfinavir, page 200
    Contraceptives, oral - See Contraceptives, oral with Nelfinavir, page 215
    Delavirdine - See Delavirdine with Nelfinavir, page 244
    Indinavir - See Indinavir with Nelfinavir, page 308
    Narcotics: methadone and congeners - See Narcotics: methadone and congeners with Nelfinavir, page 358
    Nevirapine
        Possible decrease in nelfinavir effect (mechanism not established)
            C Merry et al, The pharmacokinetics of combination therapy with nelfinavir plus nevirapine. AIDS, 12:1163, 1998; G Skowron et al, Lack of pharmacokinetic interaction between nelfinavir and nevirapine. AIDS 12:1243, 1998
        Conflicting results; larger study found no interaction
    Phenytoin
        Possible decreased nelfinavir effect (increased metabolism; CYP3A)
            Manufacturer's package insert (nelfinavir)
        Clinical significance remains to be established

NELFINAVIR, with: *(continued)*
  Rifabutin
    Possible rifabutin toxicity (decreased metabolism; CYP3A)
      Manufacturer's package insert (nelfinavir)
    Monitor rifabutin concentration; manufacturer recommends reducing rifabutin dosage by half
  Rifampin
    Possible decreased nelfinavir effect (increased metabolism; CYP3A)
      Manufacturer's package insert (nelfinavir)
    Avoid concurrent use
  Ritonavir
    Possible nelfinavir toxicity (decreased metabolism; CYP3A)
      Manufacturer's package insert (nelfinavir); AL Tseng and MM Foisy, Significant interactions with new antiretrovirals and psychotropic drugs. Ann Pharmacother, 33:461, 1999; M Barry et al, Pharmacokinetics and potential interactions amongst antiretroviral agents used to treat patients with HIV infection. Clin Pharmacokinet, 36:289, 1999
    Clinical significance remains to be established
  Saquinavir
    Possible saquinavir toxicity (decreased metabolism)
      Manufacturer's package insert; C Merry et al, Saquinavir pharmacokinetics alone and in combination with nelfinavir in HIV-infected patients. AIDS, 11:F117, 1997
    Interaction may be therapeutically useful, but adverse effects may increase; effect highly variable from patient to patient
  Tacrolimus
    Possible tacrolimus toxicity (decreased metabolism; probably CYP3A4; decreased transport; probably P-glycoprotein)
      AM Sheikh et al, Concomitant human immunodeficiency virus protease inhibitor therapy markedly reduces tacrolimus metabolism and increases blood levels. Transplantation, 68:307, 1999; R Schvarcz et al, Interaction between nelfinavir and tacrolimus after orthoptic liver transplantation in a patient coinfected with HIV and hepatitis C virus (HCV). Transplantation, 69:2194, 2000
    Two case reports (1999; 2000); one case required dramatic reduction in tacrolimus dose; monitor tacrolimus concentrations and clinical status

Neomycin, see Aminoglycoside antibiotics
Neostigmine, see Anticholinesterases
Netilmicin, see Aminoglycoside antibiotics
NEUROMUSCULAR BLOCKING AGENTS, with:
  Alkylating agents - See Alkylating agents with Neuromuscular blocking agents, page 23
  Aminoglycoside antibiotics - See Aminoglycoside antibiotics with Neuromuscular blocking agents, page 32
  Anabolic and androgenic steroids - See Anabolic and androgenic steroids with Neuromuscular blocking agents, page 42

(continued)

NEUROMUSCULAR BLOCKING AGENTS, with: *(continued)*

Antifungals, Amphotericin B - See Antifungals, Amphotericin B with Neuromuscular blocking agents, page 94

Antihistamines, H_2-blockers - See Antihistamines, H_2-blockers with Neuromuscular blocking agents, page 121

Benzodiazepines - See Benzodiazepines with Neuromuscular blocking agents, page 146

Beta-adrenergic blockers - See Beta-adrenergic blockers with Neuromuscular blocking agents, page 158

Carbamazepine - See Carbamazepine with Neuromuscular blocking agents, page 182

Clindamycin - See Clindamycin with Neuromuscular blocking agents, page 203

Corticosteroids - See Corticosteroids with Neuromuscular blocking agents, page 221

Cyclosporine - See Cyclosporine with Neuromuscular blocking agents, page 235

Digitoxin - See Digitoxin with Neuromuscular blocking agents, page 250

Digoxin - See Digoxin with Neuromuscular blocking agents, page 254

Disopyramide - See Disopyramide with Neuromuscular blocking agents, page 263

Donepezil - See Donepezil with Neuromuscular blocking agents, page 266

Doxapram - See Doxapram with Neuromuscular blocking agents, page 266

Furosemide - See Furosemide with Neuromuscular blocking agents, page 286

Lincomycin - See Lincomycin with Neuromuscular blocking agents, page 323

Lithium - See Lithium with Neuromuscular blocking agents, page 324

Magnesium sulfate - See Magnesium sulfate with Neuromuscular blocking agents, page 335

Malathion - See Malathion with Neuromuscular blocking agents, page 335

Metoclopramide - See Metoclopramide with Neuromuscular blocking agents, page 343

Monoamine oxidase inhibitors - See Monoamine oxidase inhibitors with Neuromuscular blocking agents, page 350

Narcotics: morphine-like - See Narcotics: morphine-like with Neuromuscular blocking agents, page 360

Penicillins

Recurrent neuromuscular blockade with IV piperacillin and vecuronium (mechanism not established)

> K Mackie and EG Pavlin, Recurrent paralysis following piperacillin administration. Anesthesiology, 72:561, 1990

Single case report (1990)

Phenytoin

Decreased neuromuscular blockade with doxacurium, pancuronium, metocurine, rocuronium or vecuronium with chronic use of phenytoin (mechanism not established)

> DL Callanan, Development of resistance to pancuronium in adult respiratory distress syndrome. Anesth Analg, 64:1126 1985; FH Norris, Jr et al, Effect of diphenylhydantoin on neuromuscular synapse. Neurology, 14:869, 1964; E Ornstein et al, Resistance to metocurine-induced neuromuscular blockade in patients receiving phenytoin. Anesthesiology,

NEUROMUSCULAR BLOCKING AGENTS, with: *(continued)*

> 63:294, 1985; E Ornstein et al, The effect of phenytoin on the magnitude and duration of neuromuscular block following atracurium or vecuronium. Anesthesiology, 67:191, 1987; DR Hickey et al, Phenytoin-induced resistance to pancuronium. Anaesthesia, 43:757, 1988; PR Platt and NM Thackray, Phenytoin-induced resistance to vecuronium. Anaesth Intens Care, 21:185, 1993; J Szenohradszky et al, Interaction of recuronium (ORG 9426) and phenytoin in a patient undergoing cadaver renal transplantation: a possible pharmacokinetic mechanism? Anesthesiology, 80:1167, 1994; manufacturer's package insert for doxacurium; PB Loan et al, Neuromuscular effects of rocuronium in patients receiving beta-adrenoreceptor blocking, calcium entry blocking and anticonvulsant drugs. Br J Anaesth, 78:90, 1997; RE Haas and JE Masters, Comparative recovery from three nondepolarizing neuromuscular blockers in a patient before and after chronic anticonvulsant therapy: a case report. J Am Assoc Nurse Anesth, 65:475, 1997

> *Monitor clinical status; not reported with atracurium or tubocurarine; only two cases with rocuronium (1994, 1997)*

> Possible neuromuscular blockade with vecuronium when phenytoin is first given (mechanism not established)
>> JE Baumgardner and R Bagshaw, Acute versus chronic phenytoin therapy and neuromuscular blockade. Anaesthesia, 45:493, 1990
>
> *Several case reports (1990)*

Polymyxins

> Prolonged neuromuscular blockade with pancuronium and polymyxin B (additive)
>> MM Giala and AG Paradelis, Two cases of prolonged respiratory depression due to interaction of pancuronium with colistin and streptomycin. J Antimicrob Chemother, 5:234, 1979
>
> *Monitor neuromuscular status*

Quinidine

> Prolonged neuromuscular blockade (additive)
>> JL Schmidt et al, The effect of quinidine on the action of muscle relaxants. JAMA, 183:669, 1963; WL Way et al, Recurarization with quinidine. JAMA, 200:153, 1967; JR Kambam et al, Effect of quinidine on plasma cholinesterase activity and succinylcholine neuromuscular blockade. Anesthesiology, 67:858, 1987
>
> *May require respiratory support postoperatively; use with caution*

Quinine

> Prolonged neuromuscular blockade with pancuronium (mechanism not established)
>> MH Sher and PA Mathews, Recurarization with quinine administration after reversal from anaesthesia. Anaesth Intensive Care, 11:241, 1983
>
> *Single report (1983); blockade was reversed with neostigmine and atropine, but recurarization followed IV quinine*

(continued)

NEUROMUSCULAR BLOCKING AGENTS, with: *(continued)*

Sympathomimetic bronchodilators
Prolonged neuromuscular blockade with vecuronium and IV salbutamol (mechanism not established)
> Y Salib and F Donati, Potentiation of pancuronium and vecuronium neuromuscular blockade by intravenous salbutamol. Can J Anaesth, 40:50, 1993

Single case report; patient had bronchospasm during anesthesia

Tamoxifen
Prolonged neuromuscular blockade with atracurium (mechanism not established)
> M Naguib and HK Gyasi, Antiestrogenic drugs and atracurium – a possible interaction? Can Anaesthesiol Soc J, 33:682, 1986

Monitor closely

Theophyllines
Arrhythmias with pancuronium (possibly additive effect on adrenergic cardiac mechanisms); also decreased neuromuscular blockade
> KG Belani et al, Adverse drug interaction involving pancuronium and aminophylline. Anesth Analg, 61:473, 1982; JA Daller et al, Aminophylline antagonizes the neuromuscular blockade of pancuronium but not vecuronium. Crit Care Med, 19:983, 1991

Avoid concurrent use

Thiazide diuretics
Prolonged neuromuscular blockade (hypokalemia)
> JE Goddard, Jr and OC Phillips, The influence of non-anesthetic drugs on the course of anesthesia. Penn Med J, 68:43, 1965

Monitor neuromuscular status; monitor potassium concentration and discontinue diuretic if time allows

Vancomycin
Increased succinylcholine and vecuronium effect (probably additive)
> KC Huang et al, Vancomycin enhances the neuromuscular blockade of vecuronium. Anesth Analg, 71:194, 1990; RF Albrecht, II et al, Potentiation of succinylcholine-induced phase II block by vancomycin. Anesth Analg, 77:1300, 1993

Monitor neuromuscular status; single case reports (1990, 1993)

Verapamil
Prolonged neuromuscular blockade with vecuronium, pancuronium or tubocurarine (mechanism not established)
> RM Jones et al, Verapamil potentiation of neuromuscular blockade: failure of reversal with neostigmine but prompt reversal with edrophonium. Anesth Analg, 64:1021, 1985; JF van Poorten et al, Verapamil and reversal of vecuronium neuromuscular blockade. Anesth Analg, 63:155, 1984

Two case reports (1984, 1985); reversal of one with edrophonium, neither with neostigmine

NEVIRAPINE, with:
Contraceptives, oral - See Contraceptives, oral with Nevirapine, page 215

NEVIRAPINE, with: *(continued)*
  Indinavir - See Indinavir with Nevirapine, page 308
  Lopinavir/Ritonavir - See Lopinavir/Ritonavir with Nevirapine, page 329
  Narcotics: methadone and congeners - See Narcotics: methadone and congeners with Nevirapine, page 358
  Nelfinavir - See Nelfinavir with Nevirapine, page 362
  Rifabutin
    Possible rifabutin toxicity (decreased metabolism; CYP3A)
      Manufacturer's package insert (nevirapine)
    Theoretical; manufacturer recommends avoiding concurrent use if possible
  Rifampin
    Possible decreased nevirapine effect (increased metabolism)
      P Robinson et al, Pharmacokinetic (PK) interaction between nevirapine (NVP) and rifampin (RMP). Int Conf AIDS, 12:1115, 1998, abstract 60623; GL Dean et al, Effect of tuberculosis therapy on nevirapine trough plasma concentrations. AIDS, 13:2489, 1999
    Monitor clinical status: nevirapine dose may need to be increased; some have used the combination with good results
  Ritonavir
    Possible decreased ritonavir effect (increased metabolism; CYP3A)
      Manufacturer's package insert (nevirapine)
    Combination has been used successfully with dosage adjustment
  Saquinavir
    Possible decreased protease inhibitor effect (increased metabolism)
      Manufacturer's package insert
    Combination has been used successfully with dosage adjustment
Niacin, see Nicotinic acid
NICARDIPINE, with:
  Beta-adrenergic blockers - See Beta-adrenergic blockers with Nicardipine, page 159
  Carbamazepine - See Carbamazepine with Nicardipine, page 183
  Cyclosporine - See Cyclosporine with Nicardipine, page 235
NICOTINE GUM, with:
  Adenosine - See Adenosine with Nicotine gum, page 12
  Caffeine - See Caffeine with Nicotine gum, page 174
NICOTINIC ACID, with:
  Alcohol - See Alcohol with Nicotinic acid, page 20
  Cholestyramine - See Cholestyramine with Nicotinic acid, page 197
  Colestipol - See Colestipol with Nicotinic acid, page 212
  HMG-CoA reductase inhibitors - See HMG-CoA reductase inhibitors with Nicotinic acid, page 301
NIFEDIPINE, with:
  Alcohol - See Alcohol with Nifedipine, page 20
  Angiotensin-converting enzyme (ACE) inhibitors - See Angiotensin-converting enzyme (ACE) inhibitors with Nifedipine, page 47
  Antidepressants, tricyclic - See Antidepressants, tricyclic with Nifedipine, page 88

(continued)

NIFEDIPINE, with: *(continued)*

Antifungals, imidazoles and triazoles - See Antifungals, imidazoles and triazoles with Nifedipine, page 104

Antihistamines, H$_1$-blockers: astemizole, terfenadine - See Antihistamines, H$_1$-blockers: astemizole, terfenadine with Nifedipine, page 111

Antihistamines, H$_2$-blockers - See Antihistamines, H$_2$-blockers with Nifedipine, page 121

Beta-adrenergic blockers - See Beta-adrenergic blockers with Nifedipine, page 159

Cisapride - See Cisapride with Nifedipine, page 201

Cyclosporine - See Cyclosporine with Nifedipine, page 235

Digoxin - See Digoxin with Nifedipine, page 254

Diltiazem - See Diltiazem with Nifedipine, page 261

Magnesium sulfate - See Magnesium sulfate with Nifedipine, page 335

Narcotics: meperidine and congeners - See Narcotics: meperidine and congeners with Nifedipine, page 356

Nonsteroidal anti-inflammatory drugs

Possible decreased antihypertensive effect with indomethacin (mechanism not established)

UM Thatte et al, Acute drug interaction between indomethacin and nifedipine in hypertensive patients. J Assoc Physicians India, 36:695, 1988

Clinical significance not established; monitor blood pressure

Phenytoin

Phenytoin toxicity (mechanism not established)

S Ahmad, Nifedipine-phenytoin interaction. J Am Coll Cardiol, 3:1582, 1984

Single case report (1984)

Prazosin

Severe hypotension (mechanism not established)

LD Jee and LH Opie, Acute hypotensive response to nifedipine added to prazosin in treatment of hypertension. Br Med J, 287:1574, 1983

Avoid concurrent use

Quinidine

Decreased quinidine effect (mechanism not established)

MA Munger et al, Elucidation of the nifedipine-quinidine interaction. Clin Pharmacol Ther, 45:411, 1989

Appears to be relatively rare; study in healthy subjects failed to confirm

Possible nifedipine toxicity (decreased metabolism)

SK Bowles et al, Evaluation of the pharmacokinetic and pharmacodynamic interaction between quinidine and nifedipine. J Clin Pharmacol, 33:727, 1993

Based on study in healthy subjects; monitor quinidine and nifedipine concentrations

Quinupristin/dalfopristin

Possible nifedipine toxicity (decreased metabolism; CYP3A4)

Manufacturer's package insert (quinupriston/dalfopristin)

NIFEDIPINE, with: *(continued)*
Based on study in healthy volunteers; monitor clinical status

Rifampin

Decreased antihypertensive effect of nifedipine (probably increased metabolism)

> Y Tada et al, Case report: Nifedipine-rifampicin interaction attenuates the effect on blood pressure in a patient with essential hypertension. Am J Med Sci, 303:25, 1992; H Yoshimoto et al, Influence of rifampicin on antihypertensive effects of dihydropiridine calcium-channel blockers in four elderly patients. Jpn J Geriat, 33:692, 1996

Reports of several cases; monitor clinical response

Selective serotonin reuptake inhibitors (SSRIs)

Nifedipine toxicity with fluoxetine (probably decreased metabolism)

> H Sternbach, Fluoxetine-associated potentiation of calcium-channel blockers. J Clin Psychopharmacol, 11:390, 1991; TLT Azaz-Livshits and HD Danenberg, Tachycardia, orthostatic hypotension and profound weakness due to concomitant use of fluoxetine and nifedipine. Pharmacopsychiatry, 30:274, 1997

Two case reports (1991, 1997)

Tacrolimus

Reduced dosage requirements for tacrolimus (probably decreased metabolism)

> RA Seifeldin et al, Nifedipine interaction with tacrolimus in liver transplant recipients. Ann Pharmacother, 31:571, 1997

Based on study in liver transplant recipients; monitor tacrolimus concentrations

Theophyllines

Possible theophylline toxicity (possibly decreased metabolism)

> SHD Jackson et al, The interaction between i.v. theophylline and chronic oral dosing with slow release nifedipine in volunteers. Br J Clin Pharmacol, 21:389, 1986; SR Smith et al, The influence of nifedipine and diltiazem on serum theophylline concentration-time profiles. J Clin Pharm Ther, 14:403, 1989

Questionable clinical significance at usual doses

Vincristine

Possible vincristine toxicity (decreased metabolism)

> L Fedeli et al, Pharmacokinetics of vincristine in cancer patients treated with nifedipine. Cancer, 64:1805, 1989

Monitor clinical status

NIMODIPINE, with:

Grapefruit juice - See Grapefruit juice with Nimodipine, page 290

NISOLDIPINE, with:

Antifungals, imidazoles and triazoles - See Antifungals, imidazoles and triazoles with Nisoldipine, page 104

Antihistamines, H_2-blockers - See Antihistamines, H_2-blockers with Nisoldipine, page 121

(continued)

NISOLDIPINE, with: *(continued)*

Beta-adrenergic blockers - See Beta-adrenergic blockers with Nisoldipine, page 159

Grapefruit juice - See Grapefruit juice with Nisoldipine, page 291

Phenytoin

Possible decreased nisoldipine effect (probably decreased metabolism)

R Michelucci et al, Reduced plasma nisoldipine concentrations in phenytoin-treated patients with epilepsy. Epilepsia, 37:1107, 1996

Monitor clinical status; other calcium-channel blockers may be similarly affected

Rifampin

Decreased antihypertensive effect of nisoldipine (possibly increased metabolism)

Y Tada et al, Case report: Nifedipine-rifampicin interaction attenuates the effect on blood pressure in a patient with essential hypertension. Am J Med Sci, 303:25, 1992 [nisoldipine also studied]

Single case report (1991)

NITRATES, with:

Alcohol - See Alcohol with Nitrates, page 20

Antidepressants, tricyclic - See Antidepressants, tricyclic with Nitrates, page 88

Diazoxide - See Diazoxide with Nitrates, page 246

Digoxin - See Digoxin with Nitrates, page 255

Diltiazem - See Diltiazem with Nitrates, page 261

Disopyramide - See Disopyramide with Nitrates, page 263

Heparins - See Heparins with Nitrates, page 298

Sildenafil

Hypotension (probably additive)

Manufacturer's package insert; DJ Webb et al, Sildenafil citrate and blood-pressure-lowering drugs: results of drug interaction studies with an organic nitrate and a calcium antagonist. Am J Cardiol, 83:21C, 1999; MD Cheitlin et al, Use of sildenafil (Viagra) in patients with cardiovascular disease. Circulation, 99:168, 1999; RA Kloner et al, Cardiovascular effects of sildenafil citrate and recommendations for its use. Am J Cardiol, 84:11N, 1999; RR Arora et al, Acute myocardial infarction after the use of sildenafil. N Engl J Med, 341:700, 1999; M O'Rourke and J Xiong-Jing, Sildenafil/nitrate interaction. Circulation, 101:E90, 2000; DJ Webb et al, Sildenafil citrate potentiates the hypotensive effects of nitric oxide donor drugs in male patients with stable angina. J Am Coll Cardiol, 36:25, 2000

Deaths have been reported; avoid concurrent use

Nitrazepam, see Benzodiazepines

NITRENDIPINE, with:

Digoxin - See Digoxin with Nitrendipine, page 255

NITROFURANTOIN, with:

Antacids - See Antacids with Nitrofurantoin, page 54

Nitrofurazone, no documented interactions, see page 4, Criteria for Listing Interactions

Nitroglycerin, see Nitrates

Nitroprusside, see Nitrates
NITROUS OXIDE, with:
  Angiotensin-converting enzyme (ACE) inhibitors - See Angiotensin-converting enzyme (ACE) inhibitors with Nitrous oxide, page 47
  Reserpine
    Hypotension (additive)
      CS Coakley et al, Circulatory responses during anesthesia of patients on rauwolfia therapy. JAMA, 161:1143, 1958; RL Katz et al, Anesthesia, surgery and rauwolfia. Anesthesiology, 25:142, 1964
    Monitor blood pressure
Nizatidine, see Antihistamines, H$_2$-blockers
Nonoxynol-9, no documented interactions, see page 4, Criteria for Listing Interactions
NONSTEROIDAL ANTI-INFLAMMATORY DRUGS, with:
  Alcohol - See Alcohol with Nonsteroidal anti-inflammatory drugs, page 21
  Alkylating agents - See Alkylating agents with Nonsteroidal anti-inflammatory drugs, page 24
  Aminoglycoside antibiotics - See Aminoglycoside antibiotics with Nonsteroidal anti-inflammatory drugs, page 32
  Angiotensin-converting enzyme (ACE) inhibitors - See Angiotensin-converting enzyme (ACE) inhibitors with Nonsteroidal anti-inflammatory drugs, page 47
  Antacids - See Antacids with Nonsteroidal anti-inflammatory drugs, page 54
  Anticoagulants, oral - See Anticoagulants, oral with Nonsteroidal anti-inflammatory drugs, page 72
  Antidepressants, tricyclic - See Antidepressants, tricyclic with Nonsteroidal anti-inflammatory drugs, page 88
  Antifungals, Griseofulvin - See Antifungals, Griseofulvin with Nonsteroidal anti-inflammatory drugs, page 95
  Antihistamines, H$_2$-blockers - See Antihistamines, H$_2$-blockers with Nonsteroidal anti-inflammatory drugs, page 121
  Barbiturates - See Barbiturates with Nonsteroidal anti-inflammatory drugs, page 135
  Benzodiazepines - See Benzodiazepines with Nonsteroidal anti-inflammatory drugs, page 146
  Beta-adrenergic blockers - See Beta-adrenergic blockers with Nonsteroidal anti-inflammatory drugs, page 159
  Bumetanide - See Bumetanide with Nonsteroidal anti-inflammatory drugs, page 168
  Carbonic anhydrase inhibitors - See Carbonic anhydrase inhibitors with Nonsteroidal anti-inflammatory drugs, page 189
  Cephalosporins - See Cephalosporins with Nonsteroidal anti-inflammatory drugs, page 191
  Cholestyramine - See Cholestyramine with Nonsteroidal anti-inflammatory drugs, page 197
  Clopidogrel - See Clopidogrel with Nonsteroidal anti-inflammatory drugs, page 205

(continued)

NONSTEROIDAL ANTI-INFLAMMATORY DRUGS, with: *(continued)*
- **Cocaine** - See Cocaine with Nonsteroidal anti-inflammatory drugs, page 210
- **Colestipol** - See Colestipol with Nonsteroidal anti-inflammatory drugs, page 212
- **Corticosteroids** - See Corticosteroids with Nonsteroidal anti-inflammatory drugs, page 222
- **COX-2 inhibitors** - See COX-2 inhibitors with Nonsteroidal anti-inflammatory drugs, page 225
- **Cyclosporine** - See Cyclosporine with Nonsteroidal anti-inflammatory drugs, page 235
- **Diazoxide** - See Diazoxide with Nonsteroidal anti-inflammatory drugs, page 246
- **Digoxin** - See Digoxin with Nonsteroidal anti-inflammatory drugs, page 255
- **Dimethyl sulfoxide** - See Dimethyl sulfoxide with Nonsteroidal anti-inflammatory drugs, page 262
- **Dipyridamole** - See Dipyridamole with Nonsteroidal anti-inflammatory drugs, page 262
- **Furosemide** - See Furosemide with Nonsteroidal anti-inflammatory drugs, page 286
- **Gold sodium thiomalate** - See Gold sodium thiomalate with Nonsteroidal anti-inflammatory drugs, page 290
- **Haloperidol** - See Haloperidol with Nonsteroidal anti-inflammatory drugs, page 295
- **Heparins** - See Heparins with Nonsteroidal anti-inflammatory drugs, page 299
- **HMG-CoA reductase inhibitors** - See HMG-CoA reductase inhibitors with Nonsteroidal anti-inflammatory drugs, page 301
- **Hydralazine** - See Hydralazine with Nonsteroidal anti-inflammatory drugs, page 302
- **Hypoglycemics, sulfonylurea** - See Hypoglycemics, sulfonylurea with Nonsteroidal anti-inflammatory drugs, page 304
- **Insulin** - See Insulin with Nonsteroidal anti-inflammatory drugs, page 310
- **Lithium** - See Lithium with Nonsteroidal anti-inflammatory drugs, page 324
- **Losartan** - See Losartan with Nonsteroidal anti-inflammatory drugs, page 330
- **Metformin** - See Metformin with Nonsteroidal anti-inflammatory drugs, page 338
- **Methotrexate** - See Methotrexate with Nonsteroidal anti-inflammatory drugs, page 339
- **Misoprostol** - See Misoprostol with Nonsteroidal anti-inflammatory drugs, page 347
- **Nifedipine** - See Nifedipine with Nonsteroidal anti-inflammatory drugs, page 368
- **Omeprazole**

Possible salicylate toxicity (disruption of enteric coating due to increased gastric pH)

FZ Nefesoglu et al, Interaction of omeprazole with enteric-coated salicylate tablets. Int J Clin Pharmacol Ther, 36:549, 1998; P Iñarrea et al, Omeprazole does not interfere with the antiplatelet effect of low-dose aspirin in man. Scand J Gastroenterol, 35:242, 2000

Based on study in healthy subjects; omeprazole does not appear to interfere with the antiplatelet effect of aspirin

NONSTEROIDAL ANTI-INFLAMMATORY DRUGS, with: *(continued)*

Penicillamine
Possible penicillamine toxicity with indomethacin (mechanism not established)
> P Seideman and B Lindström, Pharmacokinetic interactions of penicillamine in rheumatoid arthritis. J Rheumatol, 16:473, 1989

Monitor penicillamine concentration

Pentosan
Increased bleeding risk (additive)
> Manufacturer's package insert

Avoid concurrent use

Phenytoin
Possible decreased bromfenac effect (probably increased metabolism)
> K Gumbhir-Shah et al, Evaluation of pharmacokinetic interaction between bromfenac and phenytoin in healthy males. J Clin Pharmacol, 37:160, 1997

Monitor analgesia

Potassium
Hyperkalemia with indomethacin (inhibition of renal prostaglandin synthesis)
> F Akbarpour et al, Severe hyperkalemia caused by indomethacin and potassium supplementation. South Med J, 78:756, 1985; JW Findling et al, Indomethacin-induced hyperkalemia in three patients with gouty arthritis. JAMA 244:1127, 1980; MG Nicholls and EA Espiner, Indomethacin induced azotemia and hyperkalaemia: a case study. N Z Med J, 94:377, 1981; DE Meier et al, Indomethacin associated hyperkalemia in the elderly, J Am Geriatr Soc, 31:371, 1983

Has occurred with indomethacin alone; avoid concurrent use, if possible; monitor potassium concentration

Prazosin
Decreased hypotensive effect with indomethacin (possibly decreased adrenergic receptor activity)
> P Rubin et al, Studies on the clinical pharmacology of prazosin. II The influence of indomethacin and of propranolol on the action and disposition of prazosin. Br J Clin Pharmacol, 10:33, 1980

Occurs only in some patients, who may need increased prazosin dosage

Probenecid
Possible NSAIDs toxicity (decreased renal excretion)
> ES Waller, The effect of probenecid on the disposition of meclofenamate sodium. Drug Intell Clin Pharm, 17:453, 1983; United States Pharmacopeial Convention, *Drug Information for the Health Care Provider* (USP DI), vol I, 18th ed., Rockville, MD:Authors, 1998, p 385; R Runkel et al, Naproxen-probenecid interaction. Clin Pharmacol Ther, 24:706, 1978; RA Upton et al, Effects of probenecid on ketoprofen kinetics. Clin Pharmacol Ther, 3:705, 1982; H Sinclair and T Gibson, Interaction between probenecid and indomethacin. Br J Rheumatol, 25:316, 1986; EJ Mroszczak et al, The effect of probenecid (P) on ketorolac (K) pharmacokinetics after oral dosing of ketorolac tromethamine (KT). Clin Pharmacol Ther, 51:154, 1992 abs PII-34

Monitor clinical status

(continued)

NONSTEROIDAL ANTI-INFLAMMATORY DRUGS, with: *(continued)*
  Decreased uricosuric effect of probenecid with salicylates (mechanism not established)
    JE Seegmiller and Al Grayzel, Use of the newer uricosuric agents in the management of gout. JAMA, 173:1076, 1960; AB Gutman and TF Yu, Benemid (p-di-n-propylsulfamyl)-benzoic acid) as uricosuric agent in chronic gouty arthritis. Trans Assoc Am Physicians, 64:279, 1951
  Avoid salicylates except in occasional small doses

Quinidine
  Bleeding with aspirin (additive antiplatelet effect)
    D Lawson et al, Cumulative effects of quinidine and aspirin on bleeding time and platelet alpha$_2$-adrenoceptors: potential mechanism of bleeding diathesis in patients receiving this combination. J Lab Clin Med, 108:581, 1986
  Avoid concurrent use

Ritonavir
  Possible piroxicam toxicity (decreased metabolism)
    Manufacturer's package insert (ritonavir)
  Theoretical; listed as contraindicated in product information

Salicylates, topical
  Possible salicylate toxicity from topical use (mechanism not established)
    DL Shupp and AL Schroeter, An unusual case of salicylate toxicity. J Am Acad Dermatol, 15:300, 1986
  Monitor salicylate concentration

Spironolactone
  Decreased diuretic effect with indomethacin (inhibition of renal prostaglandin synthesis)
    HJ Kramer et al, Interaction of conventional and antikaliuretic diuretics with the renal prostaglandin system. Clin Sci, 59:67, 1980
  Avoid concurrent use, if possible

  Decreased diuretic effect with aspirin (interference with renal tubular excretion of spironolactone metabolite)
    MG Tweeddale and RI Ogilvie, Antagonism of spironolactone-induced natriuresis by aspirin in man. N Engl J Med, 289:198, 1973
  Clinical significance not established

Sucralfate
  Decreased diclofenac effect (probably decreased absorption)
    J Pedrazzoli Júnior et al, Short-term sucralfate administration alters potassium diclofenac absorption in healthy male volunteers. Br J Clin Pharmacol, 43:104, 1997
  Based on study in healthy subjects; give diclofenac 2 hours before or 6 hours after sucralfate

Sulfinpyrazone
  Decreased uricosuric effect with salicylates (mechanism not established)
    TF Yu et al, Mutual suppression of the uricosuric effects of sulfinpyrazone and salicylate: a study in interactions between drugs. J Clin Invest,

NONSTEROIDAL ANTI-INFLAMMATORY DRUGS, with: *(continued)*
42:1330, 1963
Avoid salicylates except in occasional small doses

Thiazide diuretics

Decrease in diuretic and antihypertensive effects (inhibition of renal prostaglandin synthesis); hyponatremia (additive decrease in free water excretion)

E Steiness and S Waldorff, Different interactions of indomethacin and sulindac with thiazides in hypertension. Br Med J, 285:1702, 1982; PP Koopmans et al, Influence of non-steroidal anti-inflammatory drugs on diuretic treatment of mild to moderate essential hypertension. Br Med J, 289:1492, 1984; PP Koopmans et al, The effects of sulindac and indomethacin on the antihypertensive and diuretic action of hydrochlorothiazide in patients with mild to moderate essential hypertension. Br J Clin Pharmacol, 21:417, 1986; JJ Dixey et al, The effects of naproxen and sulindac on renal function and their interaction with hydrochlorothiazide and piretanide in man. Br J Clin Pharmacol, 23:55, 1987; JT Wright, Jr et al, The effect of high-dose short-term ibuprofen on antihypertensive control with hydrochlorothiazide. Clin Pharmacol Ther, 46:440, 1989; D Klassen et al, Assessment of blood pressure during treatment with naproxen or ibuprofen in hypertensive patients treated with hydrochlorothiazide. J Clin Pharmacol, 33:971, 1993; DM Clive and JS Stoff, Renal syndromes associated with nonsteroidal antiinflammatory drugs. N Engl J Med, 310:563, 1984 (p 568); GK Goodenough and LJ Lutz, Hyponatremic hypervolemia caused by a drug – drug interaction mistaken for syndrome of inappropriate ADH. J Am Geriatr Soc, 36:285, 1988; EBD Ripley et al, The effect of nonsteroidal agents (NDAIDs) on the pharmacokinetics and pharmacodynamics of metolazone. Int J Clin Pharmacol Ther, 32:12, 1994; J Matte and B Martineau, Hypertensive crisis a case report. Can Pharm J, 122:545, 1989; ER Heerdink et al, NSAIDs associated with increased risk of congestive heart failure in elderly patients taking diuretics. Arch Intern Med, 158:1108, 1998

Monitor blood pressure, diuretic effect, and sodium concentration; effect on blood pressure usually small and may be delayed for several weeks; single case report of hypertensive crises with naproxen and hydrochlorothiazide (1989); exacerbation of CHF, due to decreased diuretic effect, especially during first month of NSAID therapy

Thrombolytics

Possible increase in risk of cerebral hemorrhage with aspirin (additive)

A Ciccone et al, Negative interaction of aspirin and streptokinase in acute ischemic stroke: further analysis of the Multicenter Acute Stroke Trial-Italy. Cerebrovasc Dis, 10:61, 2000

Avoid aspirin during streptokinase treatment of acute ischemic stroke

Tiludronate

Possible tiludronate toxicity with indomethacin (mechanism not established)

Manufacturer's package insert

Tiludronate bioavailability increased 2-4 fold; diclofenac may not interact

(continued)

NONSTEROIDAL ANTI-INFLAMMATORY DRUGS, with: *(continued)*
　Possible decreased tiludronate effect (mechanism not established)
　　Manufacturer's package insert
　Clinical significance not established

Tirofiban
　Increased bleeding with aspirin (additive)
　　Manufacturer's package insert
　Monitor prothrombin time

Triamterene
　Renal failure and triamterene toxicity with indomethacin or diclofenac (inhibition of prostaglandin synthesis)
　　L Favre et al, Reversible acute renal failure from combined triamterene and indomethacin. Ann Intern Med, 96:317, 1982; MS Weinberg et al, Anuric renal failure precipitated by indomethacin and triamterene. Nephron, 40:216, 1985; M Härkönen and S Ekblom-Kullberg, Reversible deterioration of renal function after diclofenac in patient receiving triamterene. Br Med J, 293:698, 1986
　Avoid concurrent use, if possible

Valproate
　Possible valproate toxicity with salicylates (displacement from binding and possibly decreased metabolism)
　　K Farrell et al, The effect of acetylsalicylic acid on serum free valproate concentrations and valproate clearance in children. J Pediatr, 101:142, 1982; JM Orr et al, Interaction between valproic acid and aspirin in epileptic children: serum protein binding and metabolic effects. Clin Pharmacol Ther, 31:642, 1982; KJ Goulden et al, Clinical valproate toxicity induced by acetylsalicylic acid. Neurology, 37:1392, 1987
　Use alternative analgesic or antipyretic drugs

　Possible decrease in valproate serum concentrations with ibuprofen (possibly displacement from binding)
　　KP Mankin and M Scanlon, Side effect of ibuprofen and valproic acid. Orthopedics, 21:264, 1998
　Single case report (1998); clinical significance not established

Vancomycin
　Possible vancomycin toxicity in neonates with indomethacin (probably decreased renal clearance)
　　JM Spivey and P Gal, SH Naqvi et al, Vancomycin pharmacokinetics in neonates. Am J Dis Child, 140:859, 1986
　Monitor vancomycin concentration

Verapamil
　Possible decreased verapamil effect with diclofenac (increased metabolism)
　　C Peterson et al, Differential effects of naproxen and diclofenac on verapamil pharmacokinetics. Clin Pharmacol Ther, 49:129, 1991 abs PI-25; MC Houston et al, The effects of nonsteroidal anti-inflammatory drugs on blood pressures of patients with hypertension controlled by verapamil. Arch Intern Med, 155:1049, 1995

NONSTEROIDAL ANTI-INFLAMMATORY DRUGS, with: *(continued)*
Based on a study in hypertensive volunteers; did not occur with naproxen or ibuprofen

Increased bruising or petechiae with aspirin (antiplatelet effect)
ME Ring et al, Clinically significant antiplatelet effects of calcium-channel blockers. J Clin Pharmacol, 26:719, 1986; E Verzino et al, Verapamil-aspirin interaction. Ann Pharmacother, 28:536, 1994
Three case reports (1986, 1994)

Zafirlukast
Possible zafirlukast toxicity with aspirin (decreased metabolism CYP3A1)
Manufacturer's package insert
Avoid concurrent use if zafirlukast concentration can not be monitored

Zidovudine
Possible bleeding in hemophiliacs with ibuprofen or possibly other non-steroidal anti-inflammatory drugs (mechanism not established)
MV Ragni et al, Bleeding tendency, platelet function, and pharmacokinetics of ibuprofen and zidovudine in HIV(+) hemophilic men. Am J Hematol, 40:176, 1992
Monitor clinical status

Norepinephrine, see Sympathomimetic amines
Norethindrone, see Contraceptives, oral; Progestins
Norethynodrel, see Progestins
Norfloxacin, see Fluoroquinolones
Norgestimate, see Contraceptives, oral; Progestins
Norgestrel, see Progestins
Nortriptyline, see Antidepressants, tricyclic

NUTRIENTS, ENTERAL PREPARATIONS, with:
Antacids - See Antacids with Nutrients, enteral preparations, page 55
Anticoagulants, oral - See Anticoagulants, oral with Nutrients, enteral preparations, page 73

Phenytoin
Decreased phenytoin effect (decreased absorption)
JJ Saklad et al, Interaction of oral phenytoin with enteral feedings. JPEN J Parenter Enteral Nutr, 10:322, 1986; LY Nishimura et al, Influence of enteral feedings on phenytoin sodium absorption from capsules. Drug Intell Clin Pharm, 22:130, 1988; KA Krueger et al, Effect of two administration schedules of an enteral nutrient formula on phenytoin bioavailability. Epilepsia, 28:706, 1987; J Weinryb and R Cogen, Interaction of nasogastric phenytoin and enteral feeding solution. JAGS, 37:195, 1989; KM Olsen et al, Effect of enteral feedings on oral phenytoin absorption. Nutr Clin Pract, 4:176, 1989
Give 2 hours apart, if possible; monitor phenytoin concentration; single-dose studies of phenytoin after Ensure showed no interaction

Theophyllines
Decreased theophylline effect (mechanism not established)
RC Ziegenbein, Theophylline clearance increase from increased amino acid

(continued)

NUTRIENTS, ENTERAL PREPARATIONS, with: *(continued)*
>in a CPN regimen. Drug Intell Clin Pharm, 21:220, 1987; VO Bhargava et al, Effect of an enteral nutrient formula on sustained-release theophylline absorption. Ther Drug Monit, 11:515, 1989; PM Plezia et al, The influence of enteral feedings on sustained-release theophylline absorption. Pharmacotherapy, 10:356, 1990

Single case report (1987); amino acid concentration in enteral feeding was high and carbohydrate low; sustained-release theophylline showed no interaction with Ensure

NUTRIENTS, LIQUID CONCENTRATES, with:

Phenytoin

Decreased phenytoin suspension effect with *Fresubin* food concentrate (probably decreased absorption)
>DM Taylor et al, Lowered serum phenytoin concentrations during therapy with liquid food concentrates. Ann Pharmacother, 27:369, 1993

Single case report (1993); monitor phenytoin concentration

NUTRIENTS, PARENTERAL, with:

Phenytoin

Decreased IV phenytoin effect (mechanism not established)
>FM Messahel et al, Does total parenteral nutrition lower serum phenytoin levels? A case report. Curr Ther Res, 47:1017, 1990

Single case report (1990)

Nystatin, no documented interactions, see page 4, Criteria for Listing Interactions

OAT BRAN, with:

HMG-CoA reductase inhibitors - See HMG-CoA reductase inhibitors with Oat bran, page 301

OCTREOTIDE, with:

Narcotics: morphine-like - See Narcotics: morphine-like with Octreotide, page 360

Ofloxacin, see Fluoroquinolones

Oil of wintergreen, see Salicylates, topical

OKT3, see Muromonab-CD3

OLANZAPINE, with:

Alcohol - See Alcohol with Olanzapine, page 21

Antidepressants, tricyclic - See Antidepressants, tricyclic with Olanzapine, page 88

Benzodiazepines - See Benzodiazepines with Olanzapine, page 146

Carbamazepine - See Carbamazepine with Olanzapine, page 183

Fluoroquinolones - See Fluoroquinolones with Olanzapine, page 280

Haloperidol - See Haloperidol with Olanzapine, page 295

Olopatadine, no documented interactions, see page 4, Criteria for Listing Interactions

Olsalazine, no documented interactions, see page 4, Criteria for Listing Interactions

OMEPRAZOLE, with:

Anticoagulants, oral - See Anticoagulants, oral with Omeprazole, page 74

Antifungals, imidazoles and triazoles - See Antifungals, imidazoles and triazoles with Omeprazole, page 104

OMEPRAZOLE, with: *(continued)*
- **Artemisinin** - See Artemisinin with Omeprazole, page 128
- **Benzodiazepines** - See Benzodiazepines with Omeprazole, page 146
- **Carbamazepine** - See Carbamazepine with Omeprazole, page 183
- **Cilostazol** - See Cilostazol with Omeprazole, page 199
- **Corticosteroids** - See Corticosteroids with Omeprazole, page 222
- **Cyclosporine** - See Cyclosporine with Omeprazole, page 236
- **Digoxin** - See Digoxin with Omeprazole, page 255
- **Disulfiram** - See Disulfiram with Omeprazole, page 264
- **Methotrexate** - See Methotrexate with Omeprazole, page 340
- **Nonsteroidal anti-inflammatory drugs** - See Nonsteroidal anti-inflammatory drugs with Omeprazole, page 372
- **Phenytoin**

    Possible oral or IV phenytoin toxicity (decreased metabolism)

    R Gugler and JC Jensen, Omeprazole inhibits oxidative drug metabolism; studies with diazepam and phenytoin in vivo and 7-ethoxycoumarin in vitro. Gastroenterology, 89:1235, 1985; PJ Prichard et al, Oral phenytoin pharmacokinetics during omeprazole therapy. Br J Clin Pharmacol, 24:543, 1987; T Andersson et al, A study of the interaction between omeprazole and phenytoin in epileptic patients. Ther Drug Monit, 12:329, 1990; MV Middle et al, No influence of pantoprazole on the pharmacokinetics of phenytoin. Int J Clin Pharmacol Ther, 33:304, 1995

    Monitor phenytoin concentration; based on studies in healthy men; negative study in 5 patients taking oral phenytoin; may be dose-dependent; pantoprazole does not appear to affect phenytoin

- **Proguanil**

    Possible decreased proguanil effect (decreased formation of active metabolite of proguanil)

    C Funck-Brentano et al, Inhibition by omeprazole of proguanil metabolism: mechanism of the interaction *in vitro* and prediction of *in vivo* results from the *in vitro* experiments. J Pharmacol Exper Ther, 280:730, 1997

    Avoid concurrent use if possible; clinical significance remains to be established

ONDANSETRON, with:
- **Alkylating Agents** - See Alkylating Agents with Ondansetron, page 24
- **Cisplatin** - See Cisplatin with Ondansetron, page 202
- **Rifampin**

    Decreased ondansetron effect (increased metabolism; CYP3A4)

    K Villikka et al, The effect of rifampin on the pharmacokinetics of oral and intravenous ondansetron. Clin Pharmacol Ther, 65:377, 1999

    Based on study in healthy subjects; effect seen with both oral and intravenous ondansetron; monitor clinical status

Opium alkaloids, see Narcotics: morphine-like
Oral contraceptives, see Contraceptives, oral
Orciprenaline, see Sympathomimetic amines
ORLISTAT, with:
- **Cyclosporine** - See Cyclosporine with Orlistat, page 236

ORPHENADRINE, with:
    Levodopa - See Levodopa with Orphenadrine, page 320

Oseltamivir, no documented interactions, see page 4, Criteria for Listing Interactions

Oxacillin, see Penicillins

OXALIPLATIN, with:
    Irinotecan - See Irinotecan with Oxaliplatin, page 311

Oxandrolone, see Anabolic and androgenic steroids

Oxaprozin, see Nonsteroidal anti-inflammatory drugs

Oxazepam, see Benzodiazepines

OXCARBAZEPINE, with:
    Barbiturates - See Barbiturates with Oxcarbazepine, page 135
    Carbamazepine - See Carbamazepine with Oxcarbazepine, page 183
    Contraceptives, oral - See Contraceptives, oral with Oxcarbazepine, page 215
    Felodipine - See Felodipine with Oxcarbazepine, page 276
    Lamotrigine - See Lamotrigine with Oxcarbazepine, page 316
    Phenytoin

        Possible decreased oxcarbazepine effect (increased metabolism)
            Manufacturer's package insert (oxcarbazepine)

        Active metabolite decreased 30%; monitor clinical status and serum concentration

        Possible phenytoin toxicity with oxcarbazepine doses of 1200/day or more (decreased metabolism)
            Manufacturer's package insert (oxcarbazepine)

        Monitor phenytoin concentration especially when oxcarbazepine dosage is ≥1200 mg/day

    Verapamil

        Decreased oxcarbazepine effect (possible increased metabolism of active metabolite (MHD); CYP450)
            Manufacturer's package insert (oxcarbazepine)

        Plasma concentrations of MHD decreased 20%; monitor MHD concentration

Oxprenolol, see Beta-adrenergic blockers

Oxtriphylline, see Theophyllines

OXYBUTYNIN, with:
    Antidepressants, tricyclic - See Antidepressants, tricyclic with Oxybutynin, page 88

Oxycodone, see Narcotics: morphine-like

OXYGEN, with:
    Bleomycin - See Bleomycin with Oxygen, page 166

Oxymetholone, see Anabolic and androgenic steroids

Oxymorphone, see Narcotics: morphine-like

Oxytetracycline, see Tetracyclines

PACLITAXEL, with:
    Antifungals, imidazoles and triazoles - See Antifungals, imidazoles and triazoles with Paclitaxel, page 105

PACLITAXEL, with: *(continued)*
   Cisplatin - See Cisplatin with Paclitaxel, page 202
   Corticosteroids - See Corticosteroids with Paclitaxel, page 222
   Delavirdine - See Delavirdine with Paclitaxel, page 245
   Saquinavir
      Possible paclitaxel toxicity (probably decreased metabolism; CYP3A4)
         JD Schwartz et al, Potential interaction of antiretroviral therapy with paclitaxel in patients with AIDS-related Kaposi's sarcoma. AIDS, 13:283, 1999
      Two case reports (1999); patients also received delavirdine and fluconazole
   Trastuzumab
      Possible trastuzumab toxicity; increased serum concentration (mechanism not established)
         Manufacturer's package insert (trastuzumab)
      Based on studies in patients; clinical significance not established

Palivizumab, no documented interactions, see page 4, Criteria for Listing Interactions

Pamidronate, no documented interactions, see page 4, Criteria for Listing Interactions

Pancuronium, see Neuromuscular blocking agents

PANIPENEM-BETAMIPRON, with:
   Valproate
      Decreased valproate effect (mechanism not established)
         T Yamagata et al, Panipenem-betamipron and decreases in serum valproic acid concentration. Ther Drug Monit, 20:396, 1998
      Based on a study in three patients (1998); two developed seizures; avoid concurrent use

Pantoprazole, no documented interactions, see page 4, Criteria for Listing Interactions

PAPAVERINE, with:
   Benzodiazepines - See Benzodiazepines with Papaverine, page 147
   Levodopa - See Levodopa with Papaverine, page 320

Para-aminosalicylic acid, see Aminosalicylic acid

Paramethasone, see Corticosteroids

Paregoric, see Narcotics: morphine-like

Parenteral nutrition, see Nutrients, parenteral

Pargyline, see Monoamine oxidase inhibitors

Paromomycin, no documented interactions, see page 4, Criteria for Listing Interactions

Paroxetine, see Selective serotonin reuptake inhibitors (SSRIs)

PAS, see Aminosalicylic acid

PECTIN, with:
   HMG-CoA reductase inhibitors - See HMG-CoA reductase inhibitors with Pectin, page 301

Pefloxacin, see Fluoroquinolones

Pegaspargase, no documented interactions, see page 4, Criteria for Listing Interactions

Pemirolast, no documented interactions, see page 4, Criteria for Listing Interactions
Pemoline, no documented interactions, see page 4, Criteria for Listing Interactions
Penbutolol, see Beta-adrenergic blockers
Penciclovir, no documented interactions, see page 4, Criteria for Listing Interactions

PENICILLAMINE, with:
  Antacids - See Antacids with Penicillamine, page 55
  Chloroquine - See Chloroquine with Penicillamine, page 194
  Contraceptives, oral - See Contraceptives, oral with Penicillamine, page 215
  Digoxin - See Digoxin with Penicillamine, page 255
  Iron - See Iron with Penicillamine, page 312
  Nonsteroidal anti-inflammatory drugs - See Nonsteroidal anti-inflammatory drugs with Penicillamine, page 373

PENICILLINS, with:
  Allopurinol - See Allopurinol with Penicillins, page 25
  Amiloride - See Amiloride with Penicillins, page 28
  Aminoglycoside antibiotics - See Aminoglycoside antibiotics with Penicillins, page 32
  Anticoagulants, oral - See Anticoagulants, oral with Penicillins, page 74
  Beta-adrenergic blockers - See Beta-adrenergic blockers with Penicillins, page 160
  Cephalosporins - See Cephalosporins with Penicillins, page 191
  Contraceptives, oral - See Contraceptives, oral with Penicillins, page 215
  Cyclosporine - See Cyclosporine with Penicillins, page 236
  Fluoroquinolones - See Fluoroquinolones with Penicillins, page 280
  Lithium - See Lithium with Penicillins, page 325
  Methotrexate - See Methotrexate with Penicillins, page 340
  Neuromuscular blocking agents - See Neuromuscular blocking agents with Penicillins, page 364
  Phenytoin
    Possible increased phenytoin toxicity with high-dose intravenous oxacillin (displacement from binding)
      A Dasgupta et al, Phenytoin-oxacillin interactions in normal and uremic sera. Pharmacotherapy, 17:375, 1997
    Based on single case report in hypoalbuminemic patient (1997) and in vitro study; total phenytoin levels may be misleading

Pentaerythritol tetranitrate, see Nitrates

PENTAGASTRIN, with:
  Antihistamines, H$_2$-blockers - See Antihistamines, H$_2$-blockers with Pentagastrin, page 122

PENTAMIDINE, with:
  Fluoroquinolones - See Fluoroquinolones with Pentamidine, page 280
  Foscarnet - See Foscarnet with Pentamidine, page 285

Pentazocine, see Narcotics: pentazocine
Pentobarbital, see Barbiturates

PENTOSAN, with:
  Anticoagulants, oral - See Anticoagulants, oral with Pentosan, page 74

PENTOSAN, with: *(continued)*
    Heparins - See Heparins with Pentosan, page 299
    Nonsteroidal anti-inflammatory drugs - See Nonsteroidal anti-inflammatory drugs with Pentosan, page 373
    Thrombolytics
        Increased bleeding risk (additive)
            Manufacturer's package insert
        Avoid concurrent use

Pentostatin, no documented interactions, see page 4, Criteria for Listing Interactions

PENTOXIFYLLINE, with:
    Antihistamines, H_2-blockers - See Antihistamines, H_2-blockers with Pentoxifylline, page 122
    Cephalosporins - See Cephalosporins with Pentoxifylline, page 191
    Fluoroquinolones - See Fluoroquinolones with Pentoxifylline, page 280
    Theophyllines
        Possible theophylline toxicity with sustained-release pentoxifylline (mechanism not established)
            MJ Ellison et al, Pentoxifylline-induced elevated steady-state theophylline serum concentrations from sustained-release formulations. Pharmacotherapy, 10:255, 1990; MJ Ellison et al, Influence of pentoxifylline on steady-state theophylline serum concentrations from sustained-release formulations. Pharmacotherapy, 10:383, 1990
        Variable effect in healthy subjects; monitor theophylline concentration
    Tobacco, smoking
        Possible decreased pentoxifylline effect (probably increased metabolism)
            VF Mauro et al, Comparison of pentoxifylline pharmacokinetics between smokers and nonsmokers. J Clin Pharmacol, 32:1054, 1992
        Based on a study in young healthy men; clinical significance not established

PERGOLIDE, with:
    Angiotensin-converting enzyme (ACE) inhibitors - See Angiotensin-converting enzyme (ACE) inhibitors with Pergolide, page 48
    Valproate
        Lethargy, somnolence and confusion (mechanism not established)
            R Malcolm et al, Pergolide Mesylate, Adverse events occurring in the treatment of cocaine dependence. Am J Addict, 6:117, 1997
        Single case report (1997)

Perindopril, see Angiotensin-converting enzyme (ACE) inhibitors
Permethrin, no documented interactions, see page 4, Criteria for Listing Interactions
Perphenazine, see Phenothiazines
Pethidine, see Narcotics: meperidine and congeners
PETN, see Nitrates
Phendimetrazine, see Sympathomimetic amines
Phenelzine, see Monoamine oxidase inhibitors

PHENFORMIN, with:
    Alcohol - See Alcohol with Phenformin, page 21
    Anticoagulants, oral - See Anticoagulants, oral with Phenformin, page 74
    Clofibrate - See Clofibrate with Phenformin, page 203
    Monoamine oxidase inhibitors - See Monoamine oxidase inhibitors with Phenformin, page 350
    Tetracyclines
       Lactic acidosis (possibly decreased phenformin excretion)
          A Aro et al, Phenformin-induced lactic acidosis precipitated by tetracycline. Lancet, 1:673, 1978
       Avoid concurrent use

Phenindione, see Anticoagulants, oral

Phenmetrazine, see Sympathomimetic amines

Phenobarbital, see Barbiturates

PHENOTHIAZINES, with:
    Alcohol - See Alcohol with Phenothiazines, page 21
    Amodiaquine - See Amodiaquine with Phenothiazines, page 38
    Anticholinergics - See Anticholinergics with Phenothiazines, page 59
    Antidepressants, tricyclic - See Antidepressants, tricyclic with Phenothiazines, page 88
    Antihistamines, H_2-blockers - See Antihistamines, H_2-blockers with Phenothiazines, page 122
    Barbiturates - See Barbiturates with Phenothiazines, page 135
    Beta-adrenergic blockers - See Beta-adrenergic blockers with Phenothiazines, page 160
    Bethanidine - See Bethanidine with Phenothiazines, page 165
    Bromocriptine - See Bromocriptine with Phenothiazines, page 167
    Bupropion - See Bupropion with Phenothiazines, page 169
    Cabergoline - See Cabergoline with Phenothiazines, page 172
    Carbamazepine - See Carbamazepine with Phenothiazines, page 183
    Chloroquine - See Chloroquine with Phenothiazines, page 194
    Clozapine - See Clozapine with Phenothiazines, page 207
    Debrisoquine - See Debrisoquine with Phenothiazines, page 243
    Diazoxide - See Diazoxide with Phenothiazines, page 247
    Disulfiram - See Disulfiram with Phenothiazines, page 264
    Dofetilide - See Dofetilide with Phenothiazines, page 265
    Enflurane - See Enflurane with Phenothiazines, page 269
    Fluoroquinolones - See Fluoroquinolones with Phenothiazines, page 281
    Guanadrel - See Guanadrel with Phenothiazines, page 292
    Guanethidine - See Guanethidine with Phenothiazines, page 292
    Haloperidol - See Haloperidol with Phenothiazines, page 295
    Levodopa - See Levodopa with Phenothiazines, page 320
    Lithium - See Lithium with Phenothiazines, page 325
    Metoclopramide - See Metoclopramide with Phenothiazines, page 344
    Naltrexone - See Naltrexone with Phenothiazines, page 354

PHENOTHIAZINES, with: *(continued)*
- **Narcotics: meperidine and congeners** - See Narcotics: meperidine and congeners with Phenothiazines, page 356

Phenytoin

Decreased mesoridazine or thioridazine effect (increased metabolism)
> M Linnoila et al, Effect of anticonvulsants on plasma haloperidol and thioridazine levels. Am J Psychiatry, 137:7, 1980; AW Marcoux, A phenytoin – thioridazine medication interaction. Hosp Pharm, 21:889, 1986

Avoid concurrent use

Decreased phenytoin effect with phenothiazines (mechanism not established)
> JH Siris et al, Anticonvulsant drug-serum levels in psychiatric patients with seizure disorders. NY State J Med, 74:1554, 1974

Rare

Pramipexole

Possible reduced pramipexole effect (dopamine antagonism)
> Manufacturer's package insert

Avoid concurrent use

Pyrimethamine

Possible chlorpromazine toxicity (decreased metabolism)
> ROA Makanjuola et al, Effects of antimalarial agents on plasma levels of chlorpromazine and its metabolites in schizophrenic patients. Trop Geographic Med, 40:31, 1988

Monitor chlorpromazine concentration

Quetiapine

Decreased qeutiapine effect with thioridazine (mechanism not established)
> Manufacturer's package insert

Monitor quetiapine response and increase dosage as needed

Ropinirole

Possible decrease in ropinirole effect (dopamine antagonism)
> Manufacturer's package insert

Avoid concurrent use

Selective serotonin reuptake inhibitors (SSRIs)

Dystonia, seizures with fluoxetine and fluphenazine, or paroxetine and perphenazine (possibly additive and/or decreased metabolism)
> R Ketai, Interaction between fluoxetine and neuroleptics. Am J Psychiatry, 150:836, 1993; V Özdemir et al, Paroxetine potentiates CNS side-effects of perphenazine. Clin Pharmacol Ther, 59:188, 1996

Monitor clinical status; case reports (1993); case report of seizures with levomepromazine plus fluvoxamine (1993)

Possible thioridazine toxicity with fluvoxamine, fluoxetine or paroxetine or other CYP2D6 inhbitors (probably decreased metabolism)
> JA Carrillo et al, Pharmacokinetic interaction of fluvoxamine and thioridazine in schizophrenic patients. J Clin Psychopharmacol, 19:494, 1999; Manufacturer's package insert (thioridazine)

(continued)

PHENOTHIAZINES, with: *(continued)*
> *Based on sudy in schizophrenic patients; concurrent use with fluvoxamine, fluoxetine, paroxetine or other known CYP2D6 inhibitors is contraindicated*

Trazodone
> Hypotension (additive)
>> K Asayesh, Combination of trazodone and phenothiazines: a possible additive hypotensive effect. Can J Psychiatry, 31:857, 1986
>
> *Monitor blood pressure*

Valproate
> Possible valproate toxicity with chlorpromazine (decreased metabolism)
>> T Ishizaki et al, The effects of neuroleptics (haloperidol and chlorpromazine) on the pharmacokinetics of valproic acid in schizophrenic patients. J Clin Psychopharmacol, 4:254, 1984
>
> *Clinical significance not established; monitor valproate concentration*
>
> Severe hepatotoxicity with chlorpromazine (synergism)
>> N Bach et al, Exaggerated cholestasis and hepatic fibrosis following simultaneous administration of chlorpromazine and sodium valproate. Dig Dis Sci, 34:1303, 1989
>
> *Single case report (1989)*

Venlafaxine
> Possible neurotoxicity (mechanism not established)
>> SR Nimmagadda et al, Neuroleptic malignant syndrome after venlafaxine. Lancet, 354:289, 2000
>
> *Single case report with venlafaxine and trifluoperazine (2000); causal relationship not established; monitor clinical status*

Vitamin C
> Decreased phenothiazine effect (increased metabolism)
>> VG Zannoni and MM Lynch, The role of ascorbic acid in drug metabolism. Drug Metab Rev, 2:57, 1973; MW Dysken et al, Drug interaction between ascorbic acid and fluphenazine. JAMA, 241:2008, 1979
>
> *Occurs only after vitamin C deficiency when normal concentration restores depressed drug metabolism*

Phenoxybenzamine, see Alpha-adrenergic blockers

Phenprocoumon, see Anticoagulants, oral

Phentermine, see Sympathomimetic amines

Phentolamine, no documented interactions, see page 4, Criteria for Listing Interactions

PHENYLBUTAZONE, with:
> **Alcohol** - See Alcohol with Phenylbutazone, page 21
>
> **Anticoagulants, oral** - See Anticoagulants, oral with Phenylbutazone, page 75
>
> **Hypoglycemics, sulfonylurea** - See Hypoglycemics, sulfonylurea with Phenylbutazone, page 305
>
> **Methotrexate** - See Methotrexate with Phenylbutazone, page 340
>
> **Misoprostol** - See Misoprostol with Phenylbutazone, page 348

PHENYLBUTAZONE, with: *(continued)*
Phenytoin
Phenytoin toxicity (decreased metabolism)
  B Andreasen et al, Diphenylhydantoin half-life in man and its inhibition by phenylbutazone: the role of genetic factors. Acta Med Scand, 193:561, 1973
  Monitor phenytoin concentration
Tobacco, smoking
Possible decreased phenylbutazone effect (increased metabolism)
  SK Garg and TN Ravi Kiran, Effect of smoking on phenylbutazone disposition. Int J Clin Pharmacol Ther Toxicol, 20:289, 1982
  Monitor clinical status

Phenylephrine, see Sympathomimetic amines; Sympathomimetic bronchodilators
Phenylpropanolamine, see Sympathomimetic amines

PHENYTOIN, with:
  Acetaminophen - See Acetaminophen with Phenytoin, page 9
  Alcohol - See Alcohol with Phenytoin, page 22
  Alkylating agents - See Alkylating agents with Phenytoin, page 24
  Amiodarone - See Amiodarone with Phenytoin, page 36
  Antacids - See Antacids with Phenytoin, page 55
  Anticoagulants, oral - See Anticoagulants, oral with Phenytoin, page 75
  Antidepressants, tricyclic - See Antidepressants, tricyclic with Phenytoin, page 89
  Antifungals, imidazoles and triazoles - See Antifungals, imidazoles and triazoles with Phenytoin, page 105
  Antihistamines, H_2-blockers - See Antihistamines, H_2-blockers with Phenytoin, page 122
  Benzodiazepines - See Benzodiazepines with Phenytoin, page 147
  Carbamazepine - See Carbamazepine with Phenytoin, page 184
  Carboplatin - See Carboplatin with Phenytoin, page 189
  Chloramphenicol - See Chloramphenicol with Phenytoin, page 193
  Cisplatin - See Cisplatin with Phenytoin, page 202
  Clofazimine - See Clofazimine with Phenytoin, page 203
  Clozapine - See Clozapine with Phenytoin, page 207
  Contraceptives, implant - See Contraceptives, implant with Phenytoin, page 212
  Contraceptives, oral - See Contraceptives, oral with Phenytoin, page 216
  Corticosteroids - See Corticosteroids with Phenytoin, page 222
  Cyclosporine - See Cyclosporine with Phenytoin, page 237
  Delavirdine - See Delavirdine with Phenytoin, page 245
  Diazoxide - See Diazoxide with Phenytoin, page 247
  Digoxin - See Digoxin with Phenytoin, page 255
  Disopyramide - See Disopyramide with Phenytoin, page 263
  Disulfiram - See Disulfiram with Phenytoin, page 264
  Estrogens - See Estrogens with Phenytoin, page 272
  Felbamate - See Felbamate with Phenytoin, page 275
  Fluoroquinolones - See Fluoroquinolones with Phenytoin, page 281
  Folic acid - See Folic acid with Phenytoin, page 284
  Furosemide - See Furosemide with Phenytoin, page 286

(continued)

PHENYTOIN, with: *(continued)*
- **Gabapentin** - See Gabapentin with Phenytoin, page 287
- **Haloperidol** - See Haloperidol with Phenytoin, page 296
- **HMG-CoA reductase inhibitors** - See HMG-CoA reductase inhibitors with Phenytoin, page 301
- **Hypoglycemics, sulfonylurea** - See Hypoglycemics, sulfonylurea with Phenytoin, page 305
- **Immune Globulin, Intravenous** - See Immune Globulin, Intravenous with Phenytoin, page 307
- **Influenza vaccine** - See Influenza vaccine with Phenytoin, page 309
- **Isoniazid** - See Isoniazid with Phenytoin, page 313
- **Lamotrigine** - See Lamotrigine with Phenytoin, page 317
- **Levodopa** - See Levodopa with Phenytoin, page 320
- **Lithium** - See Lithium with Phenytoin, page 326
- **Losartan** - See Losartan with Phenytoin, page 330
- **Macrolide antibiotics** - See Macrolide antibiotics with Phenytoin, page 331
- **Mercaptopurine** - See Mercaptopurine with Phenytoin, page 338
- **Methotrexate** - See Methotrexate with Phenytoin, page 340
- **Methoxsalen** - See Methoxsalen with Phenytoin, page 342
- **Methsuximide** - See Methsuximide with Phenytoin, page 342
- **Metronidazole** - See Metronidazole with Phenytoin, page 345
- **Mexiletine** - See Mexiletine with Phenytoin, page 345
- **Molindone** - See Molindone with Phenytoin, page 348
- **Narcotics: meperidine and congeners** - See Narcotics: meperidine and congeners with Phenytoin, page 356
- **Narcotics: methadone and congeners** - See Narcotics: methadone and congeners with Phenytoin, page 358
- **Nelfinavir** - See Nelfinavir with Phenytoin, page 362
- **Neuromuscular blocking agents** - See Neuromuscular blocking agents with Phenytoin, page 364
- **Nifedipine** - See Nifedipine with Phenytoin, page 368
- **Nisoldipine** - See Nisoldipine with Phenytoin, page 370
- **Nonsteroidal anti-inflammatory drugs** - See Nonsteroidal anti-inflammatory drugs with Phenytoin, page 373
- **Nutrients, enteral preparations** - See Nutrients, enteral preparations with Phenytoin, page 377
- **Nutrients, liquid concentrates** - See Nutrients, liquid concentrates with Phenytoin, page 378
- **Nutrients, parenteral** - See Nutrients, parenteral with Phenytoin, page 378
- **Omeprazole** - See Omeprazole with Phenytoin, page 379
- **Oxcarbazepine** - See Oxcarbazepine with Phenytoin, page 380
- **Penicillins** - See Penicillins with Phenytoin, page 382
- **Phenothiazines** - See Phenothiazines with Phenytoin, page 385
- **Phenylbutazone** - See Phenylbutazone with Phenytoin, page 387
- **Praziquantel**

    Decreased praziquantel effect (increased metabolism)
    > PRM Bittencourt et al, Phenytoin and carbamazepine decrease oral

PHENYTOIN, with: *(continued)*
>> bioavailability of praziquantel. Neurology, 42:492, 1992
> *Monitor for decreased response to praziquantel*

> **Primidone**
>> Decreased primidone effect and possible phenobarbital toxicity (increased conversion of primidone to phenobarbital)
>>> EH Reynolds et al, Interaction of phenytoin and primidone. Br Med J, 2:594, 1975; D Battino et al, Plasma levels of primidone and its metabolite phenobarbital: effect of age and associated therapy. Ther Drug Monit, 5:73, 1983
>> *Monitor primidone and phenobarbital concentrations*

> **Pyridoxine**
>> Decreased phenytoin effect (possibly increased metabolism)
>>> O Hansson and M Sillanpaa, Pyridoxine and serum concentration of phenytoin and phenobarbitone. Lancet, 1:256, 1976
>> *Occurs only occasionally; monitor phenytoin concentration*

> **Quetiapine**
>> Decreased quetiapine effect (increased metabolism; CYP3A4)
>>> Manufacturer's package insert; YWJ Wong et al, The effect of phenytoin and cimetidine on the pharmacokinetics of Seroquel. Schizophr Res, 24:200, 1997
>> *Avoid concurrent use; other enzyme inducers may produce similar effect*

> **Quinidine**
>> Decreased quinidine effect (increased metabolism)
>>> JL Data et al, Interaction of quinidine with anticonvulsant drugs. N Engl J Med, 294:699, 1976
>> *Monitor quinidine concentration*

> **Rifampin**
>> Decreased phenytoin effect (increased metabolism)
>>> L Kay et al, Influence of rifampicin and isoniazid on the kinetics of phenytoin. Br J Clin Pharmacol, 20:323, 1985; HH Zhou et al, Induction of polymorphic 4'-hydroxylation of S-mephenytoin by rifampicin. Br J Clin Pharmacol, 30:471, 1990
>> *Monitor phenytoin concentration; although isoniazid has the opposite metabolic effect, the rifampin effect tends to predominate when both drugs are used*

> **Selective serotonin reuptake inhibitors (SSRIs)**
>> Phenytoin toxicity with fluoxetine and possible toxicity with sertraline (decreased metabolism)
>>> P Jalil, Toxic reaction following the combined administration of fluoxetine and phenytoin: two case reports. J Neurol Neurosurg Psychiatry, 55:412, 1992; DJ Woods et al, Interaction of phenytoin and fluoxetine. NZ Med J, 107:19, 1994; MB Haselberger et al, Elevated serum phenytoin concentrations associated with coadministration of sertraline. J Clin Psychopharmacol, 17:107, 1997; MU Shad and SH Preskorn, Drug-drug interaction in reverse: possible loss of phenytoin efficacy as a result of fluoxetine discontinuation. J Clin Psychopharmacol, 19:472, 1999

(continued)

PHENYTOIN, with: *(continued)*

Monitor phenytoin concentration; four case reports with fluoxetine (1992, 1994, 1999) and two with sertraline (1997)

Streptozocin

Decreased streptozocin effect (mechanism not established)

L Koranyi and L Gero, Influence of diphenylhydantoin on the effect of streptozotocin. Br Med J, 1:127, 1979

Use alternative anticonvulsant

Sucralfate

Possible decreased phenytoin effect (decreased absorption)

TG Hall et al, Effect of sucralfate on phenytoin bioavailability. Drug Intell Clin Pharm, 20:607, 1986; R Malli et al, The effect of sucralfate on the steady-state serum concentrations of phenytoin. Drug Metab Drug Interact, 7:287, 1989

Monitor phenytoin concentration; study in healthy subjects failed to confirm

Sulfonamides

Possible phenytoin toxicity, except possibly with sulfisoxazole (decreased metabolism)

JM Hansen et al, The effect of different sulfonamides on phenytoin metabolism in man. Acta Med Scand, suppl 624:106, 1979

Monitor phenytoin concentration

Sympathomimetic amines

Possible phenytoin toxicity with methylphenidate (decreased metabolism)

M Ghofrani, Possible phenytoin-methylphenidate interaction. Dev Med Child Neurol, 30:267, 1988; LK Garrettson et al, Methylphenidate interaction with both anticonvulsants and ethyl biscoumacetate. JAMA, 207:2053, 1969

Appears to be rare; monitor phenytoin concentration

Hypotension with IV phenytoin in patients maintained on dopamine (mechanism not established)

BA Bivins et al, Dopamine-phenytoin interaction: a cause of hypotension in the critically ill. Arch Surg, 113:245, 1978; RP Rapp et al, Dopamine-phenytoin interaction. Drug Intell Clin Pharm, 12:429, 1978

Use another anticonvulsant

Tacrolimus

Decreased tacrolimus effect (increased metabolism; CYP3A4)

M Moreno et al, Clinical management of tacrolimus drug interactions in renal transplant patients. Transplant Proc, 31:2252, 1999

Single case report (1999); consistent with known interactive properties of drugs; monitor tacrolimus concentrations and clinical status

Teniposide

Possible decreased teniposide effect (increased metabolism)

DK Baker et al, Increased teniposide clearance with concomitant anticonvulsant therapy. J Clin Oncol, 10:311, 1992; MV Relling et al, Adverse effect of anticonvulsants on efficacy of chemotherapy for acute lymphoblastic leukaemia. Lancet, 356:285, 2000

PHENYTOIN, with: *(continued)*
> *Evidence of reduced teniposide efficacy in children with acute lymphoblastic leukemia; monitor clinical status and teniposide concentration if available*

Tetracyclines
> Decreased doxycycline effect (increased metabolism)
>> O Penttila et al, Interaction between doxycycline and some antiepileptic drugs. Br Med J, 2:470, 1974; PJ Neuvonen et al, Effect of antiepileptic drugs on the elimination of various tetracycline derivatives. Eur J Clin Pharmacol, 9:147, 1975
>
> *Choose another antibiotic*

Theophyllines
> Decreased theophylline and phenytoin effects (probably increased metabolism)
>> J-F Marquis et al, Phenytoin-theophylline interaction. N Engl J Med, 307:1189, 1982; L Hendeles et al, Decreased oral phenytoin absorption following concurrent theophylline administration. J Allergy Clin Immunol, 63:156, 1979; M Miller et al, Influence of phenytoin on theophylline clearance. Clin Pharmacol Ther, 35:666, 1984; SJ Sklar and JC Wagner, Enhanced theophylline clearance secondary to phenytoin therapy. Drug Intell Clin Pharm, 19:34, 1985
>
> *Monitor theophylline and phenytoin concentrations*

Thyroid hormones
> Decreased T_3 and T_4 concentrations (increased metabolism)
>> JL Blackshear et al, Thyroxine replacement requirements in hypothyroid patients receiving phenytoin. Ann Intern Med, 99:341, 1983; MI Surks and CR DeFesi, Normal serum free thyroid hormone concentrations in patients treated with phenytoin or carbamazepine. JAMA, 275:1495, 1996
>
> *Monitor clinical status and thyroid function; serum TSH may be more reliable than free thyroxine determinations*

Tiagabine
> Decreased tiagabine effect (increased tiagabine metabolism)
>> Manufacturer's package insert
>
> *Based on patient studies; monitor clinical status*

Ticlopidine
> Phenytoin toxicity (decreased metabolism; CYP2C19)
>> JP Rindone and G Bryan II et al, Phenytoin toxicity associated with ticlopidine administration. Arch Intern Med, 156:1113, 1996; M Privitera and TE Welty, Acute phenytoin toxicity followed by seizure breakthrough from a ticlopidine-phenytoin interaction. Arch Neurol, 53:1191, 1996; R Riva et al, Ticlopidine impairs phenytoin clearance: a case report. Neurology, 46:1172, 1996; SR Donahue et al, Ticlopidine inhibition of phenytoin metabolism mediated by potent inhibition of CYP2C19. Clin Pharmacol Ther, 62:572, 1997; SL Klaassen, Ticlopidine-induced phenytoin toxicity. Ann Pharmacother, 32:1295, 1998; S Donahue et al, Ticlopidine inhibits phenytoin clearance. Clin Pharmacol Ther, 66:563, 1999
>
> *Several case reports and pharmacokinetic study in healthy subjects; monitor phenytoin concentration*

(continued)

PHENYTOIN, with: *(continued)*

Tizanidine

Phenytoin toxicity (probably decreased metabolism)
> K Ueno et al, Phenytoin-tizanidine interaction. DICP, 25:1273, 1991

Single case report; monitor phenytoin concentrations

Topiramate

Possible decreased topiramate effect (mechanism not established)
> Manufacturer's package insert (topiramate)

Monitor topiramate concentration

Possible phenytoin toxicity (mechanism not established)
> Manufacturer's package insert (topiramate)

Monitor phenytoin concentration

Topotecan

Possible decreased topotecan effect (probably increased metabolism)
> WC Zambont et al, Phenytoin alters the disposition of topotecan and N-desmethyl topotecan in a patient with medulloblastoma. Clin Cancer Res, 4:783, 1998

Single case report (1998); monitor clinical response and adjust topotecan dose if necessary

Trazodone

Phenytoin toxicity (possibly decreased metabolism)
> JM Dorn, A case of phenytoin toxicity possibly precipitated by trazodone. J Clin Psychiatry, 47:89, 1986

Monitor phenytoin concentration

Trimethoprim-sulfamethoxazole

Phenytoin toxicity (decreased metabolism)
> MA Gillman and R Sandyk, Phenytoin toxicity and co-trimoxazole. Ann Intern Med, 102:559, 1985

Single case in a child (1985) after adding trimethoprim-sulfamethoxazole to a regimen that included sulthiame, which also inhibits hepatic phenytoin metabolism; clinical significance not established; sulfonamides with the possible exception of sulfisoxazole interact

Valproate

Phenytoin toxicity (displacement from binding)
> C Knott et al, Phenytoin-valproate interaction: importance of saliva monitoring in epilepsy. Br Med J, 284:13, 1982; LM Tsanaclis et al, Effect of valproate on free plasma phenytoin concentrations. Br J Clin Pharmacol, 18:17, 1984; R Riva et al, Time-dependent interaction between phenytoin and valproic acid. Neurology, 35:510, 1985; T May and B Rambeck, Fluctuations of unbound and total phenytoin concentrations during the day in epileptic patients on valproic acid comedication. Ther Drug Monit, 12:124, 1990

Conflicting reports; monitor phenytoin concentration (unbound concentration may be more helpful than total) and clinical status; saliva and free serum concentration may be helpful

PHENYTOIN, with: *(continued)*
>Possible decreased valproate effect (probably due to phenytoin induced enzyme induction)
>>H Cohen et al, Lack of high-dose valproic acid efficacy due to a drug interaction with phenytoin. ASHP Midyear Clinical Meeting, 34:P-169D, 1999
>
>*Single case report (1999); monitor clinical status and valproate serum concentrations*

>**Verapamil**
>
>Decreased verapamil effect (probably increased metabolism)
>>BG Woodcock et al, A reduction in verapamil concentrations with phenytoin. N Engl J Med, 325:1179, 1991
>
>*Single case report (1991)*

>**Vigabatrin**
>
>Decreased phenytoin effect (mechanism not established)
>>G Gatti et al, Vigabatrin-induced decrease in serum phenytoin concentration does not involve a change in phenytoin bioavailability.
>
>*Monitor phenytoin concentration and clinical status*

>**Vincristine**
>
>Decreased phenytoin effect with prednisone, methotrexate, mercaptopurine, and vincristine combination therapy (increased metabolism)
>>PF Jarosinski et al, Altered phenytoin clearance during intensive chemotherapy for acute lymphoblastic leukemia. J Pediatr, 112:996, 1988
>
>*Single well-studied case (1988); monitor*
>
>Decreased vincristine effect (enzyme induction; CYP3A4)
>>K Villikka et al, Cytochrome P450-inducing antiepileptics increase the clearance of vincristine in patients with brain tumors. Clin Pharmacol Ther, 66:589, 1999
>
>*Based on study in patients with brain tumors; monitor clinical status*

>**Zonisamide**
>
>Decreased zonisamide effect (increased metabolism; CYP3A4)
>>Manufacturer's package insert (zonisamide)
>
>*Monitor zonisamide concentration and clinical status; zonisamide dosage may need to be adjusted*

Physostigmine, see Anticholinesterases

Phytonadione, no documented interactions, see page 4, Criteria for Listing Interactions

PILOCARPINE, with:
>**Sympathomimetic amines**
>
>Increased myopia with pilocarpine *Ocusert* (mechanism not established)
>>RJ Duffey and JG Ferguson, Jr, Interaction of dipivefrin and epinephrine with the pilocarpine ocular therapeutic system (*Ocusert*). Arch Ophthalmol, 104:1135, 1986
>
>*Monitor for change in refraction*

PIMOZIDE, with:
  Antifungals, imidazoles and triazoles - See Antifungals, imidazoles and triazoles with Pimozide, page 105
  Lopinavir/Ritonavir - See Lopinavir/Ritonavir with Pimozide, page 329
  Macrolide antibiotics - See Macrolide antibiotics with Pimozide, page 332
  Selective serotonin reuptake inhibitors (SSRIs)
    Bradycardia with fluoxetine (mechanism not established)
      I Ahmed et al, Possible interaction between fluoxetine and pimozide causing sinus bradycardia. Can J Psychiatry, 38:62, 1993
    Single case report (1993)

    Stupor and hypersalivation with fluoxetine (mechanism not established)
      S Hansen-Grant et al, Fluoxetine-pimozide interaction. Am J Psychiatry, 150:1751, 1993
    Single case report (1993)
  Trimethoprim-sulfamethoxazole
    Decreased pimozide effect (mechanism not established)
      PAJ Speth et al, Interactie tussen pimozide en co-trimoxazol. Tijdschr Ther Geneesmdl, 11:20, 1985
    Single case report (1985)

Pindolol, see Beta-adrenergic blockers
Pioglitazone, no documented interactions, see page 4, Criteria for Listing Interactions
Pipecuronium, see Neuromuscular blocking agents
Piperacetazine, see Phenothiazines
Piperacillin, see Penicillins
Piperazine, no documented interactions, see page 4, Criteria for Listing Interactions
Pirbuterol, no documented interactions, see page 4, Criteria for Listing Interactions
Pirmenol, no documented interactions, see page 4, Criteria for Listing Interactions
Piroxicam, see Nonsteroidal anti-inflammatory drugs
Plicamycin, no documented interactions, see page 4, Criteria for Listing Interactions
Podofilox, no documented interactions, see page 4, Criteria for Listing Interactions
POLYETHYLENE GLYCOL AND ELECTROLYTES, with:
  Cyclosporine - See Cyclosporine with Polyethylene glycol and electrolytes, page 237

Polymyxin B, see Polymyxins
POLYMYXINS, with:
  Aminoglycoside antibiotics - See Aminoglycoside antibiotics with Polymyxins, page 33
  Neuromuscular blocking agents - See Neuromuscular blocking agents with Polymyxins, page 365
  Vancomycin
    Nephrotoxicity (additive)
      Manufacturer's package insert
    Avoid concurrent use

Polystyrene, see Sodium polystyrene sulfonate
Polythiazide, see Thiazide diuretics

POTASSIUM, with:
   Amiloride - See Amiloride with Potassium, page 28
   Angiotensin-converting enzyme (ACE) inhibitors - See Angiotensin-converting enzyme (ACE) inhibitors with Potassium, page 48
   Antidepressants, tricyclic - See Antidepressants, tricyclic with Potassium, page 89
   Nonsteroidal anti-inflammatory drugs - See Nonsteroidal anti-inflammatory drugs with Potassium, page 373
   Spironolactone
      Hyperkalemia (additive)
         DJ Greenblatt and J Koch-Weser, Adverse reactions to spironolactone. JAMA, 225:40, 1973; V Yap et al, Hyperkalemia with cardiac arrhythmia: induction by salt substitutes, spironolactone, and azotemia. JAMA, 236:2775, 1976
      Avoid potassium supplements
   Triamterene
      Hyperkalemia (additive)
         DH Lawson, Adverse reactions to potassium chloride. Q J Med, 43:433, 1974
      Avoid potassium supplements

Potassium citrate, see Citrates; Potassium

Pralidoxime, no documented interactions, see page 4, Criteria for Listing Interactions

PRAMIPEXOLE, with:
   Antihistamines, H$_2$-blockers - See Antihistamines, H$_2$-blockers with Pramipexole, page 123
   Haloperidol - See Haloperidol with Pramipexole, page 296
   Metoclopramide - See Metoclopramide with Pramipexole, page 344
   Phenothiazines - See Phenothiazines with Pramipexole, page 385

PRANIDIPINE, with:
   Grapefruit juice - See Grapefruit juice with Pranidipine, page 291

Pravastatin, see HMG-CoA Reductase Inhibitors

Prazepam, see Benzodiazepines

PRAZIQUANTEL, with:
   Antihistamines, H$_2$-blockers - See Antihistamines, H$_2$-blockers with Praziquantel, page 123
   Carbamazepine - See Carbamazepine with Praziquantel, page 184
   Chloroquine - See Chloroquine with Praziquantel, page 194
   Corticosteroids - See Corticosteroids with Praziquantel, page 223
   Phenytoin - See Phenytoin with Praziquantel, page 388

PRAZOSIN, with:
   Alcohol - See Alcohol with Prazosin, page 22
   Barbiturates - See Barbiturates with Prazosin, page 135
   Beta-adrenergic blockers - See Beta-adrenergic blockers with Prazosin, page 160
   Bupivacaine - See Bupivacaine with Prazosin, page 168
   Diazoxide - See Diazoxide with Prazosin, page 247

(continued)

PRAZOSIN, with: *(continued)*
  Digoxin - See Digoxin with Prazosin, page 256
  Nifedipine - See Nifedipine with Prazosin, page 368
  Nonsteroidal anti-inflammatory drugs - See Nonsteroidal anti-inflammatory drugs with Prazosin, page 373
  Verapamil
    Hypotension (synergism)
      PA Meredith and HL Elliott, An additive or synergistic drug interaction: application of concentration-effect modeling. Clin Pharmacol Ther, 51:708, 1992
    Monitor blood pressure

Prednisolone, see Corticosteroids
Prednisone, see Corticosteroids
PRILOCAINE, with:
  Trimethoprim-sulfamethoxazole
    Methemoglobinemia (probably additive)
      B Jakobson and A Nilsson, Methemoglobinemia associated with a prilocaine – lidocaine cream and trimethoprim-sulphamethoxazole. A case report. Acta Anaesthesiol Scand, 29:453, 1985
    Single case report in an infant with prilocaine-lidocaine cream (1985)

PRIMAQUINE, with:
  Dapsone - See Dapsone with Primaquine, page 242

PRIMIDONE, with:
  Carbamazepine - See Carbamazepine with Primidone, page 184
  Contraceptives, oral - See Contraceptives, oral with Primidone, page 216
  Corticosteroids - See Corticosteroids with Primidone, page 223
  Lamotrigine - See Lamotrigine with Primidone, page 317
  Phenytoin - See Phenytoin with Primidone, page 389
  Quinidine
    Decreased quinidine effect (increased metabolism)
      AM Urbano, Phenytoin-quinidine interaction in a patient with recurrent ventricular tachyarrhythmias. N Engl J Med, 308:225, 1983; JL Data et al, Interaction of quinidine with anticonvulsant drugs. N Engl J Med, 294:699, 1976
    Monitor quinidine concentration
  Sympathomimetic amines
    Possible primidone toxicity with methylphenidate (decreased metabolism)
      Manufacturer's package insert *(Ritalin)*
    Monitor primidone concentration; dosage adjustment may be necessary
  Tiagabine
    Decreased tiagabine effect (increased tiagabine metabolism)
      Manufacturer's package insert
    Based on patient studies; monitor clinical status

PROBENECID, with:
  Acetaminophen - See Acetaminophen with Probenecid, page 9
  Acyclovir - See Acyclovir with Probenecid, page 11

PROBENECID, with: (continued)
  Aminosalicylic acid - See Aminosalicylic acid with Probenecid, page 33
  Angiotensin-converting enzyme (ACE) inhibitors - See Angiotensin-converting enzyme (ACE) inhibitors with Probenecid, page 48
  Antihistamines, H_2-blockers - See Antihistamines, H_2-blockers with Probenecid, page 123
  Barbiturates - See Barbiturates with Probenecid, page 135
  Benzodiazepines - See Benzodiazepines with Probenecid, page 147
  Bumetanide - See Bumetanide with Probenecid, page 168
  Clofibrate - See Clofibrate with Probenecid, page 204
  Fluoroquinolones - See Fluoroquinolones with Probenecid, page 281
  Furosemide - See Furosemide with Probenecid, page 286
  Methotrexate - See Methotrexate with Probenecid, page 341
  Nalidixic acid - See Nalidixic acid with Probenecid, page 354
  Nonsteroidal anti-inflammatory drugs - See Nonsteroidal anti-inflammatory drugs with Probenecid, page 373
  Theophyllines
    Toxicity with dyphylline (decreased renal excretion)
      M Acara et al, Probenecid inhibition of the renal excretion of dyphylline in chicken, rat and man. J Pharm Pharmacol, 39:526, 1987; ED Marquardt et al, Ineffectiveness of probenecid in theophylline kinetics and excretion. Drug Intell Clin Pharm, 19:840, 1985
    Avoid concurrent use, if possible; may not occur with theophylline
  Zidovudine
    Rash (mechanism not established)
      BG Petty et al, Zidovudine with probenecid: a warning. Lancet, 335:1044, 1990
    In men; zidovudine dosage had been halved when probenecid was added; rash subsided after probenecid was stopped; probenecid inhibits zidovudine metabolism

PROBUCOL, with:
  Clofibrate - See Clofibrate with Probucol, page 204
  Cyclosporine - See Cyclosporine with Probucol, page 237

PROCAINAMIDE, with:
  Amiodarone - See Amiodarone with Procainamide, page 37
  Antihistamines, H_2-blockers - See Antihistamines, H_2-blockers with Procainamide, page 123
  Fluoroquinolones - See Fluoroquinolones with Procainamide, page 281
  Quinidine
    Procainamide toxicity (decreased metabolism)
      B Hughes et al, Increased procainamide plasma concentrations caused by quinidine: a new drug interaction. Am Heart J, 114:908, 1987
    Single case report (1987)
  Trimethoprim
    Possible procainamide toxicity (decreased renal clearance)
      T Kosoglou et al, Trimethoprim alters the disposition of procainamide and N-acetylprocainamide. Clin Pharmacol Ther, 44:467, 1988; PH Vlasses et al,

PROCAINAMIDE, with: *(continued)*
>Trimethoprim inhibition of the renal clearance of procainamide and N-acetylprocainamide. Arch Intern Med, 149:1350, 1989

Based on studies in healthy subjects; monitor procainamide concentration

PROCARBAZINE, with:
- **Digoxin** - See Digoxin with Procarbazine, page 256
- **Methotrexate** - See Methotrexate with Procarbazine, page 341

Prochlorperazine, see Phenothiazines

Progesterone, see Progestins

PROGESTINS, with:
- **Acitretin** - See Acitretin with Progestins, page 11
- **Cyclosporine** - See Cyclosporine with Progestins, page 237
- **Rifampin**

  Decreased norethindrone effect (increased metabolism)
  > Editor, Rifampicin, "pill" do not go well together. JAMA, 227:608, 1974; DJ Back et al, The effect of rifampicin on norethisterone pharmacokinetics. Eur J Clin Pharmacol, 15:193, 1979; JL Skolnick et al, Rifampin, oral contraceptives, and pregnancy. JAMA, 236:1382, 1976

  Use alternative contraceptive; higher doses may be needed for other uses

PROGUANIL, with:
- **Anticoagulants, oral** - See Anticoagulants, oral with Proguanil, page 75
- **Antihistamines, H$_2$-blockers** - See Antihistamines, H$_2$-blockers with Proguanil, page 123
- **Omeprazole** - See Omeprazole with Proguanil, page 379
- **Selective serotonin reuptake inhibitors (SSRIs)**

  Possible decreased proguanil effect with fluvoxamine (decreased conversion to active metabolite; CYP2C19)
  > U Jeppesen et al, The CYP2C19 catalyzed bioactivation of proguanil is abolished during fluvoxamine intake. Eur J Clin Pharmacol, 52:A134, 1997

  Monitor clinical status; based on study in healthy subjects; may be less likely with other selective serotonin reuptake inhibitors

Promazine, see Phenothiazines

PROMETHAZINE, with:
- **Chloroquine** - See Chloroquine with Promethazine, page 195

PROPAFENONE, with:
- **Anticoagulants, oral** - See Anticoagulants, oral with Propafenone, page 75
- **Antidepressants, tricyclic** - See Antidepressants, tricyclic with Propafenone, page 89
- **Beta-adrenergic blockers** - See Beta-adrenergic blockers with Propafenone, page 161
- **Cyclosporine** - See Cyclosporine with Propafenone, page 237
- **Digoxin** - See Digoxin with Propafenone, page 256
- **Lidocaine** - See Lidocaine with Propafenone, page 322
- **Lopinavir/Ritonavir** - See Lopinavir/Ritonavir with Propafenone, page 329
- **Mexiletine** - See Mexiletine with Propafenone, page 345

PROPAFENONE, with: *(continued)*
Quinidine
Possible propafenone toxicity in extensive metabolizers (decreased metabolism)
> KE Mörike and DM Roden, Quinidine-enhanced β-blockade during treatment with propafenone in extensive metabolizer human subjects. Clin Pharmacol Ther, 55:28, 1994

Monitor clinical status

Rifampin
Decreased propafenone effect (increased metabolism)
> JM Castel et al, Rifampicin lowers plasma concentrations of propafenone and its antiarrhythmic effect. Br J Clin Pharmacol, 30:155, 1990; K Dilger et al, Consequences of rifampicin treatment on propafenone disposition in extensive and poor metabolizers of CYP2D6. Pharmacogenetics, 9:551, 1999; K Dilger et al, Enzyme induction in the elderly: effect of rifampin on the pharmacokinetics and pharmacodynamics of propafenone. Clin Pharmacol Ther, 67:512, 2000

Monitor propafenone concentration and/or clinical status; single, well-documented case report (1990) and studies in healthy subjects (1999, 2000)

Ritonavir
Possible propafenone toxicity (decreased metabolism)
> Manufacturer's package insert (ritonavir)

Theoretical; listed as contraindicated in product information

Selective serotonin reuptake inhibitors (SSRIs)
Possible propafenone toxicity with fluoxetine or paroxetine (decreased metabolism; CYP2D6)
> WM Cai et al, Fluoxetine impairs the CYP2D6-mediated metabolism of propafenone enantiomers in healthy Chinese volunteers. Clin Pharmacol Ther, 66:516, 1999; A Hemeryck et al, Effect of selective serotonin reuptake inhibitors on the oxidative metabolism of propafenone: *In vitro* studies using human liver microsomes. J Clin Psychopharmacol, 20:428, 2000

Based on study in healthy subjects; monitor clinical status

Theophyllines
Theophylline toxicity (possibly decreased metabolism)
> BL Lee and ML Dohrmann, Theophylline toxicity after propafenone treatment: evidence for drug interaction. Clin Pharmacol Ther, 51:353, 1992; SA Spinler et al, Propafenone-theophylline interaction. Pharmacotherapy, 13:68, 1993

Two case reports (1992,1993); monitor theophylline concentration

Propantheline, see Anticholinergics

PROPOFOL, with:
  Benzodiazepines - See Benzodiazepines with Propofol, page 148
  Clonidine - See Clonidine with Propofol, page 205
  Cocaine - See Cocaine with Propofol, page 210
  Maprotiline - See Maprotiline with Propofol, page 335

Propoxyphene, see Narcotics: methadone and congeners

Propranolol, see Beta-adrenergic blockers

PROPYLTHIOURACIL, with:
    Anticoagulants, oral - See Anticoagulants, oral with Propylthiouracil, page 75

Protamine, no documented interactions, see page 4, Criteria for Listing Interactions

Protriptyline, see Antidepressants, tricyclic

Pseudoephedrine, see Sympathomimetic amines

PSYLLIUM, with:
    Lithium - See Lithium with Psyllium, page 326

PYRANTEL PAMOATE, with:
    Theophyllines
        Possible theophylline toxicity (mechanism not established)
            L Hecht et al, Theophylline – pyrantel pamoate interaction. DICP, 23:258, 1989
        Single case report (1989)

PYRAZINAMIDE, with:
    Allopurinol - See Allopurinol with Pyrazinamide, page 25
    Cyclosporine - See Cyclosporine with Pyrazinamide, page 237

Pyrethrins with piperonyl butoxide, no documented interactions, see page 4, Criteria for Listing Interactions

Pyridostigmine, no documented interactions, see page 4, Criteria for Listing Interactions

PYRIDOXINE, with:
    Barbiturates - See Barbiturates with Pyridoxine, page 136
    Levodopa - See Levodopa with Pyridoxine, page 321
    Phenytoin - See Phenytoin with Pyridoxine, page 389

Pyrilamine, no documented interactions, see page 4, Criteria for Listing Interactions

PYRIMETHAMINE, with:
    Antacids - See Antacids with Pyrimethamine, page 55
    Dapsone - See Dapsone with Pyrimethamine, page 242
    Halofantrine - See Halofantrine with Pyrimethamine, page 293
    Kaolin or Kaolin-pectin - See Kaolin or Kaolin-pectin with Pyrimethamine, page 315
    Phenothiazines - See Phenothiazines with Pyrimethamine, page 385

Quazepam, see Benzodiazepines

QUETIAPINE, with:
    Alcohol - See Alcohol with Quetiapine, page 22
    Anticoagulants, oral - See Anticoagulants, oral with Quetiapine, page 75
    Levodopa - See Levodopa with Quetiapine, page 321
    Phenothiazines - See Phenothiazines with Quetiapine, page 385
    Phenytoin - See Phenytoin with Quetiapine, page 389

Quinapril, see Angiotensin-converting enzyme (ACE) inhibitors

Quinestrol, see Estrogens

Quinethazone, see Thiazide diuretics

QUINIDINE, with:
    Amiloride - See Amiloride with Quinidine, page 28
    Amiodarone - See Amiodarone with Quinidine, page 37
    Amprenavir - See Amprenavir with Quinidine, page 40

QUINIDINE, with: *(continued)*

Antacids - See Antacids with Quinidine, page 55

Anticoagulants, oral - See Anticoagulants, oral with Quinidine, page 75

Antidepressants, tricyclic - See Antidepressants, tricyclic with Quinidine, page 89

Antifungals, imidazoles and triazoles - See Antifungals, imidazoles and triazoles with Quinidine, page 105

Antihistamines, H_2-blockers - See Antihistamines, H_2-blockers with Quinidine, page 124

Arbutamine - See Arbutamine with Quinidine, page 128

Barbiturates - See Barbiturates with Quinidine, page 136

Beta-adrenergic blockers - See Beta-adrenergic blockers with Quinidine, page 161

Carbonic anhydrase inhibitors - See Carbonic anhydrase inhibitors with Quinidine, page 189

Digitoxin - See Digitoxin with Quinidine, page 250

Digoxin - See Digoxin with Quinidine, page 256

Diltiazem - See Diltiazem with Quinidine, page 261

Encainide - See Encainide with Quinidine, page 268

Flecainide - See Flecainide with Quinidine, page 278

Fluoroquinolones - See Fluoroquinolones with Quinidine, page 281

Haloperidol - See Haloperidol with Quinidine, page 296

Macrolide antibiotics - See Macrolide antibiotics with Quinidine, page 332

Mefloquine - See Mefloquine with Quinidine, page 336

Metoclopramide - See Metoclopramide with Quinidine, page 344

Narcotics: dextromethorphan - See Narcotics: dextromethorphan with Quinidine, page 355

Narcotics: morphine-like - See Narcotics: morphine-like with Quinidine, page 360

Neuromuscular blocking agents - See Neuromuscular blocking agents with Quinidine, page 365

Nifedipine - See Nifedipine with Quinidine, page 368

Nonsteroidal anti-inflammatory drugs - See Nonsteroidal anti-inflammatory drugs with Quinidine, page 374

Phenytoin - See Phenytoin with Quinidine, page 389

Primidone - See Primidone with Quinidine, page 396

Procainamide - See Procainamide with Quinidine, page 397

Propafenone - See Propafenone with Quinidine, page 399

Rifampin

Decreased quinidine effect (increased metabolism)

A Schwartz and JR Brown, Quinidine-rifampin interaction. Am Heart J, 107:789, 1984; Y Twum-Barima and SG Carruthers, Evaluation of rifampin-quinidine interaction. Clin Pharmacol Ther, 27:290, 1980

Monitor quinidine concentration

Ritonavir

Possible quinidine toxicity (decreased metabolism)

Manufacturer's package insert (ritonavir)

Theoretical; listed as contraindicated in product information

(continued)

QUINIDINE, with: *(continued)*

Selective serotonin reuptake inhibitors (SSRIs)

Possible quinidine toxicity (probably decreased metabolism; probably CYP3A4)

P Damkier et al, Effect of fluvoxamine on the pharmacokinetics of quinidine. Eur J Clin Pharmacol, 55:451, 1999

Based on study in healthy subjects; monitor clinical status and quinidine concentrations

Verapamil

Hypotension with IV verapamil (additive alpha-adrenergic receptor blockade)

AS Maisel et al, Hypotension after quinidine plus verapamil. N Engl J Med, 312:167, 1985

Avoid concurrent use of IV verapamil

Possible quinidine toxicity (decreased metabolism)

RG Trohman et al, Increased quinidine plasma concentrations during administration of verapamil: a new quinidine – verapamil interaction. Am J Cardiol, 57:706, 1986; DJ Edwards et al, The effect of coadministration of verapamil on the pharmacokinetics and metabolism of quinidine. Clin Pharmacol Ther, 41:68, 1987

Single case report (1986); monitor quinidine concentration

QUININE, with:

Antacids - See Antacids with Quinine, page 55

Anticoagulants, oral - See Anticoagulants, oral with Quinine, page 76

Antihistamines, H$_1$-blockers: astemizole, terfenadine - See Antihistamines, H$_1$-blockers: astemizole, terfenadine with Quinine, page 111

Antihistamines, H$_2$-blockers - See Antihistamines, H$_2$-blockers with Quinine, page 124

Barbiturates - See Barbiturates with Quinine, page 136

Carbamazepine - See Carbamazepine with Quinine, page 184

Cyclosporine - See Cyclosporine with Quinine, page 238

Digoxin - See Digoxin with Quinine, page 257

Mefloquine - See Mefloquine with Quinine, page 337

Neuromuscular blocking agents - See Neuromuscular blocking agents with Quinine, page 365

Rifampin

Decreased quinine effect (increased metabolism)

S Wanwimolruk et al, Marked enhancement by rifampicin and lack of effect of isoniazid on the elimination of quinine in man. Br J Clin Pharmacol, 40:87, 1995

Based on study in healthy subjects

QUINUPRISTIN/DALFOPRISTIN, with:

Benzodiazepines - See Benzodiazepines with Quinupristin/dalfopristin, page 148

Cyclosporine - See Cyclosporine with Quinupristin/dalfopristin, page 238

Nifedipine - See Nifedipine with Quinupristin/dalfopristin, page 368

RABEPRAZOLE, with:
    Antifungals, imidazoles and triazoles - See Antifungals, imidazoles and triazoles with Rabeprazole, page 106
    Digoxin - See Digoxin with Rabeprazole, page 257

RABIES VACCINE, with:
    Chloroquine - See Chloroquine with Rabies vaccine, page 195

RALOXIFENE, with:
    Anticoagulants, oral - See Anticoagulants, oral with Raloxifene, page 76
    Cholestyramine - See Cholestyramine with Raloxifene, page 197
    Estrogens - See Estrogens with Raloxifene, page 272

Ramipril, see Angiotensin-converting enzyme (ACE) inhibitors

Ranitidine, see Antihistamines, H_2-blockers

REBOXETINE, with:
    Antifungals, imidazoles and triazoles - See Antifungals, imidazoles and triazoles with Reboxetine, page 106

Repaglinide, no documented interactions, see page 4, Criteria for Listing Interactions

RESERPINE, with:
    Barbiturates - See Barbiturates with Reserpine, page 136
    Cyclopropane - See Cyclopropane with Reserpine, page 226
    Diazoxide - See Diazoxide with Reserpine, page 247
    Ether - See Ether with Reserpine, page 274
    Halothane - See Halothane with Reserpine, page 297
    Isoflurane - See Isoflurane with Reserpine, page 313
    Monoamine oxidase inhibitors - See Monoamine oxidase inhibitors with Reserpine, page 350
    Nitrous oxide - See Nitrous oxide with Reserpine, page 371

Reteplase, see Thrombolytics

RETINOIC ACID, with:
    Tranexamic acid
        Fatal thromboembolism with all-trans retinoic acid (mechanism not established)
            S Hashimoto et al, Fatal thromboembolism in acute promyelocytic leukemia during all-trans retinoic acid therapy combined with antifibrinolytic therapy for prophylaxis of hemorrhage. Leukemia, 8:1113, 1994
        Single case report; patient with acute promyelocytic leukemia (1994)

RIBAVIRIN, with:
    Zidovudine
        Antagonistic *in vitro*
            Manufacturer's package insert (zidovudine)
        Avoid concurrent use

RIFABUTIN, with:
    Amprenavir - See Amprenavir with Rifabutin, page 40
    Antifungals, imidazoles and triazoles - See Antifungals, imidazoles and triazoles with Rifabutin, page 106

(continued)

RIFABUTIN, with: *(continued)*
    Contraceptives, oral - See Contraceptives, oral with Rifabutin, page 216
    Delavirdine - See Delavirdine with Rifabutin, page 245
    Indinavir - See Indinavir with Rifabutin, page 308
    Lopinavir/Ritonavir - See Lopinavir/Ritonavir with Rifabutin, page 329
    Macrolide antibiotics - See Macrolide antibiotics with Rifabutin, page 332
    Nelfinavir - See Nelfinavir with Rifabutin, page 363
    Nevirapine - See Nevirapine with Rifabutin, page 367
    Ritonavir
        Rifabutin toxicity (decreased metabolism)
            Manufacturer's package insert (ritonavir); A Cato III et al, The effect of multiple doses of ritonavir on the pharmacokinetics of rifabutin. Clin Pharmacol Ther, 63:414, 1998
        Manufacturer recommends decreasing rifabutin dose by at least 3/4 (further dosage reduction may be necessary)
    Saquinavir
        Possible decreased saquinavir effect (mechanism not established)
            Manufacturer's package insert (saquinavir)
        Monitor saquinavir concentration
Rifampicin, see Rifampin
RIFAMPIN, with:
    Aminosalicylic acid - See Aminosalicylic acid with Rifampin, page 33
    Amiodarone - See Amiodarone with Rifampin, page 37
    Amprenavir - See Amprenavir with Rifampin, page 40
    Anticoagulants, oral - See Anticoagulants, oral with Rifampin, page 76
    Antidepressants, tricyclic - See Antidepressants, tricyclic with Rifampin, page 90
    Antifungals, imidazoles and triazoles - See Antifungals, imidazoles and triazoles with Rifampin, page 106
    Atovaquone - See Atovaquone with Rifampin, page 129
    Barbiturates - See Barbiturates with Rifampin, page 136
    Benzodiazepines - See Benzodiazepines with Rifampin, page 148
    Beta-adrenergic blockers - See Beta-adrenergic blockers with Rifampin, page 161
    Buspirone - See Buspirone with Rifampin, page 171
    Chloramphenicol - See Chloramphenicol with Rifampin, page 193
    Clofibrate - See Clofibrate with Rifampin, page 204
    Clozapine - See Clozapine with Rifampin, page 207
    Contraceptives, oral - See Contraceptives, oral with Rifampin, page 216
    Corticosteroids - See Corticosteroids with Rifampin, page 223
    COX-2 inhibitors - See COX-2 inhibitors with Rifampin, page 226
    Cyclosporine - See Cyclosporine with Rifampin, page 238
    Dapsone - See Dapsone with Rifampin, page 242
    Delavirdine - See Delavirdine with Rifampin, page 245
    Digitoxin - See Digitoxin with Rifampin, page 250
    Digoxin - See Digoxin with Rifampin, page 257
    Diltiazem - See Diltiazem with Rifampin, page 261
    Disopyramide - See Disopyramide with Rifampin, page 263

RIFAMPIN, with: *(continued)*
- **Dolasetron** - See Dolasetron with Rifampin, page 265
- **Efavirenz** - See Efavirenz with Rifampin, page 268
- **Fexofenadine** - See Fexofenadine with Rifampin, page 277
- **Haloperidol** - See Haloperidol with Rifampin, page 296
- **HMG-CoA reductase inhibitors** - See HMG-CoA reductase inhibitors with Rifampin, page 301
- **Hydroxychloroquine** - See Hydroxychloroquine with Rifampin, page 303
- **Hypoglycemics, sulfonylurea** - See Hypoglycemics, sulfonylurea with Rifampin, page 305
- **Indinavir** - See Indinavir with Rifampin, page 308
- **Isoniazid** - See Isoniazid with Rifampin, page 313
- **Lamotrigine** - See Lamotrigine with Rifampin, page 317
- **Leflunomide** - See Leflunomide with Rifampin, page 319
- **Lopinavir/Ritonavir** - See Lopinavir/Ritonavir with Rifampin, page 329
- **Losartan** - See Losartan with Rifampin, page 330
- **Mephenytoin** - See Mephenytoin with Rifampin, page 337
- **Mexiletine** - See Mexiletine with Rifampin, page 346
- **Narcotics: methadone and congeners** - See Narcotics: methadone and congeners with Rifampin, page 358
- **Narcotics: Morphine-like** - See Narcotics: Morphine-like with Rifampin, page 360
- **Nelfinavir** - See Nelfinavir with Rifampin, page 363
- **Nevirapine** - See Nevirapine with Rifampin, page 367
- **Nifedipine** - See Nifedipine with Rifampin, page 369
- **Nisoldipine** - See Nisoldipine with Rifampin, page 370
- **Ondansetron** - See Ondansetron with Rifampin, page 379
- **Phenytoin** - See Phenytoin with Rifampin, page 389
- **Progestins** - See Progestins with Rifampin, page 398
- **Propafenone** - See Propafenone with Rifampin, page 399
- **Quinidine** - See Quinidine with Rifampin, page 401
- **Quinine** - See Quinine with Rifampin, page 402
- **Ritonavir**

    Possible decreased ritonavir effect (probably increased metabolism)
    Manufacturer's package insert (ritonavir)
    Avoid concurrent use; alternative agents should be considered

- **Saquinavir**

    Decreased saquinavir effect (mechanism not established)
    Manufacturer's package insert; AI Veldkamp et al, Ritonavir enables combined therapy with rifampin and saquinavir. Clin Infect Dis, 29:1586, 1999
    Monitor clinical status; adding ritonavir may allow therapeutic concentrations of saquinavir to be achieved

- **Selective serotonin reuptake inhibitors (SSRIs)**

    Decreased sertraline effect (probably enzyme induction; CYP3A4)
    JS Markowitz and CL DeVane, Rifampin-induced selective serotonin reuptake inhibitor withdrawal syndrome in a patient treated with sertraline. J Clin Psychopharmacol, 20:109, 2000

(continued)

RIFAMPIN, with: *(continued)*
Single case report (2000); monitor clinical status; avoid concomittant therapy if possible

Sirolimus

Decreased sirolimus effect (increased metabolism)

Manufacturer's package insert (sirolimus)

In one study in 14 healthy volunteers, sirolimus clearance decreased by more than 5-fold; avoid concurrent use

Tacrolimus

Decreased tacrolimus effect (increased metabolism; CYP3A4; possibly enhanced transport; glycoprotein)

V Furlan et al, Interactions between FK506 and rifampicin or erythromycin in pediatric liver recipients. Transplantation, 59:1217, 1995; T Kiuchi et al, Experience of tacrolimus-based immunosuppression in living-related liver transplantation complicated with graft tuberculosis: interaction with rifampicin and side effects. Transplant Proc, 28:3171, 1996; MF Hebert et al, Effects of rifampin on tacrolimus pharmacokinetics in healthy volunteers. J Clin Pharmacol, 39:91, 1999; M Moreno et al, Clinical management of tacrolimus drug interactions in renal transplant patients. Transplant Proc, 31:2252, 1999; R-Y Chenhsu et al, Renal allograft dysfunction associated with rifampin-tacrolimus interaction. Ann Pharmacother, 34:27, 2000

Avoid concurrent use if possible; if combination used, monitor tacrolimus concentrations and clinical status

Tamoxifen

Possible reduced tamoxifen effect (increased metabolism; CYP3A4)

KT Kivistö et al, Tamoxifen and toremifene concentrations in plasma are greatly decreased by rifampin. Clin Pharmacol Ther, 64:648, 1998

Marked reduction in tamoxifen plasma concentrations in healthy subjects; avoid concurrent use; barbiturates, carbamazepine, phenytoin, primidone, and rifabutin would also be expected to reduce tamoxifen effect

Tetracyclines

Possible decreased doxycycline effect (increased metabolism)

R Garraffo et al, Effet de la rifampicine sur la pharmacocinétique de la doxycycline. Pathol Biol, 35:746, 1987

Monitor doxycycline concentration

Theophyllines

Decreased theophylline effect (increased metabolism)

RA Robson et al, Theophylline – rifampicin interaction: non-selective induction of theophylline metabolic pathways. Br J Clin Pharmacol, 18:445, 1984; DR Brocks et al, Theophylline – rifampin interaction in a pediatric patient. Clin Pharm, 5:602, 1986; EG Boyce et al, The effect of rifampin on theophylline kinetics. J Clin Pharmacol, 26:696, 1986

Monitor theophylline concentration

Theophylline toxicity when used with both rifampin and isoniazid (decreased metabolism possibly due to hepatotoxicity of rifampin-isoniazid)

R Dal Negro et al, Rifampicin-isoniazid and delayed elimination of

RIFAMPIN, with: *(continued)*
> theophylline: a case report. Int J Clin Pharm Res, 8:275, 1988

Single case report (1988); monitor theophylline concentration

Thyroid hormones
Reduced thyroid hormone effect (probably increased metabolism)
> SR Nolan et al, Interaction between rifampin and levothyroxine. South Med J, 92:529, 1999

Single case report (1999); monitor clinical status and TSH concentrations

Tocainide
Possible decreased tocainide effect (increased metabolism)
> TL Rice et al, Influence of rifampin on the pharmacokinetics of tocainide in humans. Presented at ASHP Midyear Clin Meet, 23:CR-6, 1988; Int Pharm Abs, 26:527, 1989

Based on study in healthy volunteers; monitor tocainide concentration

Toremifene
Possible reduced toremifene effect (increased metabolism; CYP3A4)
> KT Kivistö et al, Tamoxifen and toremifene concentrations in plasma are greatly decreased by rifampin. Clin Pharmacol Ther, 64:648, 1998

Marked reduction in toremifene plasma concentrations in healthy subjects; avoid concurrent use; barbiturates, carbamazepine, phenytoin, primidone, and rifabutin would also be expected to reduce toremifene effect

Trimethoprim-sulfamethoxazole
Possible rifampin toxicity (possibly decreased metabolism)
> RS Bhatia et al, Drug interaction between rifampicin and cotrimoxazole in patients with tuberculosis. Hum Exp Toxicol, 10:419, 1991

Monitor clinical status or rifampin concentration

Verapamil
Decreased oral verapamil effect (increased metabolism in the gut wall)
> RA Barbarash et al, Near-total reduction in verapamil bioavailability by rifampin; electrocardiographic correlates. Chest, 94:954, 1988; MF Fromm et al, Gut wall metabolism of verapamil in older people: effects of rifampicin-mediated enzyme induction. Br J Clin Pharmacol, 45:247, 1998

Monitor verapamil concentration

Zaleplon
Decreased zaleplon effect (increased metabolism; CYP3A4)
> Manufacturer's package insert (zaleplon)

Based on study in healthy volunteers; serum concentration decreased by 80%; monitor clinical status

Zidovudine
Possible decreased zidovudine effect (increased metabolism)
> DM Burger et al, Pharmacokinetic interaction between rifampin and zidovudine. Antimicrob Agents Chemother, 37:1426, 1993; KD Gallicano et al, Induction of zidovudine glucuronidation and amination pathways by rifampicin in HIV-infected patients. Br J Clin Pharmacol, 48:168, 1999

Clinical importance not established; monitor clinical status

(continued)

RIFAMPIN, with: *(continued)*
  Zolpidem
    Decreased zolpidem effect (increased metabolism; CYP3A4)
        K Villikka et al, Rifampin reduces plasma concentrations and effects of zolpidem. Clin Pharmacol Ther, 62:629, 1997
    Avoid concurrent use; based on study in healthy subjects; marked decrease in zolpidem serum concentrations

Rifamycin, see Rifampin

RIFAPENTINE, with:
  Indinavir - See Indinavir with Rifapentine, page 308

Riluzole, no documented interactions, see page 4, Criteria for Listing Interactions
Rimantadine, no documented interactions, see page 4, Criteria for Listing Interactions

RISEDRONATE, with:
  Antacids - See Antacids with Risedronate, page 56
  Calcium - See Calcium with Risedronate, page 175

RISPERIDONE, with:
  Clozapine - See Clozapine with Risperidone, page 207
  Donepezil - See Donepezil with Risperidone, page 266
  Selective serotonin reuptake inhibitors (SSRIs)
    Possible decrease in fluoxetine effect (mechanism not established)
        C Andrade, Risperidone may worsen fluoxetine-treated OCD. J Clin Psychiatry, 59:255, 1998; R Mahendran, Obsessive-compulsive symptoms with risperidone. J Clin Psychiatry, 60:261, 1999; KD Fitzgerald et al, Risperidone augmentation of serotonin reuptake inhibitor treatment of pediatric obsessive compulsive disorder. J Child Adolesc Psychopharmacol, 9:115, 1999
    Single case report in patient with obsessive-compulsive disorder (1998); other patients with OCD have received risperidone plus SSRIs with good results

    Enuresis (mechanism not established)
        KJ Took and BL Buck, Enuresis with combined risperidone and SSRI use. J Am Acad Child Adolesc Psychiatry, 35:840, 1996
    Report of five patients (1996)

    Possible serotonin syndrome (additive)
        S Hamilton and K Malone, Serotonin syndrome during treatment with paroxetine and risperidone. J Clin Psychopharmacol, 20:103, 2000
    Single case report with paroxetine (2000); monitor clinical status

  Tetracyclines
    Possible decreased risperidone effect (mechanism not established)
        M Steele and J Couturier, A possible tetracycline-risperidone-sertraline interaction in an adolescent. Can J Clin Pharmacol, 6:15, 1999
    Single case report (1999); monitor for reduced risperidone effect

  Valproate
    Generalized edema (possible additive effect)
        CF Baldassano and SN Ghaemi, Generalized edema with risperidone: divalproex sodium treatment. J Clin Psychiatry, 57:9, 1996; RD Sanders and DS Lehrer, Edema associated with addition of risperidone to valproate

RISPERIDONE, with: *(continued)*
  treatment. J Clin Psychiatry, 59:689, 1998
  Two case reports (1996, 1998)

Ritodrine, see Sympathomimetic amines

RITONAVIR, with:
  Amiodarone - See Amiodarone with Ritonavir, page 37
  Amprenavir - See Amprenavir with Ritonavir, page 40
  Anticoagulants, oral - See Anticoagulants, oral with Ritonavir, page 76
  Antidepressants, tricyclic - See Antidepressants, tricyclic with Ritonavir, page 90
  Antifungals, imidazoles and triazoles - See Antifungals, imidazoles and triazoles with Ritonavir, page 107
  Antihistamines, H$_1$-blockers: astemizole, terfenadine - See Antihistamines, H$_1$-blockers: astemizole, terfenadine with Ritonavir, page 112
  Benzodiazepines - See Benzodiazepines with Ritonavir, page 148
  Bepridil - See Bepridil with Ritonavir, page 152
  Bupropion - See Bupropion with Ritonavir, page 169
  Carbamazepine - See Carbamazepine with Ritonavir, page 184
  Cisapride - See Cisapride with Ritonavir, page 201
  Clozapine - See Clozapine with Ritonavir, page 207
  Contraceptives, oral - See Contraceptives, oral with Ritonavir, page 217
  Corticosteroids - See Corticosteroids with Ritonavir, page 224
  Delavirdine - See Delavirdine with Ritonavir, page 245
  Didanosine - See Didanosine with Ritonavir, page 249
  Encainide - See Encainide with Ritonavir, page 268
  Ergot alkaloids - See Ergot alkaloids with Ritonavir, page 271
  Flecainide - See Flecainide with Ritonavir, page 278
  Indinavir - See Indinavir with Ritonavir, page 308
  Isotretinoin - See Isotretinoin with Ritonavir, page 315
  Lopinavir/Ritonavir - See Lopinavir/Ritonavir with Ritonavir, page 329
  Macrolide antibiotics - See Macrolide antibiotics with Ritonavir, page 333
  Methylenedioxymethamphetamine - See Methylenedioxymethamphetamine with Ritonavir, page 343
  Narcotics: meperidine and congeners - See Narcotics: meperidine and congeners with Ritonavir, page 356
  Narcotics: methadone and congeners - See Narcotics: methadone and congeners with Ritonavir, page 358
  Nelfinavir - See Nelfinavir with Ritonavir, page 363
  Nevirapine - See Nevirapine with Ritonavir, page 367
  Nonsteroidal anti-inflammatory drugs - See Nonsteroidal anti-inflammatory drugs with Ritonavir, page 374
  Propafenone - See Propafenone with Ritonavir, page 399
  Quinidine - See Quinidine with Ritonavir, page 401
  Rifabutin - See Rifabutin with Ritonavir, page 404
  Rifampin - See Rifampin with Ritonavir, page 405
  Saquinavir
    Possible saquinavir toxicity (decreased metabolism; CYP3A4)
      C Merry et al, Saquinavir pharmacokinetics alone and in combination with

(continued)

RITONAVIR, with: *(continued)*
>ritonavir in HIV-infected patients. AIDS, 11:F29, 1997; O Witzke et al, Side-effects of ritonavir and its combination with saquinavir with special regard to renal function. AIDS, 11:836, 1997; AL Tseng and MM Foisy, Significant interactions with new antiretrovirals and psychotropic drugs. Ann Pharmacother, 33:461, 1999; M Barry et al, Pharmacokinetics and potential interactions amongst antiretroviral agents used to treat patients with HIV infection. Clin Pharmacokinet, 36:289, 1999; C Michelet et al, Safety and efficacy of ritonavir and saquinavir in combination with zidovudine and lamivudine. Clin Pharmacol Ther, 65:661, 1999; RPG van Heeswijk et al, Once-daily dosing of saquinavir and low-dose ritonavir in HIV-1-infected individuals: a pharmacokinetic pilot study. AIDS, 16:F103, 2000; N Buss, Effect of ritonavir on saquinavir metabolism. JAMA, 283:2936, 2000

Marked increase in saquinavir concentrations, in some HIV(+) patients; monitor serum concentration and clinical status; combination including reduced dose of saquinavir (400 mg BID) may be an effective way for increasing plasma level of saquinavir; ritonavir and saquinavir combinations are increasingly being used

Selective Serotonin Reuptake Inhibitors (SSRIs)
>Possible ritonavir toxicity (probably decreased metabolism)
>>D Ouellet et al, Effect of fluoxetine on pharmacokinetics of ritonavir. Antimicrob Agents Chemother, 42:3107, 1998; SE Bellibas, Ritonavir-fluoxetine interaction. Antimicrob Agents Chemother, 43:1815, 1999
>
>*Based on study in healthy subjects; clinical significance not established*

Sildenafil
>Possible sildenafil toxicity (probably decreased metabolism; CYP3A4)
>>MCS Hall and S Ahmad, Interaction between sildenafil and HIV-1 combination therapy. Lancet, 353:2071, 1999; GJ Muirhead et al, Pharmacokinetic interactions between sildenafil and saquinavir/ritonavir. Br J Clin Pharmacol, 50:99, 2000
>
>*Single fatal case report (1999); patient taking ritonavir and saquinavir; pharmacokinetic interaction confirmed in study of healthy subjects; avoid concurrent use*

Tacrolimus
>Possible tacrolimus toxicity (decreased metabolism; probably CYP3A4; decreased transport; probably P-glycoprotein)
>>AM Sheikh et al, Concomitant human immunodeficiency virus protease inhibitor therapy markedly reduces tacrolimus metabolism and increases blood levels. Transplantation, 68:307, 1999
>
>*Single case report (1999); monitor tacrolimus concentrations and clinical status*

Theophyllines
>Possible decreased theophylline effect (mechanism not established)
>>Manufacturer's package insert (ritonavir)
>
>*Monitor theophylline concentration*

RITONAVIR, with: *(continued)*
  Thyroid Hormones
    Possible decreased thyroxine effect (possible increased metabolism; glucuronidation)
      A Tseng and D Fletcher, Interaction between ritonavir and levothyroxine. AIDS, 12:2235, 1998
    Single case report (1998)
  Zidovudine
    Possible decreased zidovudine effect (mechanism not established)
      A Cato et al, Multidose pharmacokinetics of ritonavir and zidovudine in human immunodeficiency virus-infected patients. Antimicrob Agents Chemother, 42:1788, 1998
    Based on study in HIV-positive men; clinical significance not established
  Zolpidem
    Possible zolpidem toxicity (decreased metabolism)
      Manufacturer's package insert (ritonavir); DJ Greenblatt et al, Differential impairment of triazolam and zolpidem clearance by ritonavir. J Acquir Immune Defic Syndr, 24:129, 2000
    Based on pharmacokinetic study in healthy subjects; listed as contraindicated in product information, but effect in healthy subjects was modest; monitor clinical status

Rituximab, no documented interactions, see page 4, Criteria for Listing Interactions

Rivastigmine, no documented interactions, see page 4, Criteria for Listing Interactions

Rizatriptan, see Triptans

Rocuronium bromide, no documented interactions, see page 4, Criteria for Listing Interactions

Rofecoxib, see COX-2 inhibitors

Rolitetracycline, see Tetracyclines

ROPINIROLE, with:
  Estrogens - See Estrogens with Ropinirole, page 272
  Fluoroquinolones - See Fluoroquinolones with Ropinirole, page 282
  Haloperidol - See Haloperidol with Ropinirole, page 296
  Metoclopramide - See Metoclopramide with Ropinirole, page 344
  Phenothiazines - See Phenothiazines with Ropinirole, page 385

ROPIVACAINE, with:
  Selective Serotonin Reuptake Inhibitors (SSRIs)
    Possible ropivacaine toxicity (probably decreased metabolism; CYP1A2)
      E Arlander et al, Metabolism of ropivacaine in humans is mediated by CYP1A2 and to a minor extent by CYP3A4: an interaction study with fluvoxamine and ketoconazole as in vivo inhibitors. Clin Pharmacol Ther, 64:484, 1998
    Based on study in healthy subjects; monitor clinical status

Rosiglitazone, no documented interactions, see page 4, Criteria for Listing Interactions

Rotavirus vaccine, no documented interactions, see page 4, Criteria for Listing Interactions

SAINT JOHN'S WORT, with:
   Anticoagulants, oral - See Anticoagulants, oral with Saint John's wort, page 76
   Contraceptives, oral - See Contraceptives, oral with Saint John's wort, page 217
   Cyclosporine - See Cyclosporine with Saint John's wort, page 238
   Digoxin - See Digoxin with Saint John's wort, page 257
   Indinavir - See Indinavir with Saint John's wort, page 308
   Lopinavir/Ritonavir - See Lopinavir/Ritonavir with Saint John's wort, page 329
   Narcotics: meperidine and congeners - See Narcotics: meperidine and congeners with Saint John's wort, page 357
   Nefazodone - See Nefazodone with Saint John's wort, page 362
   Selective Serotonin Reuptake Inhibitors (SSRIs)
      Possible excessive sedation (mechanism not established)
         JB Gordon, SSRIs and St. John's Wort: possible toxicity? Am Fam Physician, 57:950, 1998
      Single case report (1998)

      Possible nausea, vomiting, confusion and anxiety with sertraline and nefazodone (mechanism not established; possibly enhanced SSRI effect)
         MS Lantz et al, St. John's wort and antidepressant drug interactions in the elderly. J Geriatr Psychiatry Neurol, 12:7, 1999
      Four case reports (1999); monitor clinical status; avoid St. John's wort in patients taking SSRIs
   Theophyllines
      Possible decreased theophylline effect (mechanism not established)
         A Nebel et al, Potential metabolic interaction between St. John's wort and theophylline. Ann Pharmacother, 33:502, 1999
      Single case report (1999); monitor clinical status and theophylline concentration

Salbutamol, see Sympathomimetic bronchodilators
Salicylates, oral, see Nonsteroidal anti-inflammatory drugs
SALICYLATES, TOPICAL, with:
   Nonsteroidal anti-inflammatory drugs - See Nonsteroidal anti-inflammatory drugs with Salicylates, topical, page 374
Salmeterol, no documented interactions, see page 4, Criteria for Listing Interactions
SAMe, s-adenosyl-methionine, no documented interactions, see page 4, Criteria for Listing Interactions
SAQUINAVIR, with:
   Amprenavir - See Amprenavir with Saquinavir, page 40
   Anticoagulants, oral - See Anticoagulants, oral with Saquinavir, page 76
   Antifungals, imidazoles and triazoles - See Antifungals, imidazoles and triazoles with Saquinavir, page 107
   Antihistamines, H$_1$-blockers: astemizole, terfenadine - See Antihistamines, H$_1$-blockers: astemizole, terfenadine with Saquinavir, page 112
   Benzodiazepines - See Benzodiazepines with Saquinavir, page 148
   Cisapride - See Cisapride with Saquinavir, page 201
   Cyclosporine - See Cyclosporine with Saquinavir, page 239

SAQUINAVIR, with: *(continued)*
  Delavirdine - See Delavirdine with Saquinavir, page 245
  Efavirenz - See Efavirenz with Saquinavir, page 268
  Grapefruit juice - See Grapefruit juice with Saquinavir, page 291
  Indinavir - See Indinavir with Saquinavir, page 309
  Lopinavir/Ritonavir - See Lopinavir/Ritonavir with Saquinavir, page 329
  Nelfinavir - See Nelfinavir with Saquinavir, page 363
  Nevirapine - See Nevirapine with Saquinavir, page 367
  Paclitaxel - See Paclitaxel with Saquinavir, page 381
  Rifabutin - See Rifabutin with Saquinavir, page 404
  Rifampin - See Rifampin with Saquinavir, page 405
  Ritonavir - See Ritonavir with Saquinavir, page 409
  Sildenafil
    Possible sildenafil toxicity (probably decreased metabolism; CYP3A4)
      GJ Muirhead et al, Pharmacokinetic interactions between sildenafil and saquinavir/ritonavir. Br J Clin Pharmacol, 50:99, 2000
    Based on pharmacokinetic study of healthy subjects; avoid concurrent use
  Tacrolimus
    Possible tacrolimus toxicity (decreased metabolism; probably CYP3A4; decreased transport; probably P-glycoprotein)
      AM Sheikh et al, Concomitant human immunodeficiency virus protease inhibitor therapy markedly reduces tacrolimus metabolism and increases blood levels. Transplantation, 68:307, 1999
    Single case report (1999); monitor tacrolimus concentrations and clinical status
  Scopolamine, see Anticholinergics
  Secobarbital, see Barbiturates
SELECTIVE SEROTONIN REUPTAKE INHIBITORS (SSRIS), with:
  Anticholinergics - See Anticholinergics with Selective serotonin reuptake inhibitors (SSRIs), page 59
  Anticoagulants, oral - See Anticoagulants, oral with Selective serotonin reuptake inhibitors (SSRIs), page 76
  Antidepressants, tricyclic - See Antidepressants, tricyclic with Selective serotonin reuptake inhibitors (SSRIs), page 90
  Antifungals, imidazoles and triazoles - See Antifungals, imidazoles and triazoles with Selective serotonin reuptake inhibitors (SSRIs), page 107
  Antihistamines, H_1-blockers: astemizole, terfenadine - See Antihistamines, H_1-blockers: astemizole, terfenadine with Selective serotonin reuptake inhibitors (SSRIs), page 112
  Antihistamines, H_2-blockers - See Antihistamines, H_2-blockers with Selective serotonin reuptake inhibitors (SSRIs), page 124
  Benzodiazepines - See Benzodiazepines with Selective serotonin reuptake inhibitors (SSRIs), page 149
  Beta-adrenergic blockers - See Beta-adrenergic blockers with Selective serotonin reuptake inhibitors (SSRIs), page 161
  Bupropion - See Bupropion with Selective serotonin reuptake inhibitors (SSRIs), page 170

(continued)

SELECTIVE SEROTONIN REUPTAKE INHIBITORS (SSRIS), with: *(continued)*

Buspirone - See Buspirone with Selective serotonin reuptake inhibitors (SSRIs), page 171

Caffeine - See Caffeine with Selective serotonin reuptake inhibitors (SSRIs), page 174

Carbamazepine - See Carbamazepine with Selective serotonin reuptake inhibitors (SSRIs), page 185

Chloral hydrate - See Chloral hydrate with Selective serotonin reuptake inhibitors (SSRIs), page 192

Cisapride - See Cisapride with Selective serotonin reuptake inhibitors (SSRIs), page 201

Clozapine - See Clozapine with Selective serotonin reuptake inhibitors (SSRIs), page 207

Cyclobenzaprine - See Cyclobenzaprine with Selective serotonin reuptake inhibitors (SSRIs), page 226

Cyclosporine - See Cyclosporine with Selective serotonin reuptake inhibitors (SSRIs), page 239

Cyproheptadine - See Cyproheptadine with Selective serotonin reuptake inhibitors (SSRIs), page 241

Delavirdine - See Delavirdine with Selective serotonin reuptake inhibitors (SSRIs), page 245

Digoxin - See Digoxin with Selective serotonin reuptake inhibitors (SSRIs), page 257

Donepezil - See Donepezil with Selective serotonin reuptake inhibitors (SSRIs), page 266

Ergot alkaloids - See Ergot alkaloids with Selective serotonin reuptake inhibitors (SSRIs), page 271

Grapefruit juice - See Grapefruit juice with Selective serotonin reuptake inhibitors (SSRIs), page 291

Haloperidol - See Haloperidol with Selective serotonin reuptake inhibitors (SSRIs), page 296

Hypoglycemics, sulfonylurea - See Hypoglycemics, sulfonylurea with Selective serotonin reuptake inhibitors (SSRIs), page 305

Interferon - See Interferon with Selective serotonin reuptake inhibitors (SSRIs), page 311

Lamotrigine - See Lamotrigine with Selective serotonin reuptake inhibitors (SSRIs), page 317

Lithium - See Lithium with Selective serotonin reuptake inhibitors (SSRIs), page 326

Macrolide antibiotics - See Macrolide antibiotics with Selective serotonin reuptake inhibitors (SSRIs), page 333

Marijuana, smoking - See Marijuana, smoking with Selective serotonin reuptake inhibitors (SSRIs), page 336

Melatonin - See Melatonin with Selective serotonin reuptake inhibitors (SSRIs), page 337

SELECTIVE SEROTONIN REUPTAKE INHIBITORS (SSRIS), with: *(continued)*

Metoclopramide - See Metoclopramide with Selective serotonin reuptake inhibitors (SSRIs), page 344

Mirtazapine - See Mirtazapine with Selective serotonin reuptake inhibitors (SSRIs), page 347

Monoamine oxidase inhibitors - See Monoamine oxidase inhibitors with Selective serotonin reuptake inhibitors (SSRIs), page 350

Narcotics: dextromethorphan - See Narcotics: dextromethorphan with Selective serotonin reuptake inhibitors (SSRIs), page 355

Narcotics: methadone and congeners - See Narcotics: methadone and congeners with Selective serotonin reuptake inhibitors (SSRIs), page 359

Narcotics: pentazocine - See Narcotics: pentazocine with Selective serotonin reuptake inhibitors (SSRIs), page 361

Narcotics: tramadol - See Narcotics: tramadol with Selective serotonin reuptake inhibitors (SSRIs), page 361

Nifedipine - See Nifedipine with Selective serotonin reuptake inhibitors (SSRIs), page 369

Phenothiazines - See Phenothiazines with Selective serotonin reuptake inhibitors (SSRIs), page 385

Phenytoin - See Phenytoin with Selective serotonin reuptake inhibitors (SSRIs), page 389

Pimozide - See Pimozide with Selective serotonin reuptake inhibitors (SSRIs), page 394

Proguanil - See Proguanil with Selective serotonin reuptake inhibitors (SSRIs), page 398

Propafenone - See Propafenone with Selective serotonin reuptake inhibitors (SSRIs), page 399

Quinidine - See Quinidine with Selective serotonin reuptake inhibitors (SSRIs), page 402

Rifampin - See Rifampin with Selective serotonin reuptake inhibitors (SSRIs), page 405

Risperidone - See Risperidone with Selective serotonin reuptake inhibitors (SSRIs), page 408

Ritonavir - See Ritonavir with Selective Serotonin Reuptake Inhibitors (SSRIs), page 410

Ropivacaine - See Ropivacaine with Selective Serotonin Reuptake Inhibitors (SSRIs), page 411

Saint John's Wort - See Saint John's Wort with Selective Serotonin Reuptake Inhibitors (SSRIs), page 412

Sibutramine
Possible serotonin syndrome (additive serotonergic effect)
Manufacturer's package insert
Avoid concurrent use

Sympathomimetic amines
Increased toxicity with methylphenidate and sertraline (mechanism unknown)
DJ Feeney and WM Klykylo, Medication-induced seizures. J Am Acad Child Adolesc Psychiatry, 36:1018, 1997

(continued)

SELECTIVE SEROTONIN REUPTAKE INHIBITORS (SSRIS), with: *(continued)*
Monitor clinical status

Tacrine
Possible tacrine toxicity with fluvoxamine (decreased metabolism; CYP1A2)
> L Becquemont et al, Influence of the CYP1A2 inhibitor fluvoxamine on tacrine pharmacokinetics in humans. Clin Pharmacol Ther, 61:619, 1997; L Becquemont et al, Use of heterologously expressed human cytochrome P450 1A2 to predict tacrine-fluvoxamine drug interaction in man. Pharmacogenetics, 8:101, 1998; J Teilmann et al, Fluvoxamine is a potent inhibitor of tacrine metabolism in vivo. Eur J Clin Pharmacol, 55:375, 1999

Based on studies in healthy subjects; other selective serotonin reuptake inhibitors may be less likely to interact

Theophyllines
Theophylline toxicity with fluvoxamine (decreased metabolism)
> AD Sperber, Toxic interaction between fluvoxamine and sustained release theophylline in an 11-year-old boy. Drug Safety, 6:460, 1991; AH Thomson et al, Interaction between fluvoxamine and theophylline. Pharmaceutic J, 249:137, 1992; BB Rasmussen et al, Selective serotonin reuptake inhibitors and theophylline metabolism in human liver microsomes: potent inhibition by fluvoxamine. Br J Clin Pharmacol, 39:151, 1995; CL Devane et al, Fluvoxamine-induced theophylline toxicity. Am J Psychiatry, 154:1317, 1997; BB Rasmussen et al, Griseofulvin and fluvoxamine interactions with the metabolism of theophylline. Ther Drug Monit, 19:56, 1997

Three case reports (1991, 1992, 1997) with sustained-release theophylline; in vivo and in vitro studies show fluvoxamine is potent inhibitor of CYP1A2; a study in 12 healthy subjects found marked increase in theophylline concentrations; avoid concurrent use; a study in five normal men and women given a single dose of theophylline reported no significant clinical effect

Thyroid hormones
Possible decreased thyroxine effect with sertraline (mechanism not established)
> KC McCowen et al, Elevated serum thyrotropin in thyroxine-treated patients with hypothyroidism given sertraline. N Engl J Med, 337:1010, 1997

Monitor thyroid status

Tobacco, smoking
Possible decreased fluvoxamine effect (probably increased metabolism)
> O Spigset et al, Effect of cigarette smoking on fluvoxamine pharmacokinetics in humans. Clin Pharmacol Ther, 58:399, 1995

Monitor fluvoxamine response

Nausea after cigarette smoking with sertraline (mechanism not established)
> HB Pinkofsky et al, Serotonin, cigarettes, and nausea. J Clin Psychopharmacol, 17:492, 1997

Nausea after cigarette smoking with sertraline (mechanism not established)

Tolterodine
Possible tolterodine toxicity with fluoxetine (decreased metabolism; CYP2D6)
> Manufacturer's package insert (tolterodine); DD Short, Tolterodine, a new

SELECTIVE SEROTONIN REUPTAKE INHIBITORS (SSRIS), with: *(continued)*
> antimuscarinic drug for treatment of bladder overactivity – a comment. Pharmacotherapy, 19:1188, 1999; N Brynne et al, Fluoxetine inhibits the metabolism of tolterodine—pharmacokinetic implications and proposed clinical relevance. Br J Clin Pharmacol, 48:553, 1999
>
> *Tolterodine concentration increased; active metabolite concentration decreased; net effect usually not clinically significant*

Trazodone
> Probable trazodone toxicity with fluoxetine (probably decreased metabolism)
>> A Metz and RI Shader, Adverse interactions encountered when using trazodone to treat insomnia associated with fluoxetine. Int Clin Psychopharmacol, 5:191, 1990
>
> *Many case reports, most with increased sedation; monitor clinical response*
>
> Possible serotonin syndrome with paroxetine and trazodone (mechanism not established)
>> RR Reeves et al, Serotonin syndrome produced by aroxetine and low-dose trazodone. Psychosomatics, 36:159, 1995
>
> *Single case report (1995)*

Triptans
> Possible inhibition of sumatriptan effect (mechanism not established)
>> CP Szabo, Fluoxetine and sumatriptan: possibly a counterproductive combination. J Clin Psychiatry, 56:1, 1995; M Leung and M Ong, Lack of an interaction between sumatriptan and selective serotonin reuptake inhibitors. Headache, 35:488, 1995
>
> *Single case report (1995); study of six patients with migraine failed to confirm*
>
> Possible serotonin syndrome with sumatriptan and fluoxetine, paroxetine or sertraline (additive)
>> RT Joffe and STH Sokolov, Co-administration of fluoxetine and sumatriptan: the Canadian experience. Acta Psychiatr Scand, 95:551, 1997; NT Mathew et al, Serotonin syndrome complicating migraine pharmacotherapy. Cephalalgia, 16:323, 1996; CE Schwartz, A surfeit of serotonin: sumatriptan and serotonergic antidepressants. Arch Intern Med, 159:1141, 1999; CE Schwartz, A surfeit of serotonin: sumatriptan and serotonergic antidepressants. Arch Inern Med, 159:1141, 1999
>
> *Six cases with fluoxetine; two well documented (1997); two cases with sertraline (1996) with one patient taking other serotonergic drugs (lithium, methysergide); one case with paroxetine (1996) in patient taking other serotonergic drugs (imipramine, lithium); many patients have taken SSRIs with sumatriptan without evidence of serotonin syndrome; no clinically documented interactions have been reported with other triptans; clinical status should be monitored*

Tryptophan
> Adverse behavioral and neurological effects with fluoxetine (probably altered serotonin metabolism)
>> W Steiner and R Fontaine, Toxic reaction following the combined administration of fluoxetine and l-tryptophan: five case reports. Biol Psychiatry, 21:1067, 1986

(continued)

SELECTIVE SEROTONIN REUPTAKE INHIBITORS (SSRIS), with: *(continued)*
Avoid concurrent use

Valproate

Possible alteration in valproate effect with fluoxetine (mechanism not established)

> R Sovner and JM Davis, A potential drug interaction between fluoxetine and valproic acid. J Clin Psychopharmacol, 11:389, 1991; A Droulers et al, Decrease of valproic acid concentration in the blood when coprescribed with fluoxetine. J Clin Psychopharmacol, 17:139, 1997; Ml Lucena et al, Interaction of fluoxetine and valproic acid. Am J Psychiatry, 155:575, 1998

Two case reports of valproate toxicity, and two case reports of decreased valproate effect (1991, 1997, 1998)

Venlafaxine

Anticholinergic toxicity with fluoxetine (probably decreased metabolism; CYP2D6)

> F Benazzi, Severe anticholinergic side effects with venlafaxine-fluoxetine combination. Can J Psychiatry, 42:980, 1997; F Benazzi, Venlafaxine drug-drug interactions in clinical practice. J Psychiatry Neurosci, 23:181, 1998; F Benazzi, Venlafaxine-fluoxetine interaction. J Clin Psychopharmacol, 19:99, 1999

Several case reports; monitor clinical status

Serotonin syndrome with paroxetine or fluoxetine (additive; possible decreased metabolism)

> VS Bhatara et al, Serotonin syndrome induced by venlafaxine and fluoxetine: a case study in polypharmacy and potential pharmacodynamic and pharmacokinetic mechanisms. Ann Pharmacother, 32:432, 1998; BSH Chan et al, Serotonin syndrome resulting from drug interactions. Med J Aust, 169:523, 1998

Two case reports (1998); causal relationship not established

Verapamil

Verapamil toxicity with fluoxetine (probably decreased metabolism)

> H Sternbach, Fluoxetine-associated potentiation of calcium-channel blockers. J Clin Psychopharmacol, 11:390, 1991

Two case reports (1991)

Zolpidem

Possible zolpidem toxicity or serotonin syndrome with paroxetine, fluoxetine or sertraline (mechanism not established)

> SE Katz, Possible paroxetine-zolpidem interaction. Am J Psychiatry, 152:1689, 1995; JS Markowitz and TD Brewerton, Zolpidem-induced psychosis. Ann Clin Psychiatry, 8:89, 1996; CJ Elko et al, Zolpidem-associated hallucinations and serotonin reuptake inhibition: a possible interaction. J Toxicol Clin Toxicol, 36:195, 1998; S Allard et al, Minimal interaction between fluoxetine and multiple-dose zolpidem in healthy women. Drug Metab Dispos, 26:617, 1998; S Allard et al, coadministration of short-term zolipdem with sertraline in healthy women. J Clin Pharmacol, 39:184, 1999

SELECTIVE SEROTONIN REUPTAKE INHIBITORS (SSRIS), with: *(continued)*
    Two case reports with paroxetine (1995, 1996); two case reports with fluoxetine (1996; 1998); one case report with sertraline (1998); causal relationship not established; studies in healthy women found no significant interaction with fluoxetine (1998) or sertraline (1999)

Selegiline, see Monoamine oxidase inhibitors

Senna fruit extract, no documented interactions, see page 4, Criteria for Listing Interactions

Sermorelin, no documented interactions, see page 4, Criteria for Listing Interactions

Sertraline, see Selective serotonin reuptake inhibitors (SSRIs)

Sevoflurane, no documented interactions, see page 4, Criteria for Listing Interactions

SIBUTRAMINE, with:

    Antifungals, imidazoles and triazoles - See Antifungals, imidazoles and triazoles with Sibutramine, page 107

    Ergot alkaloids - See Ergot alkaloids with Sibutramine, page 271

    Lithium - See Lithium with Sibutramine, page 327

    Monoamine oxidase inhibitors - See Monoamine oxidase inhibitors with Sibutramine, page 351

    Narcotics: dextromethorphan - See Narcotics: dextromethorphan with Sibutramine, page 355

    Narcotics: meperidine and congeners - See Narcotics: meperidine and congeners with Sibutramine, page 357

    Selective serotonin reuptake inhibitors (SSRIs) - See Selective serotonin reuptake inhibitors (SSRIs) with Sibutramine, page 415

    Sympathomimetic amines
        Possible hypertensive reaction with ephedrine, phenylpropanolamine, pseudoephedrine (additive)
            Manufacturer's package insert
        Avoid concurrent use

    Triptans
        Possible serotonin syndrome (additive serotonergic effect)
            Manufacturer's package insert (Sibutramine)
        Avoid concurrent use

    Tryptophan
        Possible serotonin syndrome (additive serotonergic effect)
            Manufacturer's package insert
        Avoid concurrent use

SILDENAFIL, with:

    Amprenavir - See Amprenavir with Sildenafil, page 40

    Antifungals, imidazoles and triazoles - See Antifungals, imidazoles and triazoles with Sildenafil, page 107

    Antihistamines, H_2-blockers - See Antihistamines, H_2-blockers with Sildenafil, page 124

    Indinavir - See Indinavir with Sildenafil, page 309

(continued)

SILDENAFIL, with: *(continued)*
    Lopinavir/Ritonavir - See Lopinavir/Ritonavir with Sildenafil, page 329
    Macrolide antibiotics - See Macrolide antibiotics with Sildenafil, page 333
    Nitrates - See Nitrates with Sildenafil, page 370
    Ritonavir - See Ritonavir with Sildenafil, page 410
    Saquinavir - See Saquinavir with Sildenafil, page 413
    Verapamil
        Possible sildenafil toxicity (probably decreased metabolism)
            J-C Stauffer et al, Subaortic obstruction after sildenafil in a patient with hypertrophic cardiomyopathy. N Engl J Med, 341:700, 1999
        Single case report (1999); causal relationship not established; monitor clinical status

Simethicone, see Antacids

Simvastatin, see HMG-CoA Reductase Inhibitors

SIROLIMUS, with:
    Antifungals, imidazoles and triazoles - See Antifungals, imidazoles and triazoles with Sirolimus, page 107
    Cyclosporine - See Cyclosporine with Sirolimus, page 239
    Diltiazem - See Diltiazem with Sirolimus, page 261
    Grapefruit juice - See Grapefruit juice with Sirolimus, page 291
    Rifampin - See Rifampin with Sirolimus, page 406

Smoking, marijuana, see Marijuana, smoking

Smoking, tobacco, see Tobacco, smoking

Snuff, see Tobacco, smokeless

Sodium bicarbonate, see Antacids

Sodium citrate, see Citrates

Sodium phenylbutyrate, no documented interactions, see page 4, Criteria for Listing Interactions

SODIUM POLYSTYRENE SULFONATE, with:
    Antacids - See Antacids with Sodium polystyrene sulfonate, page 56
    Thyroid hormones
        Decreased thyroxine effect (decreased absorption)
            M McLean et al, Cation-exchange resin and inhibition of intestinal absorption of thyroxine. Lancet, 341:1286, 1993
        Take as far apart as possible; single case (1993)

Sodium stibogluconate, no documented interactions, see page 4, Criteria for Listing Interactions

SOMATOSTATIN, with:
    Narcotics: morphine-like - See Narcotics: morphine-like with Somatostatin, page 361

Somatropin, no documented interactions, see page 4, Criteria for Listing Interactions

SORIVUDINE, with:
    Fluorouracil - See Fluorouracil with Sorivudine, page 284

Sotalol, see Beta-adrenergic blockers

Sparfloxacin, see Fluoroquinolones

SPECTINOMYCIN, with:
   Lithium - See Lithium with Spectinomycin, page 327
SPIRAMYCIN, with:
   Levodopa - See Levodopa with Spiramycin, page 321
SPIRONOLACTONE, with:
   Angiotensin-converting enzyme (ACE) inhibitors - See Angiotensin-converting enzyme (ACE) inhibitors with Spironolactone, page 49
   Anticoagulants, oral - See Anticoagulants, oral with Spironolactone, page 77
   Cholestyramine - See Cholestyramine with Spironolactone, page 198
   Cyclopropane - See Cyclopropane with Spironolactone, page 227
   Digoxin - See Digoxin with Spironolactone, page 257
   Nonsteroidal anti-inflammatory drugs - See Nonsteroidal anti-inflammatory drugs with Spironolactone, page 374
   Potassium - See Potassium with Spironolactone, page 395
   Trimethoprim-sulfamethoxazole
      Increased risk of hyperkalemia (additive)
         MA Marinella, Severe hyperkalemia associated with trimethoprim-sulfamethoxazole and spironolactone. Infect Dis Clin Pract, 6:256, 1997
      Single case report (1997)

St John's Wort, see Saint John's Wort

Stanozolol, see Anabolic and androgenic steroids

Statin, see HMG-CoA reductase inhibitors

STAVUDINE, with:
   Didanosine - See Didanosine with Stavudine, page 249
   Isoniazid - See Isoniazid with Stavudine, page 313
   Narcotics: methadone and congeners - See Narcotics: methadone and congeners with Stavudine, page 359
   Sympathomimetic amines
      Possible hypertensive crisis (mechanism not established)
         V Khurana et al, Hypertensive crisis secondary to phenylpropanolamine interacting with triple-drug therapy for HIV prophylaxis. Am J Med, 106:118, 1999
      Single case report (1999); patient suffered from Raynaud's phenomenon and also taking indinavir and lamivudine
   Zidovudine
      Antagonistic in vitro and in vivo
         DV Havlir et al, Combination zidovudine (ZDV) and stavudine (d4T) therapy versus other nucleosides: Report of two randomized trials (ACTG 290 and 298). Conf Retrovir Opportun Infect, 5:79, 1998, abstract 2
      Avoid concurrent use

STIRIPENTOL, with:
   Carbamazepine - See Carbamazepine with Stiripentol, page 185

Streptokinase, see Thrombolytics

Streptomycin, see Aminoglycoside antibiotics

STREPTOZOCIN, with:
   Doxorubicin - See Doxorubicin with Streptozocin, page 266

(continued)

STREPTOZOCIN, with: *(continued)*
  Phenytoin - See Phenytoin with Streptozocin, page 390
Succimer, no documented interactions, see page 4, Criteria for Listing Interactions
Succinylcholine, see Neuromuscular blocking agents
SUCRALFATE, with:
  Anagrelide - See Anagrelide with Sucralfate, page 42
  Anticoagulants, oral - See Anticoagulants, oral with Sucralfate, page 77
  Antifungals, imidazoles and triazoles - See Antifungals, imidazoles and triazoles with Sucralfate, page 107
  Antihistamines, H_2-blockers - See Antihistamines, H_2-blockers with Sucralfate, page 124
  Digoxin - See Digoxin with Sucralfate, page 258
  Fluoroquinolones - See Fluoroquinolones with Sucralfate, page 282
  Lansoprazole - See Lansoprazole with Sucralfate, page 318
  Nonsteroidal anti-inflammatory drugs - See Nonsteroidal anti-inflammatory drugs with Sucralfate, page 374
  Phenytoin - See Phenytoin with Sucralfate, page 390
  Thyroid hormones
    Possible decrease in levothyroxine effect (decreased absorption)
      SI Sherman et al, Sucralfate causes malabsorption of l-thyroxine. Am J Med, 96:531, 1994; JA Campbell et al, Sucralfate and the absorption of L-thyroxine. Ann Intern Med, 121:152, 1994
    Conflicting data; may only occur in some patients; take thyroid at least 2 hours before or 6 hours after sucralfate
Sufentanil, no documented interactions, see page 4, Criteria for Listing Interactions
Sulconazole, no documented interactions, see page 4, Criteria for Listing Interactions
Sulfacetamide, see Sulfonamides
Sulfacytine, see Sulfonamides
Sulfadiazine, see Sulfonamides
Sulfameter, see Sulfonamides
Sulfamethazine, see Sulfonamides
Sulfamethizole, see Sulfonamides
Sulfamethoxazole, see Sulfonamides
Sulfanilamide, no documented interactions, see page 4, Criteria for Listing Interactions
Sulfasalazine, see Sulfonamides
SULFINPYRAZONE, with:
  Acetaminophen - See Acetaminophen with Sulfinpyrazone, page 9
  Anticoagulants, oral - See Anticoagulants, oral with Sulfinpyrazone, page 78
  Beta-adrenergic blockers - See Beta-adrenergic blockers with Sulfinpyrazone, page 162
  Mycophenolate mofetil - See Mycophenolate mofetil with Sulfinpyrazone, page 354
  Nonsteroidal anti-inflammatory drugs - See Nonsteroidal anti-inflammatory drugs with Sulfinpyrazone, page 374

SULFINPYRAZONE, with: *(continued)*
  Verapamil
    Possible decreased verapamil effect (probably increased metabolism)
      LMH Wing et al, Verapamil disposition – effects of sulphinpyrazone and cimetidine. Br J Clin Pharmacol, 19:385, 1985
    Monitor cardiovascular status
Sulfisoxazole, see Sulfonamides
SULFONAMIDES, with:
  Anticoagulants, oral - See Anticoagulants, oral with Sulfonamides, page 78
  Azathioprine - See Azathioprine with Sulfonamides, page 130
  Barbiturates - See Barbiturates with Sulfonamides, page 136
  Cyclosporine - See Cyclosporine with Sulfonamides, page 239
  Digoxin - See Digoxin with Sulfonamides, page 258
  Hypoglycemics, sulfonylurea - See Hypoglycemics, sulfonylurea with Sulfonamides, page 305
  Mercaptopurine - See Mercaptopurine with Sulfonamides, page 338
  Methotrexate - See Methotrexate with Sulfonamides, page 341
  Monoamine oxidase inhibitors - See Monoamine oxidase inhibitors with Sulfonamides, page 351
  Phenytoin - See Phenytoin with Sulfonamides, page 390
Sulindac, see Nonsteroidal anti-inflammatory drugs
Sulphadimidine, see Sulfonamides
SULPROSTONE, with:
  Acetaminophen - See Acetaminophen with Sulprostone, page 10
Sumatriptan, see Triptans
Suprofen, no documented interactions, see page 4, Criteria for Listing Interactions
Suxamethonium, see Neuromuscular blocking agents
SYMPATHOMIMETIC AMINES, with:
  Antacids - See Antacids with Sympathomimetic amines, page 56
  Anticholinergics - See Anticholinergics with Sympathomimetic amines, page 59
  Anticoagulants, oral - See Anticoagulants, oral with Sympathomimetic amines, page 78
  Antidepressants, tricyclic - See Antidepressants, tricyclic with Sympathomimetic amines, page 91
  Antihistamines, H_2-blockers - See Antihistamines, H_2-blockers with Sympathomimetic amines, page 124
  Barbiturates - See Barbiturates with Sympathomimetic amines, page 136
  Beta-adrenergic blockers - See Beta-adrenergic blockers with Sympathomimetic amines, page 162
  Bethanidine - See Bethanidine with Sympathomimetic amines, page 165
  Bretylium - See Bretylium with Sympathomimetic amines, page 166
  Bromocriptine - See Bromocriptine with Sympathomimetic amines, page 167
  Caffeine - See Caffeine with Sympathomimetic amines, page 174
  Carbamazepine - See Carbamazepine with Sympathomimetic amines, page 185
  Carbonic anhydrase inhibitors - See Carbonic anhydrase inhibitors with Sympathomimetic amines, page 189

(continued)

SYMPATHOMIMETIC AMINES, with: *(continued)*
- **Clonidine** - See Clonidine with Sympathomimetic amines, page 205
- **Cocaine** - See Cocaine with Sympathomimetic amines, page 210
- **Corticosteroids** - See Corticosteroids with Sympathomimetic amines, page 224
- **Cyclopropane** - See Cyclopropane with Sympathomimetic amines, page 227
- **Debrisoquine** - See Debrisoquine with Sympathomimetic amines, page 243
- **Desflurane** - See Desflurane with Sympathomimetic amines, page 245
- **Digoxin** - See Digoxin with Sympathomimetic amines, page 258
- **Entacapone** - See Entacapone with Sympathomimetic amines, page 269
- **Ergot alkaloids** - See Ergot alkaloids with Sympathomimetic amines, page 271
- **Furosemide** - See Furosemide with Sympathomimetic amines, page 286
- **Guanadrel** - See Guanadrel with Sympathomimetic amines, page 292
- **Guanethidine** - See Guanethidine with Sympathomimetic amines, page 292
- **Halothane** - See Halothane with Sympathomimetic amines, page 297
- **Insulin** - See Insulin with Sympathomimetic amines, page 310
- **Linezolid** - See Linezolid with Sympathomimetic amines, page 323
- **Mazindol** - See Mazindol with Sympathomimetic amines, page 336
- **Midodrine** - See Midodrine with Sympathomimetic amines, page 346
- **Monoamine oxidase inhibitors** - See Monoamine oxidase inhibitors with Sympathomimetic amines, page 351
- **Phenytoin** - See Phenytoin with Sympathomimetic amines, page 390
- **Pilocarpine** - See Pilocarpine with Sympathomimetic amines, page 393
- **Primidone** - See Primidone with Sympathomimetic amines, page 396
- **Selective serotonin reuptake inhibitors (SSRIs)** - See Selective serotonin reuptake inhibitors (SSRIs) with Sympathomimetic amines, page 415
- **Sibutramine** - See Sibutramine with Sympathomimetic amines, page 419
- **Stavudine** - See Stavudine with Sympathomimetic amines, page 421
- **Theophyllines**

    Arrhythmias and myocardial infarction (mechanism not established)
    A Szczeklik et al, Myocardial infarction in status asthmaticus. Lancet, 1:658, 1977; GW Josephson et al, Cardiac dysrhythmias during the treatment of acute asthma. Chest, 78:429, 1980; G Kurland et al, Fatal myocardial toxicity during continuous infusion intravenous isoproterenol therapy of asthma. J Allergy Clin Immunol, 63:407, 1979
    Monitor cardiac status

    Possible decreased theophylline effect with isoproterenol (possibly increased metabolism)
    PP O'Rourke and RH Crone, Effect of isoproterenol on measured theophylline levels. Crit Care Med, 12:373, 1984
    Monitor theophylline concentration

- **Thiazide diuretics**

    Hypokalemia with epinephrine (intracellular uptake of potassium)
    JG Meechan and MD Rawlins, The effects of two different local anaesthetic solutions administered for oral surgery on plasma potassium levels in patients taking kaliuretic diuretics. Eur J Clin Pharmacol, 42:155, 1992

SYMPATHOMIMETIC AMINES, with: *(continued)*
Occurs with local anesthesia for oral surgery; use local anesthetic, such as prilocaine, without epinephrine

Tolazoline
Severe hypotension with dopamine (unopposed beta-adrenergic stimulation)
> GC Carlon, Fatal association of tolazoline and dopamine. Chest, 76:336, 1979

Single case report (1979)

Valproate
Possible increased risk of dyskinesia with methylphenidate (mechanism not established)
> L Gara and W Roberts, Adverse response to methylphenidate in combination with valproic acid. J Child Adolesc Psychopharmacol, 10:39, 2000

Based on two case reports (2000); monitor clinical status

SYMPATHOMIMETIC BRONCHODILATORS, with:

Beta-adrenergic blockers - See Beta-adrenergic blockers with Sympathomimetic bronchodilators, page 163

Corticosteroids - See Corticosteroids with Sympathomimetic bronchodilators, page 224

Digoxin - See Digoxin with Sympathomimetic bronchodilators, page 258

Entacapone - See Entacapone with Sympathomimetic bronchodilators, page 270

Furosemide - See Furosemide with Sympathomimetic bronchodilators, page 287

Halothane - See Halothane with Sympathomimetic bronchodilators, page 297

Monoamine oxidase inhibitors - See Monoamine oxidase inhibitors with Sympathomimetic bronchodilators, page 351

Neuromuscular blocking agents - See Neuromuscular blocking agents with Sympathomimetic bronchodilators, page 366

Theophyllines
Possible decreased theophylline effect with terbutaline or albuterol (increased metabolism)
> M Garty et al, Increased theophylline clearance in asthmatic patients due to terbutaline. Eur J Clin Pharmacol, 36:25, 1989; Y Amitai et al, Enhancement of theophylline clearance by oral albuterol. Chest, 102:786, 1992

Monitor theophylline concentration

Hypokalemia with terbutaline or salbutamol and mild hyperglycemia with IV terbutaline (mechanism not established)
> KP Dawson and DM Fergusson, Effects of oral theophylline and oral salbutamol in the treatment of asthma. Arch Dis Child, 57:674, 1982; SR Smith and MJ Kendall, Potentiation of the adverse effects of intravenous terbutaline by oral theophylline. Br J Clin Pharmacol, 21:451, 1986; KF Whyte et al, Salbutamol induced hypokalaemia: the effect of theophylline alone and in combination with adrenaline. Br J Clin Pharmacol, 25:571, 1988

Monitor potassium and glucose concentrations

Possible cardiovascular toxicity with inhaled fenoterol (mechanism not established)
> A Flatt et al, The cardiovascular effects of inhaled fenoterol alone and

(continued)

SYMPATHOMIMETIC BRONCHODILATORS, with: *(continued)*
    during treatment with oral theophylline. Chest, 96:1317, 1989
  Based on study in healthy subjects; monitor cardiovascular status
  Thiazide diuretics
    Possible cardiovascular toxicity with bendroflumethiazide and albuterol (decreased potassium)
      BJ Lipworth et al, Prior treatment with diuretic augments the hypokalemic and electrocardiographic effects of inhaled albuterol. Am J Med, 86:653, 1989
    Monitor potassium and cardiovascular status

TACRINE, with:
  Antihistamines, H_2-blockers - See Antihistamines, H_2-blockers with Tacrine, page 125
  Estrogens - See Estrogens with Tacrine, page 273
  Haloperidol - See Haloperidol with Tacrine, page 297
  Selective serotonin reuptake inhibitors (SSRIs) - See Selective serotonin reuptake inhibitors (SSRIs) with Tacrine, page 416
  Theophyllines
    Possible theophylline toxicity (decreased metabolism)
      Manufacturer's package insert
    Monitor theophylline concentration

TACROLIMUS, with:
  Anabolic and androgenic steroids - See Anabolic and androgenic steroids with Tacrolimus, page 42
  Antifungals, imidazoles and triazoles - See Antifungals, imidazoles and triazoles with Tacrolimus, page 107
  Chloramphenicol - See Chloramphenicol with Tacrolimus, page 193
  Cyclosporine - See Cyclosporine with Tacrolimus, page 240
  Diltiazem - See Diltiazem with Tacrolimus, page 262
  Lopinavir/Ritonavir - See Lopinavir/Ritonavir with Tacrolimus, page 330
  Macrolide antibiotics - See Macrolide antibiotics with Tacrolimus, page 333
  Metronidazole - See Metronidazole with Tacrolimus, page 345
  Mycophenolate mofetil - See Mycophenolate mofetil with Tacrolimus, page 354
  Nefazodone - See Nefazodone with Tacrolimus, page 362
  Nelfinavir - See Nelfinavir with Tacrolimus, page 363
  Nifedipine - See Nifedipine with Tacrolimus, page 369
  Phenytoin - See Phenytoin with Tacrolimus, page 390
  Rifampin - See Rifampin with Tacrolimus, page 406
  Ritonavir - See Ritonavir with Tacrolimus, page 410
  Saquinavir - See Saquinavir with Tacrolimus, page 413
  Theophyllines
    Possible tacrolimus toxicity (mechanism not established)
      S Boubenider et al, Interaction between theophylline and tacrolimus in a renal transplant patient. Nephrol Dial Transplant, 15:1066, 2000
    Single well-documented case report (2000); monitor tacrolimus serum concentrations and clinical status

Talbutal, see Barbiturates

Talinolol, see Beta-adrenergic blockers
TAMOXIFEN, with:
   Aminoglutethimide - See Aminoglutethimide with Tamoxifen, page 29
   Anticoagulants, oral - See Anticoagulants, oral with Tamoxifen, page 78
   Antidepressants, tricyclic - See Antidepressants, tricyclic with Tamoxifen, page 92
   Digitoxin - See Digitoxin with Tamoxifen, page 251
   Etoposide - See Etoposide with Tamoxifen, page 275
   Fluoride - See Fluoride with Tamoxifen, page 278
   Mitomycin C - See Mitomycin C with Tamoxifen, page 348
   Neuromuscular blocking agents - See Neuromuscular blocking agents with Tamoxifen, page 366
   Rifampin - See Rifampin with Tamoxifen, page 406
TAMSULOSIN, with:
   Antihistamines, H_2-blockers - See Antihistamines, H_2-blockers with Tamsulosin, page 125

Tazarotene, no documented interactions, see page 4, Criteria for Listing Interactions

TELMISARTAN, with:
   Digoxin - See Digoxin with Telmisartan, page 258

Temafloxacin, see Fluoroquinolones

Temazepam, see Benzodiazepines

Temozolomide, no documented interactions, see page 4, Criteria for Listing Interactions

TENIPOSIDE, with:
   Barbiturates - See Barbiturates with Teniposide, page 137
   Carbamazepine - See Carbamazepine with Teniposide, page 186
   Phenytoin - See Phenytoin with Teniposide, page 390
   Vincristine
     Increased incidence of peripheral neuropathy (mechanism not established)
       JD Griffiths et al, Vincristine neurotoxicity enhanced in combination chemotherapy including both teniposide and vincristine. Cancer Treat Rep, 70:519, 1986
     Monitor clinical status

Tenoxicam, see Nonsteroidal anti-inflammatory drugs

TERAZOSIN, with:
   Finasteride - See Finasteride with Terazosin, page 277

Terbinafine, see Antifungals, terbinafine

Terbutaline, see Sympathomimetic bronchodilators

Terconazole, no documented interactions, see page 4, Criteria for Listing Interactions

Terfenadine, see Antihistamines, H_1-blockers: Astemizole, terfenadine

Testolactone, see Anabolic and androgenic steroids

Testosterone, see Anabolic and androgenic steroids

TETRACYCLINES, with:
   Acitretin - See Acitretin with Tetracyclines, page 11

(continued)

TETRACYCLINES, with: *(continued)*
   Alcohol - See Alcohol with Tetracyclines, page 22
   Antacids - See Antacids with Tetracyclines, page 56
   Anticoagulants, oral - See Anticoagulants, oral with Tetracyclines, page 78
   Antidepressants, tricyclic - See Antidepressants, tricyclic with Tetracyclines, page 92
   Antiseptics, mercurial - See Antiseptics, mercurial with Tetracyclines, page 127
   Atovaquone - See Atovaquone with Tetracyclines, page 129
   Barbiturates - See Barbiturates with Tetracyclines, page 137
   Bismuth subsalicylate - See Bismuth subsalicylate with Tetracyclines, page 166
   Carbamazepine - See Carbamazepine with Tetracyclines, page 186
   Contraceptives, oral - See Contraceptives, oral with Tetracyclines, page 217
   Digoxin - See Digoxin with Tetracyclines, page 258
   Iron - See Iron with Tetracyclines, page 312
   Isotretinoin - See Isotretinoin with Tetracyclines, page 315
   Kaolin or Kaolin-pectin - See Kaolin or Kaolin-pectin with Tetracyclines, page 316
   Lithium - See Lithium with Tetracyclines, page 327
   Methotrexate - See Methotrexate with Tetracyclines, page 341
   Molindone - See Molindone with Tetracyclines, page 348
   Phenformin - See Phenformin with Tetracyclines, page 384
   Phenytoin - See Phenytoin with Tetracyclines, page 391
   Rifampin - See Rifampin with Tetracyclines, page 406
   Risperidone - See Risperidone with Tetracyclines, page 408
   Theophyllines
      Possible theophylline toxicity (mechanism not established)
         JS Seggev et al, Serum theophylline concentrations are not affected by co-administration of doxycycline. Ann Allergy, 56:156, 1986; JP McCormack et al, Theophylline toxicity induced by tetracycline. Clin Pharm, 9:546, 1990
      Monitor theophylline concentration; small number of subjects with large individual variation
   Zinc
      Decreased tetracycline effect (decreased absorption)
         O Penttila et al, Effect of zinc sulfate on the absorption of tetracycline and doxycycline in man. Eur J Clin Pharmacol, 9:131, 1975; K-E Andersson et al, Inhibition of tetracycline absorption by zinc. Eur J Clin Pharmacol, 10:59, 1976
      Avoid concurrent use or give as far apart as possible
Thalidomide, no documented interactions, see page 4, Criteria for Listing Interactions
THEOPHYLLINES, with:
   Acyclovir - See Acyclovir with Theophyllines, page 11
   Adenosine - See Adenosine with Theophyllines, page 12
   Allopurinol - See Allopurinol with Theophyllines, page 25
   Aminoglutethimide - See Aminoglutethimide with Theophyllines, page 29
   Amiodarone - See Amiodarone with Theophyllines, page 37
   Antacids - See Antacids with Theophyllines, page 56

THEOPHYLLINES, with: *(continued)*
- **Antifungals, Griseofulvin** - See Antifungals, Griseofulvin with Theophyllines, page 95
- **Antifungals, imidazoles and triazoles** - See Antifungals, imidazoles and triazoles with Theophyllines, page 108
- **Antihistamines, H$_2$-blockers** - See Antihistamines, H$_2$-blockers with Theophyllines, page 125
- **Auranofin** - See Auranofin with Theophyllines, page 129
- **Barbiturates** - See Barbiturates with Theophyllines, page 137
- **Benzodiazepines** - See Benzodiazepines with Theophyllines, page 150
- **Beta-adrenergic blockers** - See Beta-adrenergic blockers with Theophyllines, page 163
- **Bupropion** - See Bupropion with Theophyllines, page 170
- **Caffeine** - See Caffeine with Theophyllines, page 174
- **Carbamazepine** - See Carbamazepine with Theophyllines, page 186
- **Contraceptives, oral** - See Contraceptives, oral with Theophyllines, page 217
- **Corticosteroids** - See Corticosteroids with Theophyllines, page 224
- **Diltiazem** - See Diltiazem with Theophyllines, page 262
- **Disulfiram** - See Disulfiram with Theophyllines, page 264
- **Fluoroquinolones** - See Fluoroquinolones with Theophyllines, page 282
- **Furosemide** - See Furosemide with Theophyllines, page 287
- **Grapefruit juice** - See Grapefruit juice with Theophyllines, page 291
- **Halothane** - See Halothane with Theophyllines, page 298
- **Imipenem** - See Imipenem with Theophyllines, page 306
- **Influenza vaccine** - See Influenza vaccine with Theophyllines, page 309
- **Interferon** - See Interferon with Theophyllines, page 311
- **Isoniazid** - See Isoniazid with Theophyllines, page 314
- **Lansoprazole** - See Lansoprazole with Theophyllines, page 318
- **Lithium** - See Lithium with Theophyllines, page 327
- **Macrolide antibiotics** - See Macrolide antibiotics with Theophyllines, page 333
- **Marijuana, smoking** - See Marijuana, smoking with Theophyllines, page 336
- **Methotrexate** - See Methotrexate with Theophyllines, page 341
- **Mexiletine** - See Mexiletine with Theophyllines, page 346
- **Moricizine** - See Moricizine with Theophyllines, page 353
- **Neuromuscular blocking agents** - See Neuromuscular blocking agents with Theophyllines, page 366
- **Nifedipine** - See Nifedipine with Theophyllines, page 369
- **Nutrients, enteral preparations** - See Nutrients, enteral preparations with Theophyllines, page 377
- **Pentoxifylline** - See Pentoxifylline with Theophyllines, page 383
- **Phenytoin** - See Phenytoin with Theophyllines, page 391
- **Probenecid** - See Probenecid with Theophyllines, page 397
- **Propafenone** - See Propafenone with Theophyllines, page 399
- **Pyrantel pamoate** - See Pyrantel pamoate with Theophyllines, page 400
- **Rifampin** - See Rifampin with Theophyllines, page 406
- **Ritonavir** - See Ritonavir with Theophyllines, page 410

(continued)

THEOPHYLLINES, with: *(continued)*

Saint John's wort - See Saint John's wort with Theophyllines, page 412

Selective serotonin reuptake inhibitors (SSRIs) - See Selective serotonin reuptake inhibitors (SSRIs) with Theophyllines, page 416

Sympathomimetic amines - See Sympathomimetic amines with Theophyllines, page 424

Sympathomimetic bronchodilators - See Sympathomimetic bronchodilators with Theophyllines, page 425

Tacrine - See Tacrine with Theophyllines, page 426

Tacrolimus - See Tacrolimus with Theophyllines, page 426

Tetracyclines - See Tetracyclines with Theophyllines, page 428

Thiabendazole

Theophylline toxicity (decreased metabolism)

D Schneider et al, Theophylline and antiparasitic drug interactions: A case report and study of the influence of thiabendazole and mebendazole on theophylline pharmacokinetics in adults. Chest, 97:84, 1990

Avoid concurrent use, if possible

Ticlopidine

Possible theophylline toxicity (decreased metabolism)

A Colli et al, Ticlopidine-theophylline interaction. Clin Pharmacol Ther, 41:358, 1987

Monitor theophylline concentration; based on study in 10 healthy men

Tobacco, smokeless

Decreased theophylline effect (increased metabolism)

R Rockwood and N Henann, Smokeless tobacco and theophylline clearance. Drug Intell Clin Pharm, 20:624, 1986

Monitor theophylline concentration

Tobacco, smoking

Decreased theophylline effect (increased metabolism)

S Samaan and R Fox, The effect of smoking on theophylline kinetics in healthy and asthmatic elderly males. J Clin Pharmacol, 29:448, 1989; SK Matsunga et al, Effects of passive smoking on theophylline clearance. Clin Pharmacol Ther, 46:399, 1989; S Zevin and NL Benowitz, Drug interactions with tobacco smoking. Clin Pharmacokinet, 36:425, 1999

Monitor theophylline concentration; effect may not occur in men more than 65 years old; passive smoking can have a similar effect

Troleandomycin

Theophylline toxicity (decreased metabolism)

M Weinberger et al, Inhibition of theophylline clearance by troleandomycin. J Allergy Clin Immunol, 59:228, 1977; AK Kamada et al, Effect of low-dose troleandomycin on theophylline clearance: implications for therapeutic drug monitoring. Pharmacotherapy, 12:98, 1992

Monitor theophylline concentration

Verapamil

Possible theophylline toxicity (decreased metabolism)

JE Nielsen-Kudsk et al, Verapamil-induced inhibition of theophylline elimination in healthy humans. Pharmacol Toxicol, 66:101, 1990; KA Stringer et

THEOPHYLLINES, with: *(continued)*
>al, The effect of three different oral doses of verapamil on the disposition of theophylline. Eur J Clin Pharmacol, 43:35, 1992; L Bangura et al, Theophylline and verapamil: clinically significant drug interaction. J Pharm Technol, 13:241, 1997

>*Based on pharmacokinetic studies and isolated case reports; probably occurs rarely at usual doses*

>**Vidarabine**
>>Possible theophylline toxicity (decreased metabolism)
>>>R Gannon et al, Possible interaction between vidarabine and theophylline. Ann Intern Med, 101:148, 1984
>>
>>*Well-documented case report (1984); monitor theophylline concentration*

>**Zafirlukast**
>>Possible decreased zafirlukast effect (increased metabolism, CYP3A1)
>>>Manufacturer's package insert
>>
>>*Avoid concurrent use if zafirlukast concentration can not be monitored*
>>
>>Possible theophylline toxicity (probably decreased metabolism)
>>>RK Katial et al, A drug interaction between zafirlukast and theophylline. Arch Intern Med, 158:1713, 1998
>>
>>*Single case report with positive rechallenge (1998)*

>**Zileuton**
>>Possible theophylline toxicity (decreased metabolism)
>>>GR Granneman et al, Effect of zileuton on theophylline pharmacokinetics. Clin Pharmacokinet, 29 suppl 2:77, 1995
>>
>>*Monitor theophylline concentration*

THIABENDAZOLE, with:
>**Anticoagulants, oral** - See Anticoagulants, oral with Thiabendazole, page 78
>**Theophyllines** - See Theophyllines with Thiabendazole, page 430

Thiamylol, see Barbiturates

THIAZIDE DIURETICS, with:
>**Allopurinol** - See Allopurinol with Thiazide diuretics, page 26
>**Amantadine** - See Amantadine with Thiazide diuretics, page 27
>**Amiloride** - See Amiloride with Thiazide diuretics, page 28
>**Aminoglutethimide** - See Aminoglutethimide with Thiazide diuretics, page 29
>**Angiotensin-converting enzyme (ACE) inhibitors** - See Angiotensin-converting enzyme (ACE) inhibitors with Thiazide diuretics, page 49
>**Antacids** - See Antacids with Thiazide diuretics, page 56
>**Beta-adrenergic blockers** - See Beta-adrenergic blockers with Thiazide diuretics, page 163
>**Carbamazepine** - See Carbamazepine with Thiazide diuretics, page 186
>**Cholestyramine** - See Cholestyramine with Thiazide diuretics, page 198
>**Clofibrate** - See Clofibrate with Thiazide diuretics, page 204
>**Colestipol** - See Colestipol with Thiazide diuretics, page 212
>**Corticosteroids** - See Corticosteroids with Thiazide diuretics, page 224
>**COX-2 inhibitors** - See COX-2 inhibitors with Thiazide diuretics, page 226

(continued)

THIAZIDE DIURETICS, with: *(continued)*
  Cyclosporine - See Cyclosporine with Thiazide diuretics, page 240
  Diazoxide - See Diazoxide with Thiazide diuretics, page 247
  Digitoxin - See Digitoxin with Thiazide diuretics, page 251
  Digoxin - See Digoxin with Thiazide diuretics, page 258
  Glycyrrhiza - See Glycyrrhiza with Thiazide diuretics, page 289
  Hypoglycemics, sulfonylurea - See Hypoglycemics, sulfonylurea with Thiazide diuretics, page 306
  Lithium - See Lithium with Thiazide diuretics, page 327
  Methyldopa - See Methyldopa with Thiazide diuretics, page 343
  Neuromuscular blocking agents - See Neuromuscular blocking agents with Thiazide diuretics, page 366
  Nonsteroidal anti-inflammatory drugs - See Nonsteroidal anti-inflammatory drugs with Thiazide diuretics, page 375
  Sympathomimetic amines - See Sympathomimetic amines with Thiazide diuretics, page 424
  Sympathomimetic bronchodilators - See Sympathomimetic bronchodilators with Thiazide diuretics, page 426
  Trimethoprim
    Trimethoprim may potentiate hyponatremia caused by concomitant use of amiloride with thiazide diuretics (additive)

      R Eastell and CJ Edmonds, Hyponatraemia associated with trimethoprim and a diuretic. Br Med J, 289:1658, 1984; TL Hart et al, Hyponatremia secondary to thiazide – trimethoprim interaction. Can J Hosp Pharm, 42:243, 1989
    Monitor serum sodium

Thiethylperazine, see Phenothiazines
Thimerosal, see Antiseptics, mercurial
THIOGUANINE, with:
  Alkylating agents - See Alkylating agents with Thioguanine, page 24
Thiopental, see Barbiturates
Thiopentone, see Barbiturates
Thioridazine, see Phenothiazines
Thiotepa, see Alkylating agents
Thiothixene, see Phenothiazines
3TC, see Lamivudine
THROMBOLYTICS, with:
  Eptifibatide - See Eptifibatide with Thrombolytics, page 270
  Nonsteroidal anti-inflammatory drugs - See Nonsteroidal anti-inflammatory drugs with Thrombolytics, page 375
  Pentosan - See Pentosan with Thrombolytics, page 383
THYROID HORMONES, with:
  Amiodarone - See Amiodarone with Thyroid hormones, page 37
  Antacids - See Antacids with Thyroid hormones, page 57
  Anticoagulants, oral - See Anticoagulants, oral with Thyroid hormones, page 79
  Beta-adrenergic blockers - See Beta-adrenergic blockers with Thyroid hormones, page 163

THYROID HORMONES, with: *(continued)*
   Calcium - See Calcium with Thyroid hormones, page 175
   Chloroquine - See Chloroquine with Thyroid hormones, page 195
   Cholestyramine - See Cholestyramine with Thyroid hormones, page 198
   HMG-CoA reductase inhibitors - See HMG-CoA reductase inhibitors with Thyroid hormones, page 302
   Iron - See Iron with Thyroid hormones, page 312
   Phenytoin - See Phenytoin with Thyroid hormones, page 391
   Rifampin - See Rifampin with Thyroid hormones, page 407
   Ritonavir - See Ritonavir with Thyroid Hormones, page 411
   Selective serotonin reuptake inhibitors (SSRIs) - See Selective serotonin reuptake inhibitors (SSRIs) with Thyroid hormones, page 416
   Sodium polystyrene sulfonate - See Sodium polystyrene sulfonate with Thyroid hormones, page 420
   Sucralfate - See Sucralfate with Thyroid hormones, page 422
Thyroxine, see Thyroid hormones
TIAGABINE, with:
   Barbiturates - See Barbiturates with Tiagabine, page 137
   Carbamazepine - See Carbamazepine with Tiagabine, page 186
   Phenytoin - See Phenytoin with Tiagabine, page 391
   Primidone - See Primidone with Tiagabine, page 396
Ticarcillin, see Penicillins
TICLOPIDINE, with:
   Antacids - See Antacids with Ticlopidine, page 57
   Anticoagulants, oral - See Anticoagulants, oral with Ticlopidine, page 79
   Antihistamines, H_2-blockers - See Antihistamines, H_2-blockers with Ticlopidine, page 126
   Carbamazepine - See Carbamazepine with Ticlopidine, page 186
   Cyclosporine - See Cyclosporine with Ticlopidine, page 240
   Phenytoin - See Phenytoin with Ticlopidine, page 391
   Theophyllines - See Theophyllines with Ticlopidine, page 430
TILUDRONATE, with:
   Antacids - See Antacids with Tiludronate, page 57
   Nonsteroidal anti-inflammatory drugs - See Nonsteroidal anti-inflammatory drugs with Tiludronate, page 375
Timolol, see Beta-adrenergic blockers
Tioconazole, no documented interactions, see page 4, Criteria for Listing Interactions
Tiopronin, no documented interactions, see page 4, Criteria for Listing Interactions
TIROFIBAN, with:
   Heparins - See Heparins with Tirofiban, page 299
   Nonsteroidal anti-inflammatory drugs - See Nonsteroidal anti-inflammatory drugs with Tirofiban, page 376
TIZANIDINE, with:
   Alcohol - See Alcohol with Tizanidine, page 22
   Contraceptives, oral - See Contraceptives, oral with Tizanidine, page 218

(continued)

TIZANIDINE, with: *(continued)*
  Phenytoin - See Phenytoin with Tizanidine, page 392
TOBACCO, SMOKELESS, with:
  Theophyllines - See Theophyllines with Tobacco, smokeless, page 430
TOBACCO, SMOKING, with:
  Acetaminophen - See Acetaminophen with Tobacco, smoking, page 10
  Antidepressants, tricyclic - See Antidepressants, tricyclic with Tobacco, smoking, page 92
  Beta-adrenergic blockers - See Beta-adrenergic blockers with Tobacco, smoking, page 164
  Clozapine - See Clozapine with Tobacco, smoking, page 209
  Estrogens - See Estrogens with Tobacco, smoking, page 273
  Haloperidol - See Haloperidol with Tobacco, smoking, page 297
  Insulin - See Insulin with Tobacco, smoking, page 310
  Mexiletine - See Mexiletine with Tobacco, smoking, page 346
  Pentoxifylline - See Pentoxifylline with Tobacco, smoking, page 383
  Phenylbutazone - See Phenylbutazone with Tobacco, smoking, page 387
  Selective serotonin reuptake inhibitors (SSRIs) - See Selective serotonin reuptake inhibitors (SSRIs) with Tobacco, smoking, page 416
  Theophyllines - See Theophyllines with Tobacco, smoking, page 430
Tobramycin, see Aminoglycoside antibiotics
TOCAINIDE, with:
  Antihistamines, H$_2$-blockers - See Antihistamines, H$_2$-blockers with Tocainide, page 126
  Beta-adrenergic blockers - See Beta-adrenergic blockers with Tocainide, page 164
  Lidocaine - See Lidocaine with Tocainide, page 322
  Rifampin - See Rifampin with Tocainide, page 407
Tolazamide, see Hypoglycemics, sulfonylurea
TOLAZOLINE, with:
  Antihistamines, H$_2$-blockers - See Antihistamines, H$_2$-blockers with Tolazoline, page 126
  Clonidine - See Clonidine with Tolazoline, page 205
  Sympathomimetic amines - See Sympathomimetic amines with Tolazoline, page 425
Tolbutamide, see Hypoglycemics, sulfonylurea
TOLCAPONE, with:
  Monoamine oxidase inhibitors - See Monoamine oxidase inhibitors with Tolcapone, page 352
Tolmetin, see Nonsteroidal anti-inflammatory drugs
Tolnaftate, no documented interactions, see page 4, Criteria for Listing Interactions
TOLTERODINE, with:
  Anticoagulants, oral - See Anticoagulants, oral with Tolterodine, page 79
  Selective serotonin reuptake inhibitors (SSRIs) - See Selective serotonin reuptake inhibitors (SSRIs) with Tolterodine, page 416
TOPIRAMATE, with:
  Carbamazepine - See Carbamazepine with Topiramate, page 186

TOPIRAMATE, with: *(continued)*
    Carbonic anhydrase inhibitors - See Carbonic anhydrase inhibitors with Topiramate, page 189
    Contraceptives, oral - See Contraceptives, oral with Topiramate, page 218
    Phenytoin - See Phenytoin with Topiramate, page 392

TOPOTECAN, with:
    Phenytoin - See Phenytoin with Topotecan, page 392

TOREMIFENE, with:
    Anticoagulants, oral - See Anticoagulants, oral with Toremifene, page 79
    Rifampin - See Rifampin with Toremifene, page 407

TORSEMIDE, with:
    Digoxin - See Digoxin with Torsemide, page 259

Tramadol, see Narcotics: tramadol

Trandolapril, see Angiotensin-converting enzyme (ACE) inhibitors

TRANEXAMIC ACID, with:
    Retinoic acid - See Retinoic acid with Tranexamic acid, page 403

Transfusion, see Blood transfusion

Tranylcypromine, see Monoamine oxidase inhibitors

TRASTUZUMAB, with:
    Anticoagulants, oral - See Anticoagulants, oral with Trastuzumab, page 79
    Paclitaxel - See Paclitaxel with Trastuzumab, page 381

TRAZODONE, with:
    Anticholinergics - See Anticholinergics with Trazodone, page 59
    Anticoagulants, oral - See Anticoagulants, oral with Trazodone, page 79
    Buspirone - See Buspirone with Trazodone, page 171
    Carbamazepine - See Carbamazepine with Trazodone, page 187
    Digoxin - See Digoxin with Trazodone, page 259
    Ginkgo biloba - See Ginkgo biloba with Trazodone, page 289
    Interferon - See Interferon with Trazodone, page 311
    Nefazodone - See Nefazodone with Trazodone, page 362
    Phenothiazines - See Phenothiazines with Trazodone, page 386
    Phenytoin - See Phenytoin with Trazodone, page 392
    Selective serotonin reuptake inhibitors (SSRIs) - See Selective serotonin reuptake inhibitors (SSRIs) with Trazodone, page 417

Triamcinolone, see Corticosteroids

TRIAMTERENE, with:
    Amantadine - See Amantadine with Triamterene, page 27
    Angiotensin-converting enzyme (ACE) inhibitors - See Angiotensin-converting enzyme (ACE) inhibitors with Triamterene, page 49
    Methotrexate - See Methotrexate with Triamterene, page 341
    Nonsteroidal anti-inflammatory drugs - See Nonsteroidal anti-inflammatory drugs with Triamterene, page 376
    Potassium - See Potassium with Triamterene, page 395

Triazolam, see Benzodiazepines

Triazoles, see Antifungals, Imidazoles and Triazoles

Trichlormethiazide, see Thiazide diuretics

Trichloroacetic acid, no documented interactions, see page 4, Criteria for Listing

Interactions
TRICLOFOS SODIUM, with:
   Anticoagulants, oral - See Anticoagulants, oral with Triclofos sodium, page 79
Tricyclic antidepressants, see Antidepressants, tricyclic
Trifluoperazine, see Phenothiazines
Triflupromazine, see Phenothiazines
Trifluridine, no documented interactions, see page 4, Criteria for Listing Interactions
Trihexyphenidyl, see Anticholinergics
Triiodothyronine, see Thyroid hormones
Trimeprazine, see Phenothiazines
TRIMETHOPRIM, with:
   Amiloride - See Amiloride with Trimethoprim, page 28
   Angiotensin-converting enzyme (ACE) inhibitors - See Angiotensin-converting enzyme (ACE) inhibitors with Trimethoprim, page 49
   Azathioprine - See Azathioprine with Trimethoprim, page 130
   Contraceptives, oral - See Contraceptives, oral with Trimethoprim, page 218
   Cyclosporine - See Cyclosporine with Trimethoprim, page 240
   Dapsone - See Dapsone with Trimethoprim, page 243
   Digoxin - See Digoxin with Trimethoprim, page 259
   Dofetilide - See Dofetilide with Trimethoprim, page 265
   Procainamide - See Procainamide with Trimethoprim, page 397
   Thiazide diuretics - See Thiazide diuretics with Trimethoprim, page 432
   Zidovudine
      Possible zidovudine toxicity (decreased excretion)
         BL Lee et al, Trimethoprim decreases the renal clearance of zidovudine. Clin Pharmacol Ther, 51:183, 1992 abs PIII-51; JY Chatton et al, Trimethoprim, alone or in combination with sulphamethoxazole, decreases the renal excretion of zidovudine and its glucuronide. Br J Clin Pharmacol, 34:551, 1992
      Monitor clinical status and zidovudine concentration
TRIMETHOPRIM-SULFAMETHOXAZOLE, with:
   Alcohol - See Alcohol with Trimethoprim-sulfamethoxazole, page 22
   Amantadine - See Amantadine with Trimethoprim-sulfamethoxazole, page 27
   Anticoagulants, oral - See Anticoagulants, oral with Trimethoprim-sulfamethoxazole, page 79
   Antidepressants, tricyclic - See Antidepressants, tricyclic with Trimethoprim-sulfamethoxazole, page 92
   Contraceptives, oral - See Contraceptives, oral with Trimethoprim-sulfamethoxazole, page 218
   Dapsone - See Dapsone with Trimethoprim-sulfamethoxazole, page 243
   Dofetilide - See Dofetilide with Trimethoprim-sulfamethoxazole, page 265
   Lidocaine - See Lidocaine with Trimethoprim-sulfamethoxazole, page 322
   Mercaptopurine - See Mercaptopurine with Trimethoprim-sulfamethoxazole, page 338
   Methotrexate - See Methotrexate with Trimethoprim-sulfamethoxazole, page 341

TRIMETHOPRIM-SULFAMETHOXAZOLE, with: *(continued)*
    Narcotics: meperidine and congeners - See Narcotics: meperidine and congeners with Trimethoprim-sulfamethoxazole, page 357
    Phenytoin - See Phenytoin with Trimethoprim-sulfamethoxazole, page 392
    Pimozide - See Pimozide with Trimethoprim-sulfamethoxazole, page 394
    Prilocaine - See Prilocaine with Trimethoprim-sulfamethoxazole, page 396
    Rifampin - See Rifampin with Trimethoprim-sulfamethoxazole, page 407
    Spironolactone - See Spironolactone with Trimethoprim-sulfamethoxazole, page 421

Trimetrexate, no documented interactions, see page 4, Criteria for Listing Interactions

Trimipramine, see Antidepressants, tricyclic

Tripelennamine, no documented interactions, see page 4, Criteria for Listing Interactions

Triprolidine, no documented interactions, see page 4, Criteria for Listing Interactions

TRIPTANS, with:
    Antihistamines, H_2-blockers - See Antihistamines, H_2-blockers with Triptans, page 126
    Beta-adrenergic blockers - See Beta-adrenergic blockers with Triptans, page 164
    Ergot alkaloids - See Ergot alkaloids with Triptans, page 272
    Monoamine oxidase inhibitors - See Monoamine oxidase inhibitors with Triptans, page 352
    Selective serotonin reuptake inhibitors (SSRIs) - See Selective serotonin reuptake inhibitors (SSRIs) with Triptans, page 417
    Sibutramine - See Sibutramine with Triptans, page 419

Trisulfapyrimidines, see Sulfonamides

TROGLITAZONE, with:
    Anticoagulants, oral - See Anticoagulants, oral with Troglitazone, page 80
    Antihistamines, H_1-blockers: astemizole, terfenadine - See Antihistamines, H_1-blockers: astemizole, terfenadine with Troglitazone, page 112
    Cholestyramine - See Cholestyramine with Troglitazone, page 198
    Contraceptives, oral - See Contraceptives, oral with Troglitazone, page 218
    Cyclosporine - See Cyclosporine with Troglitazone, page 240
    Gemfibrozil - See Gemfibrozil with Troglitazone, page 288
    HMG-COA reductase inhibitors - See HMG-COA reductase inhibitors with Troglitazone, page 302

TROLEANDOMYCIN, with:
    Antidepressants, tricyclic - See Antidepressants, tricyclic with Troleandomycin, page 92
    Antihistamines, H_1-blockers: astemizole, terfenadine - See Antihistamines, H_1-blockers: astemizole, terfenadine with Troleandomycin, page 112
    Benzodiazepines - See Benzodiazepines with Troleandomycin, page 150
    Carbamazepine - See Carbamazepine with Troleandomycin, page 187
    Cisapride - See Cisapride with Troleandomycin, page 201
    Contraceptives, oral - See Contraceptives, oral with Troleandomycin, page 218

(continued)

TROLEANDOMYCIN, with: *(continued)*
   Corticosteroids - See Corticosteroids with Troleandomycin, page 225
   Ergot alkaloids - See Ergot alkaloids with Troleandomycin, page 272
   Theophyllines - See Theophyllines with Troleandomycin, page 430
Tropicamide, no documented interactions, see page 4, Criteria for Listing Interactions
Trovafloxacin, see Fluoroquinolones
TRYPTOPHAN, with:
   Monoamine oxidase inhibitors - See Monoamine oxidase inhibitors with Tryptophan, page 352
   Selective serotonin reuptake inhibitors (SSRIs) - See Selective serotonin reuptake inhibitors (SSRIs) with Tryptophan, page 417
   Sibutramine - See Sibutramine with Tryptophan, page 419
Tubocurarine, see Neuromuscular blocking agents
TYRAMINE-RICH FOODS AND BEVERAGES, with:
   Antihistamines, H_2-blockers - See Antihistamines, H_2-blockers with Tyramine-rich foods and beverages, page 126
   Isoniazid - See Isoniazid with Tyramine-rich foods and beverages, page 314
   Linezolid - See Linezolid with Tyramine-rich foods and beverages, page 323
   Monoamine oxidase inhibitors - See Monoamine oxidase inhibitors with Tyramine-rich foods and beverages, page 352
Undecylenic acids, no documented interactions, see page 4, Criteria for Listing Interactions
URSODIOL, with:
   Antacids - See Antacids with Ursodiol, page 57
   Cholestyramine - See Cholestyramine with Ursodiol, page 198
   Colestipol - See Colestipol with Ursodiol, page 212
   Fluoroquinolones - See Fluoroquinolones with Ursodiol, page 283
Vaccine, influenza, see Influenza vaccine
Vaccine, rabies, see Rabies vaccine
Valacyclovir, no documented interactions, see page 4, Criteria for Listing Interactions
VALERIAN ROOT, with:
   Narcotics: meperidine and congeners - See Narcotics: meperidine and congeners with Valerian root, page 357
VALPROATE, with:
   Acarbose - See Acarbose with Valproate, page 6
   Antacids - See Antacids with Valproate, page 57
   Anticoagulants, oral - See Anticoagulants, oral with Valproate, page 80
   Antidepressants, tricyclic - See Antidepressants, tricyclic with Valproate, page 93
   Antihistamines, H_2-blockers - See Antihistamines, H_2-blockers with Valproate, page 127
   Barbiturates - See Barbiturates with Valproate, page 137
   Benzodiazepines - See Benzodiazepines with Valproate, page 150
   Carbamazepine - See Carbamazepine with Valproate, page 187
   Cholestyramine - See Cholestyramine with Valproate, page 198

VALPROATE, with: *(continued)*
  Cisplatin - See Cisplatin with Valproate, page 202
  Clozapine - See Clozapine with Valproate, page 209
  Corticotropin - See Corticotropin with Valproate, page 225
  Epoetin - See Epoetin with Valproate, page 270
  Ethosuximide - See Ethosuximide with Valproate, page 274
  Felbamate - See Felbamate with Valproate, page 276
  Guanfacine - See Guanfacine with Valproate, page 293
  Isoniazid - See Isoniazid with Valproate, page 314
  Lamotrigine - See Lamotrigine with Valproate, page 317
  Macrolide antibiotics - See Macrolide antibiotics with Valproate, page 334
  Nonsteroidal anti-inflammatory drugs - See Nonsteroidal anti-inflammatory drugs with Valproate, page 376
  Panipenem-betamipron - See Panipenem-betamipron with Valproate, page 381
  Pergolide - See Pergolide with Valproate, page 383
  Phenothiazines - See Phenothiazines with Valproate, page 386
  Phenytoin - See Phenytoin with Valproate, page 392
  Risperidone - See Risperidone with Valproate, page 408
  Selective serotonin reuptake inhibitors (SSRIs) - See Selective serotonin reuptake inhibitors (SSRIs) with Valproate, page 418
  Sympathomimetic amines - See Sympathomimetic amines with Valproate, page 425
  Zidovudine
    Possible zidovudine toxicity (decreased metabolism - glucuronidation)
      JJL Lertora et al, Pharmacokinetic interaction between zidovudine and valpric acid in patients infected with human immunodeficiency virus. Clin Pharmacol Ther, 56:272, 1994; SK Akula et al, Valproic acid increases cerebrospinal fluid zidovudine levels in a patient with AIDS. Am J Med Sci, 313:244, 1997
    Monitor clinical status and zidovudine concentration if available
Valproic acid, see Valproate
VALPROMIDE, with:
  Antidepressants, tricyclic - See Antidepressants, tricyclic with Valpromide, page 93
  Carbamazepine - See Carbamazepine with Valpromide, page 188
Valrubicin, no documented interactions, see page 4, Criteria for Listing Interactions
Valsartan, no documented interactions, see page 4, Criteria for Listing Interactions
VANCOMYCIN, with:
  Aminoglycoside antibiotics - See Aminoglycoside antibiotics with Vancomycin, page 33
  Digoxin - See Digoxin with Vancomycin, page 259
  Furosemide - See Furosemide with Vancomycin, page 287
  Neuromuscular blocking agents - See Neuromuscular blocking agents with Vancomycin, page 366
  Nonsteroidal anti-inflammatory drugs - See Nonsteroidal anti-inflammatory drugs with Vancomycin, page 376

(continued)

VANCOMYCIN, with: *(continued)*
   Polymyxins - See Polymyxins with Vancomycin, page 394
Vecuronium, see Neuromuscular blocking agents
VENLAFAXINE, with:
   Antidepressants, tricyclic - See Antidepressants, tricyclic with Venlafaxine, page 93
   Antihistamines, H$_1$-blockers: diphenhydramine - See Antihistamines, H$_1$-blockers: diphenhydramine with Venlafaxine, page 113
   Antihistamines, H$_2$-blockers - See Antihistamines, H$_2$-blockers with Venlafaxine, page 127
   Benzodiazepines - See Benzodiazepines with Venlafaxine, page 151
   Guanfacine - See Guanfacine with Venlafaxine, page 293
   Lithium - See Lithium with Venlafaxine, page 327
   Monoamine oxidase inhibitors - See Monoamine oxidase inhibitors with Venlafaxine, page 353
   Phenothiazines - See Phenothiazines with Venlafaxine, page 386
   Selective serotonin reuptake inhibitors (SSRIs) - See Selective serotonin reuptake inhibitors (SSRIs) with Venlafaxine, page 418
   Zolpidem
      Hallucinations (additive)
            CJ Elko et al, Zolpidem-associated hallucinations and serotonin reuptake inhibition: a possible interaction. Clin Toxicol, 36:195, 1998
      Single case report (1998)
Venom, see Insect venom extracts
VERAPAMIL, with:
   Adenosine - See Adenosine with Verapamil, page 12
   Alcohol - See Alcohol with Verapamil, page 22
   Angiotensin-converting enzyme (ACE) inhibitors - See Angiotensin-converting enzyme (ACE) inhibitors with Verapamil, page 50
   Anticholinesterases - See Anticholinesterases with Verapamil, page 60
   Antidepressants, tricyclic - See Antidepressants, tricyclic with Verapamil, page 93
   Antifungals, imidazoles and triazoles - See Antifungals, imidazoles and triazoles with Verapamil, page 108
   Antihistamines, H$_1$-blockers: astemizole, terfenadine - See Antihistamines, H$_1$-blockers: astemizole, terfenadine with Verapamil, page 112
   Antihistamines, H$_2$-blockers - See Antihistamines, H$_2$-blockers with Verapamil, page 127
   Barbiturates - See Barbiturates with Verapamil, page 138
   Benzodiazepines - See Benzodiazepines with Verapamil, page 151
   Beta-adrenergic blockers - See Beta-adrenergic blockers with Verapamil, page 164
   Bupivacaine - See Bupivacaine with Verapamil, page 169
   Buspirone - See Buspirone with Verapamil, page 171
   Caffeine - See Caffeine with Verapamil, page 175
   Carbamazepine - See Carbamazepine with Verapamil, page 188
   Cephalosporins - See Cephalosporins with Verapamil, page 191

VERAPAMIL, with: *(continued)*
  Clindamycin - See Clindamycin with Verapamil, page 203
  Clonidine - See Clonidine with Verapamil, page 205
  Colesevelam - See Colesevelam with Verapamil, page 211
  Cyclosporine - See Cyclosporine with Verapamil, page 240
  Dantrolene - See Dantrolene with Verapamil, page 242
  Digitoxin - See Digitoxin with Verapamil, page 251
  Digoxin - See Digoxin with Verapamil, page 259
  Dofetilide - See Dofetilide with Verapamil, page 265
  Dolasetron - See Dolasetron with Verapamil, page 266
  Etomidate - See Etomidate with Verapamil, page 274
  Flecainide - See Flecainide with Verapamil, page 278
  Halothane - See Halothane with Verapamil, page 298
  HMG-CoA reductase inhibitors - See HMG-CoA reductase inhibitors with Verapamil, page 302
  Hypoglycemics, sulfonylurea - See Hypoglycemics, sulfonylurea with Verapamil, page 306
  Lithium - See Lithium with Verapamil, page 328
  Macrolide Antibiotics - See Macrolide Antibiotics with Verapamil, page 334
  Neuromuscular blocking agents - See Neuromuscular blocking agents with Verapamil, page 366
  Nonsteroidal anti-inflammatory drugs - See Nonsteroidal anti-inflammatory drugs with Verapamil, page 376
  Oxcarbazepine - See Oxcarbazepine with Verapamil, page 380
  Phenytoin - See Phenytoin with Verapamil, page 393
  Prazosin - See Prazosin with Verapamil, page 396
  Quinidine - See Quinidine with Verapamil, page 402
  Rifampin - See Rifampin with Verapamil, page 407
  Selective serotonin reuptake inhibitors (SSRIs) - See Selective serotonin reuptake inhibitors (SSRIs) with Verapamil, page 418
  Sildenafil - See Sildenafil with Verapamil, page 420
  Sulfinpyrazone - See Sulfinpyrazone with Verapamil, page 423
  Theophyllines - See Theophyllines with Verapamil, page 430
Verteporfin, no documented interactions, see page 4, Criteria for Listing Interactions
VIDARABINE, with:
  Allopurinol - See Allopurinol with Vidarabine, page 26
  Theophyllines - See Theophyllines with Vidarabine, page 431
VIGABATRIN, with:
  Phenytoin - See Phenytoin with Vigabatrin, page 393
Vinblastine, no documented interactions, see page 4, Criteria for Listing Interactions
VINCRISTINE, with:
  Antifungals, imidazoles and triazoles - See Antifungals, imidazoles and triazoles with Vincristine, page 109
  Carbamazepine - See Carbamazepine with Vincristine, page 188

(continued)

VINCRISTINE, with: *(continued)*
  Cyclosporine - See Cyclosporine with Vincristine, page 241
  Digoxin - See Digoxin with Vincristine, page 259
  Isoniazid - See Isoniazid with Vincristine, page 314
  Nifedipine - See Nifedipine with Vincristine, page 369
  Phenytoin - See Phenytoin with Vincristine, page 393
  Teniposide - See Teniposide with Vincristine, page 427
Vinorelbine, no documented interactions, see page 4, Criteria for Listing Interactions
VITAMIN A, with:
  Anticoagulants, oral - See Anticoagulants, oral with Vitamin A, page 80
VITAMIN C, with:
  Antacids - See Antacids with Vitamin C, page 57
  Anticoagulants, oral - See Anticoagulants, oral with Vitamin C, page 80
  Beta-adrenergic blockers - See Beta-adrenergic blockers with Vitamin C, page 165
  Contraceptives, oral - See Contraceptives, oral with Vitamin C, page 218
  Estrogens - See Estrogens with Vitamin C, page 273
  Phenothiazines - See Phenothiazines with Vitamin C, page 386
VITAMIN D, with:
  Anabolic and androgenic steroids - See Anabolic and androgenic steroids with Vitamin D, page 42
  Antacids - See Antacids with Vitamin D, page 58
  Corticosteroids - See Corticosteroids with Vitamin D, page 225
VITAMIN E, with:
  Anticoagulants, oral - See Anticoagulants, oral with Vitamin E, page 80
Warfarin, see Anticoagulants, oral
Yellow fever vaccine, no documented interactions, see page 4, Criteria for Listing Interactions
Yohimbine, no documented interactions, see page 4, Criteria for Listing Interactions
ZAFIRLUKAST, with:
  Anticoagulants, oral - See Anticoagulants, oral with Zafirlukast, page 80
  Antihistamines, H_1-blockers: astemizole, terfenadine - See Antihistamines, H_1-blockers: astemizole, terfenadine with Zafirlukast, page 113
  Nonsteroidal anti-inflammatory drugs - See Nonsteroidal anti-inflammatory drugs with Zafirlukast, page 377
  Theophyllines - See Theophyllines with Zafirlukast, page 431
ZALCITABINE, with:
  Didanosine - See Didanosine with Zalcitabine, page 249
ZALEPLON, with:
  Antihistamines, H_2-blockers - See Antihistamines, H_2-blockers with Zaleplon, page 127
  Rifampin - See Rifampin with Zaleplon, page 407
Zanamivir, no documented interactions, see page 4, Criteria for Listing Interactions
ZIDOVUDINE, with:
  Acetaminophen - See Acetaminophen with Zidovudine, page 10
  Acyclovir - See Acyclovir with Zidovudine, page 11

ZIDOVUDINE, with: *(continued)*
   Amprenavir - See Amprenavir with Zidovudine, page 40
   Antifungals, imidazoles and triazoles - See Antifungals, imidazoles and triazoles with Zidovudine, page 109
   Atovaquone - See Atovaquone with Zidovudine, page 129
   Benzodiazepines - See Benzodiazepines with Zidovudine, page 151
   Didanosine - See Didanosine with Zidovudine, page 249
   Lamivudine - See Lamivudine with Zidovudine, page 316
   Macrolide antibiotics - See Macrolide antibiotics with Zidovudine, page 334
   Narcotics: methadone and congeners - See Narcotics: methadone and congeners with Zidovudine, page 359
   Nonsteroidal anti-inflammatory drugs - See Nonsteroidal anti-inflammatory drugs with Zidovudine, page 377
   Probenecid - See Probenecid with Zidovudine, page 397
   Ribavirin - See Ribavirin with Zidovudine, page 403
   Rifampin - See Rifampin with Zidovudine, page 407
   Ritonavir - See Ritonavir with Zidovudine, page 411
   Stavudine - See Stavudine with Zidovudine, page 421
   Trimethoprim - See Trimethoprim with Zidovudine, page 436
   Valproate - See Valproate with Zidovudine, page 439

ZILEUTON, with:
   Anticoagulants, oral - See Anticoagulants, oral with Zileuton, page 80
   Antihistamines, H_1-blockers: astemizole, terfenadine - See Antihistamines, H_1-blockers: astemizole, terfenadine with Zileuton, page 113
   Beta-adrenergic blockers - See Beta-adrenergic blockers with Zileuton, page 165
   Theophyllines - See Theophyllines with Zileuton, page 431

Zimelidine, see Antidepressants, tricyclic

ZINC, with:
   Calcium - See Calcium with Zinc, page 176
   Fluoroquinolones - See Fluoroquinolones with Zinc, page 283
   Folic acid - See Folic acid with Zinc, page 284
   Iron - See Iron with Zinc, page 312
   Tetracyclines - See Tetracyclines with Zinc, page 428

Zolmitriptan, see Triptans

ZOLPIDEM, with:
   Antidepressants, tricyclic - See Antidepressants, tricyclic with Zolpidem, page 93
   Antifungals, imidazoles and triazoles - See Antifungals, imidazoles and triazoles with Zolpidem, page 109
   Bupropion - See Bupropion with Zolpidem, page 170
   Rifampin - See Rifampin with Zolpidem, page 408
   Ritonavir - See Ritonavir with Zolpidem, page 411
   Selective serotonin reuptake inhibitors (SSRIs) - See Selective serotonin reuptake inhibitors (SSRIs) with Zolpidem, page 418
   Venlafaxine - See Venlafaxine with Zolpidem, page 440

Zomepirac, see Nonsteroidal anti-inflammatory drugs

ZONISAMIDE, with:
   Barbiturates - See Barbiturates with Zonisamide, page 138
   Carbamazepine - See Carbamazepine with Zonisamide, page 188
   Phenytoin - See Phenytoin with Zonisamide, page 393
Zopiclone, see Benzodiazepines

FOODS INTERACTING WITH MAO INHIBITORS

	Comments
FOOD CONTAINING TYRAMINE	
Avocados	Particularly if overripe[1,2]
Bananas	Reactions can occur if eaten in large amounts; tyramine levels high in peel.[2,3]
Bean curd	Fermented bean curd, fermented soya bean, soya bean pastes, soy sauces and miso soup, prepared from fermented bean curd, all contain tyramine in large amounts; miso soup has caused reactions.[4,5]
Beer and ale	Major domestic bottled brands do not contain appreciable amounts; some imported brands and domestic tap lagers from local breweries have high levels.[6] Nonalcoholic beer may contain tyramine and should be avoided.[7]
Caviar	Safe if vacuum-packed and eaten fresh or refrigerated only briefly[6]
Cheese	Reactions possible with most, except unfermented varieties such as cottage cheese and possibly some other cheeses.[5,6] In others, tyramine concentration is higher near rind and close to fermentation holes.[6]
Dietary supplements (weight loss products)	May contain large amounts of yeast and/or yeast extracts, and cocoa.[8]
Figs	Particularly if overripe.[2]
Fish	Safe if fresh; dried products should not be eaten. Caution required in restaurants. Vacuum-packed products are safe if eaten promptly or refrigerated only briefly.[6]
Liver	Safe if very fresh, but rapidly accumulates tyramine; caution required in restaurants.[9]

1. JA Generali et al, Drug Intell Clin Pharm, 15:904, 1981
2. S Udenfriend et al, Arch Biochem Biophys, 85:487, 1959
3. B Blackwell and DC Taylor, Br Med J, 2:381, 1969
4. SK Sung et al, Hum Psychopharmacol, 1:103, 1986; RE Mesmer, JAMA, 258:3515, 1987
5. KI Shulman and SE Walker, J Clin Psychiatry, 60:191, 1999
6. M Da Prada et al, J Neural Transm, 26 suppl:31, 1988; P Hannah et al, Lancet, 1:879, 1988; SAN Tailor et al, J Clin Psychopharmacol, 14:5, 1994
7. JA Murray et al, Lancet, 1:1167, 1988; R Draper et al, Br Med J, 289:308, 1984; J Thakore et al, Int Clin Psychopharmacol, 7:59, 1992
8. RA Sweet et al, J Clin Psychopharmacol, 11:331, 1991
9. AA Boulton et al, Can Med Assoc J, 102:1394, 1970; ed., Biol Ther Psychiatry, 11:1, 1988

	Comments
Milk products	Milk and yogurt appear to be safe.[10]
Protein extracts	See also soups; avoid liquid and powdered protein dietary supplements.[11]
Meat	Safe if known to be fresh; caution required in restaurants.[6,9]
Sauerkraut	Contains large amounts of tyramine; no reaction has been reported[12]
Sausage	Fermented varieties such as bologna, pepperoni and salami have a high tyramine content.[6]
Shrimp paste	Contains large amounts of tyramine.[4]
Soups	May contain protein extracts and should be avoided.[11]
Soy sauce	Contains large amounts of tyramine; reactions have occurred with teriyaki.[4,5,13]
Wines	Generally do not contain tyramine, but many reactions have been reported with Chianti, champagne and other wines.
Yeast extracts	Dietary supplements, e.g. *Marmite*, contain large amounts. Yeast in baked goods, however, is safe.[14]

FOOD NOT CONTAINING TYRAMINE

Caffeine	A weak pressor agent; large amounts may cause reactions.
Chocolate	Contains phenylethylamine, a pressor agent which can cause reactions in large amounts.[2,15]
Fava beans (broad beans, "Italian" green beans)	Contain dopamine, a pressor amine, particularly when overripe.[2]
Ginseng	Some preparations have caused headache, tremulousness and manic-like symptoms.[16]
Liqueurs	Reactions reported with some, e.g. *Chartreuse* and *Drambuie*; cause unknown.
New Zealand prickly spinach	Single case report; patient ate large amounts.[17]
Whiskey	Reactions have occurred; cause unknown.[18]

10. D Horwitz et al, JAMA, 188:1108, 1964
11. M Zetin et al, J Clin Psychiatry, 48:499, 1987
12. KI Shulman et al, J Clin Psychopharmacol, 9:397, 1989
13. JH Abrams et al, N Engl J Med, 313:52, 1985
14. B Blackwell et al, Lancet, 1:940, 1965
15. DM Krikler and B Lewis, Lancet, 1:1166, 1965
16. BD Jones and AM Runikis, J Clin Psychopharmacol, 7:201, 1987; RI Shader and DJ Greenblatt, J Clin Psychopharmacol, 8:235, 1988
17. A Comfort, Lancet, 2:472, 1981
18. ed., Biol Ther Psychiatry, 11:34, Sept 1988

NOTES

NOTES

NOTES

NOTES

NOTES

NOTES

NOTES

NOTES

NOTES

NOTES

INDEX OF BRAND NAMES

(Note: Group headings under which drugs are listed are indicated in parentheses)
Items marked (•), no interactions listed, see page 4, Criteria for Listing Interactions.

A-200 — Pyrethrins with piperonyl butoxide•
Abelcet — amphotericin B (Antifungals, Amphotericin B)
Abitrexate — methotrexate
Abreva — docosanol•
Acabamate — meprobamate
Acapav — papaverine
Accolate — zafirlukast
Accupril — quinapril (Angiotensin-converting enzyme (ACE) inhibitors)
Accurbron — theophyllines
Accutane — isotretinoin
Aceon — perindopril (angiotensin-converting enzyme (ACE) inhibitors)
Acephen — acetaminophen
Aceta — acetaminophen
Aceta-Gesic — acetaminophen
Acet-Am — acetaminophen
Acetocot — triamcinolone (Corticosteroids)
Achromycin — tetracyclines
Aciphex — rabeprazole
Acon — vitamin A
Actamin — acetaminophen
Acthar — corticotropin
Acticort — hydrocortisone (Corticosteroids)
Actidil — triprolidine•
Actigall — ursodiol
Actimmune — interferon gamma (Interferon)
Actinex — masoprocol•
Actiprofen — ibuprofen (Nonsteroidal anti-inflammatory drugs)
Actiq — fentanyl (Narcotics: meperidine and congeners)
Activase — alteplase (Thrombolytics)
Actonel — risedronate
Actos — pioglitazone•
Acular — ketorolac (Nonsteroidal anti-inflammatory drugs)
Adalat — nifedipine
Adapin — doxepin (Antidepressants, tricyclic)
Adeflor — fluoride
Adenocard — adenosine
Adeno-Jec — adenosine
Adenoscan — adenosine
Adipex — phentermine (Sympathomimetic amines)
Adrenalin — epinephrine (Sympathomimetic amines)
Adrenocot — dexamethasone (Corticosteroids)
Adriamycin — doxorubicin
Adrolazine — hydralazine
Adroxazine — hydroxyzine
Adrucil — fluorouracil
Adsorbocarpine — pilocarpine
Advil — ibuprofen (Nonsteroidal anti-inflammatory drugs)
Aeroaid — thimerosal (Antiseptics, mercurial)
Aerobid — flunisolide (Corticosteroids)
Aerolate — theophyllines
Aerolone — isoproterenol (Sympathomimetic amines; Sympathomimetic bronchodilators)
Aeroseb-Dex — dexamethasone (Corticosteroids)
Aeroseb-HC — hydrocortisone (Corticosteroids)
Afrinol — pseudoephedrine (Sympathomimetic amines)

- 447 -

Agenerase — amprenavir
Aggrastat — tirofiban
Agrylin — anagrelide
A-HydroCort — hydrocortisone (Corticosteroids)
Airet — albuterol (Sympathomimetic bronchodilators)
Akarpine — pilocarpine
AK-Chlor — chloramphenicol
AK-Dex — dexamethasone (Corticosteroids)
Akineton — biperiden•
AK-Mycin — erythromycins (Macrolide antibiotics)
Akne-mycin — erythromycins (Macrolide antibiotics)
AK-Pred — prednisolone (Corticosteroids)
AK-Ramycin — doxycycline (Tetracyclines)
AK-Ratabs — doxycycline (Tetracyclines)
AK-Sulf — sulfacetamide (Sulfonamides)
AK-Tate — prednisolone (Corticosteroids)
AK-Zol — acetazolamide (Carbonic anhydrase inhibitors)
Ala-Cort — hydrocortisone (Corticosteroids)
Alamast — pemirolast•
Ala-Tet — tetracyclines
Albay — insect venom extracts
Alcomicin — gentamicin (Aminoglycoside antibiotics)
Alconefrin — phenylephrine (Sympathomimetic amines)
Aldactazide — hydrochlorothiazide; spironolactone (Thiazide diuretics; Spironolactone)
Aldactone — spironolactone
Aldara — imiquimod•
Aldomet — methyldopa
Aldoril — methyldopa; hydrochlorothiazide (Methyldopa; Thiazide diuretics)
Alertec — modafinil

Alesse — contraceptives, oral
Alfenta — alfentanil (Narcotics: meperidine and congeners)
Alka-Seltzer — sodium bicarbonate; aspirin; citric acid (Antacids; Nonsteroidal anti-inflammatory drugs; Citrates)
Alkeran — melphalan (Alkylating agents)
Alkets — magnesium carbonate (Antacids)
Allegra — fexofenadine
Allercor — hydrocortisone (Corticosteroids)
Allerest — phenylephrine (Sympathomimetic amines)
Alloprin — allopurinol
Almocarpine — pilocarpine
Alocort — hydrocortisone acetate (Corticosteroids)
Alocril — nedocromil•
Alomide — lodoxamide•
Alora — estradiol (Estrogens)
Alphagan — brimonidine
Alphalin — vitamin A
Alphatrex — betamethasone (Corticosteroids)
Altace — ramipril (Angiotensin-converting enzyme (ACE) inhibitors)
ALternaGEL — aluminum hydroxide (Antacids)
Altex — spironolactone
Alto-Pred — prednisolone (Corticosteroids)
Alu-Cap — aluminum hydroxide (Antacids)
Aludrox — aluminum, magnesium hydroxide (Antacids)
Alupent — metaproterenol (Sympathomimetic bronchodilators)
Alurate — aprobarbital (Barbiturates)
Alu-Tab — aluminum hydroxide (Antacids)
Alzapam — lorazepam (Benzodiazepines)
Amaryl — glimepiride•

Ambien — zolpidem
AmBisome — amphotericin B (Antifungals, Amphotericin B)
Amcap — ampicillin (Penicillins)
Amcill — ampicillin (Penicillins)
Amcort — triamcinolone (Corticosteroids)
Amen — medroxyprogesterone (Progestins)
Amerge — naratriptan (Triptans)
Amersol — ibuprofen (Nonsteroidal anti-inflammatory drugs)
Amer-Tet — tetracyclines
A-Methapred — methylprednisolone (Corticosteroids)
Amficot — ampicillin (Penicillins)
Amicar — aminocaproic acid•
Amidate — etomidate
Amigesic — Nonsteroidal anti-inflammatory drugs
Amikin — amikacin (Aminoglycoside antibiotics)
Aminodur — aminophylline (Theophyllines)
Aminodyne — acetaminophen
Aminophyllin — aminophylline (Theophyllines)
Amitone — calcium carbonate (Antacids)
Amitril — amitriptyline (Antidepressants, tricyclic)
Amnestrogen — estrogens
Amoxil — amoxicillin (Penicillins)
Amphocaps — ampicillin (Penicillins)
Amphojel — aluminum hydroxide (Antacids)
Amphotec — amphotericin B (Antifungals, Amphotericin B)
Ampicin — ampicillin (Penicillins)
Ampilean — ampicillin (Penicillins)
Amplin — ampicillin (Penicillins)
Amytal — amobarbital (Barbiturates)
Anabol — methandriol (Anabolic and androgenic steroids)
Anabolin — nandrolone (Anabolic and androgenic steroids)
Anacin — acetaminophen
Anadrol — oxymetholone (Anabolic and androgenic steroids)
Anafranil — clomipramine (Antidepressants, tricyclic)
Ana-Guard — epinephrine (Sympathomimetic amines)
Anapolon 50 — oxymetholone (Anabolic and androgenic steroids)
Anaprox — naproxen (Nonsteroidal anti-inflammatory drugs)
Anaspaz — hyoscyamine (Anticholinergics)
Ancef — cefazolin (Cephalosporins)
Ancobon — flucytosine
Andriol — methandriol (Anabolic and androgenic steroids)
Andro — testosterone (Anabolic and androgenic steroids)
Andro-Cyp — testosterone (Anabolic and androgenic steroids)
Androderm — testosterone (Anabolic and androgenic steroids)
AndroGel — testosterone (Anabolic and androgenic steroids)
Android — methyltestosterone (Anabolic and androgenic steroids)
Android-F — fluoxymesterone (Anabolic and androgenic steroids)
Android-T — testosterone (Anabolic and androgenic steroids)
Androlan — testosterone (Anabolic and androgenic steroids)
Androlone — nandrolone (Anabolic and androgenic steroids)
Andronaq — testosterone (Anabolic and androgenic steroids)
Andropository — testosterone (Anabolic and androgenic steroids)
Andryl — testosterone (Anabolic and androgenic steroids)
Anectine — succinylcholine (Neuromuscular blocking agents)
Anergan 25 — promethazine
Anestacon — lidocaine
Anesthacaine — lidocaine
Angijen — pentaerythritol tetranitrate (Nitrates)

Anginar — erythrityl tetranitrate (Nitrates)
Ang-O-Span — nitroglycerin (Nitrates)
Anhydron — cyclothiazide (Thiazide diuretics)
Anodynos-DHC — hydrocodone (Narcotics: morphine-like)
Anorex — phentermine (Sympathomimetic amines)
Anoxine-AM — phentermine (Sympathomimetic amines)
Ansaid — flurbiprofen (Nonsteroidal anti-inflammatory drugs)
Anspor — cephradine (Cephalosporins)
Anta Gel — aluminum hydroxide, magnesium hydroxide, simethicone (Antacids)
Antabuse — disulfiram
Antilirium — physostigmine (Anticholinesterases)
Antiminth — pyrantel pamoate
Antispas — dicyclomine (Anticholinergics)
Antivert — meclizine hydrochloride•
Antrizine — meclizine hydrochloride•
Anturane — sulfinpyrazone
Anusol-HC — hydrocortisone (Corticosteroids)
Anxanil — hydroxyzine
Anzemet — dolasetron
Aoracillin — penicillin G (Penicillins)
Aparkane — trihexyphenidyl (Anticholinergics)
Apogen — gentamicin (Aminoglycoside antibiotics)
A-poxide — chlordiazepoxide (Benzodiazepines)
Apresazide — hydralazine; hydrochlorothiazide (Hydralazine; Thiazide diuretics)
Apresoline — hydralazine
Apresrex — hydralazine
Aquachloral — chloral hydrate
Aquacot — trichlormethiazide (Thiazide diuretics)

Aquadril — hydrochlorothiazide (Thiazide diuretics)
Aquagen — estrogens
Aquamucil — psyllium
Aquaphyllin — theophyllines
Aquasol-A — vitamin A
Aquasol-E — vitamin E
Aquatag — benzthiazide (Thiazide diuretics)
Aquatensen — methyclothiazide (Thiazide diuretics)
Aquazide — trichlormethiazide (Thiazide diuretics)
Aquazide H — hydrochlorothiazide (Thiazide diuretics)
Aquest — estrogens
Aquex — trichlormethiazide (Thiazide diuretics)
Aralen — chloroquine
Aramine — metaraminol (Sympathomimetic amines)
Arava — leflunomide
Arbolic — methandriol (Anabolic and androgenic steroids)
Arcoban — meprobamate
Arcocillin — penicillin G (Penicillins)
Arcosterone — methyltestosterone (Anabolic and androgenic steroids)
Arcotrate — pentaerythritol tetranitrate (Nitrates)
Arcum R-S — reserpine
Arcylate — salicylsalicylic acid (Nonsteroidal anti-inflammatory drugs)
Ardecaine — lidocaine
Ardefem — estradiol (Estrogens)
Arderone — testosterone (Anabolic and androgenic steroids)
Arduan — pipecuronium (Neuromuscular blocking agents)
Aredia — pamidronate•
Aricept — donepezil
Arimidex — anastrozole•
Aristocort — triamcinolone (Corticosteroids)
Aristospan — triamcinolone (Corticosteroids)
Arm-A-Med — isoetharine

(Sympathomimetic amines; Sympathomimetic bronchodilators)
Aromasin — exemestane•
Artane — trihexyphenidyl (Anticholinergics)
Artha-G — salicylsalicylic acid (Nonsteroidal anti-inflammatory drugs)
Arthicare — capsaicin
Articulose-50 — prednisolone (Corticosteroids)
Articulose-L.A. — triamcinolone (Corticosteroids)
A.S.A. — aspirin (Nonsteroidal anti-inflammatory drugs)
Asacol — mesalamine
Ascorbicap — vitamin C
Ascorbineed — vitamin C
Ascriptin — aspirin (Nonsteroidal anti-inflammatory drugs)
Asendin — amoxapine (Antidepressants, tricyclic)
Asmalix — theophyllines
Asmolin — epinephrine (Sympathomimetic amines)
Aspergum — aspirin (Nonsteroidal anti-inflammatory drugs)
Aspirjen Jr — aspirin (Nonsteroidal anti-inflammatory drugs)
Aspirtab — aspirin (Nonsteroidal anti-inflammatory drugs)
Astelin — azelastine•
Asthma Meter — epinephrine (Sympathomimetic amines)
Asthmanefrin — epinephrine (Sympathomimetic amines)
Astramorph — morphine (Narcotics: morphine-like)
Astrin — aspirin (Nonsteroidal anti-inflammatory drugs)
Atacand — candesartan•
Atarax — hydroxyzine
Athrombin-K — warfarin (Anticoagulants, oral)
Ativan — lorazepam (Benzodiazepines)
ATP — adenosine
Atromid-S — clofibrate

Atropair — atropine (Anticholinergics)
Atropisol — atropine (Anticholinergics)
A/T/S — erythromycins (Macrolide antibiotics)
Augmentin — amoxicillin-clavulanic acid (Penicillins)
Aurorix — moclobemide (Monoamine oxidase inhibitors)
Avandia — rosiglitazone•
Avapro — irbesartan
Avelox — moxifloxacin (Fluoroquinolones)
Aventyl — nortriptyline (Antidepressants, tricyclic)
Axid — nizatidine (Antihistamines, H_2-blockers)
Axsain — capsaicin
Aygestin — norethindrone (Contraceptives, oral; Progestins)
Azactam — aztreonam•
Azelex — azelaic acid•
Azmacort — triamcinolone (Corticosteroids)
Azolid — phenylbutazone
Azopt — brinzolamide•
Azulfidine — sulfasalazine (Sulfonamides)

B*actrim* — trimethoprim-sulfamethoxazole
Bamate — meprobamate
Banacid — aluminum hydroxide, magnesium hydroxide & trisilicate (Antacids)
Banan — cefpodoxime (Cephalosporins)
Banesin — acetaminophen
Banflex — orphenadrine
Banthine — methantheline (Anticholinergics)
Barbita — phenobarbital (Barbiturates)
Basaljel — aluminum carbonate (Antacids)

Baycol — cerivastatin (HMG-CoA Reductase Inhibitors)
Bayer — aspirin (Nonsteroidal anti-inflammatory drugs)
Baypress — nitrendipine
BBS — butabarbital (Barbiturates)
BC — aspirin (Nonsteroidal anti-inflammatory drugs)
Beano — α-galactosidase•
Beben — betamethasone (Corticosteroids)
Beclovent — beclomethasone (Corticosteroids)
Beconase — beclomethasone (Corticosteroids)
Beepen-VK — penicillin V (Penicillins)
Beesix — pyridoxine
Bellafoline — hyoscyamine (Anticholinergics)
Benacen — probenecid
Benadryl — diphenhydramine (Antihistamines, H$_1$-blockers: diphenhydramine)
Benemid — probenecid
Benn — probenecid
Bentyl — dicyclomine (Anticholinergics)
Benuryl — probenecid
Benylin DM — dextromethorphan (Narcotics: dextromethorphan)
Bepadin — bepridil
Bestrone — estrone (Estrogens)
Betacort — betamethasone (Corticosteroids)
Betaderm — betamethasone (Corticosteroids)
Betagan — levobunolol (Beta-adrenergic blockers)
Betaloc — metoprolol (Beta-adrenergic blockers)
Betamet — metipranolol (Beta-adrenergic blockers)
Betamethacot — betamethasone (Corticosteroids)
Betapace — sotalol (Beta-adrenergic blockers)
Betapen-VK — penicillin V (Penicillins)
Betatrex — betamethasone (Corticosteroids)
Bethaprim — trimethoprim-sulfamethoxazole
Betnesol — betamethasone (Corticosteroids)
Betnovate — betamethasone (Corticosteroids)
Betoptic — betaxolol (Beta-adrenergic blockers)
Biaxin — clarithromycin (Macrolide antibiotics)
Bicillin — penicillin G (Penicillins)
Bicitra — sodium citrate, citric acid (Citrates)
BiCNU — carmustine
Bicycline — tetracyclines
Biltricide — praziquantel
Bio Dopa — levodopa
Bio-Cef — cephalexin (Cephalosporins)
Biogroton — chlorthalidone (Thiazide diuretics)
Biotic-T — penicillin G (Penicillins)
Biphetamine — amphetamine (Sympathomimetic amines)
Biquin — quinidine
Bisodol — calcium carbonate, magnesium hydroxide (Antacids)
Blenoxane — bleomycin
Bleph-10 — sulfacetamide (Sulfonamides)
Blocadren — timolol (Beta-adrenergic blockers)
Bolvidon — mianserin
Bonine — meclizine hydrochloride•
BP-Papaverine — papaverine
Bravavir — sorivudine
Brethaire — terbutaline (Sympathomimetic bronchodilators)
Brethine — terbutaline (Sympathomimetic bronchodilators)
Bretylate — bretylium
Bretylol — bretylium
Brevibloc — esmolol (Beta-

- adrenergic blockers)
- *Brevicon* — contraceptives, oral
- *Brevital* — methohexital (Barbiturates)
- *Bricanyl* — terbutaline (Sympathomimetic bronchodilators)
- *Brietal* — methohexital (Barbiturates)
- *Brigen-G* — chlordiazepoxide (Benzodiazepines)
- *Brodspec* — tetracyclines
- *Bronkodyl* — theophyllines
- *Bronkometer* — isoetharine (Sympathomimetic bronchodilators)
- *Bronkosol* — isoetharine (Sympathomimetic bronchodilators)
- *Broserpine* — reserpine
- *Bufferin* — magnesium carbonate; aspirin (Antacids; Nonsteroidal anti-inflammatory drugs)
- *Buffinol* — aspirin (Nonsteroidal anti-inflammatory drugs)
- *Bumex* — bumetanide
- *Buphenyl* — sodium phenylbutyrate•
- *Buprenex* — buprenorphine
- *Bursul* — sulfamethizole (Sulfonamides)
- *Buscopan* — hyoscine (Anticholinergics)
- *Busodium* — butabarbital (Barbiturates)
- *BuSpar* — buspirone
- *Butacaps* — butabarbital (Barbiturates)
- *Butalan* — butabarbital (Barbiturates)
- *Butatab* — phenylbutazone
- *Butatran* — butabarbital (Barbiturates)
- *Butazolidin* — phenylbutazone
- *Butisol* — butabarbital (Barbiturates)

C*afergot* — ergotamine (Ergot alkaloids)
- *Calan* — verapamil
- *Calcet* — calcium
- *Calcicaps* — calcium
- *Calcichew* — calcium
- *Calciday* — calcium
- *Calciferol* — vitamin D
- *Calcijex* — calcitriol•
- *Calcimar* — calcitonin
- *Calciparine* — heparins
- *Calcitrel* — calcium carbonate, magnesia (Antacids)
- *Caldecort* — hydrocortisone (Corticosteroids)
- *Calderol* — calcifediol (Vitamin D)
- *Cal-Plus* — calcium
- *Caltrate* — calcium
- *Camalox* — aluminum hydroxide; magnesium hydroxide; calcium carbonate (Antacids)
- *Camptosar* — irinotecan
- *Cantil* — mepenzolate bromide (Anticholinergics)
- *Capastat* — capreomycin•
- *Capoten* — captopril (Angiotensin-converting enzyme (ACE) inhibitors)
- *Capozide* — captopril; hydrochlorothiazide (Angiotensin-converting enzyme (ACE) inhibitors; Thiazide diuretics)
- *Capzasin* — capsaicin
- *Carafate* — sucralfate
- *Carbocaine* — mepivacaine
- *Carbocot* — mepivacaine
- *Cardabid* — nitroglycerin (Nitrates)
- *Cardene* — nicardipine
- *Cardilate* — erythrityl tetranitrate (Nitrates)
- *Cardioquin* — quinidine
- *Cardizem* — diltiazem
- *Cardoxin* — digoxin
- *Cardura* — doxazosin•
- *Cari-Tab* — fluoride
- *Carnitor* — levocarnitine
- *Caropen-VK* — penicillin V (Penicillins)
- *Carozide* — hydrochlorothiazide (Thiazide diuretics)

Cartrol — carteolol (Beta-adrenergic blockers)
Casodex — bicalutamide•
Cataflam — diclofenac (Nonsteroidal anti-inflammatory drugs)
Catapres — clonidine
Cavacaine — mepivacaine
Caverject — alprostadil•
C-Caps — vitamin C
C.D.P. HCl — chlordiazepoxide (Benzodiazepines)
Cecapan — dexamethasone (Corticosteroids)
Ceclor — cefaclor (Cephalosporins)
Cecon — vitamin C
Cedax — ceftibuten (Cephalosporins)
Cedocard — isosorbide dinitrate (Nitrates)
Cee-500 — vitamin C
CeeNu — lomustine (Alkylating agents)
Cefadyl — cephapirin (Cephalosporins)
Cefanex — cephalexin (Cephalosporins)
Cefizox — ceftizoxime (Cephalosporins)
Cefmax — cefmenoxime (Cephalosporins)
Cefobid — cefoperazone (Cephalosporins)
Cefotan — cefotetan (Cephalosporins)
Ceftin — cefuroxime axetil (Cephalosporins)
Cefzil — cefprozil (Cephalosporins)
Celbenin — methicillin (Penicillins)
Celebrex — celecoxib (COX-2 inhibitors)
Celestone — betamethasone (Corticosteroids)
Celexa — citalopram (Selective serotonin reuptake inhibitors (SSRIs))
CellCept — mycophenolate mofetil
Celontin — methsuximide

Cena K — potassium
Cenafed — pseudoephedrine (Sympathomimetic amines)
Cenestin — estrogens
Cenocort — triamcinolone (Corticosteroids)
Cenolate — vitamin C
Centet — tetracyclines
Centrax — prazepam (Benzodiazepines)
Cephulac — lactulose•
Ceporacin — cephalothin (Cephalosporins)
Ceptaz — ceftazidime (Cephalosporins)
Cerebid — papaverine
Ceredase — alglucerase•
Cerespan — papaverine
Cerubidine — daunorubicin•
Ces — estrogens
Cesamet — nabilone•
Cetamide — sulfacetamide (Sulfonamides)
Cetane — vitamin C
Ceticort — triamcinolone (Corticosteroids)
Cevalin — vitamin C
Cevi-bid — vitamin C
Ce-Vi-Sol — vitamin C
Chemet — succimer•
Chero-Trisulfa-V — trisulfapyrimidines (Sulfonamides)
Chlordiazachel — diazepam (Benzodiazepines)
Chlorocon — chloroquine
Chlorofair — chloramphenicol
Chloromycetin — chloramphenicol
Chloroptic — chloramphenicol
Chlorpromanyl — chlorpromazine (Phenothiazines)
Chlorulan — chlorothiazide (Thiazide diuretics)
Chlorzide — hydrochlorothiazide (Thiazide diuretics)
Chlorzine — chlorpromazine (Phenothiazines)
Choice — potassium
Choledyl — oxtriphylline

(Theophyllines)
Choloxin — dextrothyroxine
Chophylline — oxtriphylline (Theophyllines)
Chronovera — verapamil
Chronulac — lactulose•
Chymex — bentiromide
Cibacalcin — calcitonin
Cibalith-S — lithium
Cidomycin — gentamicin (Aminoglycoside antibiotics)
Cinobac — cinoxacin (Fluoroquinolones)
Cinonide — triamcinolone (Corticosteroids)
Cin-quin — quinidine
Cipro — ciprofloxacin (Fluoroquinolones)
Cirbed — papaverine
Circubid — ethaverine (Papaverine)
Citacal — calcium
Citanest — prilocaine
Citrocarbonate — sodium bicarbonate; sodium citrate (Citrates; Antacids)
Claforan — cefotaxime (Cephalosporins)
Claripex — clofibrate
Claritin — loratadine (Antihistamines, H$_1$-blockers: loratadine)
Cleocin — clindamycin
C-Lexin — cephalexin (Cephalosporins)
Climara — estradiol (Estrogens)
Clinoril — sulindac (Nonsteroidal anti-inflammatory drugs)
Cloderm — clocortolone•
Clopra — metoclopramide
Cloxapen — cloxacillin (Penicillins)
Clozaril — clozapine
Cobalasine — adenosine
Cogentin — benztropine (Anticholinergics)
Cognex — tacrine
Colace — docusate sodium•
Co-Lav — Polyethylene glycol and electrolytes

Colestid — colestipol
Coly-Mycin — colistimethate (Polymyxins)
Colyte — Polyethylene glycol and electrolytes
Comazol — prochlorperazine (Phenothiazines)
Combipres — clonidine; chlorthalidone (Clonidine; Thiazide diuretics)
Compa-Z — prochlorperazine (Phenothiazines)
Compazine — prochlorperazine (Phenothiazines)
Compocillin-V — penicillin V (Penicillins)
Comprecin — enoxacin (Fluoroquinolones)
Comtan — entacapone
Conacetol — acetaminophen
Concecol — betamethasone (Corticosteroids)
Concerta — methylphenidate (Sympathomimetic amines)
Condylox — podofilox•
Conest — estrogens
Congest — estrogens
Conray — iothalamate meglumine (Contrast media)
Constant-T — theophyllines
Copaxone — glatiramer•
Coradur — isosorbide dinitrate (Nitrates)
Coranum — talinolol (Beta-adrenergic blockers)
Cordarone — amiodarone
Cordran — flurandrenolide•
Cordrol — prednisolone (Corticosteroids)
Coreg — carvedilol (Beta-adrenergic blockers)
Corgard — nadolol (Beta-adrenergic blockers)
Coricidin — phenylephrine (Sympathomimetic amines)
Corlopam — fenoldopam
Coronex — isosorbide dinitrate (Nitrates)

Cortacet — hydrocortisone (Corticosteroids)
Cortalone — prednisolone (Corticosteroids)
Cortamed — hydrocortisone (Corticosteroids)
Cortate — hydrocortisone (Corticosteroids)
Cort-Dome — hydrocortisone (Corticosteroids)
Cortef — hydrocortisone (Corticosteroids)
Cortenema — hydrocortisone (Corticosteroids)
Cortifoam — hydrocortisone (Corticosteroids)
Cortinal — hydrocortisone (Corticosteroids)
Cortispan Forte — triamcinolone (Corticosteroids)
Cortril — hydrocortisone (Corticosteroids)
Corvert — ibutilide•
Corzide — nadolol; bendroflumethiazide (Beta-adrenergic blockers; Thiazide diuretics)
Cosmegen — dactinomycin•
Cotacort — hydrocortisone (Corticosteroids)
Cotolone — prednisolone (Corticosteroids)
Cotranzine — prochlorperazine (Phenothiazines)
Cotrim — trimethoprim-sulfamethoxazole
Cotropine — benztropine (Anticholinergics)
Coumadin — warfarin (Anticoagulants, oral)
Coversyl — perindopril (Angiotensin-converting enzyme (ACE) inhibitors)
Cozaar — losartan
Creamalin — aluminum hydroxide, magnesium carbonate, ± simethicone (Antacids)
Crestabolic — methandriol (Anabolic and androgenic steroids)
Crixivan — indinavir
Cruex — undecylenic acids•
Cryspen — penicillin G (Penicillins)
Crystapen — penicillin G (Penicillins)
Crysticillin — penicillin G (Penicillins)
Crystodigin — digitoxin
Cuprimine — penicillamine
Curretab — medroxyprogesterone (Progestins)
Cutivate — fluticasone (Corticosteroids)
Cyclocort — amcinonide•
Cycloflex — cyclobenzaprine
Cyclopar — tetracyclines
Cyklokapron — tranexamic acid
Cylert — pemoline•
Cypromar — cyproheptadine
Cystadane — betaine•
Cystagon — cysteamine•
CystoSpaz — hyoscyamine (Anticholinergics)
Cytadren — aminoglutethimide
Cytolen — levothyroxine (Thyroid hormones)
Cytomel — liothyronine (Thyroid hormones)
Cytosar-U — cytarabine
Cytotec — misoprostol
Cytovene — ganciclovir
Cytoxan — cyclophosphamide (Alkylating agents)

Dalalone — dexamethasone (Corticosteroids)
Dalcaine — lidocaine
Dalgan — dezocine•
Dalimycin — oxytetracycline (Tetracyclines)
Dalmane — flurazepam (Benzodiazepines)
Dalpro — valproate
D-Amp — ampicillin (Penicillins)

Danocrine — danazol (Anabolic and androgenic steroids)
Dantrium — dantrolene
Dapa — acetaminophen
Dapex-37.5 — phentermine (Sympathomimetic amines)
Daranide — dichlorphenamide (Carbonic anhydrase inhibitors)
Daraprim — pyrimethamine
Darbid — isopropamide iodide (Anticholinergics)
Darvocet — acetaminophen; propoxyphene (Acetaminophen; Narcotics: methadone and congeners)
Darvon — propoxyphene (Narcotics: methadone and congeners)
Da-Sed — butabarbital (Barbiturates)
Dathroid — thyroid hormones
Datril — acetaminophen
Daxolin — loxapine
Daypro — oxaprozin (Nonsteroidal anti-inflammatory drugs)
Deapril-ST — ergoloid mesylates (Ergot alkaloids)
Decadrol — dexamethasone (Corticosteroids)
Decadron — dexamethasone (Corticosteroids)
Deca-Durabolin — nandrolone (Anabolic and androgenic steroids)
Decaject — dexamethasone (Corticosteroids)
Decameth — dexamethasone (Corticosteroids)
Decarex — dexamethasone (Corticosteroids)
Decasone — dexamethasone (Corticosteroids)
Decaspray — dexamethasone (Corticosteroids)
Declinax — debrisoquine
Declomycin — demeclocycline (Tetracyclines)
Dekasol — dexamethasone (Corticosteroids)
Deladiol-40 — estradiol (Estrogens)
Delalutin — hydroxyprogesterone (Progestins)
Delapav — papaverine
Delatest — testosterone (Anabolic and androgenic steroids)
Delatestryl — testosterone (Anabolic and androgenic steroids)
Delcoid — thyroid hormones
Delestrogen — estradiol (Estrogens)
Delsym — dextromethorphan (Narcotics: dextromethorphan)
Delta-Cortef — prednisolone (Corticosteroids)
Deltalin — vitamin D
Deltapen — penicillin G (Penicillins)
Deltasone — prednisone (Corticosteroids)
Demadex — torsemide
Demerol — meperidine (Narcotics: meperidine and congeners)
Demulen — contraceptives, oral
Denavir — penciclovir•
Dep Gynogen — estradiol (Estrogens)
Depacon — valproate
Depakene — valproate
Depakote — divalproex (Valproate)
Dep-Andro — testosterone (Anabolic and androgenic steroids)
Depapred — methylprednisolone (Corticosteroids)
Depen — penicillamine
Depgynogen — estradiol (Estrogens)
Depmedalone — methylprednisolone (Corticosteroids)
Depo-Estradiol — estradiol (Estrogens)
Depoject — methylprednisolone (Corticosteroids)
Depo-Medrol — methylprednisolone (Corticosteroids)
Depo-Nandrolone — nandrolone (Anabolic and androgenic steroids)
Deponit — nitroglycerin (Nitrates)
Depopred — methylprednisolone (Corticosteroids)

Depo-Predate — methylprednisolone (Corticosteroids)
Depotest — testosterone (Anabolic and androgenic steroids)
Depo-Testosterone — testosterone (Anabolic and androgenic steroids)
Deprenyl — selegiline (Monoamine oxidase inhibitors)
Deproic — valproate
Dep-Test — testosterone (Anabolic and androgenic steroids)
Dequibolin-100 — nandrolone (Anabolic and androgenic steroids)
Desenex — undecylenic acids•
Desogen — contraceptives, oral
Desowen — desonide•
Desoxyn — methamphetamine (Sympathomimetic amines)
D-Est — estradiol (Estrogens)
Desyrel — trazodone
Detrol — tolterodine
Deursil — ursodiol
Dexacen — dexamethasone (Corticosteroids)
Dexacort — dexamethasone (Corticosteroids)
Dexair — dexamethasone (Corticosteroids)
Dexampex — dextroamphetamine (Sympathomimetic amines)
Dexasone — dexamethasone (Corticosteroids)
Dexedrine — dextroamphetamine (Sympathomimetic amines)
Dexim — dexamethasone (Corticosteroids)
Dexone — dexamethasone (Corticosteroids)
D-Feda — pseudoephedrine (Sympathomimetic amines)
D.H.E. 45 — dihydroergotamine (Ergot alkaloids)
DHEA — dehydroepiandrosterone•
Diaβeta — glyburide (Hypoglycemics, sulfonylurea)
Diabinese — chlorpropamide (Hypoglycemics, sulfonylurea)
Diagen — salicylsalicylic acid (Nonsteroidal anti-inflammatory drugs)
Dialume — aluminum hydroxide (Antacids)
Diamox — acetazolamide (Carbonic anhydrase inhibitors)
Diaqua — hydrochlorothiazide (Thiazide diuretics)
Diastat — diazepam (Benzodiazepines)
Diazma — dyphylline (Theophyllines)
Dibenzyline — phenoxybenzamine (Alpha-adrenergic blockers)
Dicarbosil — calcium carbonate (Antacids)
Dicodethal — dextromethorphan (Narcotics: dextromethorphan)
Didrex — benzphetamine (Sympathomimetic amines)
Didronel — etidronate•
Dietac — phenylpropanolamine (Sympathomimetic amines)
Differin — adapalene•
Diflucan — fluconazole (Antifungals, imidazoles and triazoles)
Di-GEL — aluminum hydroxide, magnesium carbonate (Antacids)
Digibind — digoxin immune Fab
Digitaline — digitoxin
Dihycon — phenytoin
Dihydroergotamine mesylate — ergoloid mesylates (Ergot alkaloids)
Dilac-80 — pentaerythritol tetranitrate (Nitrates)
Dilacor-XR — diltiazem
Dilantin — phenytoin
Dilatrate — isosorbide dinitrate (Nitrates)
Dilaudid — hydromorphone (Narcotics: morphine-like)
Dilocaine — lidocaine
Dilor — dyphylline (Theophyllines)
Diltia XT — diltiazem
Dimacid — calcium carbonate, magnesium carbonate (Antacids)
Dimelor — acetohexamide

(Hypoglycemics, sulfonylurea)
Diol L.A. — estradiol (Estrogens)
Dioval — estradiol (Estrogens)
Diovan — valsartan•
Dipentum — olsalazine•
Diphen — phenytoin
Diphentoin — phenytoin
Diphenylan — phenytoin
Diphylets — dextroamphetamine (Sympathomimetic amines)
Dipimol — dipyridamole
Dipridacot — dipyridamole
Dipridamole — dipyridamole
Diprivan — propofol
Diprolene — betamethasone (Corticosteroids)
Diprosone — betamethasone (Corticosteroids)
Dipyridacot — dipyridamole
Disalcid — Nonsteroidal anti-inflammatory drugs
Ditropan — oxybutynin
Diucardin — hydroflumethiazide (Thiazide diuretics)
Diuchlor H — hydrochlorothiazide (Thiazide diuretics)
Diulo — metolazone (Thiazide diuretics)
Diurese — trichlormethiazide (Thiazide diuretics)
Diuril — chlorothiazide (Thiazide diuretics)
Diu-Scrip — hydrochlorothiazide (Thiazide diuretics)
Dixarit — clonidine
Dizac — diazepam (Benzodiazepines)
Dizmiss — meclizine hydrochloride•
DMS — dexamethasone (Corticosteroids)
Doan's Backache Pills — magnesium salicylate (Nonsteroidal anti-inflammatory drugs)
Dobutrex — dobutamine (Sympathomimetic amines)
Dolanex — acetaminophen
Dolene AP-65 — propoxyphene (Narcotics: methadone and congeners)
Dolgesic — ibuprofen (Nonsteroidal anti-inflammatory drugs)
Dolicaine — lidocaine
Dolobid — diflunisal (Nonsteroidal anti-inflammatory drugs)
Dolophine — methadone (Narcotics: methadone and congeners)
Donnamar — hyoscamine (Anticholinergics)
Dopamet — methyldopa
Dopar — levodopa
Dopram — doxapram
Doral — quazepam (Benzodiazepines)
Doraphen-65 — propoxyphene (Narcotics: methadone and congeners)
Dorcol Fever and Pain Reducer — acetaminophen
Dorico — acetaminophen
Doriden — glutethimide
Dorimide — glutethimide
Dormalin — quazepam (Benzodiazepines)
Doryx — doxycycline (Tetracyclines)
Dosaflex — senna fruit extract•
Dostinex — cabergoline
Dowmycin E — erythromycins (Macrolide antibiotics)
Dox-100 — doxycycline (Tetracyclines)
Doxaphene — propoxyphene (Narcotics: methadone and congeners)
Doxy — doxycycline (Tetracyclines)
Doxy-Caps — doxycycline (Tetracyclines)
Doxychel — doxycycline (Tetracyclines)
Doxycin — doxycycline (Tetracyclines)
Doxy-D — doxycycline (Tetracyclines)
Doxygen — doxycycline (Tetracyclines)
Dralzine — hydralazine
Dramamine — dimenhydrinate•

Dramamine II — meclizine hydrochloride•
Drisdol — vitamin D
Drithrocreme — anthralin•
Drithro-scalp — anthralin•
Droxine — dyphylline (Theophyllines)
DTAP — diphtheria-tetanus-acellular pertussis vaccine•
D-Tes — testosterone (Anabolic and androgenic steroids)
D-Test — testosterone (Anabolic and androgenic steroids)
DTIC-Dome — dacarbazine
DTP — diphtheria-tetanus-pertussis vaccine•
Duo-Medihaler — phenylephrine (Sympathomimetic bronchodilators)
Duotrate — pentaerythritol tetranitrate (Nitrates)
Durabolin — nandrolone (Anabolic and androgenic steroids)
Duracillin — penicillin G (Penicillins)
Duracort 50 — prednisolone (Corticosteroids)
Duract — bromfenac (Nonsteroidal anti-inflammatory drugs)
Dura-Estradiol — estradiol (Estrogens)
Dura-Estrin — estradiol (Estrogens)
Duragen — estradiol (Estrogens)
Duragesic — fentanyl (Narcotics: meperidine and congeners)
Duralone — methylprednisolone (Corticosteroids)
Dura-Meth — methylprednisolone (Corticosteroids)
Duramorph PF — morphine (Narcotics: morphine-like)
Durandro — testosterone (Anabolic and androgenic steroids)
Durandrol — methandriol (Anabolic and androgenic steroids)
Duraphyl — theophyllines
Duraquin — quinidine
Duratest — testosterone (Anabolic and androgenic steroids)

Dura-Testosterone — testosterone (Anabolic and androgenic steroids)
Dura-Testrone — testosterone (Anabolic and androgenic steroids)
Durathate-200 — testosterone (Anabolic and androgenic steroids)
Duratrad — estradiol (Estrogens)
Duretic — methyclothiazide (Thiazide diuretics)
Duricef — cefadroxil (Cephalosporins)
Duvoid — bethanechol chloride•
D-Val — diazepam (Benzodiazepines)
D-Vi-Sol — vitamin D
Dyatoin — phenytoin
Dyazide — hydrochlorothiazide; triamterene (Thiazide diuretics; Triamterene)
Dycill — dicloxacillin (Penicillins)
Dyflex — dyphylline (Theophyllines)
Dyflex-200 — diphylline (Theophyllines)
Dyflex-400 — diphylline (Theophyllines)
Dylix — dyphylline (Theophyllines)
Dymelor — acetohexamide (Hypoglycemics, sulfonylurea)
Dynabac — dirithromycin (Macrolide antibiotics)
Dynacin — minocycline (Tetracyclines)
DynaCirc — isradipine
Dynapen — dicloxacillin (Penicillins)
Dyrenium — triamterene
Dysaps — dicyclomine (Anticholinergics)
Dysne-Inhal — epinephrine (Sympathomimetic amines)

E*aspirin* — aspirin (Nonsteroidal anti-inflammatory drugs)
E-Base — erythromycins (Macrolide antibiotics)
Econochlor — chloramphenicol
Econopred — prednisolone

(Corticosteroids)
Ecotrin — aspirin (Nonsteroidal anti-inflammatory drugs)
Ecstasy — Methylenedioxymethamphetamine
E-Cypionate — estradiol (Estrogens)
Edecrin — ethacrynic acid
Edex — alprostadil•
Edrex-25 — promethazine
E.E.S. — erythromycins (Macrolide antibiotics)
Efacin — nicotinic acid
Effer-Syllium — psyllium
Effexor — venlafaxine
Efudex — fluorouracil
Ekko — phenytoin
Elavil — amitriptyline (Antidepressants, tricyclic)
Eldepryl — selegiline (Monoamine oxidase inhibitors)
Elixicon — theophyllines
Elixomin — theophyllines
Elixophyllin — theophyllines
Ellence — epirubicin
Elmiron — pentosan
Elocon — mometasone (Corticosteroids)
Elserpine — reserpine
Elspar — asparaginase•
Eltor — pseudoephedrine (Sympathomimetic amines)
Eltroxin — levothyroxine (Thyroid hormones)
Embeline — clobetasol•
Emcyt — estramustine (Alkylating agents)
Eminase — anistreplase (Thrombolytics)
Emitrip — amitriptyline (Antidepressants, tricyclic)
Empirin — aspirin (Nonsteroidal anti-inflammatory drugs)
Emtet-500 — tetracyclines
E-Mycin — erythromycins (Macrolide antibiotics)
Enbrel — etanercept•
Endep — amitriptyline (Antidepressants, tricyclic)
Enduron — methyclothiazide (Thiazide diuretics)
Enerjets — caffeine
Enkaid — encainide
Enlon — edrophonium (Anticholinesterases)
Enovid — contraceptives, oral
Enovil — amitriptyline (Antidepressants, tricyclic)
Ensure — nutrients, enteral preparations
Ensure Plus — nutrients, enteral preparations
Entron — ferrous gluconate (Iron)
E.P. Mycin — oxytetracycline (Tetracyclines)
Ephrine — phenylephrine (Sympathomimetic amines)
Epifrin — epinephrine (Sympathomimetic amines)
Epinal — epinephrine (Sympathomimetic amines)
EpiPen — epinephrine (Sympathomimetic amines)
Epitol — carbamazepine
Epitrate — epinephrine (Sympathomimetic amines)
Epivir — lamivudine
Epogen — epoetin
Eprex — epoetin
Eprolin — vitamin E
Equanil — meprobamate
Equibolin-50 — nandrolone (Anabolic and androgenic steroids)
Ercaf — ergotamine (Ergot Alkaloids)
Ergocalciferol — calciferol (Vitamin D)
Ergomar — ergotamine (Ergot alkaloids)
Ergostat — ergotamine (Ergot alkaloids)
Ergotrate — ergonovine (Ergot alkaloids)
ERYC — erythromycins (Macrolide antibiotics)
Erycette — erythromycins (Macrolide antibiotics)

Eryderm — erythromycins (Macrolide antibiotics)
Erygel — erythromycins (Macrolide antibiotics)
Erymax — erythromycins (Macrolide antibiotics)
Erypar — erythromycins (Macrolide antibiotics)
EryPed — erythromycins (Macrolide antibiotics)
Ery-Sol — erythromycins (Macrolide antibiotics)
Ery-Tab — erythromycins (Macrolide antibiotics)
Erythro — erythromycins (Macrolide antibiotics)
Erythrocin — erythromycins (Macrolide antibiotics)
Erythrocot — erythromycins (Macrolide antibiotics)
Esdinate — estradiol (Estrogens)
Esdival — estradiol (Estrogens)
Eserine — physostigmine (Anticholinesterases)
Esidrix — hydrochlorothiazide (Thiazide diuretics)
Esimil — guanethidine; hydrochlorothiazide (Guanethidine; Thiazide diuretics)
Eskalith — lithium
Estate — estradiol (Estrogens)
Estinyl — ethinyl estradiol (Estrogens)
Estone — estradiol (Estrogens)
Estrace — estradiol (Estrogens)
Estra-D — estradiol (Estrogens)
Estraderm — estradiol (Estrogens)
Estradurin — estradiol (Estrogens)
Estra-L — estradiol (Estrogens)
Estratab — estrogens
Estrinate — estradiol (Estrogens)
Estro-A — estrogens
Estrocon — estrogens
Estro-Cyp — estradiol (Estrogens)
Estrofem — estradiol (Estrogens)
Estroject — estradiol (Estrogens)
Estro-L.A. — estradiol (Estrogens)
Estronol — estrone (Estrogens)
Estronol-LA — estradiol (Estrogens)
Estroquin — estrogens
Estrosan — estrogens
Estro-Span — estradiol (Estrogens)
Estrovis — quinestrol (Estrogens)
Etalent — ethaverine (Papaverine)
Ethaquin — ethaverine (Papaverine)
Ethatab — ethaverine (Papaverine)
Ethavas — ethaverine (Papaverine)
Ethavex — ethaverine (Papaverine)
Ethmozine — moricizine
Ethon — methyclothiazide (Thiazide diuretics)
Ethrane — enflurane
E.T.S. — erythromycins (Macrolide antibiotics)
Euglucon — glyburide (Hypoglycemics, sulfonylurea)
Euhypnos — temazepam (Benzodiazepines)
Eulexin — flutamide
Euthroid — liotrix (Thyroid hormones)
Eutonyl — pargyline (Monoamine oxidase inhibitors)
Everone — testosterone (Anabolic and androgenic steroids)
Evestrone — estrogens
Evista — raloxifene
Evoxac — cevimeline•
Excedrin — acetaminophen
Exelderm — sulconazole•
Exelon — rivastigmine•
Exna — benzthiazide (Thiazide diuretics)
Expansatol — butabarbital (Barbiturates)

***F**amvir* — famciclovir•
Fansidar — pyrimethamine, sulfadoxine (Pyrimethamine)
Fareston — toremifene
Fastin — phentermine (Sympathomimetic amines)
Faverin — fluvoxamine (Selective serotonin reuptake inhibitors

(SSRIs))
Fed-Mycin — tetracyclines
Felbatol — Felbamate
Feldene — piroxicam (Nonsteroidal anti-inflammatory drugs)
Fellobolic — methandriol (Anabolic and androgenic steroids)
Fellozine — promethazine
Felsules — chloral hydrate
Femara — letrozole•
Feminate — estradiol (Estrogens)
Feminiol — estradiol (Estrogens)
Feminone — ethinyl estradiol (Estrogens)
Femiron — ferrous fumarate (Iron)
Femogen — estrogens
Femotrone — progesterone (Progestins)
Femstat — butoconazole•
Fendon — acetaminophen
Feostat — ferrous fumarate (Iron)
Fergon — ferrous gluconate (Iron)
Fer-iron — ferrous sulfate (Iron)
Fernisolone — prednisolone (Corticosteroids)
Fero-Gradumet — ferrous sulfate (Iron)
Ferolix — ferrous sulfate (Iron)
Ferosol — ferrous sulfate (Iron)
Ferralet — ferrous gluconate (Iron)
Ferralyn — ferrous sulfate (Iron)
Ferranol — ferrous fumarate (Iron)
Ferra-TD — ferrous sulfate (Iron)
Ferretts — ferrous fumarate (Iron)
Ferrinal — ferrous fumarate (Iron)
Fesotyme — ferrous sulfate (Iron)
Flagyl — metronidazole
Flexeril — cyclobenzaprine
Flexoject — orphenadrine
Flexon — orphenadrine
Flolan — epoprostenol•
Flomax — tamsulosin
Flonase — fluticasone (Corticosteroids)
Florinef — fludrocortisone (Corticosteroids)
Flovent — fluticasone (Corticosteroids)
Floxin — ofloxacin (Fluoroquinolones)
Fludara — fludarabine•
Flumadine — rimantadine•
Fluogen — influenza vaccine
Fluor-A-Day — fluoride
Fluorigard — fluoride
Fluorineed — fluoride
Fluorinse — fluoride
Fluoritab — fluoride
Fluorodex — fluoride
Fluor-Op — fluorometholone (Corticosteroids)
Fluoroplex — fluorouracil
Fluothane — halothane
Fluotic — fluoride
Flura-Drops — fluoride
Flura-Tab — fluoride
Flurobate — betamethasone (Corticosteroids)
FluShield — influenza vaccine
Fluvirin — influenza vaccine
Fluzone — influenza vaccine
FML — fluorometholone (Corticosteroids)
Foamicon — alumina, magnesium trisilicate (Antacids)
Folex — methotrexate
Folvite — folic acid
Forane — isoflurane
Fortaz — ceftazidime (Cephalosporins)
Fortovase — saquinavir
Fosamax — alendronate•
Foscavir — foscarnet
Foygen — estrone (Estrogens)
Fragmin — dalteparin•
Fresubin — nutrients, liquid concentrates
Froben — flurbiprofen (Nonsteroidal anti-inflammatory drugs)
FUDR — floxuridine•
Fulvicin — Antifungals, griseofulvin
Fulvicin P/G — Antifungals, griseofulvin
Fulvicin U/F — Antifungals, griseofulvin
Fumasorb — ferrous fumarate (Iron)

Fumerin — ferrous fumarate (Iron)
Fumide — furosemide
Fungizone — amphotericin B (Antifungals, Amphotericin B)
Furacin — nitrofurazone•
Furadantin — nitrofurantoin
Furalan — nitrofurantoin
Furatoin — nitrofurantoin
Furocot — furosemide
Furomide — furosemide
Furoxone — furazolidone (Monoamine oxidase inhibitors)

Gabitril — tiagabine
Gamazole — sulfamethoxazole (Sulfonamides)
Gammagard S/D — Immune Globulin, Intravenous
Gammar-P — Immune Globulin, Intravenous
Ganite — gallium
Gantanol — sulfamethoxazole (Sulfonamides)
Gantrisin — sulfisoxazole (Sulfonamides)
Garamycin — gentamicin (Aminoglycoside antibiotics)
Gastrografin — diatrizoate meglumine (Contrast Media)
Gastrosed — hyoscyamine (Anticholinergics)
Gaviscon — magnesium trisilicate (Antacids)
Gel "7" — fluoride
Gel-Kam — fluoride
Gelstan — fluoride
Gelusil — aluminum hydroxide, magnesium carbonate, ± simethicone (Antacids)
Gemonil — metharbital (Barbiturates)
Gemzar — gemcitabine
Genabid — papaverine
Genapap — acetaminophen
Gen-cept — contraceptives, oral
Genebs — acetaminophen

GenEsa — arbutamine
Genisis — estrogens
Gen-K — potassium
Genoptic — gentamicin (Aminoglycoside antibiotics)
Genora — contraceptives, oral
Genostrin — estrogens
Genotropin — growth hormone, recombinant•
Gentacidin — gentamicin (Aminoglycoside antibiotics)
Gentacin — gentamicin (Aminoglycoside antibiotics)
Gentafair — gentamicin (Aminoglycoside antibiotics)
Gentak — gentamicin (Aminoglycoside antibiotics)
Gentamar — gentamicin (Aminoglycoside antibiotics)
Gentrasul — gentamicin (Aminoglycoside antibiotics)
Gen-Xene — clorazepate (Benzodiazepines)
Geocillin — carbenicillin (Penicillins)
Geopen — carbenicillin (Penicillins)
Geref — sermorelin•
Gerimal — ergoloid mesylates (Ergot alkaloids)
Gesterol 50 — progesterone (Progestins)
Gesterol L.A. 250 — hydroxyprogesterone (Progestins)
Glaucon — epinephrine (Sympathomimetic amines; Sympathomimetic bronchodilators)
Glaupax — acetazolamide (Carbonic anhydrase inhibitors)
GlucoNorm — repaglinide•
Glucophage — metformin
Glucotrol — glipizide (Hypoglycemics, sulfonylurea)
Glucovance — glyburide; metformin (Hypoglycemics, sulfonylurea; metformin)
Glu-K — potassium
Gly-Cort — hydrocortisone (Corticosteroids)
Glynase — glyburide

(Hypoglycemics, sulfonylurea)
Glyset — miglitol
G-Mycin — gentamicin
(Aminoglycoside antibiotics)
G-Myticin — gentamicin
(Aminoglycoside antibiotics)
Go-Evac — Polyethylene glycol and electrolytes
GoLYTELY — Polyethylene glycol and electrolytes
Gravigen — estrogens
G-Recillin-T — penicillin G (Penicillins)
Grifulvin V — Antifungals, griseofulvin
Grisactin — Antifungals, griseofulvin
Grisovin-FP — Antifungals, griseofulvin
Gris-PEG — Antifungals, griseofulvin
Grivate — griseofulvin (Antifungals, griseofulvin)
G-Sox — sulfisoxazole (Sulfonamides)
Gulfasin — sulfisoxazole (Sulfonamides)
G-Well — lindane•
Gynergen — ergotamine (Ergot alkaloids)
Gyne-Sulf — trisulfapyrimidines (Sulfonamides)
Gynogen — estrogens
Gynogen L.A. — estradiol (Estrogens)

Halcion — triazolam (Benzodiazepines)
Haldol — haloperidol
Haldrone — paramethasone (Corticosteroids)
Halenol — acetaminophen
Haley's M-O — magnesium hydroxide, mineral oil (Antacids)
Halfan — halofantrine
Halfprin — aspirin (Nonsteroidal anti-inflammatory drugs)
Halog — halcinonide•
Haloperon — haloperidol
Halotestin — fluoxymesterone (Anabolic and androgenic steroids)
Halotex — haloprogin•
Haltran — ibuprofen (Nonsteroidal anti-inflammatory drugs)
HC — hydrocortisone (Corticosteroids)
Hemocyte — Iron
HepaLean — heparins
Hepathrom — heparins
Heprinar — heparins
Herceptin — trastuzumab
Hexa Betalin — pyridoxine
Hexabrix — ioxaglate (Contrast media)
Hexadrol — dexamethasone (Corticosteroids)
Hexalen — altretamine
Hexavibex — pyridoxine
Hexyphen — trihexyphenidyl (Anticholinergics)
Hi-Cor — hydrocortisone (Corticosteroids)
Hismanal — astemizole (Antihistamines, H$_1$-blockers: astemizole, terfenadine)
Histerone — testosterone (Anabolic and androgenic steroids)
Hivid — zalcitabine
Homapin — homatropine (Anticholinergics)
Homogene-S — testosterone (Anabolic and androgenic steroids)
Honvol — diethylstilbestrol (Estrogens)
Hormogen — estradiol (Estrogens)
Humalog — insulin
Humatin — paromomycin•
Humatrope — growth hormone, recombinant•
Humulin — insulin
Hyalgan — hyaluronan•
Hyasorb — penicillin G (Penicillins)
Hybalergine — ergot alkaloids
Hybolin — nandrolone (Anabolic and androgenic steroids)

Hycamtin — topotecan
Hycodan — hydrocodone (Narcotics: morphine-like)
Hycort — hydrocortisone (Corticosteroids)
Hydeltrasol — prednisolone (Corticosteroids)
Hydergine — ergoloid mesylates (Ergot alkaloids)
Hydoril — hydrochlorothiazide (Thiazide diuretics)
Hydralin — hydralazine
Hydrea — hydroxyurea
Hydrex — benzthiazide (Thiazide diuretics)
Hydro Par — hydrochlorothiazide (Thiazide diuretics)
Hydroaca — hydrochlorothiazide (Thiazide diuretics)
Hydrochlor — hydrochlorothiazide (Thiazide diuretics)
Hydrochlorulan — hydrochlorothiazide (Thiazide diuretics)
Hydrocort — hydrocortisone (Corticosteroids)
Hydrocorten-A — hydrocortisone (Corticosteroids)
Hydrocortone — hydrocortisone (Corticosteroids)
Hydrocot — hydrochlorothiazide (Thiazide diuretics)
HydroDiuril — hydrochlorothiazide (Thiazide diuretics)
Hydro-Ergot — ergot alkaloids
Hydrogenat — ergot alkaloids
Hydromal — hydrochlorothiazide (Thiazide diuretics)
Hydromox — quinethazone (Thiazide diuretics)
Hydrosol — prednisolone (Corticosteroids)
Hydro-T — hydrochlorothiazide (Thiazide diuretics)
Hydro-Tex — hydrocortisone (Corticosteroids)
Hydroxacen — hydroxyzine
Hydrozide — hydrochlorothiazide (Thiazide diuretics)
Hy-Gestrone — hydroxyprogesterone (Progestins)
Hygroton — chlorthalidone (Thiazide diuretics)
Hylorel — guanadrel
Hylutin — hydroxyprogesterone (Progestins)
Hy-Pam — hydroxyzine
Hypaque — diatrizoate meglumine (Contrast media)
Hyperstat — diazoxide
Hyprogest — hydroxyprogesterone (Progestins)
Hysterone — fluoxymesterone (Anabolic and androgenic steroids)
Hytakerol — dihydrotachysterol (Vitamin D)
Hytone — hydrocortisone (Corticosteroids)
Hytrin — terazosin
Hyzaar — losartan; hydrochlorothiazide (Losartan; Thiazide diuretics)
Hyzine — hydroxyzine

Ibren — ibuprofen (Nonsteroidal anti-inflammatory drugs)
Ibuprin — ibuprofen (Nonsteroidal anti-inflammatory drugs)
Ibupro-600 — ibuprofen (Nonsteroidal anti-inflammatory drugs)
Ibuprohm — ibuprofen (Nonsteroidal anti-inflammatory drugs)
Ibu-Tab — ibuprofen (Nonsteroidal anti-inflammatory drugs)
Ibutex — ibuprofen (Nonsteroidal anti-inflammatory drugs)
I-Chlor — chloramphenicol
Idamycin — idarubicin
Ifen — ibuprofen (Nonsteroidal anti-inflammatory drugs)
Ifex — ifosfamide
I-Gent — gentamicin (Aminoglycoside antibiotics)
I-Homatrine — homatropine

(Anticholinergics)
Iletin — insulin
Ilosone — erythromycins (Macrolide antibiotics)
Ilotycin — erythromycins (Macrolide antibiotics)
Imdur — isosorbide mononitrate (Nitrates)
Imitrex — sumatriptan (Triptans)
Imodium — loperamide (Narcotics: meperidine and congeners)
Imovane — zopiclone (Benzodiazepines)
Imovax Rabies — rabies vaccine
Impril — imipramine (Antidepressants, tricyclic)
Imuran — azathioprine
Inapsine — droperidol
Indameth — indomethacin (Nonsteroidal anti-inflammatory drugs)
Inderal — propranolol (Beta-adrenergic blockers)
Inderide — propranolol; hydrochlorothiazide (Beta-adrenergic blockers; Thiazide diuretics)
Indocid — indomethacin (Nonsteroidal anti-inflammatory drugs)
Indocin — indomethacin (Nonsteroidal anti-inflammatory drugs)
Indo-Lemmon — indomethacin (Nonsteroidal anti-inflammatory drugs)
Indomethagan — indomethacin (Nonsteroidal anti-inflammatory drugs)
Inflamase — prednisolone (Corticosteroids)
Infumorph — morphine (Narcotics: morphine-like)
Ingadine — guanethidine
I.N.H. — isoniazid
Innovar — droperidol; fentanyl (Droperidol; Narcotics: meperidine and congeners)

Inocor — amrinone
Insulatard — insulin
Intal — cromolyn sodium•
Integrillin — eptifibatide
Intrabutazone — phenylbutazone
Intralipid — lipids, intravenous preparations
IntronA — interferon alfa-2b (Interferon)
Intropin — dopamine (Sympathomimetic amines)
Invirase — saquinavir
Ionamin — phentermine (Sympathomimetic amines)
I-Pilopine — pilocarpine
I-Pred — prednisolone (Corticosteroids)
Ircon — Iron
Irospan — Iron
Ismelin — guanethidine
Ismo — isosorbide mononitrate (Nitrates)
Isobec — amobarbital (Barbiturates)
Iso-Bid — isosorbide dinitrate (Nitrates)
Isocal — nutrients, enteral preparations
Iso-D — isosorbide dinitrate (Nitrates)
Isolone Forte — prednisolone (Corticosteroids)
Isonal — aprobarbital (Barbiturates)
Isonate — isosorbide dinitrate (Nitrates)
Iso-Par — isosorbide dinitrate (Nitrates)
Isopro Aerometer — isoproterenol (Sympathomimetic amines; Sympathomimetic bronchodilators)
Isoptin — verapamil
Isoptin SR — verapamil
Isopto-Atropine — atropine (Anticholinergics)
Isopto-Carpine — pilocarpine
Isopto-Cetamide — sulfacetamide (Sulfonamides)
Isopto-Eserine — physostigmine (Anticholinesterases)

- 467 -

Isopto-Homatropine — homatropine (Anticholinergics)
Isopto-Hyoscine — scopolamine (Anticholinergics)
Isorbid — isosorbide dinitrate (Nitrates)
Isordil — isosorbide dinitrate (Nitrates)
Isosorb — isosorbide dinitrate (Nitrates)
Isotamine — isoniazid
Isotrate — isosorbide dinitrate (Nitrates)
Isovex — ethaverine (Papaverine)
I-Sulfacet — sulfacetamide (Sulfonamides)
Isuprel — isoproterenol (Sympathomimetic amines; Sympathomimetic bronchodilators)
I-Tropine — atropine (Anticholinergics)
Iveegam IV — Immune Globulin, Intravenous
Izonid — isoniazid

Janimine — imipramine (Antidepressants, tricyclic)
Jenamicin — gentamicin (Aminoglycoside antibiotics)
Jenest — contraceptives, oral

K-10 — potassium
Kabikinase — streptokinase (Thrombolytics)
Kabolin — nandrolone (Anabolic and androgenic steroids)
Kaletra — lopinavir/ritonavir
Kalium Durules — potassium
Kantrex — kanamycin (Aminoglycoside antibiotics)
Kaochlor — potassium
Kaon — potassium
Kaopectate — kaolin-pectin (Kaolin or Kaolin-pectin)
Kaopectolin — kaolin-pectin (Kaolin or Kaolin-pectin)
Karidium — fluoride
Kato — potassium
Kay Ciel — potassium
Kayexalate — sodium polystyrene sulfonate
Kaylixir — potassium
K-Care — potassium
K-Cillin — penicillin G (Penicillins)
K-Dur — potassium
Keflet — cephalexin (Cephalosporins)
Keflex — cephalexin (Cephalosporins)
Keflin — cephalothin (Cephalosporins)
Keforal — cephalexin (Cephalosporins)
Keftab — cephalexin (Cephalosporins)
Kefurox — cefuroxime (Cephalosporins)
Kefzol — cefazolin (Cephalosporins)
Kemadrin — Procyclidine (Anticholinergics)
Kenacort — triamcinolone (Corticosteroids)
Kenaject — triamcinolone (Corticosteroids)
Kenalog — triamcinolone (Corticosteroids)
Keppra — levetiracetam•
Kerlone — betaxolol (Beta-adrenergic blockers)
Kestrin — estrogens
Kestrone — estrone (Estrogens)
Ketalar — ketamine•
Key-Pred — prednisolone (Corticosteroids)
Keysone — prednisone (Corticosteroids)
K-G — potassium
K-ide — potassium
Klavikordal — nitroglycerin (Nitrates)
K-LEASE — potassium
Kleer — phenylpropanolamine (Sympathomimetic amines)
K-Long — potassium

Klonopin — clonazepam (Benzodiazepines)
K-Lor — potassium
Klor-Con — potassium
Kloride — potassium
Klorvess — potassium
Klotrix — potassium
K-Lyte — potassium
K-Norm — potassium
Koffex Syrup — dextromethorphan (Narcotics: dextromethorphan)
Konakion — phytonadione•
Konsyl — psyllium
Kortrate — pentaerythritol tetranitrate (Nitrates)
K-Pen — penicillin G (Penicillins)
K-Phen — promethazine
K-Sol — potassium
K-Tab — potassium
K-Ten — potassium
Kudrox — aluminum hydroxide, magnesium hydroxide (Antacids)
Kwell — lindane•
Kytril — granisetron•

L.A.E. — estradiol (Estrogens)
Lamictal — lamotrigine
Lamisil — terbinafine (Antifungals, terbinafine)
Lamprene — clofazimine
Lanacillin VK — penicillin V (Penicillins)
Lanestrin — estrogens
Laniazid Syrup — isoniazid
Lanophyllin — theophyllines
Lanoxicaps — digoxin
Lanoxin — digoxin
Lanvis — thioguanine
Lapay — papaverine
Largactil — chlorpromazine (Phenothiazines)
Lariam — mefloquine
Larodopa — levodopa
Lasaject — furosemide
Lasimide — furosemide
Lasix — furosemide
L-Caine — lidocaine

Ledercillin — penicillin V (Penicillins)
Lente — insulin
Lescol — fluvastatin (HMG-CoA Reductase Inhibitors)
Leukeran — chlorambucil
Leukine — Sargramostim (colony stimulating factors)
Levabid — hyoscyamine (Anticholinergics)
Levaquin — levofloxacin (Fluoroquinolones)
Levate — amitriptyline (Antidepressants, tricyclic)
Levatol — penbutolol (Beta-adrenergic blockers)
Levlen — contraceptives, oral
Levo-Dromoran — levorphanol (Narcotics: morphine-like)
Levoid — levothyroxine (Thyroid hormones)
Levopa — levodopa
Levophed — norepinephrine (Sympathomimetic amines)
Levora — contraceptives, oral
Levothroid — levothyroxine (Thyroid hormones)
Levoxine — levothyroxine sodium (Thyroid hormones)
Levsin — hyoscyamine (Anticholinergics)
Lexocort — hydrocortisone (Corticosteroids)
Lexxel — felodipine; enalapril (Felodipine; Angiotensin-converting enzyme (ACE) inhibitors)
Libritabs — chlordiazepoxide (Benzodiazepines)
Librium — chlordiazepoxide (Benzodiazepines)
Lidoject — lidocaine
Lidomar — lidocaine
Lidone — molindone
Lincocin — lincomycin
Lioresal — baclofen
Lipidil Micro — fenofibrate
Lipitor — atorvastatin (HMG-CoA Reductase Inhibitors)

Lipo-Hepin — heparins
Lipo-Lutin — progesterone (Progestins)
Lipoxide — chlordiazepoxide (Benzodiazepines)
Liquaemin — heparins
Liquid Pred — prednisone (Corticosteroids)
Liquiprin — acetaminophen
Lisacort — prednisone (Corticosteroids)
Lithane — lithium
Lithizine — lithium
Lithobid — lithium
Lithonate — lithium
Lithotabs — lithium
Livostin — levocabastine•
Lixaminol — aminophylline (Theophyllines)
Lixolin — theophyllines
Lo-Aqua — furosemide
Locholest — cholestyramine
Lodine — etodolac (Nonsteroidal anti-inflammatory drugs)
Lodrane — theophyllines
Loestrin — contraceptives, oral
Loftran — ketazolam (Benzodiazepines)
Loniten — minoxidil
Lo/Ovral — contraceptives, oral
Lopid — gemfibrozil
Lopressor — metoprolol (Beta-adrenergic blockers)
Lopressor HCT — metoprolol; hydrochlorothiazide (Beta-adrenergic blockers; Thiazide diuretics)
Loprox — ciclopirox•
Lopurin — allopurinol
Loqua-50 — hydrochlorothiazide (Thiazide diuretics)
Lorabid — loracarbef•
Loraz — lorazepam (Benzodiazepines)
Lorelco — probucol
Lorol — propranolol (Beta-adrenergic blockers)
Losec — omeprazole

Lotensin — benazepril (Angiotensin-converting enzyme (ACE) inhibitors)
Lotensin HCT — benazepril; hydrochlorothiaze (Angiotensin-converting enzyme (ACE) inhibitors; Thiazide diuretics)
Lotrel — amlodipine; benazepril (Amlodipine; Angiotensin-converting enzyme (ACE) inhibitors)
Lotrimin — clotrimazole (Antifungals, Imidazoles and Triazoles)
Lotrimin AF — clotrimazole (Antifungals, Imidazoles and Triazoles)
Lotusate — talbutal (Barbiturates)
Lovenox — enoxaparin•
Loxapac — loxapine
Loxitane — loxapine
Lozol — indapamide
Ludiomil — maprotiline
Lufyllin — dyphylline (Theophyllines)
Luminal — phenobarbital (Barbiturates)
Lupron — leuprolide•
Luramide — furosemide
Luride — fluoride
Lutolin-S — progesterone (Progestins)
Luvox — fluvoxamine (Selective serotonin reuptake inhibitors (SSRIs))
LYMErix — lyme disease vaccine•
Lynoral — ethinyl estradiol (Estrogens)
Lyopine — atropine (Anticholinergics)
Lyphocin — vancomycin
Lysodren — mitotane

Maalox — aluminum hydroxide, magnesium hydroxide, simethicone (Antacids)

- 470 -

Macpac — nitrofurantoin
Macrobid — nitrofurantoin
Macrodantin — nitrofurantoin
Magan — magnesium salicylate (Nonsteroidal anti-inflammatory drugs)
Maglucate — magnesium gluconate (Antacids)
Magna-Gel — aluminum hydroxide, magnesium carbonate (Antacids)
Malarone — atovaquone; proguanil
Mallamint — calcium carbonate (Antacids)
Malogen — testosterone (Anabolic and androgenic steroids)
Malotrone — testosterone (Anabolic and androgenic steroids)
Man-Agin — testosterone (Anabolic and androgenic steroids)
Mandol — cefamandole (Cephalosporins)
Mandrax — methaqualone•
Mannest — estrogens
Marazide — benzthiazide (Thiazide diuretics)
Marazide II — trichlormethiazide (Thiazide diuretics)
Marblen — calcium carbonate, magnesium carbonate (Antacids)
Marcaine — bupivacaine
Marcillin — ampicillin (Penicillins)
Marflex — orphenadrine
Marinol — dronabinol•
Marpap — papaverine
Marplan — isocarboxazid (Monoamine oxidase inhibitors)
Mar-Pred — methylprednisolone (Corticosteroids)
Marthritic — salicylsalicylic acid (Nonsteroidal anti-inflammatory drugs)
Maso-chlora — chloral hydrate
Maso-Pred — prednisone (Corticosteroids)
Maso-Toxin — digoxin
Maso-trol — pentaerythritol tetranitrate (Nitrates)
Masoxin — digoxin

Matulane — procarbazine
Mavik — trandolapril (Angiotensin-converting enzyme (ACE) inhibitors)
Maxair — pirbuterol•
Maxalt — rizatriptan (Triptans)
Maxaquin — lomefloxacin (Fluoroquinolones)
Maxenal — pseudoephedrine (Sympathomimetic amines)
Maxeran — metoclopramide
Maxidex — dexamethasone (Corticosteroids)
Maxipime — cefepime (Cephalosporins)
Maxolon — metoclopramide
Maxzide — hydrochlorothiazide; triamterene (Thiazide diuretics; Triamterene)
Mazanor — mazindol
Mazepine — carbamazepine
Measurin — aspirin (Nonsteroidal anti-inflammatory drugs)
Mebaral — mephobarbital (Barbiturates)
Meclodium — meclofenamate (Nonsteroidal anti-inflammatory drugs)
Meclofen — meclofenamate (Nonsteroidal anti-inflammatory drugs)
Meclomen — meclofenamate (Nonsteroidal anti-inflammatory drugs)
Meda-Cap — acetaminophen
Medarsed — butabarbital (Barbiturates)
Meda-Tab — acetaminophen
Medicort 50 — prednisolone (Corticosteroids)
Medidex — dexamethasone (Corticosteroids)
Medidiol — estradiol (Estrogens)
Medigesic — acetaminophen
Medihaler-Ergotamine — ergotamine (Ergot alkaloids)
Medihaler-Iso — isoproterenol (Sympathomimetic bronchodilators)

Medilium — chlordiazepoxide (Benzodiazepines)
Medipred — methylprednisolone (Corticosteroids)
Medipren — ibuprofen (Nonsteroidal anti-inflammatory drugs)
Mediquell — dextromethorphan (Narcotics: dextromethorphan)
Medispaz — hyoscyamine (Anticholinergics)
Meditest — testosterone (Anabolic and androgenic steroids)
Meditran — meprobamate
Med-Jec-40 — methylprednisolone (Corticosteroids)
Medlone — methylprednisolone (Corticosteroids)
Medralone — methylprednisolone (Corticosteroids)
Medrex — methylprednisolone (Corticosteroids)
Medrol — methylprednisolone (Corticosteroids)
Mefoxin — cefoxitin (Cephalosporins)
Megace — megestrol acetate
Megacillin — penicillin G (Penicillins)
Melfiat — phendimetrazine (Sympathomimetic amines)
Mellaril — thioridazine (Phenothiazines)
Menaval — estradiol (Estrogens)
Menest — estrogens
Meni-D — meclizine hydrochloride•
Menolyn — ethinyl estradiol (Estrogens)
Menopak-E — estrogens
Menotabs — estrogens
Menrium — chlordiazepoxide (Benzodiazepines)
Mentax — butenafine•
Mepred — methylprednisolone (Corticosteroids)
Meprocon — meprobamate
Meprolone — methylprednisolone (Corticosteroids)
Mepron — atovaquone
Meprospan — meprobamate
Mercurochrome — merbromin (Antiseptics, mercurial)
Meridia — sibutramine
Merphol — thimerosal (Antiseptics, mercurial)
Merrem — meropenem•
Mersol — thimerosal (Antiseptics, mercurial)
Mesantoin — mephenytoin
Mesnex — mesna
Mestinon — pyridostigmine•
Metaglucina — acetohexamide (Hypoglycemics, sulfonylurea)
Metahydrin — trichlormethiazide (Thiazide diuretics)
Metalone — prednisolone (Corticosteroids)
Metandren — methyltestosterone (Anabolic and androgenic steroids)
Metaprel — metaproterenol (Sympathomimetic bronchodilators)
Metestone — methyltestosterone (Anabolic and androgenic steroids)
Methadose — methadone (Narcotics: methadone and congeners)
Methampex — methamphetamine (Sympathomimetic amines)
Methazine — promethazine
Methergine — methylergonovine (Ergot alkaloids)
Methydrol — methylprednisolone (Corticosteroids)
Methylcotolone — methylprednisolone (Corticosteroids)
Methylin — methylphenidate (Sympathomimetic amines)
Methylone — methylprednisolone (Corticosteroids)
Methylpred — methylprednisolone (Corticosteroids)
Meticorten — prednisone (Corticosteroids)
Metopirone — metyrapone

Metranil — pentaerythritol tetranitrate (Nitrates)
Metreton — prednisolone (Corticosteroids)
Metric 21 — metronidazole
Metro I.V. — metronidazole
Metrogel — metronidazole
Metronid — metronidazole
Metryl — metronidazole
Metubine — metocurine (Neuromuscular blocking agents)
Mevacor — lovastatin (HMG-CoA Reductase Inhibitors)
Meval — diazepam (Benzodiazepines)
Mexate — methotrexate
Mexitil — mexiletine
Mezlin — mezlocillin (Penicillins)
Miacalcin — calcitonin
Micardis — telmisartan
Microcort — hydrocortisone (Corticosteroids)
Micro-K — potassium
Micronase — glyburide (Hypoglycemics, sulfonylurea)
Micronor — contraceptives, oral; progestins
Microsul — sulfamethizole (Sulfonamides)
Microsulfon — sulfadiazine (Sulfonamides)
Mictrin — hydrochlorothiazide (Thiazide diuretics)
Midamor — amiloride
Milocarpine — pilocarpine
Miltown — meprobamate
Minestrin — contraceptives, oral
Minipress — prazosin
Minitran — nitroglycerin (Nitrates)
Minocin — minocycline (Tetracyclines)
Minodyl — minoxidil
Min-Ovral — contraceptives, oral
Mintezol — thiabendazole
Mio-Rel — orphenadrine
Mi-Pilo — pilocarpine
Mira Lax — Polyethylene glycol and electrolytes

Miradon — anisindione (Anticoagulants, oral)
Mirapex — pramipexole
Mithracin — plicamycin•
Mitran — chlordiazepoxide (Benzodiazepines)
Mivacron — mivacurium (Neuromuscular blocking agents)
Mixtard — insulin
Moban — molindone
Mobenol — tolbutamide (Hypoglycemics, sulfonylurea)
Mobic — meloxicam (Nonsteroidal anti-inflammatory drugs)
Modane — psyllium
Modane Versabran — psyllium
Modecate — fluphenazine (Phenothiazines)
Modicon — contraceptives, oral
Moditen — fluphenazine (Phenothiazines)
Moduretic — amiloride, hydrochlorothiazide (amiloride; Thiazide diuretics)
Mogadon — nitrazepam (Benzodiazepines)
Monistat — miconazole (Antifungals, Imidazoles and Triazoles)
Monitan — acebutolol (Beta-adrenergic blockers)
Monocid — cefonicid (Cephalosporins)
Monodox — doxycycline (Tetracyclines)
Mono-Gesic — salicylsalicylic acid (Nonsteroidal anti-inflammatory drugs)
Monoket — isosorbide mononitrate (Nitrates)
Monopril — fosinopril (Angiotensin-converting enzyme (ACE) inhibitors)
Monurol — fosfomycin
M-Orexic — diethylpropion (Sympathomimetic amines)
Morphitec — morphine (Narcotics; morphine-like)

M.O.S. — morphine (Narcotics: morphine-like)
Motilium — domperidone•
Motrin — ibuprofen (Nonsteroidal anti-inflammatory drugs)
Moxam — moxalactam (Cephalosporins)
MS Contin — morphine (Narcotics: morphine-like)
MSIR — morphine (Narcotics: morphine-like)
Ms-Med — estrogens
Mucillium — psyllium
Multifuge — piperazine•
Multipax — hydroxyzine
Murocoll — homatropine (Anticholinergics)
MUSE — alprostadil•
Mustargen — mechlorethamine (Alkylating agents)
Mutamycin — mitomycin C
Myambutol — ethambutol•
My-B-Den — adenosine
Mycelex — clotrimazole (Antifungals, Imidazoles and Triazoles)
Mycifradin — neomycin (Aminoglycoside antibiotics)
Myclopramide — metoclopramide
Mycobutin — rifabutin
Mycostatin — nystatin•
Mydfrin — phenylephrine (Sympathomimetic amines)
My-E — erythromycins (Macrolide antibiotics)
Myidone — primidone
Mykrox — metolazone (Thiazide diuretics)
Mylanta — aluminum hydroxide, magnesium hydroxide, simethicone (Antacids)
Myleran — busulfan (Alkylating agents)
Mylotarg — gemtuzumab•
Myobid — papaverine
Myochrysine — gold sodium thiomalate
Myolin — orphenadrine
Myospaz — propoxyphene (Narcotics: methadone and congeners)
Myotrol — orphenadrine
Myproic Acid — valproate
MyroSemide — furosemide
Mysoline — primidone
M-Zide — hydrochlorothiazide (Thiazide diuretics)

Nafcil — nafcillin (Penicillins)
Nafrinse — fluoride
Naftin — naftifine•
Naldegesic — pseudoephedrine (Sympathomimetic amines)
Nalfon — fenoprofen (Nonsteroidal anti-inflammatory drugs)
Nallpen — nafcillin sodium (Penicillins)
Nandrobolic — nandrolone (Anabolic and androgenic steroids)
Nandrocot — nandrolone (Anabolic and androgenic steroids)
Nandrolate — nandrolone (Anabolic and androgenic steroids)
Naprelan — naproxen (Nonsteroidal anti-inflammatory drugs)
Naprosyn — naproxen (Nonsteroidal anti-inflammatory drugs)
Naptrate — pentaerythritol tetranitrate (Nitrates)
Naqua — trichlormethiazide (Thiazide diuretics)
Narcan — naloxone
Nardil — phenelzine (Monoamine oxidase inhibitors)
Naropin — ropivacaine
Nasacort — triamcinolone (Corticosteroids)
Nasalcrom — cromolyn sodium•
Nasalide — flunisolide (Corticosteroids)
Nasarel — flunisolide (Corticosteroids)
Nasonex — mometasone (Corticosteroids)

Natulan — procarbazine
Naturetin — bendroflumethiazide (Thiazide diuretics)
Navane — thiothixene (Phenothiazines)
Navelbine — vinorelbine•
Naxen — naproxen (Nonsteroidal anti-inflammatory drugs)
Nebcin — tobramycin (Aminoglycoside antibiotics)
NebuPent — pentamidine
Necon — contraceptives, oral
N.E.E. — contraceptives, oral
NegGram — nalidixic acid
Nelova — contraceptives, oral
Nemasol — aminosalicylic acid
Nembutal — pentobarbital (Barbiturates)
Neo-Codema — hydrochlorothiazide (Thiazide diuretics)
Neocurb — phendimetrazine (Sympathomimetic amines)
Neocyten — orphenadrine
Neo-Durabolic — nandrolone (Anabolic and androgenic steroids)
Neo-Hombreol-F — testosterone (Anabolic and androgenic steroids)
Neo-Hombreol-M — methyltestosterone (Anabolic and androgenic steroids)
Neo-Medrol — methylprednisolone (Corticosteroids)
Neopap — acetaminophen
Neopasalate — aminosalicylic acid
Neopavrin — ethaverine (Papaverine)
Neoral — cyclosporine
Neosar — cyclophosphamide (Alkylating agents)
Neo-Synephrine — phenylephrine (Sympathomimetic amines)
Neothylline — dyphylline (Theophyllines)
Neotrizine — trisulfapyrimidines (Sulfonamides)
Nephronex — nitrofurantoin
Neptazane — methazolamide (Carbonic anhydrase inhibitors)

Nervocaine — lidocaine
Netromycin — netilmicin (Aminoglycoside antibiotics)
Neucalm 50 — hydroxyzine
Neupogen — Filgrastim (colony stimulating factors)
Neuromax — Doxacurium (Neuromuscular blocking agents)
Neurontin — gabapentin
Neut — sodium bicarbonate (Antacids)
Neutralca-S — aluminum hydroxide, magnesium hydroxide (Antacids)
Neutrexin — trimetrexate•
Neuvil — ibuprofen (Nonsteroidal anti-inflammatory drugs)
Niac — nicotinic acid
Niaspan — nicotinic acid
NiCard XL — nicotinic acid
Nico-400 — nicotinic acid
Nicobid — nicotinic acid
Nicolar — nicotinic acid
Niconyl — isoniazid
Nicorette — nicotine gum
Nicotinex — nicotinic acid
Niglycon — nitroglycerin (Nitrates)
Niloric — ergot alkaloids
Nilprin — acetaminophen
Nilstatin — nystatin•
Nimotop — nimodipine
Niong — nitroglycerin (Nitrates)
Nipride — nitroprusside (Nitrates)
Nisolone — prednisolone (Corticosteroids)
Ni-Span — nicotinic acid
Nitrek — nitroglycerin (Nitrates)
Nitrex — nitrofurantoin
Nitrin — pentaerythritol tetranitrate (Nitrates)
Nitro SA — nitroglycerin (Nitrates)
Nitro Trans System — nitroglycerin (Nitrates)
Nitro-Bid — nitroglycerin (Nitrates)
Nitrocap T.D. — nitroglycerin (Nitrates)
Nitrocels — nitroglycerin (Nitrates)
Nitrocine — nitroglycerin (Nitrates)
Nitrocot — nitroglycerin (Nitrates)

Nitro-Derm — nitroglycerin (Nitrates)
Nitro-Dial — nitroglycerin (Nitrates)
Nitrodisc — nitroglycerin (Nitrates)
Nitro-Dur — nitroglycerin (Nitrates)
Nitrodyl — nitroglycerin (Nitrates)
Nitrofor — nitrofurantoin
Nitrofuracot — nitrofurantoin
Nitrogard — nitroglycerin (Nitrates)
Nitroglyn — nitroglycerin (Nitrates)
Nitrojet — nitroglycerin (Nitrates)
Nitrol — nitroglycerin (Nitrates)
Nitrolan — nitroglycerin (Nitrates)
Nitrolin — nitroglycerin (Nitrates)
Nitrolingual — nitroglycerin (Nitrates)
Nitro-Lyn — nitroglycerin (Nitrates)
Nitromed — isosorbide dinitrate (Nitrates)
Nitronet — nitroglycerin (Nitrates)
Nitrong — nitroglycerin (Nitrates)
Nitropar — nitroglycerin (Nitrates)
Nitropress — nitroprusside (Nitrates)
Nitroprex — nitroglycerin (Nitrates)
Nitroquick — nitroglycerin (Nitrates)
Nitrorex — nitroglycerin (Nitrates)
Nitrospan — nitroglycerin (Nitrates)
Nitrostat — nitroglycerin (Nitrates)
Nitro-Time — nitroglycerin (Nitrates)
Nitrotransdermal — nitroglycerin (Nitrates)
Nitrotym — nitroglycerin (Nitrates)
Nizoral — ketoconazole (Antifungals, imidazoles and triazoles)
No Doz — caffeine
Nobesine — diethylpropion (Sympathomimetic amines)
Noctec — chloral hydrate
Nolvadex — tamoxifen
Noradex — orphenadrine
Norcept-E — contraceptives, oral
Norcuron — vecuronium (Neuromuscular blocking agents)
Nordette — contraceptives, oral
Norditropin — growth hormone, recombinant•

Norethin — contraceptives, oral
Norflex — orphenadrine
Norfranil — imipramine (Antidepressants, tricyclic)
Norinyl — contraceptives, oral
Norisodrine — isoproterenol (Sympathomimetic amines; Sympathomimetic bronchodilators)
Norlestrin — contraceptives, oral
Norlutate — norethindrone acetate (Progestins)
Norlutin — norethindrone (Contraceptives, oral; Progestins)
Normiflo — ardeparin•
Normodyne — labetalol (Beta-adrenergic blockers)
Normozide — labetalol (Beta-adrenergic blockers)
Norocaine — lidocaine
Noroxin — norfloxacin (Fluoroquinolones)
Norpace — disopyramide
Norpanth — propantheline (Anticholinergics)
Norphyl — aminophylline (Theophyllines)
Norplant — levonorgestrel (Contraceptives, implant)
Norpramin — desipramine (Antidepressants, tricyclic)
Nor-Pred — prednisolone (Corticosteroids)
Nor-Q.D. — contraceptives, oral
Norquen — contraceptives, oral
Nor-Tet — tetracyclines
Norvasc — amlodipine
Norvir — ritonavir
Norwich Aspirin — aspirin (Nonsteroidal anti-inflammatory drugs)
Nospaz — dicyclomine (Anticholinergics)
Novafed — pseudoephedrine (Sympathomimetic amines)
Novamobarb — amobarbital (Barbiturates)
Novantrone — mitozoxane•
Nova-Phenicol — chloramphenicol

Nova-Pred — prednisolone (Corticosteroids)
Novobetamet — betamethasone (Corticosteroids)
Novobutamide — tolbutamide (Hypoglycemics, sulfonylurea)
Novobutazone — phenylbutazone
Novocarbamaz — carbamazepine
Novochlorhydrate — chloral hydrate
Novochlorocap — chloramphenicol
Novochlorpromazine — chlorpromazine (Phenothiazines)
Novocimetidine — cimetidine (Antihistamines, H_2-blockers)
Novoclopate — clorazepate (Benzodiazepines)
Novodifenac — diclofenac (Nonsteroidal anti-inflammatory drugs)
Novo-Digoxin — digoxin
Novodiltiazem — diltiazem
Novodipam — diazepam (Benzodiazepines)
Novodipiradol — dipyridamole
Novodoxylin — doxycycline (Tetracyclines)
Novoferrogluc — ferrous gluconate (Iron)
Novoferrosulfa — ferrous sulfate (Iron)
Novofibrate — clofibrate
Novoflupam — flurazepam (Benzodiazepines)
Novoflurazine — trifluoperazine (Phenothiazines)
Novofuran — nitrofurantoin
Novohydrazide — hydrochlorothiazide (Thiazide diuretics)
Novohydrocort — hydrocortisone (Corticosteroids)
Novohydroxyzin — hydroxyzine
Novohylazin — hydralazine
Novolente-K — potassium
Novolexin — cephalexin (Cephalosporins)
Novolin — insulin
Novolorazem — lorazepam (Benzodiazepines)
Novomedopa — methyldopa
Novomepro — meprobamate
Novomethacin — indomethacin (Nonsteroidal anti-inflammatory drugs)
Novometoprol — metoprolol (Beta-adrenergic blockers)
Novonaprox — naproxen (Nonsteroidal anti-inflammatory drugs)
Novonidazol — metronidazole
Novonifedin — nifedipine
Novoperidol — haloperidol
Novopirocam — piroxicam (Nonsteroidal anti-inflammatory drugs)
Novopoxide — chlordiazepoxide (Benzodiazepines)
Novo-Pramine — imipramine (Antidepressants, tricyclic)
Novopranol — propranolol (Beta-adrenergic blockers)
Novoprofen — ibuprofen (Nonsteroidal anti-inflammatory drugs)
Novopropamide — chlorpropamide (Hypoglycemics, sulfonylurea)
Novopropanthil — propantheline (Anticholinergics)
Novopropoxyn — propoxyphene (Narcotics: methadone and congeners)
Novopurol — allopurinol
Novoquinidin — quinidine
Novoramidine — ranitidine (Antihistamines, H_2-blockers)
Novoridazine — thioridazine (Phenothiazines)
Novosalmol — albuterol (Sympathomimetic bronchodilators)
Novosemide — furosemide
Novosorbide — isosorbide dinitrate (Nitrates)
Novospiroton — spironolactone
Novosundac — sulindac (Nonsteroidal anti-inflammatory

Novotrimel — trimethoprim-sulfamethoxazole
Novotriptyn — amitriptyline (Antidepressants, tricyclic)
Novoveramil — verapamil
Novoxapam — oxazepam (Benzodiazepines)
Nu-Ampi — ampicillin (Penicillins)
Nu-Atenol — atenolol (Beta-adrenergic blockers)
Nubain — nalbuphine (Narcotics: morphine-like)
Nu-Diltiaz — diltiazem
NuLYTELY — Polyethylene glycol and electrolytes
Nu-Medopa — methyldopa
Numorphan — oxymorphone (Narcotics: morphine-like)
Nuprin — ibuprofen (Nonsteroidal anti-inflammatory drugs)
Nutramag — aluminum hydroxide, magnesium hydroxide (Antacids)
Nutranel — nutrients, enteral preparations
Nutrilyte — nutrients, parenteral
Nutropin — growth hormone, recombinant•
Nydrazid — isoniazid
Nystex — nystatin•

Obe-Mar — phentermine (Sympathomimetic amines)
Obe-Nix — phentermine (Sympathomimetic amines)
Obephen — phentermine (Sympathomimetic amines)
Obermine — phentermine (Sympathomimetic amines)
Obestat — phenylpropanolamine (Sympathomimetic amines)
Obetrol — amphetamine (Sympathomimetic amines)
Occlusal — salicylic acid (Nonsteroidal anti-inflammatory drugs)
Octamide — metoclopramide
Ocu-Carpine — pilocarpine
Ocu-Dex — dexamethasone (Corticosteroids)
Ocufen — flurbiprofen (Nonsteroidal anti-inflammatory drugs)
Ocu-Mycin — gentamicin (Aminoglycoside antibiotics)
Ocu-Pred — prednisolone (Corticosteroids)
Ocusert — pilocarpine
Ocu-Sul — sulfacetamide (Sulfonamides)
Ocusulf-10 — sulfacetamide (Sulfonamides)
Ocu-Tropine — atropine (Anticholinergics)
Ocu-Zolamide — acetazolamide (Carbonic anhydrase inhibitors)
Odor Scrip — methionine
Oestrilin — estrone (Estrogens)
O'Flex — orphenadrine
Ogen — estrone (Estrogens)
Omnicef — cefdinir (Cephalosporins)
Omniflox — temafloxacin (Fluoroquinolones)
Omnipaque — iohexol (Contrast media)
Omnipen-N — ampicillin (Penicillins)
Oncovin — vincristine
Onset — isosorbide dinitrate (Nitrates)
Ophthacet — sulfacetamide (Sulfonamides)
Opthochlor — chloramphenicol
Opticrom — cromolyn sodium•
Optimine — azatadine•
Optiphyllin — theophyllines
Orabase HCA — hydrocortisone (Corticosteroids)
Oracit — sodium citrate, citric acid (Citrates)
OraCort — triamcinolone (Corticosteroids)
Oradexon — dexamethasone (Corticosteroids)
Oradrate — chloral hydrate

Oralone — triamcinolone (Corticosteroids)
Oralphylline — theophyllines
Oramorph — morphine (Narcotics: morphine-like)
Orap — pimozide
Orapin — estrogens
Orasone — prednisone (Corticosteroids)
Ora-Testryl — fluoxymesterone (Anabolic and androgenic steroids)
Ora-VK — penicillin V (Penicillins)
Or-Bolic — methandrostenolone (Anabolic and androgenic steroids)
Or-Dex — dexamethasone (Corticosteroids)
Oretic — hydrochlorothiazide (Thiazide diuretics)
Oreton Methyl — methyltestosterone (Anabolic and androgenic steroids)
Orflagen — orphenadrine
Orfro — orphenadrine
Orgaran — danaparoid•
Oribetic — tolbutamide (Hypoglycemics, sulfonylurea)
Orinase — tolbutamide (Hypoglycemics, sulfonylurea)
Orlaam — levomethadyl•
Ormazine — chlorpromazine (Phenothiazines)
Oro-Naf — fluoride
Or-Phen-50 — promethazine
Orphenate — orphenadrine
Ortho Tri-Cyclen — ethinyl estradiol, norgestimate (Contraceptives, oral)
Ortho-Cept — contraceptives, oral
Orthoclone OKT3 — muromonab-CD3
Ortho-Cyclen — contraceptives, oral
Ortho-Est — estropipate (Estrogens)
Ortho-Novum — contraceptives, oral
Ortho-Tri-Cyclen — contraceptives, oral
Orudis — ketoprofen (Nonsteroidal anti-inflammatory drugs)
Os-Cal — calcium

Osmolite — nutrients, enteral preparations
Ostoforte — vitamin D
Ostone — methyltestosterone (Anabolic and androgenic steroids)
Ovcon — contraceptives, oral
Ovest — estrogens
Ovide Lotion — malathion
Ovlin — estrogens
Ovogyn — ethinyl estradiol (Estrogens)
Ovral — contraceptives, oral
Ovrette — contraceptives, oral
Ovulen — contraceptives, oral
Oxlopar — oxytetracycline (Tetracyclines)
Oxsoralen — methoxsalen
Oxycontin — oxycodone (Narcotics: morphine-like)
Oxydess — dextroamphetamine (Sympathomimetic amines)
Oxylone — fluorometholone (Corticosteroids)

P-200 — papaverine
Palaron — aminophylline (Theophyllines)
Palmophylline — theophyllines
Palocillin — penicillin G (Penicillins)
Paludrine — proguanil
Pamelor — nortriptyline (Antidepressants, tricyclic)
Pamine — methscopolamine (Anticholinergics)
Pan B6 — pyridoxine
Panadol — acetaminophen
Panasol — prednisone (Corticosteroids)
Panectyl — trimeprazine (Phenothiazines)
Pan-Estra LA 40 — estradiol (Estrogens)
Panex — acetaminophen
Panisolone — prednisolone (Corticosteroids)
Pan-Kloride — potassium

Panmycin — tetracyclines
Panshape M — phentermine (Sympathomimetic amines)
Pansone — prednisone (Corticosteroids)
Pantocrin-F — thyroid hormones
Pantopon — opium alkaloids (Narcotics: morphine-like)
Panwarfin — warfarin (Anticoagulants, oral)
Papacon — papaverine
Paraflex — chlorzoxazone
Parafon — chlorzoxazone
Parafon Forte DSC — chlorzoxazone
Paraplatin — carboplatin
Parcillin — penicillin G (Penicillins)
Parda — levodopa
Parlodel — bromocriptine
Parloid — thyroid hormones
Parmine — phentermine (Sympathomimetic amines)
Parnate — tranylcypromine (Monoamine oxidase inhibitors)
Pasara — aminosalicylic acid
Pasdium — aminosalicylic acid
Paser — aminosalicylic acid
Paskalium — aminosalicylic acid
Pasmex — hyoscyamine (Anticholinergics)
Patanol — olopatadine•
Pathocil — dicloxacillin (Penicillins)
Pava Par — papaverine
Pavabid — papaverine
Pavacap — papaverine
Pavacels — papaverine
Pavaclor — papaverine
Pavacot — papaverine
Pavacron — papaverine
Pavadel — papaverine
Pavadyl — papaverine
Pavagen — papaverine
Pavakey — papaverine
Pava-Lyn — papaverine
Pavased — papaverine
Pavasule — papaverine
Pavatab-200 — papaverine
Pavates — papaverine
Pavatime — papaverine
Pavatran — papaverine
Pavatym — papaverine
Paveral — codeine (Narcotics: morphine-like)
Paverine — papaverine
Paverolan — papaverine
Pavex — papaverine
Pavulon — pancuronium (Neuromuscular blocking agents)
Pax-400 — meprobamate
Paxil — paroxetine (Selective serotonin reuptake inhibitors (SSRIs))
Paxipam — halazepam (Benzodiazepines)
PBZ — tripelennamine•
PCE Dispertab — erythromycins (Macrolide antibiotics)
Pecto-Kalin — kaolin-pectin (Kaolin or Kaolin-pectin)
Pectokay — kaolin-pectin (Kaolin or Kaolin-pectin)
Pedameth — methionine
Pediaflor — fluoride
Pediamycin — erythromycins; sulfisoxazole (Macrolide antibiotics; Sulfonamides)
Pediapred — prednisolone (Corticosteroids)
Pediaprofen — ibuprofen (Nonsteroidal anti-inflammatory drugs)
Pediazole — erythromycins; sulfisoxazole (Macrolide antibiotics; Sulfonamides)
Pedi-Dent — fluoride
PemADD — pemoline•
Penagen-VK — penicillin V (Penicillins)
Penamp — ampicillin (Penicillins)
Penbritin — ampicillin (Penicillins)
Penetrex — enoxacin (Fluoroquinolones)
Pen-G — penicillin G (Penicillins)
Penlac — ciclopirox•
Pensorb — penicillin G (Penicillins)
Penta — pentobarbital (Barbiturates)
Penta-cap — pentaerythritol

tetranitrate (Nitrates)
Pentafin — pentaerythritol tetranitrate (Nitrates)
Pentam 300 — pentamidine
Pentasa — mesalamine
Pentazine — promethazine
Pentestan — pentaerythritol tetranitrate (Nitrates)
Pentet — pentaerythritol tetranitrate (Nitrates)
Pentetra — pentaerythritol tetranitrate (Nitrates)
Pentids — penicillin G (Penicillins)
Pentogen — pentobarbital (Barbiturates)
Pentol — pentaerythritol tetranitrate (Nitrates)
Pentostam — sodium stibogluconate•
Pentothal — thiopental (Barbiturates)
Pentylan — pentaerythritol tetranitrate (Nitrates)
Pen-V — penicillin V (Penicillins)
Pen-Vee K — penicillin V (Penicillins)
Pepcid — famotidine (Antihistamines, H$_2$-blockers)
Peptavlon — pentagastrin
Pepto-Bismol — bismuth subsalicylate
Peptol — cimetidine (Antihistamines, H$_2$-blockers)
Percocet — oxycodone; acetaminophen (Narcotics: morphine-like; Acetaminophen)
Percodan — oxycodone; aspirin (Narcotics: morphine-like; Nonsteroidal anti-inflammatory drugs)
Percolone — oxycodone (Narcotics: morphine-like)
Perdiem — psyllium
Periactin — cyproheptadine
Peridex — chlorhexidine•
Peridol — haloperidol
Peritrate — pentaerythritol tetranitrate (Nitrates)
Permax — pergolide

Permitil — fluphenazine (Phenothiazines)
Persantine — dipyridamole
Pertofrane — desipramine (Antidepressants, tricyclic)
Pertropin — vitamin E
P.E.T.N. — pentaerythritol tetranitrate (Nitrates)
Petro-20 — pentaerythritol tetranitrate (Nitrates)
Pfizerpen VK — penicillin V (Penicillins)
Pharbec — amobarbital (Barbiturates)
Pharmaflur — fluoride
Pharmalgen — insect venom extracts
Pharmorubicin — epirubicin
Phenameth — promethazine
Phenaphen — acetaminophen
Phenazine — perphenazine (Phenothiazines)
Phenbuff — phenylbutazone
Phencen-50 — promethazine
Phenerex — promethazine
Phenergan — promethazine
Phenerhist — promethazine
Phenerzine — promethazine
Phenoject-50 — promethazine
Phentercot — phentermine (Sympathomimetic amines)
Phenterspan — phentermine (Sympathomimetic amines)
Phentride — phentermine (Sympathomimetic amines)
Phentrol — phentermine (Sympathomimetic amines)
Phenytex — phenytoin
Phosphaljel — aluminum phosphate (Antacids)
Phyllocontin — aminophylline (Theophyllines)
Pilocar — pilocarpine
Pilokair — pilocarpine
Pilomiotin — pilocarpine
Pilopine-HS — pilocarpine
Piloptic — pilocarpine
Pilostat — pilocarpine

Pima — potassium
Pipracil — piperacillin (Penicillins)
Pirmavar — pirmenol•
Placidyl — ethchlorvynol•
Plaquenil — hydroxychloroquine
Platinol — cisplatin
Plavix — clopidogrel
Plendil — felodipine
Pletal — cilostazol
PMB — estrogens
Polocaine — mepivacaine
Polycillin — ampicillin (Penicillins)
Polycitra Syrup — potassium citrate, sodium citrate, citric acid (Citrates; Potassium)
Polycitra-K — potassium citrate, citric acid (Citrates; Potassium)
Polycitra-LC — potassium citrate, sodium citrate, citric acid (Citrates; Potassium)
Polygam S/D — Immune Globulin, Intravenous
Polymox — amoxicillin (Penicillins)
Ponderal — fenfluramine (Sympathomimetic amines)
Pondimin — fenfluramine (Sympathomimetic amines)
Ponstan — mefenamic acid (Nonsteroidal anti-inflammatory drugs)
Ponstel — mefenamic acid (Nonsteroidal anti-inflammatory drugs)
Posture — calcium
Potage — potassium
Potasalan — potassium
Potassine — potassium
Poxi — chlordiazepoxide (Benzodiazepines)
Prandase — acarbose
Prandin — repaglinide•
Pravachol — pravastatin (HMG-CoA Reductase Inhibitors)
Precorsin — tryptophan
Precose — acarbose
Pred Air A — prednisolone (Corticosteroids)
Pred Forte — prednisolone (Corticosteroids)
Predacorten — methylprednisolone (Corticosteroids)
Predair — prednisolone (Corticosteroids)
Predaject-50 — prednisolone (Corticosteroids)
Predalone 50 — prednisolone (Corticosteroids)
Predate — prednisolone (Corticosteroids)
Predcor — prednisolone (Corticosteroids)
Predicort-50 — prednisolone (Corticosteroids)
Pred-ject-50 — prednisolone (Corticosteroids)
Prednicen-M — prednisone (Corticosteroids)
Prednicot — prednisone (Corticosteroids)
Prefrin — phenylephrine (Sympathomimetic amines)
Preladron — dexamethasone (Corticosteroids)
Prelestone — betamethasone (Corticosteroids)
Prelestrin — estrogens
Prelone — prednisolone (Corticosteroids)
Preludin — phenmetrazine (Sympathomimetic amines)
Premarin — estrogens
Presamine — imipramine (Antidepressants, tricyclic)
Prevacid — lansoprazole
Prevalite — cholestyramine
Preven — contraceptives, oral
Preveon — adefovir•
Pri-Cortin — prednisolone (Corticosteroids)
Priftin — rifapentine
Prilosec — omeprazole
Primatene — epinephrine (Sympathomimetic bronchodilators)
Primaxin — imipenem
Primazine — promazine

(Phenothiazines)
Primestrin — estrogens
Primethasone — dexamethasone (Corticosteroids)
Pri-Methylate — methylprednisolone (Corticosteroids)
Primotest — methyltestosterone (Anabolic and androgenic steroids)
Primotest Depot — testosterone (Anabolic and androgenic steroids)
Principen — ampicillin (Penicillins)
Prinivil — lisinopril (Angiotensin-converting enzyme (ACE) inhibitors)
Prinzide — lisinopril; hydrochlorothiazide (Angiotensin-converting enzyme (ACE) inhibitors; Thiazide diuretics)
Priscoline — tolazoline
Pro-50 — promethazine
ProAmatine — midodrine
Proaqua — benzthiazide (Thiazide diuretics)
Probalan — probenecid
Probamide — propantheline (Anticholinergics)
Pro-Banthine — propantheline (Anticholinergics)
Probate — meprobamate
Probeta — bisoprolol (Beta-adrenergic blockers)
Probolic — methandriol (Anabolic and androgenic steroids)
Procamide SR — procainamide
Procan SR — procainamide
Procanbid — procainamide
Procapan — procainamide
Procardia — nifedipine
Proclan — promethazine
Procrit — epoetin
Proctocort — hydrocortisone (Corticosteroids)
Procytox — cyclophosphamide (Alkylating agents)
Pro-Depo — hydroxyprogesterone (Progestins)
Profen — ibuprofen (Nonsteroidal anti-inflammatory drugs)
Profenal — suprofen•

Progelan — progesterone (Progestins)
Progesic — propoxyphene (Narcotics: methadone and congeners)
Progestaject-50 — progesterone (Progestins)
Progestasert — progesterone (Progestins)
Proglycem — diazoxide
Prograf — tacrolimus
Progynon — estradiol (Estrogens)
Proklar — sulfamethizole (Sulfonamides)
Prolastin — antitrypsin
Proleukin — interleukin-2
Prolixin — fluphenazine (Phenothiazines)
Prolocaine — mepivacaine
Proloid — thyroid hormones
Proloprim — trimethoprim
Promachlor — chlorpromazine (Phenothiazines)
Promacot — promethazine
Promapar — chlorpromazine (Phenothiazines)
Promaz — chlorpromazine (Phenothiazines)
Prometa — metaproterenol (Sympathomimetic bronchodilators)
Prometh — promethazine
Promethapar — promethazine
Promethegan — promethazine
Prometrium — progestins
Promide — propantheline (Anticholinergics)
Pronestyl — procainamide
Pronto — Pyrethrins with piperonyl butoxide•
Propacet — acetaminophen; propoxyphene (Acetaminophen; Narcotics: methadone and congeners)
Propadrine — phenylpropanolamine (Sympathomimetic amines)
Propagest — phenylpropanolamine (Sympathomimetic amines)

- 483 -

Propagon-S — estrone (Estrogens)
Propan — phenylpropanolamine (Sympathomimetic amines)
Propecia — finasteride
Propine — dipivefrin (Sympathomimetic amines)
Propoxycon — propoxyphene (Narcotics: methadone and congeners)
Propulsid — cisapride
Propyl-Thyracil — propylthiouracil
Prorex — promethazine
Prorone — progesterone (Progestins)
Proscar — finasteride
ProSom — estazolam (Benzodiazepines)
Prostaphlin — oxacillin (Penicillins)
Prostigmin — neostigmine (Anticholinesterases)
Prostin — alprostadil•
Protabolin — nandrolone (Anabolic and androgenic steroids)
Proternol — isoproterenol (Sympathomimetic amines; Sympathomimetic bronchodilators)
Prothazine — promethazine
Protonix — pantoprazole•
Protopam — pralidoxime•
Protostat — metronidazole
Protrin — trimethoprim-sulfamethoxazole
Protropin — growth hormone, recombinant•
Proventil — albuterol (Sympathomimetic bronchodilators)
Provera — medroxyprogesterone (Progestins)
Provigan — promethazine
Provigil — modafinil
Prozac — fluoxetine (Selective serotonin reuptake inhibitors (SSRIs))
Prozine-50 — promazine (Phenothiazines)
Pseudofrin — pseudoephedrine (Sympathomimetic amines)

Psorian — betamethasone (Corticosteroids)
P.S.P. — prednisolone (Corticosteroids)
Pulmicort — budesonide (Corticosteroids)
Pulmozyme — deoxyribonuclease•
Purinethol — mercaptopurine
Purinol — allopurinol
P.V. Carpine — pilocarpine
Pyopen — carbenicillin (Penicillins)
Pyri — pyridoxine
Pyrohep — cyproheptadine

Q*M-260* — quinine
Q-Pam — diazepam (Benzodiazepines)
Quelicin — succinylcholine (Neuromuscular blocking agents)
Questran — cholestyramine
Quibron-T — theophyllines
Quiebar — butabarbital (Barbiturates)
Quiess — hydroxyzine
Quin-260 — quinine
Quinagen — quinidine
Quinaglute — quinidine
Quinalan — quinidine
Quin-Amino — quinine
Quinaminoph — quinine
Quinamm — quinine
Quinate — quinidine
Quinatime — quinidine
Quindan — quinine
Quine — quinine
Quin-G — quinidine
Quinicardine — quinidine
Quinidex — quinidine
Quinitime — quinidine
Quinora — quinidine
Quin-Release — quinidine
Quiphile — quinine

R*adiostol* — vitamin D

Rapamune — sirolimus
Rate — pentaerythritol tetranitrate (Nitrates)
Rauloydin — reserpine
Raurine — reserpine
Raxar — grepafloxacin (Fluoroquinolones)
Rebetrol — ribavirin
Reclomide — metoclopramide
Rectalad — aminophylline (Theophyllines)
Regitine — phentolamine•
Reglan — metoclopramide
Regranex — becaplermin•
Reithritol — pentaerythritol tetranitrate (Nitrates)
Relafen — nabumetone (Nonsteroidal anti-inflammatory drugs)
Relenza — zanamivir•
Remeron — mirtazapine
Remicade — infliximab•
Remsed — promethazine
Remular-S — cholestyramine
Renbu — butabarbital (Barbiturates)
Renese — polythiazide (Thiazide diuretics)
Renografin — diatrizoate meglumine (Contrast media)
Renoquid — sulfacytine (Sulfonamides)
Renovist — diatrizoate meglumine (Contrast Media)
ReoPro — abciximab•
Repose — promazine (Phenothiazines)
Rep-Pred — methylprednisolone (Corticosteroids)
Requip — ropinirole
Resa — reserpine
Rescriptor — delavirdine
Reserjen — reserpine
Reserpaneed — reserpine
Respbid — theophyllines
Restocort — hydrocortisone (Corticosteroids)
Restoril — temazepam (Benzodiazepines)
Retandros — testosterone (Anabolic and androgenic steroids)
Retavase — reteplase (Thrombolytics)
Retestrin — estradiol (Estrogens)
Retin-A — Tretinoin (retinoic acid)
Retrovir — zidovudine
Reverin — rolitetracycline (Tetracyclines)
Reversol — edrophonium (Anticholinesterases)
Revex — nalmefene•
Revimine — dopamine (Sympathomimetic amines)
Rexolate — salicylates (Nonsteroidal anti-inflammatory drugs; Salicylates, topical)
Rezine — hydroxyzine
Rezulin — troglitazone
Rheumatrex — methotrexate
Rhindecon — phenylpropanolamine (Sympathomimetic amines)
Rhinocort — budesonide (Corticosteroids)
Rhodis — ketoprofen (Nonsteroidal anti-inflammatory drugs)
Rhotrimine — trimipramine (Antidepressants, tricyclic)
Rhythmin-SR — procainamide
RID — Pyrethrins with piperonyl butoxide•
Ridaura — auranofin
Rifadin — rifampin
Rilutek — riluzole•
Rimactane — rifampin
Rimso-50 — dimethyl sulfoxide
Riopan — magnesium aluminate, magaldrate (Antacids)
Risperdal — risperidone
Ritalin — methylphenidate (Sympathomimetic amines)
Rituxan — rituximab•
Rivotril — clonazepam (Benzodiazepines)
RMS — morphine (Narcotics: morphine-like)
Roampicillin — ampicillin (Penicillins)

Robantaline — propantheline (Anticholinergics)
Robaxin — methocarbamol•
Robenecid — probenecid
Robese — dextroamphetamine (Sympathomimetic amines)
Robicillin VK — penicillin V (Penicillins)
Robidone — hydrocodone (Narcotics: morphine-like)
Robidrine — pseudoephedrine (Sympathomimetic amines)
Robigesic — acetaminophen
Robimycin — erythromycins (Macrolide antibiotics)
Robinul — glycopyrrolate (Anticholinergics)
Robitet — tetracyclines
Robitussin — dextromethorphan (Narcotics: dextromethorphan)
Robolic — methandriol (Anabolic and androgenic steroids)
Rocaine — lidocaine
Rocaltrol — calcitriol•
Rocephin — ceftriaxone (Cephalosporins)
Rochlomethiazide — trichlormethiazide (Thiazide diuretics)
Rodex — pyridoxine
Ro-Diet — diethylpropion (Sympathomimetic amines)
Rofact — rifampin
Ro-Fedrin — pseudoephedrine (Sympathomimetic amines)
Roferon-A — interferon alfa-2a (Interferon)
Rogaine — minoxidil
Rogenic — Iron
Ro-Hydrazide — hydrochlorothiazide (Thiazide diuretics)
Rolaids — calcium carbonate (Antacids)
Rolaphent — phentermine (Sympathomimetic amines)
Rolathimide — glutethimide
Rolazid — isoniazid

Roldiol — ethaverine (Papaverine)
Ronase — tolazamide (Hypoglycemics, sulfonylurea)
Ro-Papav — papaverine
Ro-Pox 65 — propoxyphene (Narcotics: methadone and congeners)
Ropoxy — propoxyphene (Narcotics: methadone and congeners)
Ropred — prednisone (Corticosteroids)
Rosoxol — sulfisoxazole (Sulfonamides)
Rotashield — rotavirus vaccine•
Rothav — ethaverine (Papaverine)
Roubac — trimethoprim-sulfamethoxazole
Rounox — acetaminophen
Rouphylline — oxtriphylline (Theophyllines)
Rovamycine — spiramycin
Rowasa — mesalamine
Roxanol — morphine (Narcotics: morphine-like)
Roxicodone — oxycodone (Narcotics: morphine-like)
Roxithromycin — Macrolide antibiotics
Roychlor — potassium
RP-Mycin — erythromycins (Macrolide antibiotics)
RU 486 — Mifepristone
Rubex — doxorubicin
Rufen — ibuprofen (Nonsteroidal anti-inflammatory drugs)
Rum-K — potassium
Rythmodan — disopyramide
Rythmol — propafenone

S-*60* — sodium salicylate (Nonsteroidal anti-inflammatory drugs)
Sabril — Vigabatrin
Saizen — growth hormone, recombinant•
Salazopyrin — sulfasalazine

(Sulfonamides)
Salcylic Acid — salicylates, oral (Nonsteroidal anti-inflammatory drugs)
Salflex — salicylsalicylic acid (Nonsteroidal anti-inflammatory drugs)
Salgesic — salicylsalicylic acid (Nonsteroidal anti-inflammatory drugs)
Salsalate — salicylsalicylic acid (Nonsteroidal anti-inflammatory drugs)
Salsitab — salicylsalicylic acid (Nonsteroidal anti-inflammatory drugs)
Saluron — hydroflumethiazide (Thiazide diuretics)
Sandimmune — cyclosporine
Sandoglobulin — Immune Globulin, Intravenous
Sandostatin — octreotide
Sanorex — mazindol
Sansert — methysergide (Ergot alkaloids)
Sarisol — butabarbital (Barbiturates)
Sarodant — nitrofurantoin
Sarogesic — prednisone (Corticosteroids)
S.A.S. — sulfasalazine (Sulfonamides)
Scoline — methscopolamine (Anticholinergics)
Scopace — scopolamine (Anticholinergics)
Scotrex — tetracyclines
Screen — chlordiazepoxide (Benzodiazepines)
Sebizon — sulfacetamide (Sulfonamides)
Seco-8 — secobarbital (Barbiturates)
Seconal — secobarbital (Barbiturates)
Sectral — acebutolol (Beta-adrenergic blockers)
Sedabamate — meprobamate
Sedatuss — dextromethorphan (Narcotics: dextromethorphan)
Seffin — cephalothin (Cephalosporins)
Seldane — terfenadine (Antihistamines, H_1-blockers: astemizole, terfenadine)
Selestoject — betamethasone (Corticosteroids)
Semilente — insulin
Semprex — acrivastine•
Senexon — senna fruit extract•
Senokot — senna fruit extract•
Senormin — atenolol (Beta-adrenergic blockers)
Sensorcaine — bupivacaine
Septra — trimethoprim-sulfamethoxazole
Serax — oxazepam (Benzodiazepines)
Serbina — reserpine
Sereen — chlordiazepoxide (Benzodiazepines)
Serentil — mesoridazine (Phenothiazines)
Serevent — salmeterol•
Seromycin — cycloserine
Seroquel — quetiapine
Serostim — growth hormone, recombinant•
Serpalan — reserpine
Serpanray — reserpine
Serpasil — reserpine
Serpatabs — reserpine
Sertan — primidone
Serzone — nefazodone
Shocaine — lidocaine
Shogan — promethazine
Shohl's solution — sodium citrate, citric acid (Citrates)
Sholog — triamcinolone (Corticosteroids)
Sholone — prednisolone (Corticosteroids)
Shotest — testosterone (Anabolic and androgenic steroids)
Sigazine — promethazine
Sigpred — prednisolone (Corticosteroids)

Silain-Gel — aluminum hydroxide, magnesium hydroxide, simethicone (Antacids)
Simulect — basiliximab•
Sinarest — phenylephrine (Sympathomimetic amines)
Sinemet — carbidopa-levodopa (Levodopa)
Sinequan — doxepin (Antidepressants, tricyclic)
Singulair — montelukast
Sinufed — pseudoephedrine (Sympathomimetic amines)
Skelaxin — metaxalone•
Skelid — tiludronate
Slo-bid — theophyllines
Slo-Phyllin — theophyllines
Slow-FE — ferrous sulfate (Iron)
Slow-K — potassium
Slow-Trasicor — oxprenolol (Beta-adrenergic blockers)
Sodasone — prednisolone (Corticosteroids)
Sodestrin — estrogens
Soduben — butabarbital (Barbiturates)
Sofarin — warfarin (Anticoagulants, oral)
Solazine — trifluoperazine (Phenothiazines)
Solfoton — phenobarbital (Barbiturates)
Solium — chlordiazepoxide (Benzodiazepines)
Sol-Pred — prednisolone (Corticosteroids)
Solu-Barb — phenobarbital (Barbiturates)
Solucap E — vitamin E
Solu-Cortef — hydrocortisone (Corticosteroids)
Solu-Flur — fluoride
Solu-Medrol — methylprednisolone (Corticosteroids)
Solu-Phyllin — theophyllines
Solurex — dexamethasone (Corticosteroids)
Soma — carisoprodol•
Somnol — flurazepam (Benzodiazepines)
Somnos — chloral hydrate
Somophylline — theophyllines
Sonata — zaleplon
Sonazide — hydroflumethiazide (Thiazide diuretics)
Sonazine — chlorpromazine (Phenothiazines)
Sopamycetin — chloramphenicol
Sorbitrate — isosorbide dinitrate (Nitrates)
Soriatane — acitretin
Sorquad — isosorbide dinitrate (Nitrates)
Sotacor — sotalol (Beta-adrenergic blockers)
Soxa — sulfisoxazole (Sulfonamides)
Span Niacin — nicotinic acid
Spancap No. 1 — dextroamphetamine (Sympathomimetic amines)
Span-Est — estradiol (Estrogens)
Span-FF — Iron
Span-Test — testosterone (Anabolic and androgenic steroids)
Sparine — promazine (Phenothiazines)
Spasdel — hyoscyamine (Anticholinergics)
Spasodil — ethaverine (Papaverine)
Spastil — propantheline (Anticholinergics)
Spectazole — econazole•
Spectro-Atropine — atropine (Anticholinergics)
Spectro-Chlor — chloramphenicol
Spectro-Dex — dexamethasone (Corticosteroids)
Spectro-Erythromycin — erythromycins (Macrolide antibiotics)
Spectro-Genta — gentamicin (Aminoglycoside antibiotics)
Spectro-Homatropine — homatropine (Anticholinergics)
Spectro-Pilo — pilocarpine

Spectro-Pred — prednisolone (Corticosteroids)
Spectro-Sulf — sulfacetamide (Sulfonamides)
Spectro-Tate — prednisolone (Corticosteroids)
Spersacarpine — pilocarpine
Spersadex — dexamethasone (Corticosteroids)
Spersanicol — chloramphenicol
Spersaphrine — phenylephrine (Sympathomimetic amines)
Sporanox — itraconazole (Antifungals, imidazoles and triazoles)
SPS — sodium polystyrene sulfonate
S-P-T — thyroid hormones
S-T Cort — hydrocortisone (Corticosteroids)
St Joseph Aspirin — aspirin (Nonsteroidal anti-inflammatory drugs)
St Joseph Cough Syrup — dextromethorphan (Narcotics: dextromethorphan)
Stadol — butorphanol•
Stanacaine — lidocaine
Staphcillin — methicillin (Penicillins)
Statex — morphine (Narcotics: morphine-like)
Staticin — erythromycins (Macrolide antibiotics)
Stelazine — trifluoperazine (Phenothiazines)
Stemetil — prochlorperazine (Phenothiazines)
Ster-5 — prednisolone (Corticosteroids)
Steraject — prednisolone (Corticosteroids)
Sterane — prednisolone (Corticosteroids)
Sterapred — prednisone (Corticosteroids)
Stilphostrol — diethylstilbestrol (Estrogens)
Stim 250 — caffeine

Storz-G — gentamicin (Aminoglycoside antibiotics)
Strema — quinine
Streptase — streptokinase (thrombolytics)
Stromba — stanozolol (Anabolic and androgenic steroids)
Stromectol — ivermectin
Sublimaze — fentanyl (Narcotics: meperidine and congeners)
Sucostrin — succinylcholine (Neuromuscular blocking agents)
Sudafed — pseudoephedrine (Sympathomimetic amines)
Sufenta — sufentanil•
Sular — nisoldipine
Sulcolon — sulfasalazine (Sulfonamides)
Sulf-10 — sulfacetamide (Sulfonamides)
Sulfacet-R — sulfacetamide (Sulfonamides)
Sulfagan — sulfisoxazole (Sulfonamides)
Sulfa-Gyn — trisulfapyrimidines (Sulfonamides)
Sulfair — sulfacetamide (Sulfonamides)
Sulfair Forte — sulfacetamide (Sulfonamides)
Sulfamar — trimethoprim-sulfamethoxazole
Sulfamethoprim — trimethoprim-sulfamethoxazole
Sulfamide — sulfacetamide (Sulfonamides)
Sulfaprim — trimethoprim-sulfamethoxazole
Sulfasol — sulfamethizole (Sulfonamides)
Sulfatrim — trimethoprim-sulfamethoxazole
Sulfex — sulfacetamide (Sulfonamides)
Sulfizin — sulfisoxazole (Sulfonamides)
Sulfoxaprim — trimethoprim-sulfamethoxazole

Sulfstat — sulfamethizole (Sulfonamides)
Sulfurine — sulfamethizole (Sulfonamides)
Sulnac — trisulfapyrimidines (Sulfonamides)
Sulten — sulfacetamide (Sulfonamides)
Sultrin — trisulfapyrimidines (Sulfonamides)
Sumycin — tetracyclines
Sunkist — vitamin C
Supeudol — oxycodone (Narcotics: morphine-like)
Suppap — acetaminophen
Suprane — desflurane
Suprax — cefixime (Cephalosporins)
Suprazine — trifluoperazine (Phenothiazines)
Surital — thiamylal (Barbiturates)
Surmontil — trimipramine (Antidepressants, tricyclic)
Suspen — penicillin V (Penicillins)
Sus-Phrine — epinephrine (Sympathomimetic amines)
Sustaire — theophyllines
Sustiva — efavirenz
Sux-Cert — succinylcholine (Neuromuscular blocking agents)
Symadine — amantadine
Symmetrel — amantadine
Synacort — hydrocortisone (Corticosteroids)
Synagis — palivizumab•
Syn-Captopril — captopril (Angiotensin-converting enzyme (ACE) inhibitors)
Syn-Diltiazem — diltiazem
Synercid — quinupristin/dalfopristin
Synflex — naproxen (Nonsteroidal anti-inflammatory drugs)
Synkayvite — menadione•
Synophylate — theophyllines
Synphasic — contraceptives, oral
Syntetrin — rolitetracycline (Tetracyclines)
Synthroid — levothyroxine (Thyroid hormones)
Synthrox — levothyroxine (Thyroid hormones)
Synvisc — hyaluronan•

Tac 3 — triamcinolone (Corticosteroids)
TACE — estrogens
Tag-39 — estrogens
Tagamet — cimetidine (Antihistamines, H_2-blockers)
Talwin — pentazocine (Narcotics: pentazocine)
Tambocor — flecainide
Tamiflu — oseltamivir•
Tamofen — tamoxifen
Tamone — tamoxifen
TAO — troleandomycin
Tapanol — acetaminophen
Tarabine — cytarabine
Taractan — chlorprothixene (Phenothiazines)
Tarasan — chlorprothixene (Phenothiazines)
Targretin — bexarotene
Tarka — verapamil; trandolapril (Verapamil; Angiotensin-converting enzyme (ACE) inhibitors)
Taside — potassium
Tasmar — tolcapone
Taxol — paclitaxel
Taxotere — docetaxel•
Tazicef — ceftazidime (Cephalosporins)
Tazidime — ceftazidime (Cephalosporins)
Tazol — tolazoline
Tazorac — tazarotene•
Tc-99m teboroxime — cardiotech•
T-CAIN — lidocaine
T-Cypionate — testosterone (Anabolic and androgenic steroids)
T-Diet — phentermine (Sympathomimetic amines)
Teczem — diltiazem; enalapril (Diltiazem; Angiotensin-converting enzyme (ACE) inhibitors)
Teebacin — aminosalicylic acid

Teebaconin — isoniazid
Tega-C — vitamin C
Tega-Cort — hydrocortisone (Corticosteroids)
Tega-Cycline — tetracyclines
Tega-E — vitamin E
Tega-Flex — orphenadrine
Tegison — etretinate
Tegopen — cloxacillin (Penicillins)
Tegretol — carbamazepine
Teline — tetracyclines
Temaril — trimeprazine (Phenothiazines)
Temaz — temazepam (Benzodiazepines)
Temergan 50 — promethazine
Temodar — temozolomide•
Temovate — clobetasol propionate•
Tempra — acetaminophen
Tenex — guanfacine
Ten-K — potassium
Tenol — acetaminophen
Tenoretic — atenolol; chlorthalidone (Beta-adrenergic blockers; Thiazide diuretics)
Tenormin — atenolol (Beta-adrenergic blockers)
Tensilon — edrophonium (Anticholinesterases)
Tensin — reserpine
Tentrate — pentaerythritol tetranitrate (Nitrates)
Tenuate — diethylpropion (Sympathomimetic amines)
Tepanil — diethylpropion (Sympathomimetic amines)
Tequin — gatifloxacin (Fluoroquinolones)
Teramin — phentermine (Sympathomimetic amines)
Terazol — terconazole•
Terpium — chlorpromazine (Phenothiazines)
Terramycin — oxytetracycline (Tetracyclines)
Teslac — testolactone (Anabolic and androgenic steroids)
Tessalon — benzonatate•

Testa-C — testosterone (Anabolic and androgenic steroids)
Testamone-100 — testosterone (Anabolic and androgenic steroids)
Testaqua — testosterone (Anabolic and androgenic steroids)
Testaspan — testosterone (Anabolic and androgenic steroids)
Testate — testosterone (Anabolic and androgenic steroids)
Testex — testosterone (Anabolic and androgenic steroids)
Testoderm — testosterone (Anabolic and androgenic steroids)
Testoject — testosterone (Anabolic and androgenic steroids)
Testolin — testosterone (Anabolic and androgenic steroids)
Testone L.A. — testosterone (Anabolic and androgenic steroids)
Testred — methyltestosterone (Anabolic and androgenic steroids)
Testred Cypionate — testosterone (Anabolic and androgenic steroids)
Testrin-P.A. — testosterone (Anabolic and androgenic steroids)
Testro — testosterone (Anabolic and androgenic steroids)
Testrone — testosterone (Anabolic and androgenic steroids)
Tet-Cy — tetracyclines
Tetra-C — tetracyclines
Tetrachlor — tetracyclines
Tetracon — tetracyclines
Tetracyn — tetracyclines
Tetralan — tetracyclines
Tetram — tetracyclines
Tetramax — tetracyclines
Tetraneed — pentaerythritol tetranitrate (Nitrates)
Tetratab — pentaerythritol tetranitrate (Nitrates)
Teveten — eprosartan•
Texacort — hydrocortisone (Corticosteroids)
Thalitone — chlorthalidone (Thiazide diuretics)
Thalomid — thalidomide•

Theelin — estrone (Estrogens)
Theo — theophyllines
Theo-24 — theophyllines
Theobid — theophyllines
Theochron — theophyllines
Theoclear — theophyllines
Theocot — theophyllines
Theo-Dur — theophyllines
Theogen — estrone (Estrogens)
Theolair — theophyllines
Theomar — theophyllines
Theon — theophyllines
Theospan — theophyllines
Theo-SR — theophyllines
Theostat — theophyllines
Theo-Time — theophyllines
Theovent — theophyllines
Thermoloid — thyroid hormones
Thiosulfil — sulfamethizole (Sulfonamides)
Thiuretic — hydrochlorothiazide (Thiazide diuretics)
Thoradol — chlorpromazine (Phenothiazines)
Thorazine — chlorpromazine (Phenothiazines)
Thoronil — chlorpromazine (Phenothiazines)
Thor-Prom — chlorpromazine (Phenothiazines)
Thylline — dyphylline (Theophyllines)
Thyrar — thyroid hormones
Thyrobrom — thyroid hormones
Thyrocrine — thyroid hormones
Thyrolar — liotrix (Thyroid hormones)
Thyro-teric — thyroid hormones
Thytropar — thyrotropin (Thyroid hormones)
Tiazac — diltiazem
Ticar — ticarcillin (Penicillins)
Ticlid — ticlopidine
Ticlodix — ticlopidine
Tidex — dextroamphetamine (Sympathomimetic amines)
Tija — oxytetracycline (Tetracyclines)

Tikosyn — dofetilide
Tilade — nedocromil•
Timacor — timolol (Beta-adrenergic blockers)
Timolide — timolol; hydrochlorothiazide (Beta-adrenergic blockers; Thiazide diuretics)
Timoptic — timolol (Beta-adrenergic blockers)
Tinactin — tolnaftate•
Tindal — acetophenazine (Phenothiazines)
Tipramine — imipramine (Antidepressants, tricyclic)
Tirend — caffeine
Tobrex — tobramycin (Aminoglycoside antibiotics)
Tocopheryl — vitamin E
Tofranil — imipramine (Antidepressants, tricyclic)
Tolamide — tolazamide (Hypoglycemics, sulfonylurea)
Tolectin — tolmetin (Nonsteroidal anti-inflammatory drugs)
Tolinase — tolazamide (Hypoglycemics, sulfonylurea)
Toloxan — tolazoline
Tolzol — tolazoline
Tone-Tes — testosterone (Anabolic and androgenic steroids)
Tonocard — tocainide
Topamax — topiramate
Topicort — desoximetasone•
Topicycline — tetracyclines
Toprol XL — metoprolol (Beta-adrenergic blockers)
Tora — phentermine (Sympathomimetic amines)
Toradol — ketorolac (Nonsteroidal anti-inflammatory drugs)
Torecan — thiethylperazine (Phenothiazines)
Tornalate — bitolterol
Totacillin — ampicillin (Penicillins)
T-Phyl — theophyllines
T-Quil — diazepam (Benzodiazepines)

Tracilon — triamcinolone (Corticosteroids)
Tracrium — atracurium (Neuromuscular blocking agents)
Tramacort 40 — triamcinolone (Corticosteroids)
Trancot — meprobamate
Trandate — labetalol (Beta-adrenergic blockers)
Tranite — pentaerythritol tetranitrate (Nitrates)
Tranmep — meprobamate
Tranquiline — meprobamate
Transderm-Nitro — nitroglycerin (Nitrates)
Transderm-Scop — scopolamine (Anticholinergics)
Transderm-V — scopolamine (Anticholinergics)
Trans-Ver-Sal — salicylic acid (Nonsteroidal anti-inflammatory drugs)
Trantoin — nitrofurantoin
Tranxene — clorazepate (Benzodiazepines)
Trasicor — oxprenolol (Beta-adrenergic blockers)
Trasylol — aprotinin
Trates — nitroglycerin (Nitrates)
Trazon — trazodone
Trecator — ethionamide•
Trental — pentoxifylline
Trexal — naltrexone
Trexan — naltrexone
Trexin — tetracyclines
Triacet — triamcinolone (Corticosteroids)
Triacilon — triamcinolone (Corticosteroids)
Triadapin — doxepin (Antidepressants, tricyclic)
Trialodine — trazodone
Triam Acet — triamcinolone (Corticosteroids)
Triam-A — triamcinolone (Corticosteroids)
Triam-Forte — triamcinolone (Corticosteroids)

Triamolone 40 — triamcinolone (Corticosteroids)
Triamonide 40 — triamcinolone (Corticosteroids)
Trianide — triamcinolone (Corticosteroids)
Triazole — trimethoprim-sulfamethoxazole
Trichlorex — trichlormethiazide (Thiazide diuretics)
Tricor — fenofibrate
Tricosal — choline magnesium salicylate (Nonsteroidal anti-inflammatory drugs)
Tridil — nitroglycerin (Nitrates)
Trihexane — trihexyphenidyl (Anticholinergics)
Trihexy — trihexyphenidyl (Anticholinergics)
Trikacide — metronidazole
Tri-Kort — triamcinolone (Corticosteroids)
Trilafon — perphenazine (Phenothiazines)
Trileptal — oxcarbazepine
Tri-Levlen — contraceptives, oral
Trilisate — choline magnesium salicylate (Nonsteroidal anti-inflammatory drugs)
Trilog — triamcinolone (Corticosteroids)
Trilone — triamcinolone (Corticosteroids)
Tri-Med — triamcinolone (Corticosteroids)
Trimeth-Sulfa — trimethoprim-sulfamethoxazole
Trimox — amoxicillin (Penicillins)
Trimpex — trimethoprim
Tri-Norinyl — contraceptives, oral
Triphasil — contraceptives, oral
Triptil — protriptyline (Antidepressants, tricyclic)
Triquilar — contraceptives, oral
Tristoject — triamcinolone (Corticosteroids)
Trisulfam — trimethoprim-sulfamethoxazole

Tritane — trihexyphenidyl (Anticholinergics)
Trivora — contraceptives, oral
Trobicin — spectinomycin
Trofan — tryptophan
Trovan — trovafloxacin (Fluoroquinolones)
Truphylline — aminophylline (Theophyllines)
Trusopt — dorzolamide•
Truxacaine — lidocaine
Truxazole — sulfisoxazole (Sulfonamides)
Truxcillin — penicillin G (Penicillins)
Truxophyllin — theophyllines
Trylone — triamcinolone (Corticosteroids)
Tryptacin — tryptophan
Tryptan — tryptophan
Trypto-Som — tryptophan
Trysul — trisulfapyrimidines (Sulfonamides)
T-Serp — reserpine
T-Stat — erythromycins (Macrolide antibiotics)
Tubarine — tubocurarine (Neuromuscular blocking agents)
Tu-Cillin — penicillin G (Penicillins)
Tuinal — amobarbital, secobarbital (Barbiturates)
Tums — calcium carbonate (Antacids)
T-Vibra — doxycycline (Tetracyclines)
Ty-Caplets — acetaminophen
Ty-Caps — acetaminophen
Tylenol — acetaminophen
Ty-Pap — acetaminophen
Ty-Tabs — acetaminophen

Uendex — dextran sulfate
Ulacort — prednisolone (Corticosteroids)
Ultane — sevoflurane•
Ultracef — cefadroxil (Cephalosporins)
Ultracortenol — prednisolone (Corticosteroids)
Ultragris — Antifungals, griseofulvin
Ultram — Narcotics: tramadol
Ultravate — halobetasol propionate•
Ultrazine-10 — prochlorperazine (Phenothiazines)
Unasyn — ampicillin/sulbactam (Penicillins)
Unicort — hydrocortisone (Corticosteroids)
Uni-Dur — theophyllines
Unigen — estrogens
Uni-Gine — ergot alkaloids
Unipen — nafcillin (Penicillins)
Uni-Phyl — theophyllines
Unisom — doxylamine•
Univasc — moexipril (Angiotensin-converting enzyme (ACE) inhibitors)
Uracel — salicylates, oral (Nonsteroidal anti-inflammatory drugs)
Uranap — methionine
Urazide — benzthiazide (Thiazide diuretics)
Urecholine — bethanechol chloride•
Urestrin — estrogens
Uridon — chlorthalidone (Thiazide diuretics)
Urifon — sulfamethizole (Sulfonamides)
Urispas — flavoxate•
Uri-tet — oxytetracycline (Tetracyclines)
Uritol — furosemide
Urobak — sulfamethoxazole (Sulfonamides)
Urobiotic — oxytetracycline (Tetracyclines)
Urocit-K — Potassium citrate (Citrates; Potassium)
Uroplus — trimethoprim-sulfamethoxazole
Urotoin — nitrofurantoin
Ursinus — pseudoephedrine (Sympathomimetic amines)
Uticillin VK — penicillin V (Penicillins)

Uticort — betamethasone (Corticosteroids)

Vagistat — tioconazole•
Valadol — acetaminophen
Valergen — estradiol (Estrogens)
Valesco — estradiol (Estrogens)
Valisone — betamethasone (Corticosteroids)
Valium — diazepam (Benzodiazepines)
Valnac — betamethasone (Corticosteroids)
Valorin — acetaminophen
Valrelease — diazepam (Benzodiazepines)
Valstar — valrubicin•
Valtrex — valacyclovir•
Vanatrip — amitriptyline (Antidepressants, tricyclic)
Vancerase — beclomethasone (Corticosteroids)
Vanceril — beclomethasone (Corticosteroids)
Vancocin — vancomycin
Vancoled — vancomycin
Vaniqa — eflornithine•
Vantin — cefpodoxime (Cephalosporins)
Vapo-Iso — isoproterenol (Sympathomimetic bronchodilators)
Vaponefrin — epinephrine (Sympathomimetic bronchodilators)
Vascor — bepridil
Vaseretic — enalapril; hydrochlorothiazide (Angiotensin-converting enzyme (ACE) inhibitors; Thiazide diuretics)
Vasobid — ethaverine (Papaverine)
Vasocap — papaverine
Vasoglyn — nitroglycerin (Nitrates)
Vasolate — pentaerythritol tetranitrate (Nitrates)
Vasotec — enalapril (Angiotensin-converting enzyme (ACE) inhibitors)
Vasotec I.V. — enalaprilat (Angiotensin-converting enzyme (ACE) inhibitors)
Vasotherm — nicotinic acid
Vazepam — diazepam (Benzodiazepines)
Vazosan — papaverine
V-Cillin K — penicillins
Vectrin — minocycline (tetracyclines)
Veetids — penicillin V (Penicillins)
Velacycline — rolitetracycline (Tetracyclines)
Velban — vinblastine•
Velmatrol — sulfisoxazole (Sulfonamides)
Velosef — cephradine (Cephalosporins)
Velosulin — insulin
Venoglobulin — Immune Globulin, Intravenous
Ventolin — albuterol (Sympathomimetic bronchodilators)
Vepesid — etoposide
Verelan — verapamil
Vergon — meclizine hydrochloride•
Vermidol — piperazine•
Vermizine — piperazine•
Vermox — mebendazole•
Versed — midazolam (Benzodiazepines)
Versenate — calcium disodium edetate•
Vesprin — triflupromazine (Phenothiazines)
Vestra — reboxetine
Vestran — prazepam (Benzodiazepines)
V-Gan — promethazine
Viagra — sildenafil
Vibramycin — doxycycline (Tetracyclines)
Vibra-Tabs — doxycycline (Tetracyclines)
Videx — didanosine
Vi-Dom-A — vitamin A

Vigorex — methyltestosterone (Anabolic and androgenic steroids)
Vincasar — vincristine
Vincrex — vincristine
Vioxx — rofecoxib (COX-2 inhibitors)
Vira-A — vidarabine
Viracept — nelfinavir
Viramune — nevirapine
Virazole — ribavirin
Virilon — methyltestosterone (Anabolic and androgenic steroids)
Virilon IM — testosterone (Anabolic and androgenic steroids)
Viroptic — trifluridine•
Visa — hydroxyzine
Visken — pindolol (Beta-adrenergic blockers)
Visrex — hydroxyzine
Vistacon-50 — hydroxyzine
Vistacot — hydroxyzine
Vistaject — hydroxyzine
Vistaril — hydroxyzine
Vistazine — hydroxyzine
Vistide — cidofovir•
Visudyne — verteporfin•
Vitabee 6 — pyridoxine
VitaCarn — levocarnitine
Vitrasert — ganciclovir
Vivactil — protriptyline (Antidepressants, tricyclic)
Vivarin — caffeine
Vivelle — estradiol (Estrogens)
Vivol — diazepam (Benzodiazepines)
Vivox — doxycycline (Tetracyclines)
Volmax — albuterol (Sympathomimetic bronchodilators)
Voltaren — diclofenac (Nonsteroidal anti-inflammatory drugs)
V-Pen — penicillin V (Penicillins)
Vumon — teniposide

Warfilone — warfarin (Anticoagulants, oral)

Wasocaps — nicotinic acid
W.D.D. — imipramine (Antidepressants, tricyclic)
Wehgen — estrogens
Welchol — colesevelam
Wellbutrin — bupropion
Wesmycin — tetracyclines
Westcort — hydrocortisone (Corticosteroids)
Westhroid — thyroid hormones
Wigraine — ergotamine (Ergot Alkaloids)
Wilpowr — phentermine (Sympathomimetic amines)
Win-Cillin VK — penicillins
WinGel — aluminum hydroxide, magnesium hydroxide (Antacids)
Winpred — prednisone (Corticosteroids)
Winstrol — stanozolol (Anabolic and androgenic steroids)
Wintrocin — erythromycins (Macrolide antibiotics)
Wyamycin — erythromycins (Macrolide antibiotics)
Wycillin — penicillin G (Penicillins)
Wygesic — acetaminophen; propoxyphene (Acetaminophen; Narcotics: methadone and congeners)
Wytensin — guanabenz acetate•

Xalatan — latanoprost•
Xanax — alprazolam (Benzodiazepines)
Xeloda — capecitabine (Fluorouracil)
Xenical — orlistat
Xopenex — levalbuterol (Sympathomimetic amines)
Xylocaine — lidocaine
Xylocard — lidocaine

Yocon — yohimbine•